T0179052

RESPIRATORY CONTROL AND DISORDERS IN THE NEWBORN

Edited by

Oommen P. Mathew

Brody School of Medicine at East Carolina University
Greenville, North Carolina, U.S.A.

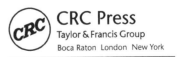

CRC Press
Taylor & Francis Group
Boca Raton London New York

CRC Press is an imprint of the
Taylor & Francis Group, an **informa** business

CRC Press
Taylor & Francis Group
6000 Broken Sound Parkway NW, Suite 300
Boca Raton, FL 33487-2742

First issued in paperback 2019

© 2003 by Taylor & Francis Group, LLC
CRC Press is an imprint of Taylor & Francis Group, an Informa business

ISBN-13: 978-0-8247-0984-6 (hbk)
ISBN-13: 978-0-367-39552-0 (pbk)

Visit the Taylor & Francis Web site at
http://www.taylorandfrancis.com

and the CRC Press Web site at
http://www.crcpress.com

LUNG BIOLOGY IN HEALTH AND DISEASE

Executive Editor

Claude Lenfant
Director National Heart Lung and Blood Institute
National Institutes of Health
Bethesda Maryland

The opinions expressed in these volumes do not necessarily represent the views of the National Institutes of Health

I want to note with sadness the passing of my former colleague, Giuseppe Sant'Ambrogio, M.D. He was not only an inspiration to many but, above all, a friend in the truest sense. His presence in the scientific community will be sorely missed. I dedicate this book to his memory.

INTRODUCTION

Newborn and infant mortality has been a plague of public health for centuries. However, during the 1900s, an extraordinary effort began to correct this disgraceful situation. Especially remarkable have been the accomplishments of the last 30 years or so. Although many challenges remain, very noticeable progress has been made relative to some specific causes of death in babies.

In the United States, neonatal respiratory distress syndrome (NRDS) was one of the main causes of death in premature newborns. However, an intensive research effort led to a major reduction of the number of deaths due to this condition—from about 55,000 per year in the 1960s to less than 5000 per year at the end of the twentieth century—and the number is still going down.

Paralleling the NRDS epidemic was that of sudden infant death syndrome (SIDS). Although some successes had occurred during the twentieth century, we really had to wait for a public health campaign, the "Back to Sleep" campaign, to witness more rapid declines.

In a way, NRDS and SIDS have some commonalities. NRDS relates to lung development and its respiratory function (i.e., gas exchange), whereas SIDS is one expression of dysfunction of the respiratory control system.

The respiratory machinery is one of the most complex of the human body. It has fascinated philosophers, teleologists, and biologists for a very long time, maybe beginning with the Chinese as far back as 2000 B.C. Erasistratus (around 304 B.C.) and then Gallen (around 130 A.D.) were the first to connect the lungs to the brain through "hollow" nerves, in which the blood was charged with "animal spirit." Since then, a long line of biologists have studied this machinery and its control. All this work led to the realization that the "hollow" nerves were not blood conduits at all, but "real" nerves conducting commands from the brain in response to stimuli from various parts of the body.

The first chapter of this new volume gives a panoramic view of respiratory control in the newborn. It is only the beginning of a journey that will show the reader how this control works and what it does in health and disease—from gasping to apnea, from feeding to gastroesophageal reflux, and many more newborn respiratory control disorders. This is a book for investigators, but also for clinical practitioners.

As the Executive Editor of the Lung Biology in Health and Disease series, I cannot overstate how enthusiastic my response was to Dr. Oommen Mathew's expression of interest in editing this volume. I knew this would be an important contribution, as well as a source of invaluable information and inspiration, for researchers and for clinicians. I am grateful to him and to the contributors for the opportunity to introduce this volume to the readership of the series.

Claude Lenfant, M.D.
Bethesda, Maryland, U.S.A.

PREFACE

Since the inception of this series, several volumes have been devoted to respiratory control. These contributions have critically reviewed the experimental evidence (beginning with the observation by LeGallois) that the respiratory center is located in the medulla. Until now, respiratory control in the newborn has been a small part of the general discussion of respiratory control. In recent years, the increasing interest in developmental neurobiology—more specifically, our quest for understanding the cellular mechanisms involved in the control of breathing—has put our knowledge of respiratory control disorders on a firmer footing. These cellular events are complex and often show marked developmental changes. Interpretation and integration of these cellular events into the system levels are necessary for better understanding of the pathophysiology of various respiratory control disorders, and, in turn, targeted therapeutic interventions can be developed. An excellent example of this undertaking is the discovery of surfactant deficiency as the underlying cause of respiratory distress syndrome in premature infants, and the subsequent development of natural and synthetic surfactants to treat this "developmental disorder." We hopefully anticipate the development of drugs specifically targeted to enhance maturation of respiratory control in premature infants and the rectification of abnormal cellular properties through molecular genetics technology.

This volume is devoted to the disorders of respiratory control in the newborn. To refresh and enhance our understanding of respiratory control, the first part deals with respiratory control in the normal newborn. Several chapters in this section address the relevant topics critically, in the fetus and the newborn, at both the system and cellular levels. These include chapters on development of respiratory control, gasping, and neural and chemical control of breathing. This section also features chapters on development of sleep states and metabolism—two vitally important factors in determining respiratory output.

The second part, which focuses on respiratory control disorders, begins with an overview. The diagnosis of these disorders in the neonate often begins with cardiorespiratory monitoring in the neonatal intensive care unit. An examination of the pros and cons of the cardiopulmonary monitoring techniques used in the neonate follows. The main focus of this part is apnea of prematurity; several chapters are dedicated to this clinically important topic. Congenital central hypoventilation and neuromuscular syndromes are examined next, followed by chapters on control of breathing in acute and chronic respiratory failure. A discussion of the maturational aspect of the respiratory control mechanisms sets the stage for the final chapter, which addresses modifiable risk factors in sudden infant death syndrome.

I would like to thank this outstanding group of international contributors for their comprehensive, critical, and up-to-date chapters.

Oommen P. Mathew

CONTRIBUTORS

Lilia Curzi-Dascalova, M.D., Ph.D.   INSERM, Hôpital Robert Debré, Paris, France

Eric C. Eichenwald, M.D.   Assistant Professor of Pediatrics, Harvard Medical School, and Department of Newborn Medicine, Brigham and Women's Hospital, Boston, Massachusetts, U.S.A

Neil N. Finer, M.D., F.R.C.P.C   Professor, Department of Pediatrics, and Director, Division of Neonatology, University of California, San Diego, San Diego, California, U.S.A.

John T. Fisher, Ph.D.   Departments of Physiology, Paediatrics, and Medicine, Queen's University, Kingston, Ontario, Canada

Estelle B. Gauda, M.D.   Associate Professor, Department of Pediatrics, The Johns Hopkins University, Baltimore, Maryland, U.S.A.

Alison Graham, D.O.   Division of Neonatology, University of California, San Diego, San Diego, California, U.S.A.

Anne Greenough, M.D., F.R.C.P., F.R.C.P.C.H., D.C.H. Children Nationwide Professor of Neonatology and Clinical Respiratory Physiology, Guy's, King's and St Thomas' School of Medicine, and Children Nationwide Regional Neonatal Intensive Care Centre, King's College Hospital, London, England

Gabriel G. Haddad, M.D.* Professor of Pediatrics and Cellular and Molecular Physiology, Department of Pediatrics, Yale University School of Medicine, New Haven, Connecticut, U.S.A.

Musa A. Haxhiu, M.D., Ph.D Director, Department of Physiology and Biophysics, Howard University College of Medicine, Washington, D.C., U.S.A.

Miriam Katz-Salamon, Ph.D. Associate Professor, Department of Women's and Children's Health, Karolinska Institute, and Department of Neonatology, Karolinska Hospital, Stockholm, Sweden

Edward E. Lawson, M.D. Professor, Department of Pediatrics, John Hopkins University School of Medicine, Baltimore, Maryland, U.S.A.

Richard J. Martin, M.D. Professor of Pediatrics, Reproductive Biology, Biophysics, and Physiology, Case Western Reserve University, Cleveland, Ohio, U.S.A.

Oommen P. Mathew, M.D. Professor of Pediatrics, Department of Pediatrics, Brody School of Medicine at East Carolina University, Greenville, North Carolina, U.S.A.

Martha Jane Miller, M.D., Ph.D. Associate Professor, Department of Pediatrics, Case Western Reserve University, Cleveland, Ohio, U.S.A.

Jacopo P. Mortola, M.D. Professor, Department of Physiology, McGill University, Montreal, Quebec, Canada

Taher Omari, Ph.D. Senior Research Officer, Department of Pediatrics, University of Adelaide, and Gastroenterology Unit, Women's and Children's Hospital, Adelaide, South Australia, Australia

Christian F. Poets, M.D. Department of Neonatology, University of Tübingen, Tübingen, Germany

---

*Current affiliation: Albert Einstein College of Medicine and Children's Hospital at Montefiore, Bronx, New York, U.S.A.

Henrique Rigatto, M.D. Professor of Pediatrics, Physiology, and Reproductive Medicine, Department of Pediatrics, University of Manitoba, Winnipeg, Manitoba, Canada

Cyril E. Schweitzer, M.D. Department of Physiology, Queen's University, Kingston, Ontario, Canada

Jean M. Silvestri, M.D. Associate Professor, Department of Pediatrics, Rush Children's Hospital, Chicago, Illinois, U.S.A.

Malcolm P. Sparrow, Ph.D. Asthma and Allergy Research Institute, Department of Medicine, University of Western Australia, Nedlands, Western Australia, Australia

Ann R. Stark, M.D. Associate Clinical Professor of Pediatrics, Harvard Medical School, and Department of Newborn Medicine, Brigham and Women's Hospital, Boston, Massachusetts, U.S.A.

Walter M. St.-John, Ph.D. Department of Physiology, Dartmouth Medical School and Dartmouth-Hitchcock Medical Center, Lebanon, New Hampshire, U.S.A.

Debra E. Weese-Mayer, M.D. Professor of Pediatrics and Director of Pediatric Respiratory Medicine, Rush Children's Hospital, Chicago, Illinois, U.S.A.

Markus Weichselbaum, Ph.D. Asthma and Allergy Research Institute, Department of Medicine, University of Western Australia, Nedlands, Western Australia, Australia

CONTENTS

1

Respiratory Control in the Newborn
Comparative Physiology and Clinical Disorders

GABRIEL G. HADDAD*

Yale University School of Medicine
New Haven, Connecticut, U.S.A.

I. Introduction

The control of respiration is one of the most fascinating phenomena in physiology, along with the genesis of heart pacing and rhythm, diurnal rhythm, and other cyclical phenomena. Indeed, there are amazing short-term and long-term cyclic phenomena that take place in nature from plants to humans. Consider, for example, the diurnal cyclicity of gene expression that occurs in plants being activated in the morning to protect plants from the heat of the sun and others being activated in the evening to protect them from cold temperatures and freezing! Cyclic phenomena are clearly intriguing, and it is well recognized that cyclic phenomena occur in all tissues of the body, whether they are related to regions of the brain that are responsible for diurnal rhythms (suprachiasmatic nucleus) or not. Respiration is a short-term cyclical phenomenon that involves the brain, lungs, heart, circulation, carotid bodies, and other sensors and interconnections among these various organs. This is clearly a crucial act for air-breathing mammals; hence its regulation is of paramount importance.

Current affiliation: Albert Einstein College of Medicine and Children's Hospital at Montefiore, Bronx, New York, U.S.A.

The control of respiration is not mature at birth in full-term infants, and it is certainly not mature in premature infants. Keeping in mind that ~10% of births in the United States are premature, the basic understanding of respiration in the immature infant takes on added significance. Although there are a number of elements of the control system that are likely to be immature in the newly born, especially in the premature infant, the aims of this chapter will be [1] to review some of the salient features of respiratory control in the mature individual, [2] highlight some of the major differences between the newly born and the mature subject, and [3] illustrate how certain defects and/or abnormalities in the control system lead to disease and clinical manifestations.

II. Overall Concepts of Respiratory Control

To describe the respiratory control system and highlight its main features, I present below six concepts or main ideas that characterize the respiratory control system. These concepts constitute a distillation of a considerable amount of work done over more than two centuries, ever since LeGallois's experiments. In these experiments, done at the turn of the 19th century, he described the *noeud vital* in famous rabbit experiments when he discovered that no breathing efforts occurred when he severed the spinal cord from the *noeud vital*, located at the level of "origin of the nerves of the eighth pair" (1).

> **CONCEPT I:** *Respiration is controlled via a negative feedback system with a controller present in the central nervous system (CNS) and a controlled organ composed of respiratory muscles and lungs.*

Animal models and humans have been studied extensively and these investigations have clearly shown that the CNS integrates the drive and generates the oscillatory respiratory motor pattern, depending on inputs from a variety of feedback elements. This controller then adjusts the output of the system such as to optimize the function desired. Inputs from the carotid bodies, airway receptors, muscle receptors, and other sensors converge onto the CNS, which integrates and formulates the output to the respiratory muscles. Therefore, this feedback loop depends on several elements including sensors, comparators, integrators, and effectors. With every disturbance sensed, the feedback system tries to change its output to minimize the effect of the disturbance on the overall function of the system and to attempt to return it to baseline.

> **CONCEPT II:** *The central neuronal processing and integration in the brainstem is hierarchical in nature.*

This idea is important from the point of view of neuronal network as well as the "decision-making process" in the CNS when faced with competing inputs. For example, many experiments have shown that the laryngeal afferent input into the brainstem is an extraordinarily potent inhibitory reflex to breathing and its effect on the CNS integrator/pattern generator is instantaneous, taking place in milliseconds (2,3) (Fig. 1)! This reflex is even more powerful during anesthesia, when cortical input onto the brainstem is attenuated. We and others have performed a variety of experiments in animal models and shown that, although there is a major interplay between anesthesia and this reflex, laryngeal input overwhelms other inputs coming to the brainstem (2,3).

> **CONCEPT III:** *The respiratory rhythm generation in central neurons is most likely a result of an integration among network, synaptic, cellular, and molecular characteristics of brainstem and other neurons involved.*

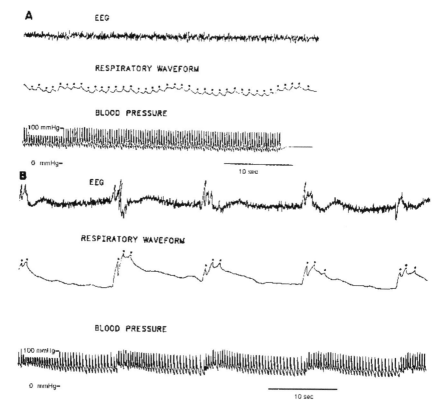

Figure 1 Original record in an experiment in which the superior laryngeal nerve (SLN) was chronically instrumented and the animal (piglet) was awake and unrestrained. Note the potent respiratory inhibition (compare A, which is at rest, with B, 10 min after the stimulation of the SLN) and the intermittent breakthough or respiration when the SLN was stimulated.

This idea has been developed in the past decade, as we have been able to utilize reduced preparations and study the membrane properties of individual neurons (4–6). The nature of the rhythm generator is not well delineated, but there are two potential scenarios. The respiratory controller may be a group of neurons that either form an *emergent network* or are *endogenous* or *conditional burster* neurons. In the first case, respiratory neurons would not have any special inherent membrane properties (e.g., bursting properties) that would make their membrane potential spontaneously oscillate (6). Rather, the output of the network they form would oscillate because of the special synaptic interactions among these respiratory neurons (6). In the second case, respiratory neurons, similar to those forming the sinus node of the heart, would have properties that make them individually "burst" or oscillate, even if they are *not* connected to any other neuron. This is termed an endogenous burster, or pacemaker neuron. A conditional burster is a neuron that oscillates only when exposed to certain chemicals (e.g., neurotransmitters). The properties of these neurons are also very critical in shaping the output of the network itself, irrespective of the properties of the respiratory network as a whole.

Although the exact nature of how these respiratory neurons operate is not known, more recent data have suggested that the respiratory rhythm is generated by an oscillating network in the ventrolateral formation of the medulla oblongata (7). The region that seems to be essential for the rhythm is the pre-Botzinger complex, as all cranial nerve activity ceases totally after this region is separated from lower brainstem levels (7–9). A number of questions clearly remain to be answered: [1] what are properties of individual neurons in this area? [2] how interconnected are these with others? and [3] what is the nature of their synapses with neurons in the brainstem and other more rostral regions? Recently, Feldman and colleagues have attempted to answer a number of these questions. For example, we know now that glutamatergic receptors (AMPA) and glutamate as a ligand play an important role in inducing the respiratory rhythm (10–12).

We and others have discovered a number of impressive membrane currents that may shape their repetitive firing activity (6). These include not only the classic sodium and potassium currents responsible for the action potential, but also an A-current, two types of calcium currents, calcium-activated potassium currents, inward rectifier currents, ATP-sensitive K^+ currents, and other currents (6,13). There seems to be little disagreement about the presence of these channels in respiratory neurons, since after their initial demonstration in brain slices, many of these channels were studied in identified respiratory neurons in vivo (6). Although the evidence is still insufficient, it has been suggested that delayed excitation may be responsible for the firing activity of "late" inspiratory neurons in the dorsal respiratory group (DRG) (6). If this is true, it is possible that the A-current in these neurons works in conjunction with processes, such as synaptic facilitation, to shape a ramp excitatory drive to phrenic motoneurons. Assignment of a role for this current in forming the activity of the dorsal group (DRG) neurons is subject to study and speculation, and will ultimately require further investigation in vivo. However, we should emphasize that one of the important observations of the past several years is that these pre-Botzinger neurons do not seem to have special membrane properties. They seem to have receptors, ion channels, and transporters similar to those in other neurons in the CNS. Neurons in the brainstem do not seem to have properties similar to those that oscillate by themselves, i.e., oscillate by virtue of specific membrane properties, without the need of input from surrounding neurons. It is therefore very likely that the oscillations of brainstem respiratory neurons are based not on membrane properties alone but also on the integration of membrane, synaptic, and network properties.

CONCEPT IV: *Afferent information to the CNS is not essential for neuronal rhythmicity but is important for modulation of respiration.*

A considerable number of afferent messages converge on the brainstem at any one time. For example, chemoreceptors and mechanoreceptors in the upper airways constantly sense stretch, air temperature, and chemical changes over the mucosa and relay this information to the brainstem. Afferent impulses from these areas travel through the superior laryngeal nerve and the 10th cranial nerve (vagus). Changes in O_2 or CO_2 tensions are also sensed at the carotid and aortic bodies, and afferent impulses travel through the carotid and aortic sinus nerves. Thermal or metabolic changes are sensed by superficial receptors or by hypothalamic neurons and are carried through spinal tracts to the brainstem. Furthermore, afferent information to the controller in the brainstem need not be only formulated and sensed by the peripheral nervous system. As an example, sensors of CO_2 lie on the ventral surface of the medulla oblongata and constitute a major feedback regarding CO_2 homeostasis.

It is well known that afferent information is not a prerequisite for the generation and maintenance of respiration. When the brainstem and spinal cord are removed from the body of the rat and maintained in vitro, rhythmic phrenic activity can be detected for hours (7). Other experiments on chronically instrumented dogs in vivo in which several sensory systems are simultaneously blocked (cold vagal block, 100% O_2 breathing to eliminate carotid discharges, sleep to eliminate wakeful stimuli, and diuretics to alkalinize the blood) indicate that afferent information is not necessary to generate the inherent respiratory rhythm. However, both in vitro and in vivo studies demonstrate that, in the absence of afferent information, the inherent rhythm of the central generator (respiratory frequency) is slowed down considerably. Hence chemoreceptor afferents can play an important role in modulating respiration and rhythmic behavior. Furthermore, cortical and other central inputs are important afferent inputs onto the brainstem. They have a major impact on the regulation of respiration, although they do not participate in rhythmogenesis. Consider for example, the effect of emotions, the wake state, sight, hearing, etc., on breathing (14).

>   **CONCEPT V:** *The efferent limb of the respiratory control system (i.e., respiratory musculature) is a possible site of respiratory failure due to neuromuscular failure.*

Ventilation requires the coordinated interaction between the respiratory muscles of the chest and those of the upper airways and neck. For example, the activation of upper airway muscles occurs prior to and during the initial part of inspiration; the genioglossus contracts to move the tongue forward and thus increase the patency of the airways; and the vocal cords abduct to reduce laryngeal resistance. Indeed, we have learned considerably about the efferent limb and the respiratory muscles and the neuromuscular junction as potential sites for failure of the whole system. Extramuscular (e.g., respiratory nerves, neuro-muscular junction) and intramuscular (e.g., ionic homeostasis, energy stores, fiber types, blood flow in the muscle) factors can play major roles in either contributing to or precipitating the failure of ventilation (15).

>   **CONCEPT VI:** *The output of the respiratory control system is distributed among a number of respiratory muscles located in the airways, chest wall, and abdomen.*

This is an important idea since it is often considered that the diaphragm is the only muscle of respiration. Whereas the diaphragm is the major muscle, the best illustration for the importance of the other respiratory muscles, such as those in the upper airways, is related to the pathogenesis of upper airway obstruction/hypoventilation during sleep (OSAH) in children as well as in adults. The coordination, tone, and activation of upper-airway muscles are very important because it is the "uncoordinated" interactions between the diaphragm and upper airway muscles that can lead to hypoventilation or obstruction in the upper airways during sleep. It is therefore very essential to consider the functional state of all respiratory muscles and their synchronization; it is their coordinated activation that keeps the airways patent, especially under stress.

III. The Newborn's Respiratory Control in Perspective

A. Peripheral Sensory Aspects

In this section, I shall review data on the primary O_2 sensor in the body, the carotids. I will show that there are major differences between the newborn and the adult vis-à-vis the response of the carotids to low O_2 and with respect to the importance of this organ in overall respiratory function and survival in early life.
    Recordings from single fiber afferents have demonstrated major differences between the fetus and the newborn and between the newborn and the adult (Fig. 2). Chemoreceptor activity is present in the fetus and a large increase in

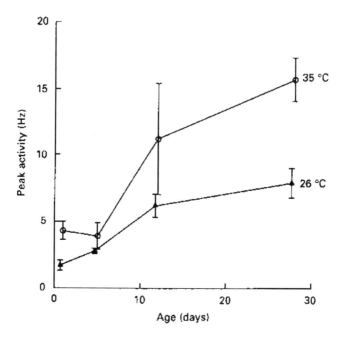

Figure 2 Peak discharge from single units of a carotid body in vitro. Note the effect of age on peak activity.

activity may be evoked by decreasing the PO_2 of the ewe (16). The estimated response curve was left-shifted such that PaO_2 values below 20 torr were required to initiate an increase in carotid sinus discharge. Furthermore, the large increase in PaO_2 at the time of birth virtually shuts off chemoreceptor activity. However, this decreased activity does not last long, and a normal, adultlike sensitivity is achieved after a few weeks (16,17). The mechanisms for the maturation of these peripheral sensors are not all worked out, but there are a number of factors, external or endogenous, that probably play a role in this process. For example, arterial chemoreceptors are subject to hormonal influences, which may affect the sensor or alter tissue PO_2 within the organ. Neurochemicals may also play a major role as they modulate chemosensitivity. For example, endorphins decrease in the newborn period, and the effect of exogenous endorphin is inhibition of chemoreceptor-mediated hypoxia sensitivity (18).

Even in studies in which hormonal or neural effects are minimized such as in in vitro experiments, the chemosensitivity of the newborn carotid is less than the adult. Nerve activity of rat carotid bodies, in vitro, following transition from normoxia to hypoxia is about fourfold greater in carotid bodies harvested from 20-day-old rats as compared to 1 to 2-day-old rats (19). This corresponds well with the maturational pattern of the respiratory response to hypoxia in the intact animal (20) and suggests that major maturational changes occur *within* the carotid body itself. For example, the maturational increase in chemosensitivity may be attributed to a maturational change in the biophysical properties of glomus cells. In one model, it seems that hypoxia directly inhibits a membrane-localized K^+ channel which is active at rest, and the resulting depolarization leads to calcium influx, secretion of neurotransmitter, and increased neural activity in adult carotid cells (21). In comparison, glomus cells harvested from immature rats show a decrease in whole-cell K^+ current during hypoxia but the decrease in K^+ current is attributed to a decreased activation of a Ca^{+2}-dependent K^+ current rather than to a specialized K^+ channel sensitive to PO_2 (22). How this leads to reduced sensitivity and reduced firing is not well understood.

What role do the carotid bodies play in growing animals? And is this role tied to O_2 sensing? In comparison to the adult, peripheral chemoreceptors are believed to assume a greater role in the newborn period. Peripheral chemo-receptor denervation in the newborn results in severe respiratory impairments and high probability of sudden death. This has been demonstrated in a number of animal models. Lambs following denervation fail to develop a mature respiratory pattern (23,24) and suffer 30% mortality rate, days, weeks, or months following surgery. In other species, denervation also leads to lethal respiratory disturbances (2,25). For instance, denervated rats suffer from severe desaturation during REM sleep (25), and piglets suffer from profound apnea during quiet sleep (3). Of particular interest is that these lethal impairments only occur during a fairly narrow developmental window. Denervation before or after this window period in early life results in only relatively minor alterations in respiratory function (3).

B. Central Neurophysiologic Aspects

Although recent studies in the neonatal rat in vitro (whole brainstem preparation) were not targeted at understanding the neonate in particular, these studies have shed light on basic fundamental issues pertaining to control mechanisms of respiration in the newborn (7). In fact, we know now from several such studies that the young rat (in the first week of life) does not need any external or peripheral drive for the oscillator to discharge. The inherent respiratory rate (as judged by cranial nerve output) is markedly downregulated. These studies corroborate the idea that peripheral or central (rostral to the medulla and pons) inputs are needed to maintain the respiratory output at a much higher frequency.

Another interesting observation is that the discharge pattern of each neuronal unit in the neonate seems, from extracellular recordings, to be different from that in the adult in two major ways. First, the inspiratory discharge is not ramp in shape, but increases and decreases very fast within the same breath. The second is that it is extremely brief, sometimes limited to even a few action potentials (26). In addition to differences in inspiratory discharge, expiratory units discharge weakly and appear often only after the imposition of an expiratory load (27,28).

Since the discharge pattern of central neurons in the adult or neonate (as discussed above) is affected by peripheral input, including input from the vagus nerve, one question that has been raised is whether the lack of myelination in the neonatal nerve fibers affects function. This is indeed the case, because of lack of myelination and potential delays in signaling. It is also because inspiratory and expiratory discharge periods are so fast or short that they preclude the effect of peripheral information on the CNS within the same breath. Therefore, one important issue that can be raised is whether breath-by-breath feedback is as potent in the young as in the adult.

Differences between neonates and adults are also observed in response to neurotransmitters or modulators. Young animals respond differently to neurotransmitters than adult animals do; this has been mostly documented by work on the opossum (29). Glutamate injected in various locations in the brainstem, even in large doses, induces respiratory pauses while it is clearly stimulatory in the older mature animal (29). Inhibitory neurotransmitters such as GABA have also been used, and these have age-dependent effects in the opossum. GABA has also been shown to be an excitatory neurotransmitter (Fig. 3) in the newborn but an inhibitory one in the mature adult neuron (30). These differences between newborns and adults are not quite understood at the fundamental level since there are many variables that have not been controlled for such as the size of the extracellular space, receptor development, and ability for sensitization, to name a few.

C. The Efferent System

There is a multitude of neuromuscular and skeletal changes that take place early in life. These include alterations in muscle cells, the neuromuscular junction, the nerve terminals and synapses, and the chest wall properties. Therefore, since muscle and chest wall properties change with age, it is likely that neural responses can be influenced by pump properties, especially that these muscles execute neural commands. One of the important maturational aspects of respiratory muscles is their pattern of innervation. In the adult, one muscle fiber is innervated by one motoneuron. In the newborn, however, each fiber is innervated by two or more motoneurons, and the axons of different motoneurons can synapse on the same muscle fiber; thus, the term polyneuronal innervation. Synapse elimination takes place postnatally, and in the case of the diaphragm, the adult type of innervation is reached by several weeks postnatally, depending on the animal species. The time course of polyneuronal innervation of the diaphragm in the human newborn is not known (15).

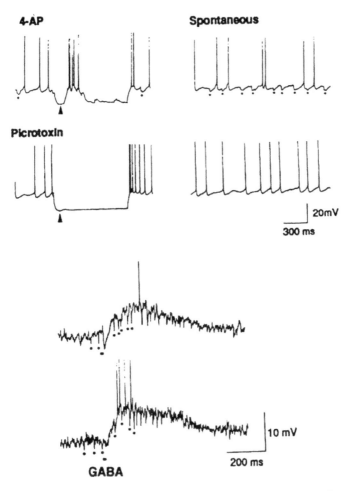

Figure 3 *Top panel of four records.* Left, above and below: Compare action potential discharge from one nerve cell in vitro after a hyperpolarization in the presence of 4-AP (I_A current blocker) or picrotoxin ($GABA_A$ receptor blocker). Note the lack of excitatory discharge in the presence of picrotoxin. Right panel shows spontaneous discharge. *Bottom panel.* Action potential discharge with depolarization with and without GABA agonist.

The neuromuscular junctional folds, postsynaptic membranes, and acetylcholine receptors and metabolism undergo major postnatal maturational changes. The acetylcholine quantal content per end plate potential is lower in the newborn than in the adult rat diaphragm (15). The newborn diaphragm is also more susceptible to neuromuscular transmission failure than that in the adult, especially at higher frequencies of stimulation (15). The reason for this is not clear.

IV. Disease States

A. Respiratory Pauses and Apneas

Although there are numerous studies on apnea in the newborn and adult human, there are still major controversies. The length of the respiratory pause, usually defined as apnea, varies and has been subject to debate. Statistically, apnea can be defined as a respiratory pause that exceeds 3 standard deviations of the mean breath time at any particular age. This definition requires data from a population of subjects, lacks physiologic value, and does not differentiate between relatively shorter or longer respiratory pauses. This definition may therefore not be the best from a functional viewpoint. Alternatively, the definition of apnea may be based on the sequelae of pauses, such as associated cardiovascular or neurophysiologic changes. Such definition relies on the functional assessment of pauses and is therefore more relevant clinically. It is important to note here that, because infants have a higher O_2 consumption (per unit weight) than the adult and relatively smaller lung volumes and O_2 stores, it is possible that relatively shorter (e.g., seconds) respiratory pauses, which may not be clinically important in the adult, can be serious in the very young or premature infant. Furthermore, independent of age, respiratory pauses are more prevalent during sleep than during wakefulness. And the frequency and duration of respiratory pauses depend on sleep state. Respiratory pauses are more frequent and shorter in REM than in quiet sleep, and more frequent in the younger than in the older child or adult.

Although there is a controversy regarding the pathogenesis of respiratory pauses, there is a consensus about certain observations. Normal full-term infants, children, and adult humans exhibit respiratory pauses during sleep. It is also believed that the presence of respiratory pauses and breathing irregularity is a "healthy" sign and that the complete absence of such pauses may be indicative of abnormalities. This parallels well the concept of heart rate variability, and a lack of short-term or long-term variability in heart rate can be a sign of disease or immaturity. Prolonged apneas, however, can be life-threatening, and the pathogenesis of these apneas may relate to the clinical condition of the patient at the time of the apneas, associated cardiovascular (systemic or pulmonary) changes, the chronicity of the clinical condition, and whether the etiology is central or peripheral. Prolonged apneic spells require therapy, but optimally, treatment should be targeted to the underlying pathophysiology.

The pathogenesis of apneas can vary considerably. The etiology can be in the CNS, in the periphery, such as in the airways, or in the coordination between peripheral and central events. Upper-airway obstruction (UAO), for example, is an entity that is characterized by having lack of normal airflow (or complete lack of airflow) not because of lack of phrenic output but because of obstruction in the airways. This is very different from abnormal (or lack of) airflow on the basis of absent phrenic impulses coming to the diaphragm. One reason for distinguishing the two conditions is to provide the optimal form of therapy.

Upper-airway obstruction during sleep is recognized with increasing frequency in children and adults. In contrast to adults with UAO in whom the etiology of obstruction often remains obscure, many children have anatomic abnormalities. A common cause of UAO in children is tonsillar and adenoidal hypertrophy, partly due to repeated upper respiratory infections. Other associated abnormalities include craniofacial malformations, micrognathia, and muscular hypotonia from a variety of causes. The usual site of obstruction of UAO in both infants and adults is the oropharynx, between the posterior pharyngeal wall, the soft palate, and the genioglossus. During sleep (especially REM sleep), upper-airway muscles, including those of the oropharynx, lose tone, and trigger an episode of UAO.

B. O_2 Deprivation and Cell Injury

A number of pathophysiologic conditions lead to respiratory failure with hypercapnia and tissue O_2 deprivation. Practically, all cardiorespiratory diseases can potentially produce failure of this system. This outcome may be deleterious to other organs because of the ensuing acidosis and hypoxia. However, it is the hypoxia that should be avoided at all cost since human tissues, especially the CNS, have relatively low tolerance to a microenvironment that is devoid of O_2 (31,32).

In the past decade, we have learned a great deal about the effect of lack of oxygenation on various mammalian and nonmammalian (vertebrate and non-vertebrate) tissues and at various ages, including fetal, postnatal, and adult. There is a vast array of cellular and molecular responses to lack of O_2. From an organismal point of view, the carotid bodies would seem to discharge and have an effect on ventilation when the PaO_2 reaches below 50 torr. It is probably the case that, in general, other tissues in the body do not respond or react to PaO_2 above 50 torr. Indeed, most tissues would start "sensing" a decrease in PaO_2 only below 35–40 torr. For example, the brain, which is one of the very sensitive tissues to lack of O_2, has a resting (no hypoxia induced) interstitial O_2 tension probably in the range of 20–35 torr depending on age, area (white vs. gray matter), neuronal metabolism, temperature, proximity to blood vessels, etc.

Although advances have been made in understanding the effect of lack of oxygenation on tissue metabolism, excitability, and function, major questions remain unanswered with respect to the mechanisms that lead to injury or those that protect tissues from it. This area of research is very complex, and we and others have focused on it for a number of years. In the case of the nervous system, for example, a number of mechanisms are activated during O_2 deprivation. Membrane biophysical events such as those pertaining to Na^+ and K^+ channels, and others such as increased anaerobic metabolism, increased intracellular levels of H^+ and Ca^{2+}, increased concentrations in extracellular neurotransmitters (e.g., glutamate and aspartate), radical production, activation of kinases, protease, and lipase; injury and destruction of important cytoskeletal proteins; gene regulation of a number of proteins (e.g., c-fos, NGF, HSP-70, -actin) are just some events that take place during lack of O_2 (32–40).

V. Summary

The newborn seems to have either different mechanisms of control of respiration or an immature set of mechanisms that, with differentiation, arrive at the adult respiratory mechanisms. However, it is important to stress that it is not clear from studies that have been done at either the sensory limb, the central controller, or the efferent limb that the newborn is at an overall increased risk for injury. In fact, there is a considerable amount of data to demonstrate that the young are at an advantage from the viewpoint of stress-related hypoxic injury.

References

1. LeGallois JJC. Experiments on the Principle of Life, 1813:12–16. As cited in: Comroe JH Jr, ed. Pulmonary and Respiratory Physiology Part II. Stroudsburg, PA: Dowden, Hutchinson & Ross, 1976.
2. Donnelly DF, Haddad GG. Respiratory changes induced by prolonged laryngeal stimulation in unanesthetized piglets. J Appl Physiol 1986; 61:1018–1024.
3. Donnelly DF, Haddad GG. Prolonged apnea and impaired survival in piglets after sinus and aortic nerve section. J Appl Physiol 1990; 68:1048–1052.
4. Haddad GG, Getting PA. Repetitive firing properties of neurons in the ventral region of the nucleus tractus soliarius. In-vitro studies in the adult and neonatal rat. J Neurophysiol 1989; 62:1213–1224.
5. Haddad GG, Donnelly DF, Getting PA. Biophysical membrane properties of hypoglossal neurons in-vitro: intracellular studies in adult and neonatal rats. J Appl Physiol 1990; 69:1509–1517.
6. Dekin MS, Haddad GG. Membrane and cellular properties in oscillating networks: implications for respiration. J Appl Physiol 1990; 69:809–821.
7. Smith JC, Ellenberger H, Ballanyi K, Richter DW, Feldman JL. Pre-Botzinger complex: a brainstem region that may generate respiratory rhythm in mammals. Science 1991; 254:726–729.
8. Feldman JL, Smith JC, Ellenberger HH, Connelly CA, Greer JJ, Lindsay AD, Otto MR. Neurogenesis of respiratory rhythm and pattern: emerging concepts. Am J Physiol 1990; 259:879–886.

9. Richter DW, Ballanyi K, Schwarzacher S. Mechanisms of respiratory rhythm generation. Curr Opin Neurobiol 1992; 2:788–793.

10. Rekling JC, Feldman JL. PreBotzinger complex and pacemaker neurons: hypothesized site and kernel for respiratory rhythm generation. Annu Rev Physiol 1990; 60:385–405.

11. Ge Q, Feldman JL. AMPA receptor activation and phosphatase inhibition affect neonatal rat respiratory rhythm generation. J Physiol 1998; 509(1):255–266.

12. Funk GD, Feldman JL. Generation of respiratory rhythm and pattern in mammals: insights from developmental studies. Curr Opin Neurobiol 1995; 6:778–785.

13. Jiang C, Haddad GG. The effect of anoxia on intracellular and extracellular K^+ in hypoglossal neurons in-vitro. J Neurophysiol 1991; 66:103–111.

14. Von Euler C. Brain stem mechanisms for generation and control of breathing pattern. In: Fishman AP, Cherniack NS, Widdicombe, Geiger SR, eds. Handbook of Physiology (Section 3: The Respiratory System). Bethesda, MD: APS, 1986:1–67.

15. Sieck GC, Fournier M. Developmental aspects of diaphragm muscle cells. In: Haddad GG, Farber JP, eds. Developmental Neurobiology of Breathing, Lung Biology in Health and Disease. New York: Marcel Dekker, 1991:375–428.

16. Blanco CE, Hanson MA, McCooke HB. Studies of chemoreceptor resetting after hyperoxic ventilation of the fetus in utero. In: Riberio JA, Pallot DJ, eds. Chemoreceptors in Respiratory Control. London: Croom Helm, 1988:221–227.

17. Hanson MA, Kumar P, McCooke HB. Post-natal resetting of carotid chemoreceptor sensitivity in the lamb. J. Physiol (Lond) 1987; 382:57P.

18. Pokorski M, Lahiri S. Effects of naloxone on carotid body chemoreception and ventilation in the cat. J Appl Physiol 1981; 51:1533–1538.

19. Kholwadwala D, Donnelly DF. Maturation of carotid chemoreceptor sensitivity to hypoxia: in vitro studies in the newborn rat. J Physiol (Lond) 1992; 453:461–473.

20. Eden GJ, Hanson MA. Maturation of the respiratory response to acute hypoxia in the newborn rat. J Physiol (Lond) 1987; 392:1–9.

21. Gonzalez C, Almaraz L, Obeso A, Rigual R. Oxygen and acid chemoreception in the carotid body chemoreceptors. TINS 1992; 15:146–153.

22. Ganfornina MD, Lopez-Barneo J. Single K^+ channels in membane patches of arterial chemoreceptor cells are modulated by O_2 tension. Proc Natl Acad Sci USA 1991; 88:2927–2930.

23. Bureau MA, Lamarche J, Foulon P, Dalle D. Postnatal maturation of respiration in intact and carotid body chemodenervated lambs. J Appl Physiol 1985; 59:869–874.

24. Bureau MA, Lamarche J, Foulon P, Dalle D. The ventilatory response to hypoxia in the newborn lamb after carotid body denervation. Respir Physiol 1985; 60:109–119.

25. Hofer MA. Lethal respiratory disturbance in neonatal rats after arterial chemoreceptor denervation. Life Sci 1984; 34:489–496.

26. Farber JP. Medullary inspiratory activity during opossum development. Am J Physiol 1988; R578–R584.

27. Farber JP. Motor responses to positive pressure breathing in the developing opossum. J Appl Physiol 1985; 58:1489–1495.

28. Farber JP. Medullary expiratory activity during opossum development. J Appl Physiol 1989; 66:1606–1612.

29. Farber JP. Effects on breathing of rostral pons glutamate injection during opossum development. J Appl Physiol 1990; 69:189–195.
30. Michelson HB, Wong RK. Excitatory synaptic responses mediated by GABAA receptors in the hippocampus. Science 1991; 253(5026):1420–1423.
31. Haddad GG, Jiang C. O_2 deprivation in the central nervous system: on mechanisms of neuronal response, differential sensitivity and injury. Proj Neurobiol 1993; 40:277–318.
32. Banasiak KJ, Haddad GG. Hypoxia-induced apoptosis: effect of hypoxic severity and role of p53 in neuronal cell death. Brain Res 1998; 797:295–304.
33. Haddad GG, Jiang C. O_2-sensing mechanisms in excitable cells: role of plasma membrane K^+ channels. Annu Rev Physiol 1997; 59:23–43.
34. Fung ML, Haddad GG. Anoxia-induced depolarization in CA1 hippocampal neurons: role of Na^+-dependent mechanisms. Brain Res 1997; 762:97–102.
35. O'Reilly JP, Cummins TR, Haddad GG. Oxygen deprivation inhibits Na^+ current in rat hippocampal neurons. J Physiol 1997; 503.3:479–488.
36. Ma E, Haddad GG. Anoxia regulates gene expression in the central nervous system of *Drosophila melanogaster*. Mol Brain Res 1997; 46:325–328.
37. Mironov SL, Richter DW. L-type Ca^{2+} channels in inspiratory neurones of mice and their modulation by hypoxia. J Physiol (Lond) 1998; 512(1):75–87.
38. Friedman JE, Chow EJ, Haddad GG. State of actin filaments is changed by anoxia in cultured rat neocortical neurons. Neuroscience 1998; 82(2):421–427.
39. Mironov SL, Richter DW. Cytoskelton mediates inhibition of the fast Na^+ current in respiratory brainstem neurons during hypoxia. Eur J Neurosci 1999; 11(5):1831–1834.
40. Ma E, Xu T, Haddad GG. Gene regulation by O_2 deprivation: an anoxia-regulated novel gene in *Drosophila melanogaster*. Mol Brain Res 1999; 63:217–224.

2

Gasping and Autoresuscitation

WALTER M. ST.-JOHN

Dartmouth Medical School and Dartmouth-Hitchcock Medical Center
Lebanon, New Hampshire, U.S.A.

I. Introduction

Gasping is the first and last breaths of life. At birth, initial breaths appear to represent the brief and maximal inspiratory efforts characteristic of gasps. Such maximal inspiratory efforts, which may be induced by the asphyxia present at birth, serve to inflate the lungs. With the establishment of adequate oxygenation, gasps are superseded by normal eupneic ventilatory activity. The supersedure of gasping by brainstem mechanisms which generate eupnea is so complete that gasping may not again emerge for many years, with the agonal gasping prior to death being the extreme for reemergence. However, gasping may also reemerge at any time when a failure of eupnea results in severe hypoxia or when severe hypoxia or ischemia has itself caused an elimination of eupnea (Fig. 1). Once recruited, gasping provides a powerful mechanism for "autoresuscitation," with a return to eupnea and normal cardiac function. Such autoresuscitation is much more effective in the neonate than in the adult (1,2).

Inherent to the above is the concept that neuronal mechanisms underlying the generation of the gasp may differ from those generating eupnea (3–5). If this concept is valid, then the question arises as to the status of these neuronal mechanisms for gasping during most of life. It appears improbable that these neuronal mechanisms would be quiescent for years and only emerge when

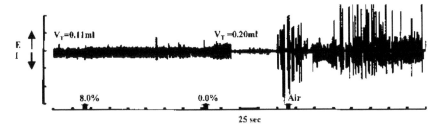

Figure 1 Autoresuscitation in the newborn. Tracing represents airflow from a plethysmograph in which an unanaesthetized 1-day-old rat had been placed. Animal was breathing 100% oxygen. At the first arrow, the inspired gas was altered to 8% oxygen in nitrogen. At the second arrow, 100% nitrogen was introduced. Note transient increase in ventilatory activity and then apnea. Apnea was succeeded by gasping, as evidenced by large excursions. Air was then re-introduced and the animal recovered a eupneic ventilatory pattern. (From Ref. 49.)

activated in severe hypoxia or ischemia. Rather, these neuronal mechanisms for gasping are incorporated into and function as part of the brainstem neuronal circuit generating eupnea. Severe hypoxia or ischemia suppresses components of this brainstem neuronal circuit and/or activates mechanisms for gasping. The mechanism of this activation and the relatively greater efficiency of "autoresuscitation" in the neonate than in the adult are also topics for consideration.

II. Elicitation of Gasping

A systematic comparison of gasping with normal eupneic ventilation was first performed by Thomas Lumsden in a series of papers in 1923 and 1924 (6–9). In addition to exposure to severe hypoxia or ischemia, Lumsden found that eupnea was replaced by gasping following a brainstem transection at the pontomedullary junction. Hence, hypoxia-induced gasping was envisaged to result from the suppression of mesencephalic and pontile components of the brainstem ventilatory control system and a freeing of mechanisms for gasping within the medulla.

Many subsequent investigators have confirmed and extended Lumsden's observations (see 3–5 for reviews). Concerning the elicitation of gasping in severe hypoxia, a stereotypical pattern of changes precedes the replacement of eupnea by gasping. Upon exposure to severe hypoxia, ventilatory activity increases, with tidal volume and frequency being progressively elevated. Both variables then decline to a "primary apnea" which is ultimately succeeded by the large, but somewhat infrequent inspiratory efforts of gasping. If hypoxia is continued, the frequency and peak height of gasps ultimately decline to a "secondary" or "terminal" apnea (1–5). Importantly, however, periodic gasps may continue for minutes or, in neonates, for hours before terminal apnea (10). If during this extended period of gasping, hypoxia is removed and normoxia or hyperoxia is reintroduced, the frequency of gasps progressively increases and they are gradually replaced by eupneic ventilatory activity. This process is termed "autoresuscitation" (1,2) (Fig. 1).

Inherent to the above considerations is the observation that eupnea and gasping are distinctive patterns of automatic ventilatory activity from the day of birth. However, in the transition from eupnea to gasping, the duration of the period of "primary apnea" is exceedingly variable. In fact, this period may be entirely absent, with the augmented eupneic ventilatory activity being replaced by gasping. With such a transition, a distinction between the last eupneic inspirations and the first gasp is not obvious (11–15). This lack of distinction has led to the concept that eupnea and gasping might be variants of a single respiratory rhythm (11,14). While this concept remains possible, there is substantial evidence that different neuronal mechanisms underlie the neurogenesis of eupnea and gasping. Most prominent upon this evidence is the finding that destruction of neurons in a discrete region of medulla irreversibly eliminates gasping but not eupnea (see Sec. VI below). Mechanisms that may underlie the neurogenesis of gasping, and the relationship of these mechanisms to those generating eupnea, will be considered in Section IV.

In addition to exposure to severe hypoxia, eupnea is replaced by gasping following a brainstem transaction at the pontomedullary junction (see 3–5 for reviews) (Fig. 2). Hence, gasping represents the pattern of ventilatory activity which can be generated by the isolated medulla. Analyses of gasping resulting from brainstem transactions with hypoxia-induced gasping has revealed a virtual identity of characteristics; these characteristics are detailed in Section III.

III. Characteristics of Gasping

A. Neural Activities

Compared to eupnea, gasping might be considered as a greatly simplified pattern of ventilatory activity. As described in detail in a number of recent reviews (5,17,18), the eupneic ventilatory cycle consists of three phases: inspiration, and phases I and II of expiration. The eupneic inspiratory phase is typically defined as the "ramplike" rise of activity of the phrenic nerve. Bursts of activity, concomitant with that of the phrenic nerve, are recorded from spinal intercostals nerves and the facial, vagal, and hypoglossal nerves.

20   *St.-John*

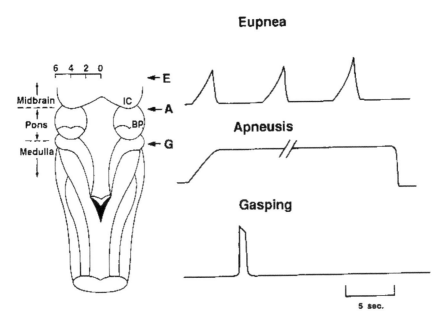

Figure 2 Patterns of automatic ventilatory activity after transections of the brainstem. Drawing is of the brainstem of the cat, with the cerebellum removed. IC, inferior colliculus; BP, brachium pontis; scale is in millimeters. Schematic records are of integrated activity of the phrenic nerve. Eupnea is recorded after a midcollicular transection (level E). After a rostral pontile transection (level A), apneusis is obtained. Gasping is recorded after a transection at the pontomedullary junction (level G). (From Ref. 4.)

Phase I of expiration is marked by the burst of activity of the branch of the recurrent laryngeal nerve innervating the thyroarytenoid muscle of the larynx (Fig. 3). Activity may also be recorded during phase I of expiration from the mylohyoid branch of the trigeminal nerve, as well as the facial and hypoglossal nerves. After phase I activities have terminated, activities of spinal nerves typically commence or augment greatly. These activities of spinal nerves define phase II of expiration.

The gasping ventilatory cycle consists of two phases: inspiration and expiration. In fact, the expiratory phase of gasping might be characterized as the "absence of inspiration" (Fig. 3).

A hallmark of gasping is the extremely rapid rise of inspiratory activity, as evidenced by the rate of rise of phrenic activity (see 3–5 for review). As opposed to the ramplike rise of phrenic activity in eupnea, phrenic activity in gasping reaches a peak value soon after onset and then declines. Hence, phrenic activity may be "decrementing" in gasping (Fig. 3).

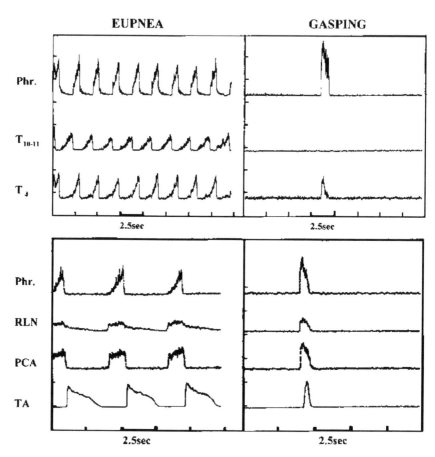

Figure 3 Activities of spinal and cranial nerves in eupnea and gasping in the adult cat. In upper panel, integrated activities of the phrenic nerve (Phr.), "expiratory" intercostal nerve (T_{10-11}), and "inspiratory" intercostal nerve (T_4) are shown. Note alteration of pattern of integrated phrenic activity from "incrementing" in eupnea to "decrementing" in gasping. Expiratory intercostal activity was eliminated. In lower panel, integrated activities of the phrenic nerve (Phr.), recurrent laryngeal nerve (RLN), and branches of the RLN innervating the posterior cricoarytenoid muscle (PCA) and thyroarytenoid muscle (TA) are shown. Note that activities during neural expiration of eupnea were eliminated in gasping. (From Ref. 28.)

Activities of spinal and cranial nerves are like that of the phrenic in gasping, with all exhibiting a decrementing discharge pattern. Compared to eupnea, activities during neural expiration, synonymous with the period between phrenic bursts, are greatly reduced or totally eliminated. Such a reduction of expiratory activities requires some clarification as, in recovery from severe hypoxia or ischaemia, appreciable activities may be observed in the periods between gasps (19,20). This observation is perhaps not surprising since, as discussed below, eupnea and gasping share some common medullary neuronal circuits. However, this reduction or absence of expiratory activities in hypoxia-induced gasping strongly implies that a neuronal circuit, including expiratory activities, does not play an essential role in the neurogenesis of the gasp.

B. Response to Chemoreceptor Stimuli

Again, responses in eupnea and gasping differ fundamentally. In eupnea, it is well accepted that exposure to hypercapnia causes an increase in peak phrenic activity and the frequency of phrenic bursts and, hence, in both the tidal volume and frequency of ventilation. Both variables likewise increase upon exposure to hypoxia. This response is dependent upon the peripheral chemoreceptors. Following sectioning of the carotid sinus nerves and vagi, hypoxia causes a fall in eupneic ventilatory activity in decerebrate or anesthetized preparations (5,21).

In gasping, following transection of the brainstem at the pontomedullary junction, neither the peak height of phrenic activity nor the frequency of gasping is systematically altered in hypercapnia. In these preparations, hypoxia does cause a transient increase in the frequency, but not the height, of gasps. However, these transient changes in hypoxia are the same in preparations having intact and those with sectioned carotid sinus nerve and vagi (22). Hence, the characteristics of the gasping ventilatory pattern appear to be defined by conditions in the environment of the medulla. Fitting with this concept is the finding that, in paralyzed preparations, variables of hypoxia-induced gasping are independent of the concomitant levels of carbon dioxide (23). Moreover, in these same paralyzed preparations, various levels of hypoxia result in gasping having the same peak height and frequency (23).

C. Responses to Mechanoreceptor and Other Afferent Stimulation

A classic reflex in respiratory physiology is the Hering-Breuer reflex, in which inflation of the lungs causes a premature termination of the eupneic inspiration. Following bilateral vagotomy, the duration of the inspiratory and expiratory phases is greatly prolonged, the respiratory frequency is greatly reduced, and the tidal volume is augmented (24). Such changes following bilateral vagotomy are most marked in the neonate. Following vagotomy, the decline of respiratory frequency is so severe that some newborns are unable to maintain a level of ventilatory activity which is sufficient for adequate oxygenation (25–27). Hence, feedbacks from mechanoreceptors of the lungs can markedly influence eupneic ventilatory activity.

Whether activation of mechanoreceptors of the lung alters the gasping ventilatory cycle has not been adequately examined. A number of investigators, beginning with Lumsden, have reported that the pattern of gasping appears the same before and after bilateral vagotomy and that lung inflation appeared not to alter the gasping pattern (6,27–29). Concerning Lumsden's work, the vagi were apparently inadvertently damaged during dissections in some of his preparations (see discussion in Ref. 4). In other studies, values before and after vagotomy or in the presence or absence of lung inflation were obtained during severe hypoxia or ischaemia (27–29). Hence, any influence of vagal mechanisms upon the gasping pattern may have been overshadowed.

Some reports do imply an influence, albeit subtle, of activation of pulmonary stretch receptors upon gasping. In one study (28), gasping was produced by ligation of the basilar artery, and the lungs were inflated by a servorespirator, in parallel with activity of the phrenic nerve. Phrenic activity was modestly altered when these lung inflations were withheld. However, given the modest frequency of phrenic bursts in gasping, withholding lung inflation would certainly cause an alteration in blood oxygenation. Two other studies (30,31) were performed using an in vitro mammalian preparation, which exhibits a pattern of rhythmic activity which is identical to gasping (4,5). In this preparation, with attached lungs, lung inflation did produce modest alterations in the duration of the phrenic burst and interval between bursts. The peak height of bursts was not altered (30,31). Using an in situ perfused rat preparation, we have reproduced the findings from the in vitro mammalian preparation during gasping (unpublished observation). Hence, in this preparation, in which oxygenation is maintained by an extracorporeal circuit, lung inflation alters the respiratory cycle in gasping, primarily by changing the period between phrenic bursts.

As in eupnea, gasping was markedly altered by stimulation of the superior laryngeal nerves (14). Such stimulation altered the duration of the gasp, its peak height, and the period between gasps. In this same context, gasping is inhibited by elicitation of a laryngeal chemoreflex, by placement of water or saline in the larynx (32).

It is perhaps not surprising that the activation of laryngeal and pulmonary receptors would alter both eupnea and gasping since afferents from both sets of receptors terminate in the region of the nucleus of tractus solitarius (33–35). It is well accepted that neurons in this region, termed the dorsomedullary respiratory nucleus, constitute a portion of the pontomedullary circuit responsible for defining activity of the phrenic nerve in eupnea and the medullary circuit which defines the gasp. However, neuronal activities in this region do not play a fundamental role in the genesis of either the gasp or eupneic inspiration. As discussed in Section V below, eupnea is generated by a pontomedullary neuronal circuit and gasping is generated by a neuronal activities within a discrete region of the ventrolateral medulla.

IV. Effectiveness of Gasping in Autoresuscitation

In every mammalian species examined, gasping has been found to be a potent physiological mechanism for restoring ventilatory and also cardiovascular activity following a severe depression of these activities (1–6,10,11,13,36–38). Hence, gasping can be a critical mechanism for ensuring survival of the organism. Such survival mechanisms are most rigorous in the newborn. It is well established that, within the first few days after birth, many species can successfully "autoresuscitate" after being in an environment of complete anoxia for more than an hour. This maximal period of anoxia declines markedly with development such that, in the adult, this period is minutes or even seconds (2,10,36,39).

Without doubt, the major factor promoting the exceeding long survival of neonates in anoxia is the marked reduction in metabolic rate (see 40 for review). Concomitant with the onset of hypoxia, metabolic rate and, hence, consumption of oxygen and production of carbon dioxide fall dramatically in the neonate, but to a much lesser degree in the adult. Evidence of this marked reduction in metabolic rate is the reduction in core temperature. Also, during this period, cardiovascular activity is greatly altered with a profound bradycardia and hypotension (41–43). In addition, there is a redistribution of blood flow, with preferential maintenance of perfusion to vital organs, including the heart and brain, and a reduction in perfusion to skin and viscera. With this reduction of metabolism, gasps become infrequent, even in the newborn. However, if oxygen becomes available, gasps become more frequent, heart rate and arterial blood pressure rise, and eupnea gradually replaces gasping (37,41,44).

In addition to a single incidence of anoxia, gasping is very effective in promoting multiple autoresuscitations from multiple exposures to anoxia. Again, such autoresuscitation is more effective in the newborn, with animals surviving numerous exposures to anoxia over limited intervals (45).

V. Failure of Gasping in Autoresuscitation

The corollary of the above discussion is that gasping is ultimately unsuccessful in autoresuscitation, and such failure is more prevalent in the adult than the newborn. Since the metabolic energy during periods of anoxia is derived primarily from glycolysis, a depletion of energy substrates appears to represent the initial factor accounting for a failure of autoresuscitation. This depletion of energy substrates occurs in the cardiovascular system before the central nervous system. Hence, even though the brainstem ventilatory control system may generate gasps, in terms of activities of the diaphragm and other "respiratory muscles," animals may not survive because of a failure of the heart to recover its normal functioning (2,42). In this context, such a failure of the cardiovascular system, before the brainstem ventilatory control system, is also observed in decerebrate, paralyzed, and ventilated preparation in which "fictive gasping" is monitored by activity of the phrenic nerve. Following a period of anoxia or asphyxia, the failure of heart rate to recover from bradycardia after the reintroduction of oxygen always precedes the failure to reestablish an eupneic pattern of phrenic activity (unpublished observation). Ultimately, however, the brainstem ventilatory control system fails and gasping ceases. Such a cessation is also observed in fictive gasping, recorded from activities of the phrenic nerve in paralyzed and ventilated preparations or, indeed, in a preparation in which the cardiovascular system has been replaced by an extracorporeal circuit (16,46). Again, such a failure of gasping doubtless reflects a failure to provide sufficient energy for maintenance of neuronal function.

This consideration of a "failure of gasping" should not obscure rigorousness of gasping, especially in the newborn. Indeed, it is difficult to induce a failure of gasping. In this context, a failure of gasping has been proposed as the basis of the "sudden infant death syndrome" (3,4,38,42,47). Based on this proposal, a number of risk factors for SIDS in humans have been reproduced in experimental preparations. Included in such risk factors are maternal use of nicotine and cocaine. However, even after prenatal exposure to relatively massive doses of nicotine and cocaine, newborn rats were still very successful in autoresuscitation in response to anoxia. The maximum number of successful autoresuscitations was reduced after exposure to nicotine, but multiple successes were still present (48–50).

VI. Critical Region for Neurogenesis of Gasping

Since gasping is expressed following a transection of the brainstem between pons and medulla (Fig. 2), gasping must be generated within the medulla. In a series of experiments, we found that gasping was irreversibly eliminated following physical lesions or injections of neurotoxins into a region of the rostral medulla. These lesions, which eliminated gasping following unilateral placement, did not disrupt the eupneic rhythm. This critical region for gasping has been termed the "gasping center" (2–5,51–56) (Fig. 4).

The gasping center lies medial and dorsal to the ventral medullary respiratory nucleus, in the region of the nucleus ambiguus. At its ventrolateral margin, the gasping center overlaps with a region of the ventral nucleus termed the "pre-Botzinger" complex (Fig. 4). Neuronal activities within this pre-

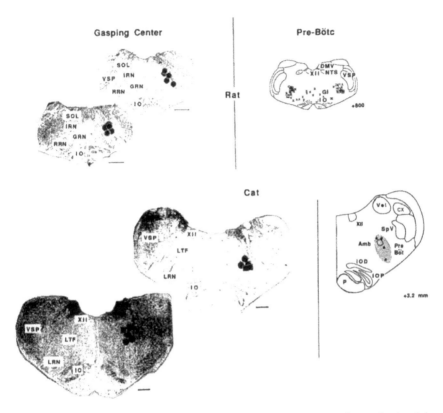

Figure 4 Locations of the gasping center and pre-Botzinger (pre-Botc) complex in adult
rat and cat. Circles and squares in left panels designate regions in which injections of
neurotoxins or physical lesions eliminated gasping, but not eupnea. Right panels show
location of neurons—designated by cross, filled circles, and shading—taken to be within
the pre-Botzinger complex. Scale is 1 mm. Amb, nucleus ambiguus; CX, nucleus cuneatus
externus; DMV, dorsal motor nucleus of vagus; GI, gigantocellular reticular nucleus; IOD,
nucleus dorsalis olivaris inferioris; IOP, nucleus principalis olivaris inferioris; IVN, inferior
vestibular nucleus; NTS, nucleus of solitary tract; p and py, medullary pyramid; PP,
nucleus prepositus; RFN, retrofacial nucleus; SpV, nucleus spinalis nervi trigemini; STN,
spinal trigeminal nucleus; STT, spinal trigeminal tract; VeI, nucleus vestublaris inferior;
VII, facial nucleus; XII, hypoglossal nucleus; 5SP, spinal trigeminal nucleus. (From
Ref. 4.)

Botzinger complex have been shown to be responsible for the neurogenesis of
rhythmic "respiratory" activities of in vitro preparations of neonatal rodents.
However, as discussed in detail in a number of reviews, this "respiratory" activity
in vitro differs markedly from eupnea in vivo but is very similar to gasping
(4,5,56a). Indeed, it is very probable that these preparations are exhibiting

gasping and, as detailed in Section VII below, mechanisms of respiratory rhythm generation in vitro provide important insights into the neurogenesis of gasping in vivo.

Given the above, the question arises as to the relationship between the gasping center and pre-Botzinger complex. In a recent review, these regions are presented as two separate entities, both of which are essential for the neurogenesis of gasping (58). However, based on neuroanatomical and physiological evidence, it appears that these adjoining regions may contain elements of the same neurons, with soma in the pre-Botzinger complex and dendrites and/or axons in the gasping center. Anatomical evidence in support of this concept is the finding that filling of neurons of the pre-Botzinger complex with various dyes reveals extensive dendritic arborizations in the region of the gasping center (59,60). In a complementary study, injections of dyes into the region of the gasping center results in labeling of soma in the pre-Botzinger complex (61).

Physiological evidence that the gasping center and pre-Botzinger complex represent the same neurons is derived from studies involving injections of neurotoxins into the regions. Hence, as noted above, injections of such toxins into the gasping center irreversibly eliminates gasping (51–54). Similar injections into the pre-Botzinger complex, if performed bilaterally, transiently interrupt eupnea but irreversibly eliminate gasping (55,56). However, the volume of neurotoxin which must be injected into the pre-Botzinger complex to eliminate gasping is greater than if injected into the gasping center. This greater "efficiency" for the gasping center is perhaps reflective of the extensive dendritic arborizations of neurons of the pre-Botzinger complex into the gasping center. In any case, it appears probable that neurons of the gasping center–pre-Botzinger complex represent one component of the pontomedullary neuronal circuit which is necessary for the neurogenesis and expression of eupnea. However, these same neurons represent a unique source for the neurogenesis and expression of gasping.

VII. Mechanisms for the Neurogenesis of Gasping

A. Neuronal Activities Which May Generate the Gasp

Ablation of neurons in a circumscribed region of the rostral medulla irreversibly eliminates gasping in vivo and its analogue, the "rhythmic activity" of en bloc and slice preparations in vitro (see discussion in 4,5). Neuronal activities in this region must therefore be essential for the neurogenesis of gasping. An initial enigma arises concerning these neuronal activities which might generate the gasp. Since gasping is elicited only under conditions of extreme hypoxia or asphyxia, neuronal activities that generate the gasp might be quiescent for most of life. This concept of neuronal quiescence for many years seems improbable. More probable is the incorporation of these neuronal activities which generate the gasp into the pontomedullary neuronal circuit responsible for the genesis and expression of eupnea. This pontomedullary circuit is reduced and reorganized in hypoxia, in ischemia, or following brainstem transactions at the pontomedullary junction, and neuronal mechanisms for gasping are released.

If a neuronal activity is responsible for generating inspiratory activity, its activity must commence before the start of activity of the phrenic nerve. For in vitro preparations, which exhibit gasping, a group of neuronal activities, termed preinspiratory, commence activity in late neural expiration and fire through the initial portion of the phrenic burst. These neuronal activities thus have a discharge consonant with generating the "burst" in vitro. The preinspiratory discharge of these neurons is by an intrinsic pacemaker mechanism (60–64).

During eupnea in vivo, the closest analogs to the preinspiratory activities in vitro are expiratory-inspiratory phase spanning neuronal activities (59,65). However, such activities cannot play an essential role in the neurogenesis of gasping, since, in fact, these activities cease in gasping. However, one group of neuronal activities, which discharge during all or the last portion of the phrenic burst in eupnea, acquires preinspiratory discharges in gasping (Fig. 5) (20,66). Thus, these neuronal activities, which have discharge characteristics that are compatible with generating the gasp, have markedly different discharges in eupnea. Such a change in discharge characteristics fits with the concept that neuronal activities that generate the gasp are superseded and captured by the pontomedullary neuronal circuit generating eupnea.

B. Release of Medullary Mechanisms for Gasping

The question obviously arises as to how severe hypoxia or ischemia or brainstem transactions between pons and medulla suppress components of the pontomedullary neuronal circuit for eupnea such that proposed medullary pacemaker mechanisms for gasping are released. Again, evidence as to the release of medullary mechanisms for gasping is derived from studies using in vitro preparations.

Evidence is now substantial that the rhythmic activity of in vitro en bloc or slice preparations is generated by the discharge of pacemaker neurons in the rostral medullary gasping center–pre-Botzinger complex. Fitting with a pacemaker mechanism for rhythm generation is the finding that in vitro rhythmic activities are only modestly altered following a blockade of inhibitory synaptic transmission within the preparation (61,62,64,67,68). This in vitro finding has been considered as enigmatic as a similar blockade of inhibitory synaptic transmission severely distorts the eupneic rhythmic activity of in situ preparations (69). Moreover, injections of blockers of inhibitory neurotransmitter into the region of the gasping center–pre-Botzinger complex of in vivo preparations

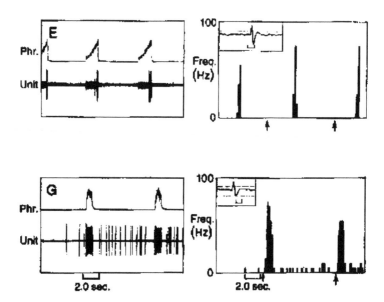

Figure 5   Neuronal activity of pre-Botzinger complex in eupnea and gasping. Left panels show integrated activity of the phrenic nerve (Phr.) and discharge of neuron (Unit) in eupnea (E) and gasping (G). Right panels show instantaneous discharge frequency of the neuron during ventilatory cycles of left panels. Arrows designate onsets of phrenic bursts. Insert is waveform of activity on extended time scale (1 msec). Note neuronal activity which commenced "late" in neural inspiration in eupnea began before the phrenic burst in gasping (From Ref. 20.)

causes an alteration of the eupneic rhythm to apneusis (70) or a "gasplike pattern" (57). This enigma concerning inhibitory synaptic transmission has been resolved by the finding that a blockade of this transmission causes a profound distortion of the eupneic rhythm of in situ preparations but only minimal changes of the gasping rhythm of this same preparation (71). The lack of sensitivity of medullary mechanisms for gasping to a blockade of inhibitory synaptic transmission fits with concept that, as in vitro, the discharge of pacemaker neurons in the gasping center–pre-Botzinger complex underlies the neurogenesis of the gasp.

Following the blockade of inhibitory synaptic transmission in situ, the eupneic rhythm was severed distorted but gasping was not elicited (71). However, as noted above, "gasplike" discharges have been recruited in some preparations following microinjections of bicuculline, a blocker of $GABA_A$ into the pre-Botzinger complex (57). Thus, in general, it would appear that a blockade of inhibitory synaptic transmission alone is not sufficient to release gasping. In this context, however, it is recognized that inhibitory synaptic transmission within the brainstem fails in mild hypoxia (72). Likewise, pontile elements are recognized as one primary source of neurons whose discharge inhibits activities of medullary respiratory neurons (5,35,70,73,74). Thus, hypoxia or brainstem transactions would remove one element suppressing medullary mechanisms for gasping, the element being inhibitory synaptic transmission, largely of pontile origin.

In contrast to the reduction in inhibitory synaptic transmission, hypoxia is reported to cause an additional release of glutamate in some regions of the brain (57,75,76). Such a release might contribute to activation of persistent sodium channels of neurons in the gasping center–pre-Botzinger complex. As considered below, activation of these persistent sodium channels may be necessary to release pacemaker activities of these neurons. Such an activation by glutamate might underlie the finding that microinjections of the potent glutamate analog DL-homocysteic acid into the pre-Botzinger complex elicit an alteration from eupnea to gasping in some preparation (77).

Concerning ionic mechanisms underlying the release of medullary mechanisms for gasping, hypoxia causes an increase in the extracellular concentration of potassium (78). This augmentation probably results from the increased neuronal activity and occurs immediately prior to and immediately after the onset of gasping (14,78). In computational models, such an augmentation shifts the reversal potential for potassium to more positive values of voltage and, hence, reduces all potassium currents (79). This reduction of potassium currents is significant since computational studies have demonstrated that the activity of certain potassium channels may affect the conductance state of persistent sodium channels. Conductances through such persistent sodium channels are necessary for the intrinsic bursting behavior of some medullary neurons to be expressed (79), and are considered to play a major role in the generation of pacemaker-driven oscillations in vitro (80,81). Thus, reducing potassium currents may release intrinsic busting behavior in conditional pacemaker neurons and hence create necessary conditions, along with the elimination of inhibitory synaptic transmission, for pacemaker-driven gaspinglike oscillations in respiratory motor outflows (79).

The augmentation in the extracellular concentration of potassium is not the only mechanism by which conductances of potassium channels are reduced. Hence, hypoxia per se suppresses several types of potassium channels and activates low- and high-voltage calcium channels and also persistent sodium channels in neurons located in many brain regions (e.g., 82–91). The exact mechanisms intermediating the hypoxia-induced changes in the functioning of ionic channels and other intrinsic neuronal properties are not well defined. These mechanisms may involve signaling pathways, such as a change in nitric oxide (92), and second-messenger systems at the intracellular level. Moreover, hypoxia may modify channel conductances and neuronal firing properties through multiple cellular/intracellular mechanisms (92).

The hypoxia-induced processes, such as alteration of the ionic/metabolic extracellular environment, modulation of the intrinsic neuronal properties, and suppression of synaptic inhibition, cannot of course be limited to the region for neurogenesis of gasping in the rostral ventrolateral medulla. Rather, hypoxia-induced processes would be altered in many regions of the brainstem and, in intact animals, in the rest of the brain as well. However, recent studies have demonstrated that neurons in the rostral ventrolateral medulla have a high intrinsic chemosensitivity to hypoxia (87,93). It is unknown what intrinsic properties of these neurons define their special role in genesis of pacemaker-driven gaspinglike oscillations.

In summary, based on both theoretical and experimental studies, it is proposed that hypoxia or ischemia suppresses the pontomedullary neuronal circuit and releases medullary mechanisms for gasping by four interrelated changes: [1] a suppression of inhibitory synaptic transmission; [2] an augmentation in extracellular potassium concentration; [3] a decreased conductance through potassium channels; [4] an increased conductance through persistent sodium channels. These hypothesized mechanisms for the release of medullary mechanisms for gasping have been validated in an experimental study using an in situ preparation of the juvenile rat. In this preparation, a blockade of glycinergic transmission with strychnine, an augmentation in extracellular potassium concentration, and a block of potassium channels with 4-aminopyridine resulted in an elimination of eupnea and elicitation of gasping. Importantly, such an elicitation of gasping occurred under conditions of hyperoxia (94).

Gasping is also elicited under conditions of hyperoxia following micro-injections of sodium cyanide into the region of the gasping center–pre-Botzinger complex (93). However, such injections would induce a region of localized "hypoxia" and thus might cause a release of gasping by mechanisms similar to those in generalized hypoxia or ischemia.

The basis for the release of gasping following several other perturbations is undefined. Hence, brainstem transactions at the pontomedullary junction would obviously remove any inhibitory synaptic transmission of pontile origin. Yet, as noted above, a blockade of inhibitory synaptic transmission alone is typically not sufficient to release gasping. For in vivo preparations, brainstem transactions result in a marked fall in arterial blood pressure and, of course, a varying region of tissue necrosis (22,95–97). Thus, the local environment in the region of the gasping center–pre-Botzinger complex might be hypoxic and/or acidotic follow-ing a brainstem transection. Yet, gasping also follows a transection at the pontomedullary junction of perfused in situ preparations of the neonatal and juvenile rat (46,94). In such preparations, perfusion of the brainstem should be relatively constant. Thus, in addition to inhibitory synaptic transmission, another "factor" of pontile origin appears capable of suppressing medullary mechanisms for gasping. In this context, removal of all pontile influences cannot reasonably be equated simply with a removal of synaptic inhibition upon medullary neurons. As shown in many studies, apneusis follows removal of the rostral pontile pneumotaxic center whereas a complete removal of caudal pons is necessary to release gasping (see discussions in 3,4). Indeed, the pneumotaxic center alone exerts multiple functions in the control of ventilatory activity (98). It is obviously unknown whether removal of all pontile influences causes a switch to gasping by removal of synaptic inhibition upon neurons of the gasping center–pre-Botzinger complex, combined with depolarization of these neurons and activation of persistent sodium channels.

The mechanism by which another procedure releases gasping is undefined. Hence, under conditions of hyperoxia, eupneic ventilatory is replaced by gasping following elicitation of the "aspiration reflex" by stimulation of the pharyngeal mucosa (99). A series of studies have validated that gasping following pharyngeal stimulation is identical to that following brainstem transactions or exposure to severe hypoxia (54,100,101).

VIII. Summary

Thomas Lumsden's papers in 1923 and 1924 (6–9) formed the foundation for contemporary studies of the neurogenesis of automatic ventilatory activity. Lumsden considered that gasping was a "relic of some transitory primitive respiratory process" which "does not appear to influence true rhythmic breathing of normal type." Yet, presaging the concept of "autoresuscitation," Lumsden notes that he "feels no surprise that the facility has persisted in the evolutional struggle" since "gasping has been sufficient to revive animals whose higher respiratory centres have temporarily failed." Gasping represents the expression of a fundamental respiratory rhythm, generated by the discharge of pacemaker neurons in the rostral medullary gasping center–pre-Botzinger complex. For most of life, these pacemaker mechanisms are suppressed, and these rostral medullary neuronal activities are incorporated into the pontomedullary neuronal circuit responsible for the neurogenesis of eupnea. Under conditions of severe hypoxia or ischemia, many components of this pontomedullary neuronal circuit, including inhibitory synaptic transmission, are depressed. These depressions release the latent medullary pacemaker discharge and the gasp is generated.

Acknowledgments

Studies from my laboratory cited in this manuscript were supported by grants 20574 and 26091 from the National Heart, Lung and Blood Institute, National Institutes of Health. Some studies were also performed in the Department of Physiology, School of Biomedical Science of the University of Bristol, England,

and were supported by a Senior International Fellowship from the Fogarty Center of the National Institutes of Health. I thank my colleagues at the Dartmouth Medical School and the University of Bristol for their helpful discussions concerning this work. Also, the helpful ideas and comments of Dr. Ilya Rybak of Drexel University, Philadelphia, are gratefully acknowledged.

References

1. Guntheroth WG, Kawabori I. Hypoxic apnea and gasping. J Clin Invest 1975; 56:1371–1377.
2. Thach BT, Jacobi MS, Gershan WM. Control of breathing during asphyxia and autoresuscitation. In: Haddad GG, Farber JP, eds. Developmental Neurobiology of Breathing. New York: Marcel Dekker, 1991:681–699.
3. St.-John WM. Neurogenesis, control and functional significance of gasping. J Appl Physiol 1990; 68:1305–1315.
4. St.-John WM. Medullary regions for neurogenesis of gasping: noeud vital or noeuds vitals? J Appl Physiol 1996; 81:1865–1877.
5. St.-John WM. Neurogenesis of patterns of automatic ventilatory activity. Prog Neurobiol 1998; 56:97–117.
6. Lumsden T. Observations on the respiratory centres in the cat. J Physiol (Lond) 1923; 57:153–160.
7. Lumsden T. Observations on the respiratory centres J Physiol (Lond) 1923; 57:354–367.
8. Lumsden T. The regulation of respiration I. J Physiol (Lond) 1923; 58:81–91.
9. Lumsden T. Effects of bulbar anaemia on respiratory movements. J Physiol (Lond) 1924; 59:LVIII-LX.
10. Adolph EF. Regulations during survival without oxygen in infant mammals. Respir Physiol 1969; 7:356–368.
11. Lawson EE, Thach BT. Respiratory patterns during progressive asphyxia in newborn rabbits. J Appl Physiol 1977; 43:468–474.
12. Davis PJ, Macefield G, Nail BS. Respiratory muscle activity during asphyxic apnoea and opisthotonos in the rabbit. Respir Physiol 1986; 65:285–294.
13. Macefield G, Nail B. Phrenic and external intercostals motoneuron activity during progressive asphyxia. J Appl Physiol 1987; 63:1413–1420.
14. Melton JE, Oyer Chae L, Edelman NH, Effects of respiratory afferent stimulation on phrenic neurogram during hypoxic gasping in the cat. J Appl Physiol 1991; 75:2091–2098.
15. Fukuda Y. Respiratory neural activity responses to chemical stimuli in newborn rats: reversible transition from normal to 'secondary' rhythm during asphyxia and its implication for 'respiratory like' activity of isolated medullary preparation. Neurosci Res 2000; 38:407–417.
16. St.-John WM, Paton JFR. Characterizations of eupnea, apneusis and gasping in a perfused rat preparation. Respir Physiol 2000; 123:201–213.

17. Richter DW. Generation and maintenance of the respiratory rhythm. J Exp Biol 1982; 100:93–107.
18. Bianchi AL, Denavit-Saubie M, Champagnat J. Central control of breathing in mammals: neuronal circuitry, membrane properties, and neurotransmitters. Physiol Rev 1995; 75:1–45.
19. Zhou D, Wasicko MS, Hu J-M, St.-John, WM. Differing activities of medullary respiratory neurons in eupnea and gasping. J Appl Physiol 1991; 70:1265–1270.
20. St.-John WM. Rostral medullary respiratory neuronal activities of decerebrate cats in eupnea, apneusis and gasping. Respir Physiol 1999; 116:47–65.
21. Von Euler C. Brain stem mechanisms for generation and control of breathing pattern. In: Cherniack NS, Widdicombe JG, eds. Handbook of Physiology—The Respiratory System II. Bethesda, MD: American Physiology Society, 1986:1–67.
22. St.-John WM, Knuth KV. A characterization of the respiratory pattern of gasping. J Appl Physiol 1981; 50:984–993.
23. St.-John WM, Rybak IA. Influence of levels of carbon dioxide and oxygen upon gasping in perfused rat preparation. Respir Physiol 2002; 129:279–287.
24. Coleridge HM, Coleridge JCG. Reflexes evoked from the tracheobronchial tree and lungs. In: Cherniack NS, Widdicombe JG, eds. Handbook of Physiology—The Respiratory System. Bethesda, MD: American Physiology Society, 1986:395–430.
25. Fedorko LE, Kelley EN, England SJ. Importance of vagal afferents in determining ventilation in newborn rats. J Appl Physiol 1988; 65:1033–1039.
26. Smith JC, Greer JJ, Liu G, Feldman JL. Neural mechanisms generating respiratory pattern in mammalian brain stem-spinal cord in vitro. I. Spatiotemporal patterns of motor and medullary neuron activity. J Neurophysiol 1990; 64:1149–1169.
27. Wang W, Fung M-L, Darnall RA, St.-John WM. Characterizations and comparisons of eupnea and gasping in neonatal rats. J Physiol (Lond) 1996; 490:277–292.
28. St. John WM, Zhou D, Fregosi RF. Expiratory neural activities in gasping. J Appl Physiol 1989; 66:223–231.
29. Plura R, Romaniuk JR. Recovery of breathing pattern after 15 minutes of cerebral ischaemia in rabbits. J Appl Physiol 1990; 69:1676–1681.
30. Mellen NM, Feldman JL. Vagal stimulation induces expiratory lengthening in the in vitro neonatal rat. J Appl Physiol 1997; 83:1607–1611.
31. Mellen NM, Feldman JL. Phasic lung inflation shortens inspiratory and respiratory period in the lung-attached neonate rat brain stem spinal cord. J Neurophysiol 2000; 83:3165–3168.
32. Khurana A, Thach BT. Effects of upper airway stimulation on swallowing, gasping and autoresuscitation in hypoxic mice. J Appl Physiol 1996; 80:472–477.
33. Donoghue S, Garcia M, Jordan D, Spyer KM. The brain-stem projections of pulmonary stretch afferent neurones in cats and rabbits. J Physiol (Lond) 1982; 322:353–363.
34. Berger AJ, Averill DB. Projection of single pulmonary stretch receptors to solitary tract region. J Neurophysiol 1983; 49:819–830.
35. Bonham AC, McCrimmon DR. Neurones in a discrete region of the nucleus tractus solitarius are required for the Breuer-Hering reflex in rat. J Physiol (Lond) 1990; 427:261–280.

36. Stafford A, Weatherall JAC. The survival of young rats in nitrogen. J Physiol (Lond) 1960; 153:457–472.
37. Jacobi MS, Thach BT. Effect of maturation on spontaneous recovery from hypoxic apnea by gasping. J Appl Physiol 1989; 66:2384–2390
38. Hunt CE. The cardiorespiratory control hypothesis for sudden infant death syndrome. Clin Perinatol 1992; 19:757–771.
39. Gozal D, Torres JE, Gozal YM, Nuckton TJ. Characterization and developmental aspects of anoxia-induced gasping in the rat. Biol Neonate 1996; 70:280–288.
40. Mortola JP. How newborn mammals cope with hypoxia. Respir Physiol 1999; 116:95–103.
41. Cassin, S, Swann HG, Cassin B. Respiratory and cardiovascular alterations during the process of anoxic death in the newborn. J Appl Physiol 1960; 15:249–252.
42. Gershan, WM., Jacobi MS, Thach BT. Maturation of cardiorespiratory interactions in spontaneous recovery from hypoxic apnea (autoresuscitation). Pediatr Res 1990; 28:87–93.
43. Poets CF, Meny RG, Chobanian MR, Bonofiglio RE. Gasping and other cardio-respiratory patterns during sudden infant deaths. Pediatr Res 1999; 45:350–354.
44. Sanocka UM, Donnelly DF, Haddad GG. Autoresuscitation: a survival mechanism in piglets. J Appl Physiol 1992; 73:749–753.
45. Fewell JE, Smith FG, Ng VG, Wong VH, Wang Y. Postnatal age influences the ability of rats to autoresuscitate from hypoxic-induced apnea. Am J Physiol 2000; 279:R39–R46.
46. Dutschmann M, Wilson RJA, Paton JFR. Respiratory activity in neonatal rats. Autonomic Neurosci Basic Clin 2000; 84:19–29.
47. Rigatto H. Maturation of breathing. Clin Perinatol 1992; 19:739–756.
48. Fewell JE, Smith JG. Perinatal nicotine exposure impairs ability of newborn rats to autoresuscitate from apnea during hypoxia. J Appl Physiol 1998; 85:2066–2074.
49. St.-John WM. Maternal cocaine alters eupneic ventilation but not gasping of neonatal rats. Neurosci Lett 1998; 246:137–140.
50. St.-John, WM, Leiter JC. Maternal nicotine depresses eupneic ventilation of neonatal rats. Neurosci Lett 1999; 267:206–208.
51. St.-John WM, Bledsoe TA, Sokol HW. Identification of medullary loci critical for neurogenesis of gasping. J Appl Physiol 1984; 56:1008–1019.
52. St.-John WM, Bledsoe TA, Tenney SM. Characterization by stimulation of medullary mechanisms underlying gasping neurogenesis. J Appl Physiol 1985; 58:121–128.
53. Fung M-L, Wang W, St.-John WM. Medullary loci critical for expression of gasping in adult rats. J Physiol (Lond) 1994; 480:597–611.
54. Fung M-L, St.-John WM, Tomori Z. Reflex recruitment of medullary gasping mechanisms in eupnea by pharyngeal stimulation in cats. J Physiol (Lond) 1994; 475:519–529.
55. Huang Q, Zhou D, St.-John WM. Lesions of regions for in vitro ventilatory genesis eliminates gasping but not eupnea. Respir Physiol 1997; 107:111–123.
56. St. Jacques R, St.-John WM. Transient, reversible apnea following ablation of the "pre-Botzinger" complex in rats. J Physiol (Lond) 1999; 520:303–314.

56a. Remmers JE. Central neural control of breathing. In: Altose MD, Kawakami Y, eds. Control of Breathing in Health and Disease. New York: Marcel Dekker, 1999:1–40.

57. Solomon IC. Excitation of phrenic and sympathetic output during acute hypoxia: contribution of medullary oxygen detectors. Respir Physiol 2000; 121:101–117.

58. Pilowsky PM, Jiang C, Lipski J. An intracellular study of respiratory neurons in the rostral ventrolateral medulla of the rat and their relationship to catecholamine-containing neurons. J Comp Neurol 1990; 301:604–617.

59. Schwarzacher SW, Smith JC, Richter DW. Pre-Botzinger complex in the cat. J Neurophysiol 1995; 73:1452–1461.

60. Koshiya N, Smith JC. Neuronal pacemaker for breathing visualized in vitro. Nature 1999; 400:360–363.

61. Onimaru H, Arata A, Homma I. Primary respiratory rhythm generator in the medulla of brainstem–spinal cord preparation from newborn rat. Brain Res 1988; 45:314–324.

62. Onimaru H, Arata A, Homma I. Firing properties of respiratory rhythm generating neurons in the absence of synaptic transmission in rat medulla in vitro. Exp Brain Res 1989; 76:530–536.

63. Johnson SM, Smith JC, Funk GD, Feldman JL. Pacemaker behavior of respiratory neurons in medullary slices from neonatal rat. J Neurophysiol 1994; 72:2598–2608.

64. Ballanyi K, Onimaru H, Homma I. Respiratory network function in the isolated brainstem–spinal cord of newborn rat. Prog Neurobiol 1999; 59:583–634.

65. Connelly CA, Dobbins EG, Feldman JL. Pre-Botzinger complex in cats: respiratory neuronal discharge patterns. Brain Res 1992; 590:337–340.

66. St-John WM. Alterations in respiratory neuronal activities in "pre-Bötzinger" region in hypocapnia. Respir Physiol 1998; 114:119–131.

67. Shao, XM, Feldman JL. Respiratory rhythm generation and synaptic inhibition of expiratory neurons in pre-Botzinger complex: differential roles of glycinergic and GABAergic transmission. J Neurophysiol 1997; 77:1853–1860.

68. Bou-Flores C, Berger AJ. Gap junctions and inhibitory synapses modulate inspiratory motoneuron synchronization. J Neurophysiol 2001; 85:1543–1551.

69. Hayashi F, Lipski J. The role of inhibitory amino acids in control of respiratory motor output in an arterially perfused rat. Respir Physiol 1992; 89:47–63.

70. Pierrefiche O, Schwarzacher SW, Bischoff AM, Richter DW. Blockade of synaptic inhibition within the pre-Botzinger complex in the cat suppresses respiratory rhythm generation in vivo. J Physiol (Lond) 1998; 509:245–254.

71. St.-John WM, Paton JFR. Inhibitory synaptic transmission is not required for the neurogenesis of gasping in a perfused rat preparation. Respir Physiol 2002; 132: 265–277.

72. Richter DW, Bischoff A, Anders K, Bellingham M, Windhorst U. Response of the medullary respiratory network of the rat to hypoxia. J Physiol (Lond) 1991; 443:231–256.

73. Fung M-L, Wang W, St. John WM. Involvement of pontile NMDA receptors in inspiratory termination in rat. Respir Physiol 1994; 96:177–188.

74. Fung M-L, St. John WM. Neuronal activities underlying inspiratory termination by pneumotaxic mechanisms. Respir Physiol 1994; 98:267–281.

75. Hagberg H, Lehmann A, Sandberg M, Nystrom B, Jacobsen I, Hamberger I. Ischemia-induced shift of inhibitory and excitatory amino acids from intra to extracellular compartments. J Cereb Blood Flow Metab 1985; 4:413–419.
76. Rothman S, Olney JW. Glutamate and the patho-physiology of hypoxic-ischemic brain damage. Ann Neurol 1986; 19:105–111.
77. Solomon I, Edelman NH, Neubauer J. Patterns of phrenic motor output evoked by chemical stimulation of neurons in the pre-Botzinger complex in vivo. J Neurophysiol 1999; 81:1150–1161.
78. Melton JE, Kadia SC, Yu QP, Neubauer JA, Edelman NH. Respiratory and sympathetic activity during recovery from hypoxic depression and gasping in cats. J Appl Physiol 1996; 80:1940–1948.
79. Rybak IA, St.-John WM, Paton, JFR. Models of neuronal bursting behavior: implications for in vivo versus in vitro respiratory rhythmogenesis. In: Frontiers in Modeling and Control of Breathing: Integration at Molecular, Cellular and Systems Levels. New York: Plenum/Kluwer Press, 2001:159–164.
80. Butera RJ, Rinzel J, Smith JC. Models of respiratory rhythm generation in the pre-Botzinger complex. I. Bursting pacemaker cells. J Neurophysiol 1999; 81:382–397.
81. Butera RJ, Rinzel J, Smith JC. Models of respiratory rhythm generation in the pre-Botzinger complex. II. Populations of coupled pacemaker neurons. J Neurophysiol 1999; 81:398–415.
82. Jiang C, Haddad GG. A direct mechanism for sensing low oxygen levels by central neurons. Proc Natl Acad Sci USA 1994; 91:7198–7201.
83. Lopez-Barneo J. Oxygen-sensing by ion channels and the regulation of cellular functions. Trends Neurosci 1996; 19:435–440.
84. Hammarstrom AKM, Gage PW. Inhibition of oxidative metabolism increases persistent sodium current in rat CA1 hippocampal neurons. J Physiol (Lond) 1998; 510:735–741.
85. Thompson RJ, Nurse CA. Anoxia differentially modulates multiple K^+ currents and depolarizes neonatal rat adrenal chromaffin cells. J Physiol (Lond) 1998; 512:421–434.
86. Gebhardt C, Heinemann U. Anoxic decrease in potassium outward currents of hippocampal cultured neurons in absence and presence of dithionite. Brain Res 1999; 837:270–276.
87. Kawai Y, Qi J, Comer AH, Gibbons H, Win J, Lipski J. Effects of cyanide and hypoxia on membrane currents in neurons acutely dissociated from the rostral ventrolateral medulla of the rat. Brain Res 1999; 830:246–257.
88. Liu H, Moczydlowski E, Haddad GG. O_2 deprivation inhibits Ca^{2+}-activated K^+ channels via cytosolic factors in mice neocortical neurons. J Clin Invest 1999; 104:577–588.
89. Horn EM, Waldrop TG. Hypoxic augmentation of fast-inactivating and persistent sodium currents in rat caudal hypothalamic neurons. J Neurophysiol 2000; 84:2572–2581.
90. Prabhakar NR. Oxygen sensing by the carotid body chemoreceptors. J Appl Physiol 2000; 88:2287–2295.

91. Lopez-Barneo J, Pardal R, Ortega-Saenz P. Cellular mechanisms of oxygen sensing. Annu Rev Physiol 2001; 63:259–287.

92. Gozal D, Torres JE, Gozal E, Nuckton TJ, Dixon MK, Gozal YM, Hornby PJ. Nitric oxide modulates anoxia-induced gasping in the developing rat. Biol Neonate 1998; 73:264–274.

93. Solomon IC, Edelman NH, Neubauer JA. Pre-Botzinger complex functions as a central hypoxia chemosensor for respiration in vivo. J Neurophysiol 2000; 83:2854–2868.

94. St.-John WM, Rybak I, Paton JFR. Potential switch from eupnea to fictive gasping after blockade of glycine transmission and potassium channels. Am J Physiol 2002; 283:R721–731.

95. Hoff HE, Breckenridge CG. The medullary origin of respiratory periodicity in the dog. Am J Physiol 1949; 158:157–172.

96. Wang SC, Ngai SH, Frumin MJ. Organization of central respiratory mechanisms in the brain stem of the cat: genesis of normal respiratory rhythmicity. Am J Physiol 1957; 190:333–342.

97. Breckenridge CG, Hoff HE. Pontine and medullary regulation of respiration in the cat. Am J Physiol 1958; 160:385–394.

98. Fung ML, St-John WM. Separation of multiple functions in ventilatory control of pneumotaxic mechanisms. Respir Physiol 1994; 96:83–98.

99. Tomori Z. The snifflike aspiration reflex. In: Herzog H, ed. Progress in Respiration Research, Cough and Other Respiratory Reflexes. Basel: Karger, 1991:224–250.

100. Fung M-L, Tomori Z, St.-John WM. Medullary neuronal activities in gasping induced by pharyngeal stimulation and hypoxia in cats. Respir Physiol 1995; 100:195–202.

101. Tomori Z, Fung ML, Donic V, Donicova V, St.-John WM. Power spectral analysis of respiratory responses to pharyngeal stimulation in cats: comparisons with eupnea and gasping. J Physiol (Lond) 1995; 485:551–559.

3

Ontogeny of Upper- and Lower-Airway Innervation

**JOHN T. FISHER and
CYRIL E. SCHWEITZER**

Queen's University
Kingston, Ontario, Canada

**MARKUS WEICHSELBAUM and
MALCOLM P. SPARROW**

University of Western Australia
Nedlands, Western Australia, Australia

I. Introduction

The development of lung innervation occurs during the pseudoglandular, canalicular, and saccular stages, each of which is characterized by separate milestones with respect to lung development. In the human lung, the primary pattern of lung branching is established during the pseudoglandular stage, followed by elongation of airways in the canalicular stage and the onset of development within the acinus during the saccular stage (see Sec. II). Until recently, the status of airway innervation and smooth muscle development was incompletely described during these phases, which at least to some extent reflected the limitations associated with the gross anatomical and cellular microscopic techniques employed. As a result, studies of the functional neurophysiologic behavior of airway afferents and efferent innervation preceded detailed confocal microscopy studies of airway innervation. Indeed, the seminal studies of lower airway afferents, such as those

---

This chapter is submitted in honor of Drs. Giuseppe and Franca Sant'Ambrogio, whose enthusiasm for research stimulated a generation of grateful research fellows while providing exciting advances in the understanding of upper- and lower-airway afferents.

39

described by Widdicombe and Sant'Ambrogio (for references see Sec. III), often referred to the need for detailed studies of the anatomical and cellular nature of airway innervation.

In the present chapter our purpose is twofold: first, to provide an overview of the spectacular advances in the knowledge of the development of airway innervation due to new imaging technologies, and secondly, to review the functional behavior of the afferents associated with the upper and lower airways. Interestingly, the former has not only caught up with the knowledge base of the latter, but in many respects now supersedes it.

II. Anatomy, Morphology, and Distribution

This section describes recent morphological insights into the ontogeny of the pulmonary innervation in relation to the developing airways. Neural tissue is a dominant feature of the fetal lung and undergoes dramatic morphological development during gestation. The stages of maturation have recently been graphically captured using confocal microscopy. Immunofluorescently stained whole lungs, lobes, and airway segments were scanned by optical sectioning through the entire thickness of the airway wall, using markers of neural tissue in conjunction with markers for airway smooth muscle and epithelial tubules. From the three-dimensional information obtained, overviews and detailed images of the network of nerves and forming ganglia that envelop the lung primordia have been prepared. As lung development proceeds through gestation to postnatal life, comprehensive maps of the pathways of the nerves to their target tissues have provided unique views of the airway innervation. The picture that emerges is that neural tissue and airway smooth muscle are an integral part of the lung from its inception, and persist in a dynamic state throughout gestation and into postnatal life and late adulthood. The evidence for this is relatively recent. It begins in the embryonic lung of the mouse, then proceeds through gestation in the pig and human.

A. Origin of the Innervation—The Fetal Mouse Lung

The development of the innervation of the fetal mouse lung from days 10 to 14 of gestation, the early pseudoglandular stage, is first described. In this period, branching morphogenesis is at its peak, and every 24 h of gestation sees a striking change in the lung structure and in the maturation of the innervation that accompanies branching. In mice, two lung buds begin to evaginate from the foregut at embryonic day 10 (E10) (1), whereas in humans and most mammals the lung develops from a single lung bud. Neural crest–derived cells (NCC) are present in the foregut prior to the formation of lung buds and have been assumed to migrate into the lung, where they differentiate into intrinsic pulmonary neurons (2). This migration has recently been demonstrated in the mouse lung by immunostaining whole mounts of foregut including the lung buds and imaging them using confocal laser scanning microscopy, from embryonic day 10 (E10) and thereafter (pseudoglandular stage) (3). NCC are identified with antibodies to protein gene product 9.5 (PGP 9.5; a general neural marker) and NCC-specific markers, including phox2b and p75[NTR]. Phox2b is a transcription factor located in NCC nuclei (4,5). p75[NTR] is a low-affinity trk receptor and is present in the membranes of NCC and their nerve processes (3,5,6). An antibody to the pan-neuronal marker, PGP 9.5 (7) stains mature neurons and nerve fibers but not precursors.

At E10, PGP 9.5- and p75-positive nerve fibers run along the dorsal side of the foregut. Among these fibers are many migrating NCC with phox2b-positive nuclei and p75[NTR]-positive membranes. At this early stage, the emerging lung buds are largely free of NCC, although a few solitary NCC at the base of the lung buds with occasional processes are directed into the bud. Some NCC in the foregut had matured sufficiently to show PGP 9.5 staining, whereas the cells in the lung buds remained negative for this neuronal marker.

By E11, the neural tissue along the foregut condenses into two large nerve trunks, the vagus nerves, which stained strongly for PGP 9.5 (3). Neural processes positive for PGP 9.5 and p75[NTR] reach from the vagi to the trachea and primary bronchi (Fig. 1A). The vagi comprise neural processes and many migrating NCC (Fig. 1B). These processes are likely to comprise both afferent fibers originating from vagal and spinal sensory ganglia, and preganglionic efferents that will ultimately synapse on NCC once they have completed migration. Neural processes from the vagi to the primary bronchi (Fig. 1C) and the dorsal trachea contain migrating NCC. Many NCC are present on the dorsal trachea located over the trachealis muscle, and some on the ventral surface of the proximal primary bronchi, in the process of aggregating into large ganglia.

By E12 the lobular organisation of the lung is complete, with one large left lobe and four smaller right lobes. A large nerve plexus is present on the ventral side of the lung on the hilum (Fig. 2A) which originates from the vagus (3), and comprises nerve fibers and large ganglia-like clusters of NCC, with numerous cells in each cluster. From these ganglia, nerves positive for PGP 9.5 (Fig. 2B) and p75[NTR] (Fig. 2C) extend along the bronchi, following the smooth muscle covered tubules. NCC also migrated along these nerve tracts but lag behind the growth of the nerve axons (Fig. 2C), e.g., in the left lobe, NCC are present as far as the branch point of the second lateral, whereas the nerves reached to the end of the lobar bronchus and also along the more proximal laterals to the base of the epithelial buds (Fig. 2B). In the original color figures (3), the superimposed confocal projections of both the neural tissue and the airway smooth muscle reveal their close relationship.

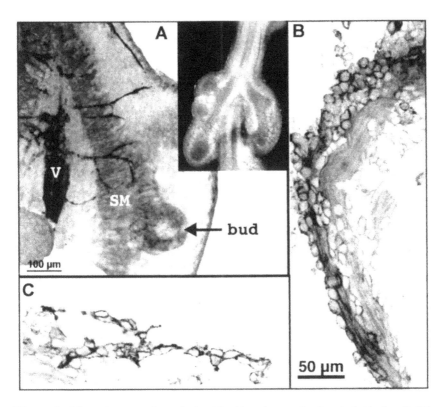

Figure 1 Mouse lung at embryonic day 11, videomicrograph of ventral side (inset). (A) A confocal projection showing a ventral view of the right upper half of an E11 mouse lung stained for nerves (black) with the protein gene product 9.5 (PGP 9.5). This also stained the undifferentiated epithelium of the tubules and growing end buds (gray). The airway smooth muscle that covers the tubules is stained with α-actin (dark gray). The carina lies at the top of the figure. The left vagus (V) sends out nerve processes to the airway smooth muscle covering the left lobar bronchus. Some extend toward the mesenchymal cap. (B) A single optical section through the vagus shows that it contains neural crest cells and many axons running between them (stained with an antibody to p75^NTR which is positive for cell membranes and axons). (C) Nerve fibers going from the vagus into the lung (see A) comprise processes and NCC cells (stained for p75^NTR). (From Ref. 3.)

By E13 the neuronal precursors lying over the dorsal trachea have matured to form a PGP 9.5–positive network of thin nerve trunks interconnected by small ganglia, giving fine fibers that penetrate the smooth muscle layer. By E14 this plexus is more extensive, comprising larger ganglia and more numerous thick nerve trunks with multiple connections to the vagi (3) (Fig. 3A). Small nerves

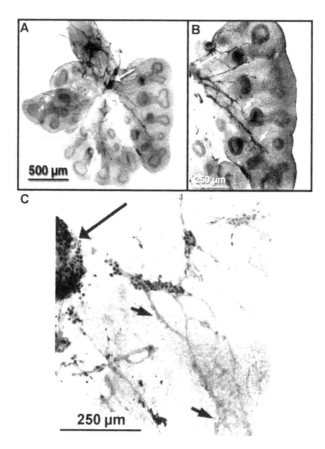

Figure 2 Mouse lung at embryonic day 12. (A) A confocal projection of the mouse lung at E12 (ventral view) shows the lobular organization (the accessory lobe and the vagi have been removed) with the epithelial tubules in longitudinal section. The first two laterals of the left lobe reveal the end buds in the process of dividing. The undifferentiated epithelium of the tubules, and particularly their end buds, are immunoreactive to PGP 9.5 (gray-black). PGP 9.5 diffusely stains ganglia connected by nerve trunks and fibers in the ventral hilum (long arrow). (B) PGP 9.5–positive nerve fibers issue from the large ganglion (long arrow) at the base of the left pulmonary bronchi and reach along the left lobar bronchus (short arrows) and along some of the laterals, but no PGP 9.5-positive cells and ganglia are present along the tubules. (C) The large ganglion at the base of the left lobar bronchus (long arrow) contains many neural crest cells (NCC) with phox2b-positive nuclei (black) and p75^{NTR}-positive membranes (gray). The NCC migrate along the p75^{NTR}-fibers (gray, short arrows) that grow along the lobar bronchus and laterals. The cells lag behind the growth of fibers; the majority have only reached as far as the first lateral and a few as far as the second lateral. (From Ref. 3.)

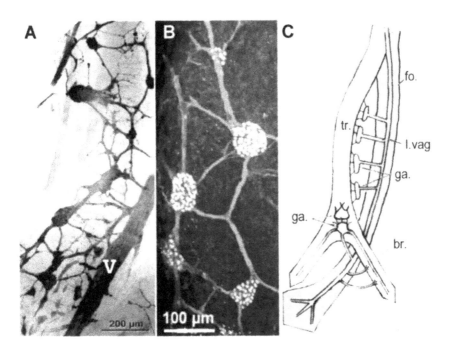

Figure 3 Mouse trachea at embryonic day 14. (A) PGP 9.5–positive (black) network of ganglia connected by thick bundles to the vagus (V). Nerves from ganglia spread over smooth muscle on the surface of trachea (upper part of panel). (B) Ganglia with phox2b-positive nuclei (white) and nerve trunks staining for GFRα1 (gray) lying over the dorsal trachea. (C) Scheme showing the innervation from the vagus to ganglia lying on the dorsal trachea and ventral hilum. Main nerve trunks to the lobes arise from the latter. Oblique ventral view. tr, trachea; fo, foregut; ga, ganglia; 1 vag., left vagus; br, bronchus. (A and B, courtesy J. Tollet, University of Western Australia.)

from the ganglia branch into many fine varicose fibers that run along the smooth muscle bundles. The ganglia vary greatly in size, and many large ganglia contain >100 cell bodies positive for PGP9.5 (Fig. 3A) and phox2b (Fig. 3B). The axons in the nerve bundles connecting the ganglia stain strongly for GFRa1, the receptor for glial-derived neurotrophic factor (see below). The innervation from the vagus to the main ganglia lying on the dorsal trachea, ventral hilum, and left lobe is schematically drawn in Figure 3C. During this early pseudoglandular phase, most nerves mainly follow the smooth muscle–covered tubules, but some nerves course through the mesenchyme toward the lung cap, where they form varicose terminal arborizations by E13 (3).

Among the first neurotransmitters to appear in the foregut is CGRP at E12 (8). By E13, nNOS can be demonstrated in the lung by NADPH-diaphorase activity in nerves associated with the airways and blood vessels. At E15, immunostaining reveals the presence of nNOS in neurons and fibers on the trachea, and from the hilum to the bronchioles (9).

Glial-derived neurotrophic factor (GDNF) has been identified as the most important neurotrophic factor in the development of the enteric nervous system (10), and there is increasing evidence to suggest that GDNF is of similar importance during lung development. In the gut of mice lacking GDNF or RET (receptor for GDNF), all neurons below the esophagus and proximal stomach are absent (11), but it is not known whether neurons of the lung are affected. In cultured explants of left lung lobes at E12, neurons survive and display proliferation, differentiation and continued migration along the developing smooth muscle–covered tubules (12,13). In the presence of serum, a characteristic of these explants is the formation of a layer of α-actin-positive cells (possibly smooth muscle precursors) that grows out from the lung periphery and attracts nerves that grow onto this layer. When cultured in GDNF-supplemented medium, the amount of neural tissue on this layer increases 14-fold. The neural tissue consists of a high density network of nerve trunks and large ganglia and is composed of many PGP 9.5–positive cells, indicating that both migration, proliferation, and differentiation of neuronal precursors as well as neurite extension have taken place as a direct result of stimulation by GDNF. This suggests that GDNF is a chemoattractant to both nerves and NCC. GDNF-impregnated beads attract nerves growing out from cultured lung explants and in some instances NCC surround the treated beads. The membranes and nerve processes of the NCC are positive for the GDNF receptor, GFRα1 (Fig. 3B), suggesting that nerves and NCC are guided by GDNF. The presence of GDNF-mRNA has been demonstrated in the mesenchyme adjacent to the fetal mouse epithelial tubules (14)—possibly in the smooth muscle, which thus may play an important role to attract nerve fibers and migrating NCC.

B. Mapping the Innervation of the Fetal Pig and Human Lung

The rapid development seen in mice during the pseudoglandular stage from 10 to 14 days of gestation contrasts with that of large mammals where the equivalent time period lasts from 3 to 8 weeks in the pig and 5 to 17 weeks in the human (15,16). In mice at E14 and thereafter, the application of confocal microscopy becomes more difficult. The signal emission is reduced at increasing depth of scanning, which is a consequence of the increased tissue thickness and density, and the associated decrease of antibody penetration. These problems can be overcome by removal of the lung cap, mesenchyme, and pulmonary vascular tissue, leaving the bronchial tree fully exposed, albeit not in mice. This dissection is feasible in fetal and postnatal lungs of larger mammals including humans, pigs, dogs, and rabbits (17–19). Thus, the entire bronchial tree, or any part of it, can be progressively scanned field by field with the confocal microscope at high resolution. Using this approach montages of near complete bronchial trees in the pseudoglandular stage ~6 mm long from fetal pigs (15,17) (Fig. 4), and smaller lengths of subsegmental airways from fetal humans (18) have been assembled. Overviews such as these clearly display the organisation of nerves and ganglia and their relationship to the airway smooth muscle (ASM), the glands, and the blood vessels. Fine detail is also shown at selected sites (Fig. 4 inset). Thus, the development of the innervation from the embryonic lung bud through to postnatal life is revealed.

The structural characteristics and distribution of the nerves are similar in the three species (mouse, pig, and human) at comparable developmental stages and, likewise, the airway smooth muscle. The muscle bundles are oriented around the airways perpendicular to their long axis from the trachea through to the base of the epithelial buds, and this arrangement persists into postnatal life. The innervation of the porcine and human bronchial tree from the adventitia to the epithelium has been reported from early gestation through to postnatal life (17–20), and it is comprehensively described by a series of confocal images on the web (21).

Pseudoglandular Stage

The main characteristics of the pseudoglandular stage are chains of forming ganglia interconnected by thick nerve trunks to each other and to the vagus lying over the ASM of the dorsal trachea and the ventral surface of the hilum. In general, two thick main nerve trunks extend from the hilum along each airway to the growing tips. These lie above the airway smooth muscle supported by the mesenchyme. In the fetal pig at 5.5 weeks' gestation, proximal trunks ~50 μm in diam. run ~40–60 μm above the ASM, progressively decreasing distally over a length of 4 mm to ~20 μm in diam. and 15–20 μm from the ASM. They terminate as thin bundles in the collar of airway smooth muscle that surrounds the epithelial buds (17,22). All along the length of the trunks, branches descend toward the smooth muscle, and break up into small bundles. From these, fine varicose fibers issue that spread over the muscle layer and exhibit arborized endings located within 1 μm distance from muscle cells, suggesting a possible functional innervation. At this stage the varicose fibers are essentially randomly distributed on and in the smooth muscle (Fig. 5), but later become oriented along the smooth muscle bundles (17,19).

Immature ganglia are present along the main trunks from which nerve branches radiate out to connect to many other smaller ganglia that form a network covering the airway wall. Figure 6 shows this innervation in the distal airways of a fetal human lung at 7.5 weeks' gestation. The mean distance between ganglia measured as the Mean Nearest Neighbor Distance (MNND) (19) is 64 ± 18 μm

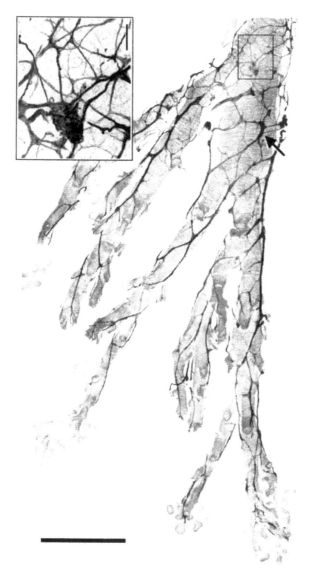

Figure 4 Montage showing the right half of the bronchial tree of a GW 5.5 (16 g body weight) fetal pig stained for nerves and ganglia with PGP 9.5 (black) and for smooth muscle with α-actin (gray). Nerve trunks run down the length of the airways and terminate at the base of the epithelial buds (scale bar 1 mm). The boxed region contains an enlarged view of a proximal area showing a network of interconnected nerve trunks and a large ganglion (scale bar: 100 μm). The large ganglion (arrow) contains ∼300 neurons. The montage was constructed from 54 single confocal images. (From Ref. 17.)

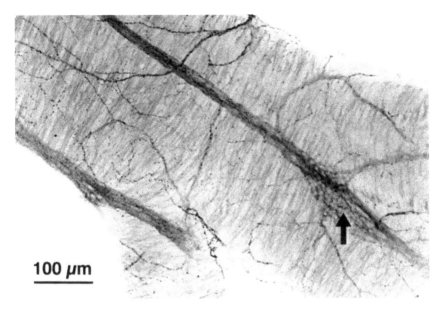

Figure 5 Two major nerve trunks stained with synaptic vesicle protein (SV2) traverse
the length of the airway, giving rise to a fine network of varicose processes overlying the
airway smooth muscle stained for smooth muscle myosin (gray). At this stage the varicose
fibers are randomly distributed on and in the smooth muscle located within 1 μm from the
muscle cells. The accumulation of cell bodies (arrow) is a precursor ganglion present at the
bifurcation point of the airway. The cell profiles in the ganglion can be distinguished by the
SV2 positive nerve fibers lying around them. (From Ref. 17.)

(n = 87), very similar to the pig (70 μm at comparable gestation). Ganglia also
lie at most airway branch points, and give rise to smaller trunks that follow the
airways as they proceed distally. Proximal ganglia are large (i.e., > 300 cell
bodies at 5.5 weeks' gestation), whereas distal ganglia are small and ultimately
comprise a few neurons. Individual neurons within the ganglia show different
intensities of staining with PGP 9.5, indicating variance in their type or maturity.

PGP 9.5 gives a diffuse staining of the nerve trunks with many unstained
cell profiles of Schwann cells (revealed using an antibody to the Schwann cell
marker S-100). Staining for synaptic vesicle protein 2 (SV2), a component of the
membranes of the vesicles in the varicosities reveals individual varicose fibers in
the nerve trunks indicating that vesicle traffic is prolific at this stage of
development (17,22). This abundance of SV2-positive fibers decreases with
ongoing maturation; by postnatal life, varicose fibers are restricted to the distal
nerve bundles and the fine fibers that lie on and in the ASM (17). Staining for

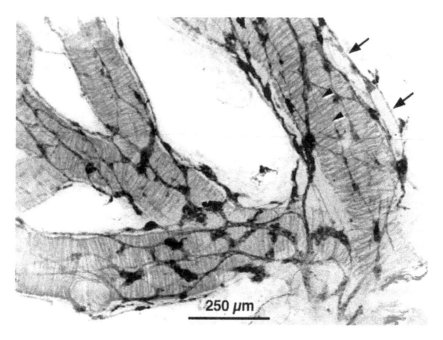

Figure 6 The innervation and airway smooth muscle in the developing airways of a fetal human lung at 58 days of gestation. The field shows branching epithelial tubules in the periphery of a lobe. Nerves and ganglia are stained for PGP 9.5 (black) and form a network overlying the airway smooth muscle stained for α-actin (gray). The bundles are arranged circumferentially around the epithelial tubule and lie essentially perpendicular to the long axis of the tubule. In some places the neural network is as much as 40 μm (arrows) from the muscle layer. Smaller nerve bundles can be discerned (arrowheads), which at higher power are seen to descend to the surface of the smooth muscle. (From Ref. 18.)

neurofilament sharply defines a small proportion of individual fibers in a trunk. These fibers can be traced along the tubules, where several terminate in the collar of smooth muscle that surrounds the base of the epithelial bud (22). The low proportion of neurofilament-positive fibers in the nerve trunks may reflect the level of maturity of these nerves, since the proportion of neurofilament-positive neural tissue increases as gestation progresses (15).

Canalicular Stage

With airway growth there is increasing spatial separation of the ganglia. The large ganglia lying on the central airways that form nodes at nerve junctions undergo a fourfold increase in MNND ~254 μm. The ganglia vary greatly in size—large ones are 120 μm at their greatest width, and contain as many as 200 neurons of average diameter 11 μm. Furthermore, many of those lying on the trunks gradually become displaced laterally to become attached by a stem, with nerves radiating out from them over the airway (15). The bronchial vasculature becomes more prominent with arterioles running adjacent to the trunks and around the ganglia. Nerve fibers penetrate the submucosal glands. By midterm, ganglia have condensed and become compact and spherical.

Figure 7 shows a large montage of the nerve tracts in the subsegmental airways of a lobe from an 18 week fetal human lung (18). It measures 11 mm in overall length with an external diameter of 2.2 mm at the proximal end, reducing to 200 μm at the distal ends, and spans seven branchings. Large nerve trunks run the entire length of airways, reducing from 45 μm to < 20 μm diam. distally, with many ganglia attached to them from which nerves issue to connect with a network of smaller ganglia lying closer to the airway surface.

A high-power view (Fig. 8) shows that a fine plexus of nerves containing many small ganglia lies close to the airway smooth muscle. Mucosal nerves are now abundant. They arise from branches of the adventitial nerves that penetrate the airway smooth muscle layer at intervals where they run in parallel bundles in the lamina propria along the length of the airway (18). The development of the mucosal vascular circulation is now well advanced (19). At this point the lung is well endowed with the beginnings of a neural network that can serve the afferent and efferent functions of the vagus nerve.

Expression of Neurotransmitters

Most neurotransmitters make their appearance in the canalicular stage (humans, 16–26 weeks (16); pigs, 7–13 weeks (15); rats, 18–19 days; and mice, 16.6–17.4 days (23). In rats at 17 days' gestation, calcitonin gene-related peptide (CGRP) is present in neuroendocrine bodies in the epithelium. At 18 days, CGRP nerve fibers are present in the trachea, stem bronchi, and proximal intrapulmonary airways, mainly lying below the epithelium, and by 19–20 days fine fibers are seen on the bronchial smooth muscle and around blood vessels in the adventitia (24). In mouse lung, nitrergic neurons can be detected in the airways as early as E13 by using the sensitive chemical assay for NADPH diaphorase. By E15, nNOS expression is immunochemically detected in airway neurons and fibers (9).

Functional cholinergic transmission has been demonstrated (as airway narrowing) in the pseudoglandular stage indicating that some fibers are already cholinergic (17). In humans, histological evidence for the presence of cholinergic neurons by 10–12 weeks was reported using acetylcholinesterase (2), which may not be a reliable marker for the presence of acetylcholine (25). Choline acetyltransferase (ChAT) is a specific marker for acetylcholine (ACh) (26), and in fetal pig lungs both ChAT-positive neurons and fibers are present in the trachea and on the airway smooth muscle of the peripheral airways at the early canalicular

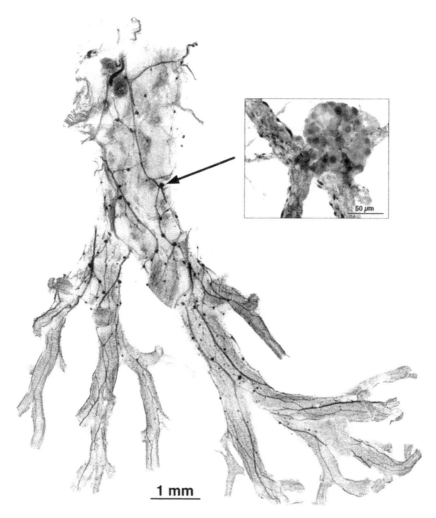

Figure 7 A montage showing the innervation of the adventitial surface of the bronchial tree of a segmental bronchus and its branches from a human fetal lung, 18 weeks' gestation. The tissue was stained for PGP 9.5 (black) and α-actin (gray) to show both nerves and smooth muscle. Nerve trunks extend to the most distal airways. Ganglia are present along the trunks and at the divisions of nerve bundles. The insert shows a higher power projection of a ganglion at the junction of several nerve trunks (arrow). (From Ref. 18.)

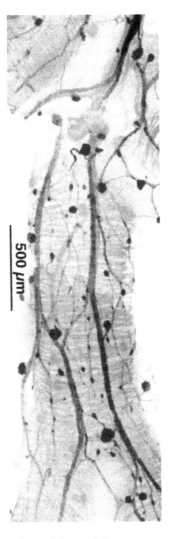

Figure 8 A higher-power view of the straight region on the right hand side of the montage in Figure 7 showing the disposition of the nerves, ganglia, airway smooth muscle, and bronchial arteries. PGP 9.5 (black) stained a plexus of fine nerves containing many small ganglia. α-Actin (gray) stained both airway smooth muscle and arterioles of the bronchial circulation that accompany the larger nerve trunks with some less distinct vessels branching off to overlie the airway smooth muscle. (From Ref. 18.)

stage. ChAT does not stain the very fine terminal varicose fibers that SV2 reveals, which may indicate that it is not sensitive enough to detect very low levels of ACh (15).

Vasoactive intestinal peptide (VIP)- and substance P (SP)-positive fibers are seen at 16 weeks in the bronchial smooth muscle, and thin fibers containing CGRP are commencing to ascend from the basement membrane of the epithelium (2). The latter are likely to be the sensory C-fibers seen in postnatal life (20,27,28). SP and CGRP are present in the axons of the nerve trunks running in the airway adventitia at midterm (19), and, by the beginning of the saccular stage VIP, TH and NPY are also present.

Saccular Stage

The saccular stage runs through most of the third trimester where further maturation of the ganglia and nerves occurs. The processes of glial cells increasingly surround the neurons in the ganglia, and the axons in nerve trunks and bundles (15). This glial ensheathement may contribute to restricting intra-ganglionic communication between adjacent neurons (29). Separation of the ganglia greatly increases as the airways lengthen and widen. Neurotransmitters are fully expressed now, with strong immunostaining of neurons and their axons (19). Neurofilament is now expressed in a great many neurons and their axons. The perikarya are located mainly in the periphery of the ganglion with many neurite structures in the center. Neurons appear to contain one major axon and therefore correspond to Dogiel type 1 neurons. Some neurons show strong PGP 9.5 staining of the nucleus only, while others exhibit a faint homogeneous staining throughout the perikaryon (15).

The bronchial mucosal circulation, which is rudimentary at the end of the pseudoglandular stage, progresses in complexity during the canalicular stage and is now a well developed network of microvessels. The mucosa is now richly innervated with nerve bundles and varicose fibers running the length of the airways, which stain for NOS, SP, CGRP, VIP, TH, and NPY in fetal pig lung (19). The presence of the neuropeptides SP and CGRP is indicative of an afferent population of nerves. Although it appears that many nerve bundles use the arterioles as conduits, our immunohistochemical evidence suggests the opposite, since the neural tissue can be stained earlier (i.e., in the pseudoglandular stage) than the bronchial vessels that are first demonstrable in the canalicular stage, where they run contiguously with the nerves.

Summary: Ontogeny of the Innervation in the Fetal Period

Neural tissue and airway smooth muscle are integral components of the primordial lung, where the epithelial tubules that constitute the future bronchial tree are enveloped in a network of precursor ganglia and loose bundles of nerve fibers. These ganglia comprise flat patches of neural crest cells that have migrated along nerve processes that issue from the vagi. They lie over the wall of the epithelial tubules supported by the mesenchyme, and are interconnected by nerve bundles. The ASM is also present, being laid down at the base of the epithelial buds that is the site of new tubule growth. This occurs through an epithelial-mesenchymal interaction (30). Thus, as the epithelial tubules elongate, the ASM forms a continuous layer that extends from the trachea to the growing tips. Small nerve bundles branch from the nerve network and descend to the smooth muscle where fine varicose fibers lie on and in the muscle bundles. This ASM is functionally mature shortly after it is formed since the terminal tubules narrow and relax spontaneously in situ (31–33).

GDNF is a likely neurotrophic factor that acts as a chemoattractant for nerves in lung explants (13), and GDNF receptors (GFRα1) are present on the nerve processes in vivo, but whether GDNF is expressed by the ASM is not known. By the end of the pseudoglandular stage, when branching is virtually complete, most precursor neural tissue has completed proliferating, and differentiation into mature neurons is progressing. In the canalicular stage ganglia develop a more compact, spherical shape, and come to lie offset from the nerve trunks and large bundles. Airway growth increases their separation. Arterioles of the bronchial circulation appear adjacent to the nerve trunks and nerve bundles. The mucosal innervation becomes established followed by the mucosal vasculature. The chemical coding of neurons and their fibers occurs during this stage. In the saccular stage (most of the third trimester), lung growth is rapid, with greater spatial separation of the ganglia, and their neurons become progressively ensheathed by glial cell processes, as do the axons in nerve trunks and bundles.

Early Postnatal Period to Adulthood

Overviews and higher-power views of the adventitial and mucosal innervation have been obtained using whole mounts of airway from rats (34), young pigs and humans (15,17,18,20), and mice (3,13). However, the classic drawings of lower airway nerves, neurons, and afferent mechanoreceptors in the ASM of an 8-month-old child, a rabbit, and a dog (35,36), and the varicose fibers in the mucosa of the epiglottis of dog (37) are a poignant reminder of the skills of these early workers.

The variety of techniques they employed is noteworthy. These include combined fixing and staining of the airways by direct instillation into the trachea after death, and the use of whole mounts and sections 50–100 μm thick. The advantages of these approaches for investigating airway innervation seem to have been overlooked later in the 20th century, when thin sections came into general use. In the past 20 years the availability of reliable, specific antibodies to most of the neurotransmitters of the autonomic nerves have seen their widespread application to characterizing the chemical coding of nerves in the airway wall. The lack of a suitable antibody to stain parasympathetic cholinergic nerves has been a major holdup. Staining for acetylcholinesterase is not specific (25). The relatively recent introduction of an antibody to acetylcholine (26) lacks the sensitivity to reveal fine varicose nerve fibers (15). More recently, an antibody to vesicular acetylcholine transporter protein has been successfully used in the intestine of rats (38). Notwithstanding this deficiency, a large body of information has been established on the neurotransmitters found in the neurons in the parasympathetic ganglia, and their efferent nerves to the component tissues of the upper and lower airways.

There are many recent specialized reviews on neurotransmitters in the nerves to airway smooth muscle (39), glands and goblets cells (40), upper respiratory tract (41), immune tissue (42), and bronchial vasculature (43), as well as reviews of their role in cotransmission and neuromodulation (44,45). In most of these studies nerves are stained in thin sections (usually ~ 7 μm thick). To show that cells are innervated requires electron microscopy, but confocal microscopy has greater utility where it can be used in conjunction with sections of up to ~ 100 μm in thickness or with whole mounts. It can show that nerves and cells lie in the same optical plane of known thickness (< 1 μm) and at the same time provides an overview of distribution of nerves. However, the morphology and distribution of the afferent nerve supply and their endings are where major deficiencies lie.

Efferent Nerves: Long Preganglionic Fibers and Short Postganglionic Fibers?

In the adult lungs of large mammals the distribution and morphology of the innervation become increasingly difficult to characterize in the lungs of adult, large mammals because of the sheer size of the lung and airway tree. The thickness of the layers of tissue, particularly connective tissue and cartilage, makes the adventitial nerves and ganglia extremely difficult to expose compared with the ease in the fetal lung. Furthermore, the density of ganglia becomes more and more diluted with growth so that the chances of finding them become very low, a point that does not seem to be widely appreciated. Ganglia are generally considered to be absent beyond the third-generation airways, a view largely based on evidence from early reports (35,46,47). From this it is assumed that long postganglionic nerves run from the ganglia in the central airways along the length of the bronchial tree to the terminal airways (29,35). The former researchers suggest that the central ganglia therefore play a key role in regulating airway function.

This view is not compatible with the studies on the development of the airway innervation reported above (15,17,18). Ganglia are shown to extend to the 9–10th generation in the canalicular stage in 18-week fetal human lungs (18) (see Fig. 7). At about this point the fine airways (100 μm diam.) break off in the parenchyma as it is dissected away, so the presence of ganglia in even smaller or more distal airways has not been documented. In the lung of midterm fetal pigs, ganglia extend to distal generations of 50 μm diam., which is the limit of the dissection employed (15,19). These ganglia are mature (proximal) or maturing (distal) ganglia, and there is no reason why they would disappear through apoptosis from the lungs at this late stage of development.

For the purposes of calculation it is reasonable to assume that ganglia lie chiefly in a thin layer surrounding the airway wall. The extent of their separation with lung growth is then a function of the increase in the surface area of the airway wall and the increase in length of the airways of the bronchial tree. It should be possible to obtain estimates for these parameters to determine ganglia separation in the adult, and thereby the probability of finding them. In summary, the view that emerges from studying the ontogeny of neural development is one of long preganglionic fibers and short postganglionic fibers (Fig. 9), which is consistent with other tissues innervated by autonomic nerves.

Density of Innervation

With the abundance of nerves reported in the fetal and postnatal airways of several species comes the need for quantifying so that comparisons can be made between tissues (e.g., ASM and epithelium), and across species (e.g., rat and pig). Nerve densities in the trachea of postnatal rats (34) and bronchi/bronchioles of pigs (17,20) have been obtained by a comparable point-counting method (Table 1). The studies show that density of the total innervation to the ASM is about twofold greater than in the epithelium, and the densities in pigs are about twice that of rats. Substance P nerves comprise 90% [rat (34)] and 94% [pig (20)] of the total epithelial nerves (stained using PGP 9.5). While nerves have not been quantified in the fetal lung, it is clear from inspection of montages of the fetal airway innervation (3,17,18) that they are as abundant in fetal life as in postnatal life. Thus, nerve density is maintained during the enormous growth that occurs during development, indicating that nerves continue to extend over the expanding surface of the airway wall as growth proceeds. These varicose fibers have, however, now become oriented in the direction of the muscle bundles, with single fibers running along most muscle bundles in the young pig (17), adult mouse (3), and human infant (18) and adult (Fig. 10, lower panel). This arrangement of a nerve fiber running along the muscle bundle is probably the main determinant of the ultimate nerve density attained (Fig. 10).

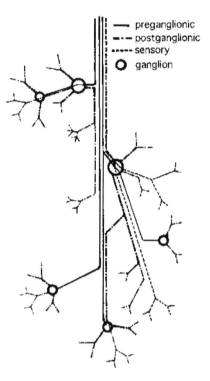

Figure 9 Proposed distribution of efferent and afferent nerves in the lung. Efferent ganglionic fibers (solid black lines) arise from the vagus and synapse on neurons in ganglia that give rise to postganglionic fibers (gray lines). Nerve endings shown as arborized branchings. From the canalicular stage onward, ganglia are separated from the nerve trunks by a short stem. Some preganglionic fibers pass through the ganglion and travel in the same trunks as the postganglionic fibers to terminate in a more distal ganglion. Postganglionic bundles branch and terminate at their respective target organs, e.g., airway smooth muscle, mucous glands. Sensory nerves (hollow lines) from receptive fields, e.g., epithelium, travel centrally through ganglia and along the vagus to their neurons in the spinal and spinal ganglia.

Orientation of Airway Smooth Muscle Bundles

The muscle bundles encircle the airways and lie perpendicular to the long axis of the airways in the fetal lungs of humans, pigs, and mice from the trachea to the terminal airways. This orientation is maintained into the postnatal and adult life of these species (3,13,15,17,18,22), as well as in postnatal rat and young dog (19). An ultrastructural study by Ebina et al. (48) reporting that ASM has a pitch of ~30° in adult humans is at variance with these wide-ranging confocal micro-

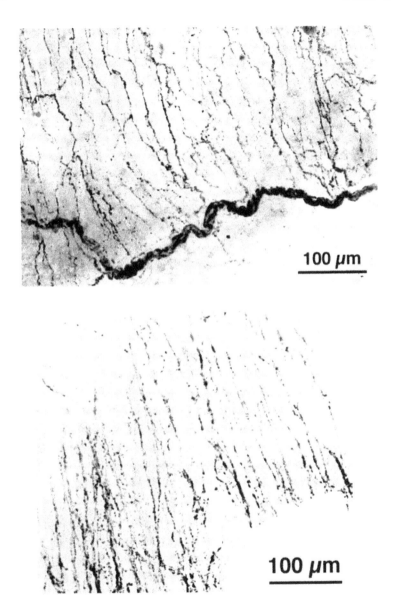

Figure 10 Confocal projection of the innervation of the airway smooth muscle viewed from the adventitial surface of the bronchus of an adult mouse (upper panel) and a 54-year-old human (lower panel). Varicose nerves run around the circumference of the airway, lying along the airway smooth muscle bundles which are arranged perpendicular to the long axis of the airway (smooth muscle bundles not shown to avoid obscuring nerves). (To view, see Refs. 2 and 19.)

Table 1 Density of Innervation of Single Axons (mm/mm²) in the Mucosa and Airway Smooth Muscle of Rat and Pig

	Rat		Pig	
	PGP 9.5	Substance P	PGP 9.5	Substance P
Airway smooth muscle				
Tracheal	96	4		
Bronchioles			210	—
Epithelium				
Apical plexus				87
Basal				21
Total	49	44	115	108
Lamina propria	17	8		
Total mucosa	66	52		

Combined area of fields counted for each tissue area: rat: 250,000 μm² (34); pig: airway smooth muscle 230,000 μm², epithelium 190,000 μm² (courtesy J. Lamb, University of Western Australia). PGP 9.5 is a pan-neuronal marker.

scopic studies, where large areas from the central and distal airways have been scanned. At branching points the perpendicular orientation of some of the ASM bundles varies to suit the local airway architecture, and occasionally one or two bundles may lie almost parallel with the length of the airway in the terminal airways region (49) (J. Lamb, unpublished).

Innervation of Pulmonary Neuroendocrine Cells

Pulmonary neuroendocrine cells are of endodermal origin and arise from the undifferentiated epithelial cells of endodermal origin that line the tubules in the fetal lung early in gestation (50). They occur as solitary cells (NEC) and as clusters in conjunction with Clara cells called neuroendocrine bodies (NEB) (51,52). They are distributed throughout the entire respiratory tract, nasal respiratory epithelium (53), laryngeal mucosa (54), and in the lung from the trachea to the terminal airways and the alveoli (52). In the fetal lung they are frequently located at the branching points of the tubules. In humans, differentiated NEC and NEB are present by 10 weeks' gestation (55,56). The NE cells are bottle- or flasklike in shape, and reach from the basement membrane to the lumen. They can be distinguished by their profile of bioactive amines and peptides—namely, serotonin, calcitonin, calcitonin gene-related peptide, chromogranin A, and bombesin (57). The NEBs may play a role as hypoxic-sensitive airway chemoreceptors (58) since an oxygen-sensitive potassium channel coupled to an oxygen sensory protein has been demonstrated in their membrane at the luminal surface in the rabbit (59). They are also considered to be involved in regulating epithelial cell growth and regeneration through a paracrine mechanism whereby their bioactive peptides are released into their environment (60).

Ultrastructural studies have shown that some NEC and NEB become innervated in fetal life (51,55,56). Nerve terminals with synaptic contacts have been described at the base of the NEC in infant bronchial epithelium (61). In fetal human lungs at 20 weeks' gestation, cholinergic axon terminals have been described deep within NEB (56). Some terminals exhibit vesicle profiles indicative of adrenergic fibres and form gap junctions with adjacent cells within the NEB (56). However, the majority of axons are sensory. This has been demonstrated by a loss of NEB innervation after unilateral nodose vagotomy (62). In rats, labeling neurons in the nodose ganglia with DiI enabled tracing of sensory afferents to NEB (63). These nerves do not contain the sensory neuropeptide CGRP, in contrast to the afferents that supply the C-fiber endings in the epithelium.

Recent studies in our laboratory (MPS) using confocal microscopy of whole mounts of adult human lungs revealed an abundance of NEC that were homogeneously distributed in the epithelium. The density was $\sim 250/mm^2$, which is several times higher than previously reported. In humans, NEB decrease in frequency with age and are rare in adult lung (64). Our data support this finding, as NEB were found only once in several hundred preparations of eight adult lungs. The solitary NEC exhibited a predominantly flasklike shape. The base of the cell bodies was located at the basement membrane and issued long processes, some neuritelike, that extended along the basement membrane and thicker processes that extended upward to the luminal surface. Nerves were present in the form of patches in the epithelium. No correlation was found between frequency of NEC and numbers of nerves. Some nerves lay in close apposition to NEC, suggestive of a possible functional innervation. CGRP was present in 20% of all NEC revealed with PGP 9.5 and bombesin. Three-dimensional animated renditions of NEC that can be viewed from multiple angles illustrate the extraordinary complexity of the processes and localized distribution of the CGRP and other markers (21).

The physiological role of the innervation to the NEC and NEB is not well understood. It has been proposed that the nerve endings at the base of the NEC subserve an axon reflex, presumably in the NEB itself and possibly to deeper tissues such as the airway smooth muscle (55). There may also be local reflex connections through peripheral ganglia. Hypoxia detected by the O_2 sensor in the NEC is presumed to release mediators that stimulate vagal afferents, but no central nervous reflexes have been identified. Whether they exert only intraganglionic effects remains to be shown. Electrophysiological recordings from single afferent fibers arising from NEB have not been made, and all studies on the effect of hypoxia on vagal afferents from C-fibers, rapidly adapting and slowly adapting receptors have been negative (66). Recent advances in microscopic techniques with increased sensitivity may shed more light on the morphological basis for many of the suggested functions of NEC innervation.

Function of the Airway Innervation During Fetal Life

Whether the innervation plays a functional role during specific events in fetal lung development is unknown. With the recent insight into the organization of the nerves in the bronchial tree, it should be feasible to carry out neurotransmission experiments on the ganglia and nerves in the lung either excised from the fetus or in situ with the fetus partially removed from the uterus. At birth a range of sensory reflexes are activated in the neonate, e.g., the Hering-Breuer reflex. It is possible that some afferent mechanoreceptors such as the slowly adapting stretch receptors located in or adjacent to the ASM of the airways may already be firing at a low discharge rate in the fetal lung, since it is inflated with liquid. It seems reasonable to assume that well before birth, afferent and efferent nerves are capable of function.

Little is known about the pathways of the afferent nerves and their receptors in the fetal airways. Afferent fibers must have been present when NCC and nerve processes migrated from the vagi at the formation of the lung bud. They doubtless represent a major component of the total fibers in the nerve trunks in the fetal lung, since >70% of the nerves in the vagus that innervate the lung are afferent (67). These are the fibers that pass through the ganglia as they extended distally (Fig. 9). Markers of C-fiber sensory nerves, viz. SP and CGRP, are seen at midterm in nerve fibers in lamina propria of rats (24) and in the epithelium in humans (2), but the apical plexus of C-fiber nerve endings in the epithelium that constitute the receptive fields in postnatal pigs and humans (20) was not observed. Surprisingly, mechanoreceptors, which are large, treelike arborizations 100–200 μm long, have not been recognized in the fetal airways, but more focused searching in the ASM and lamina propria of the trachea, bronchi, and bronchioles may remedy this.

III. Neurophysiologic Behavior of Airway Afferents

A. Upper Airway Afferents

Previous reviews of the upper and lower airways of the newborn have highlighted the apparent "choice" by the neonate to rely on what has been termed "obligatory" nasal breathing (see 68 for review). Although the latter is actually more preferential than obligatory, it highlights what appears to be a functional attempt by the neonate to separate respiratory from alimentary functions of the upper airway. The behavior of upper-airway afferents reflects this duality, since they respond to both respiratory and chemical stimuli.

The apparent importance of chemical stimuli in the upper airway of the newborn is reflected by the very powerful reflex responses to liquid stimuli reaching the upper airways (68–70; and Mathew, this volume). Studies using animal models demonstrated profound apneas in newborns exposed to various liquids in the larynx (71–73), and the key stimuli appear to be the lack of anions (70,73). In the human infant, especially preterm infants, feeding has often been associated with a dis-coordination of feeding and breathing behaviors where the former has taken precedence over the latter with deleterious impact (see Mathew, this volume). These studies highlight the importance of both qualitative and quantitative feedback from upper-airway afferents to the medulla regarding the type of media (air vs. liquid) present in the upper airway. Although studies of the impact of liquid media on respiratory reflexes of the newborn are important, this review focuses exclusively on the behavior of upper-airway (laryngeal) afferents exposed to "respiratory" stimuli (i.e., responses associated with air as the media present in the upper airway).

The reflex responses of the upper airway largely reflect the afferent feedback from the recurrent laryngeal and the superior laryngeal nerves, which are both branches of the vagus nerve (68,74). The motor and caudal afferent innervation of the larynx is provided by the recurrent laryngeal nerve (RLN), while the cranial afferent feedback from the larynx is supplied by the internal branch of the superior laryngeal nerve (75). Laryngeal reflexes are largely abolished by section of the superior laryngeal nerve (SLN), reflecting the importance of the afferent axons from this region (74,75). The SLN is composed of myelinated and unmyelinated axons, and in the newborn the former corresponds to $\sim$20% of the axons compared to almost 60% in the adult (75).

Respiratory Modulation of Upper-Airway Afferents

Initial studies of laryngeal afferents described the response of receptors to mechanical/punctate or liquid stimuli delivered to the laryngeal region (for review see 74). Although it was appreciated that stimuli of a more respiratory nature could be present, the search for a way to classify the respiratory behavior of laryngeal afferents was greatly stimulated by the observations of Mathew and coworkers (76–78). They found that application of subatmospheric pressure to the isolated upper airway caused enhancement of inspiratory genioglossus muscle activity, as well as reducing diaphragmatic discharge. This implied that receptors in the upper airway provide feedback that differentiates obstructed from normal breaths, which in turn causes strategic recruitment of respiratory muscles to reverse obstruction. Subsequently, Sant'Ambrogio and coworkers (79), whose group at this point included Mathew, provided an interpretational framework that led to a unifying classification of laryngeal respiratory afferents with respect to respiratory stimuli. This framework allowed investigators to separate the cyclical *respiratory* afferent activity, which originated from the upper airway, from that related to other stimuli. The classification of superior laryngeal receptors by Sant'Ambrogio's lab into transmural pressure, temperature/airflow, and local respiratory muscle activity or "drive" categories provided a novel classification paradigm that led to significant insight into how laryngeal afferents transduce the phase of respiration and/or the presence of upper-airway obstruction.

The typical discharge patterns of receptors sensing temperature, pressure, and laryngeal muscle contraction (or drive) are illustrated in Figure 11. The classification of laryngeal receptors into these categories relied on an ingenious series of manipulations (see Fig. 11) such that larynx afferents could be [1] subjected to normal respiration through the upper airway (Fig. 11 intact), [2] bypassed via respiration through a tracheal cannula (Fig. 11, tracheotomy), [3] exposed to subatmospheric laryngeal pressures during "occluded" respiratory efforts originating above the larynx (Fig. 1, upper AW occlusion), or [4] bypassed during "occluded" respiratory efforts originating in the lower airway (Fig. 1, lower AW occlusion). Each maneuver causes the selective removal or enhancement of one or more of the stimuli that are specific to each class of laryngeal afferents. The tracheotomy maneuver allowed for the withdrawal of pressure- and flow-related stimuli from the upper airway, leaving only respiratory drive to laryngeal muscles intact.

Occluded efforts performed below the larynx eliminated the same stimuli, except that the drive to laryngeal muscles was enhanced due to a reflex prolongation of inspiration associated with withdrawal of volume-related feedback. Occlusions performed above the larynx removed flow but enhanced subatmospheric pressure-related stimuli. By comparing the response to each maneuver receptors were classified into one of the three categories. Thus, cold-sensitive afferents discharge only when airflow is present in the upper airway, pressure-sensitive endings discharge only when exposed to subatmospheric pressure, and "respiratory drive," or laryngeal muscle contraction, afferents discharge under all conditions in which laryngeal abductors are recruited.

Further studies refined the definition of the appropriate physical stimuli for each class of afferent. For example, pressure-sensitive endings typically display a laryngeal muscle contraction- or drive-sensitive component, and laryngeal muscle drive-sensitive afferents often possess a sensitivity to subatmospheric pressure (74). The use of cold or warmed inspired air was used to confirm the temperature-sensitive nature of the cold afferents (80,81), since they fail to respond if inspired air is warmed to body temperature. Menthol acts as a chemical selective stimulant of laryngeal cold sensitive endings (81), similar to that described for other temperature-sensitive endings. The action of menthol has long been appreciated by the condiment and tobacco industry, where menthol is routinely used to produce a sensation of "coolness" or enhanced airflow in the upper airway.

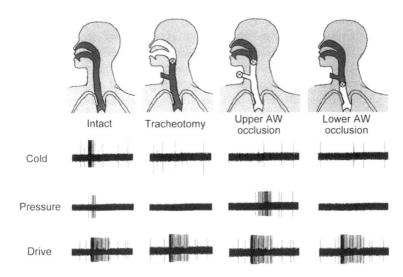

Figure 11 Cartoon illustrating the expected discharge pattern of afferent receptors recorded from the superior laryngeal nerve during a single inspiration performed during manipulations of upper-airway stimuli (left to right) in a hypothetical human subject. During normal respiration (intact), all three types of upper-airway afferents are active: temperature-sensitive endings (cold), subatmospheric pressure–sensitive endings (pressure), and endings sensing activation of laryngeal muscles due to abduction of the vocal cords (i.e., respiratory drive to laryngeal muscles). Each receptor provides phasic, inspiratory activity to the medulla (compare to other figures). If the upper airway is bypassed (tracheotomy), only Drive receptors would be expected to discharge since all other mechanical and temperature-related stimuli would be absent from the upper airway. During occlusion above the larynx (upper-AW occlusion), the larynx is subjected to enhanced subatmospheric pressure and Drive, whereas occlusion below the larynx (lower-AW occlusion) only provides Drive-related feedback. Comparison of the discharge response of the afferent receptor in each maneuver allows for classification into temperature (cold), subatmospheric pressure (pressure), and laryngeal muscle/respiratory drive receptors. Temperature/cold receptors no longer exhibit the normal inspiratory during the three experimental maneuvers due to the loss of the appropriate stimulus (compare left-hand cold receptor discharge to that seen to the right for each maneuver). Pressure-sensitive endings exhibit inspiratory discharge only during intact or occluded efforts performed above the larynx in which they are exposed to subatmospheric pressures (compare left-hand discharge and third from left for the same receptor). Laryngeal muscle/respiratory drive receptors discharge during all conditions since the laryngeal abductors always receive efferent discharge during inspiration. The "filled" shading depicts the presence of airflow. The "open" shading in the lower airways depicts the absence of airflow and presence of increased subatmospheric pressure during the occlusions. The upper-AW and lower-AW occlusion differ only in the presence or absence of subatmospheric pressure in the larynx respectively. (From Ref. 79.)

Anderson et al. (82) linked respiratory modulated laryngeal receptors to chemical stimuli. They found that respiratory modulated receptors are also acutely sensitive to a low osmolality stimulus. Interestingly, laryngeal receptors sensitive to lack of chloride ion did not possess a respiratory modulation. Thus, although some respiratory modulated receptors play a dual role, sensing air and liquid stimuli, others do not. The basis for the osmosensitivity is not clear, although it should be possible to test hypotheses that have been advanced for other osmosensitive neurons in the CNS (83). The development of an *in vitro* model in which receptor responses could be studied from an isolated larynx, similar to that employed for the lower airways (84), would allow one to directly test the molecular basis for laryngeal receptor osmosensitivity.

The collage of signals from laryngeal afferents is thought to be helpful in detecting upper-airway obstruction. Indeed, the loss of cold receptor discharge, enhanced pressure receptor discharge, and continued or enhanced respiratory drive receptor discharge provides the neurophysiological basis for the reflex responses associated with obstructive apneas. Indeed, these afferents appear to be capable of providing a signal that is graded with respect to the magnitude of upper-airway obstruction.

The same three classes of laryngeal receptors have been described in the newborn (85), although the discharge frequency of the pressure receptors in response to a range of subatmospheric pressures is reduced compared to that of the adult (86). The reflex impact of stimulation of laryngeal receptors in newborn animals appears to be amplified compared to that reported for the adult (68). For example, stimulation of cold receptors by flow or menthol through the isolated upper airway causes inhibition of breathing in newborn animals (85–88), as does subatmospheric pressure applied to the upper airway (85). Selective stimulation of laryngeal cold-sensitive endings with menthol also causes a depression of respiration in the newborn (87). Although there is a tendency in the newborn for stimulation of upper-airway afferents to cause apnea rather than simply modifying the behavior of upper-airway and respiratory muscle recruitment (68,74), this may be related to anesthesia. Indeed, inhalation of menthol in sleeping newborn animals and human infants elicits only transient effects on respiratory pattern compared to the previous studies in anesthetized animals (Anderson, Froese, and Fisher, unpublished observations).

Sant'Ambrogio and Sant'Ambrogio recently reviewed the role of laryngeal C-fiber afferents (75). Laryngeal C-fiber afferents elicit cough, changes in pattern of breathing, and bronchoconstriction, although there is considerable species variability (75). In contrast to this evidence of a role for laryngeal C-fiber afferents, Stockwell and coworkers (89) found that in adult human subjects blockade of the SLN did not reduce the response to a citric acid stimulus. Citric acid is thought to be one of many stimuli activating C-fibers, although capsaicin, the pungent ingredient from hot peppers, is typically used as a powerful and selective stimulant (90). Reconciliation of the Stockwell (89) data with other studies remains outstanding. There do not appear to be any data on the behavior of laryngeal C-fiber afferents in the fetus or newborn, and the reader is therefore referred to recent reviews of receptor behavior in the adult (75).

Future Studies of Laryngeal Afferents

Investigation of laryngeal and other upper-airway afferents has the potential to be fertile. There are no studies of the detailed ontogeny of upper-airway afferents or of their behavior in fetal life, where the larynx serves as a variable resistor that controls the egress of pulmonary fetal liquid (68). Furthermore, the morphological approach described above for the innervation of the lower airways has yet to be unleashed on laryngeal innervation. Indeed, the three-dimensional structure of laryngeal airway afferents and their ontogeny remains to be determined.

With respect to laryngeal C-fiber afferents, few studies have interpreted their findings in light of the recent advances in C-fiber afferent biology, such as the cloning of the capsaicin/vanilloid receptor (VR1) (91) or the production of a transgenic model lacking the VR1 receptor (92). Descriptions of the molecular determinants of afferent activity in other mechanoreceptor afferent systems (mutant or knockout mice) provide much promise in enhancing the understanding of upper-airway receptor behavior, as well as providing therapeutic molecular targets that could alter receptor discharge and therefore respiratory sensation.

B. Lower-Airway Afferents

The vagus nerve is a mixed nerve that is composed of myelinated and unmyelinated axons. Although the respiratory component represents a minority in terms of the total number of axons (93), respiratory discharge dominates recordings of whole vagus nerve activity in the newborn or adult. The presence of a dominant respiratory modulation in whole nerve vagal afferent recordings reflects the larger axon diameter of receptors and the associated increased amplitude of receptor signal.

Receptors having a respiratory modulation fall into two groups of myelinated afferents: slowly adapting receptors (SARs) having conduction velocities ranging from ~10–70 m/sec and rapidly adapting receptors (RARs), which are Aδ fibers, having conduction velocities ranging from 2.5 to 50 m/sec depending on the species involved (94,95). SARs are located in airway smooth muscle (96) and respond to changes in tension placed on the receptor endings as the lung is inflated (97). RARs ramify in the epithelium of the airways and may also display a respiratory modulation during inflation, but they may also respond to deflation of the lung (97). Although both types of receptors may often be treated as homogeneous groups, it is almost certain that subclassifications exist in terms of the chemical and mechanical stimuli activating them (see Table 2).

Table 2 Cell Body Properties of Respiratory Afferents in the Guinea Pig

	Cell body location	
Category	Nodose ganglion	Jugular ganglion
Aδ fibers, % of cells	95%	48%
C-fibers, % of cells	5% of fibers	52%
Mechanical sensitivity	✓✓✓	✓
Aδ fibers	15x > jugular	
C-fibers	✓	✓
Rapidly adapting receptors	✓✓✓	✓
	96%	6% of Aδ & 8% of C-fibers
Slowly adapting receptor	✓	✓✓✓
	4%	96% of Aδ & 98% of C-fibers
Cells responding to	✓✓✓	✓✓✓
hypertonic saline	92%	85% of Aδ & 88% of C-fibers
Cells responding to	No response of Aδ fibers	✓✓✓
capsaicin		73% of Aδ & C-fibers

Source: Ref. 117.

Slowly Adapting Receptors

SARs transduce transpulmonary pressure (Ptp) (97), and as a result discharge with a "phasic" component during inflation of the lung which in some receptors is also accompanied by a "tonic" discharge at functional residual capacity (Fig. 12). SARs display a slowly augmenting discharge during lung inflation and they adapt slowly to a steady state discharge frequency in response to maintained inflation (Fig. 13). The discharge frequency of neonatal SARs is reduced compared to the adult, and this appears to be a robust observation across mammalian species (74,98–101). Based on the adaptation index (AI% = peak discharge–steady-state discharge/peak discharge), the dynamic sensitivity of SARs appears to be similar for the newborn and adult (102). However, no studies have examined the sensitivity of neonatal SARs to the rate of change of applied pressure (dp/dt) or whether the relative sensitivity of the receptor to static and dynamic (dp/dt) changes of transpulmonary pressure (Ptp) is affected by hyperinflation (103).

In both the newborn and adult the activity of SARs is sensitive to underlying bronchomotor tone, and an increase in smooth muscle tone, due to reflex changes in vagal efferent activity, augments SAR discharge (104–106). This provides a feedback loop for the control of smooth muscle contraction since SAR activity reflexly reduces bronchomotor tone (107). Richardson and Mitchell

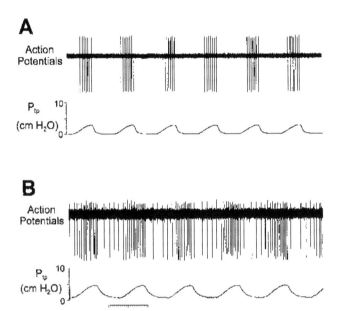

Figure 12   Respiratory modulation of slowly adapting receptor (SAR): typical recordings of a "phasic" (A) and a "tonic" (B) SAR from a newborn dog. Note the phasic slowly augmenting discharge of the SAR during inflation of the lung in both receptors. Upper trace = recording of action potentials; lower trace = transpulmonary pressure (Ptp). (From Schweitzer and Fisher, unpublished.)

(106) described the remarkably sensitive nature of this link between smooth muscle tone and SAR activity (Fig. 14). They discovered that parallel respiratory output from medullary respiratory centers was delivered to both respiratory skeletal and airway smooth muscles simultaneously, and that the phasic efferent input to smooth muscle was mechanically transduced and reflected in SAR discharge. Although SARs are capable of following very high-frequency changes in tension, airway smooth muscle responds fairly slowly to changes in vagal efferent activity, and therefore, and at high breathing frequencies, smooth muscle tone is "averaged" to a higher steady-state level (106). Thus, the accompanying SAR sensitivity to inflation may be enhanced although breath-by-breath modulation is lost (106). In the newborn, SAR activity is affected by bronchomotor tone (104,105), but the link between phrenic nerve activity and SAR discharge has not been studied directly. The input from SARs related to phrenic output in ventilated infants could help explain why some infants "fight" mechanical ventilation more than others (108–112). If so, then one would expect that muscarinic antagonists

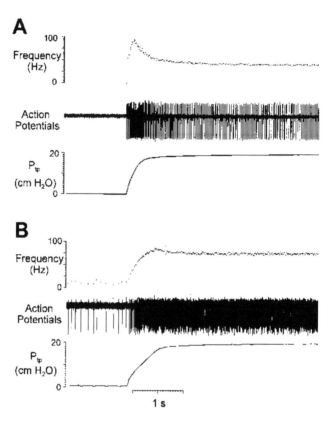

Figure 13 Adaptation of slowly adapting receptors to maintained inflation: typical adaptation of discharge frequency in a SAR from a newborn dog. Note that both phasic (A) and tonic (B) receptors display slow adaptation to the maintained lung inflation and that the speed of inflation (i.e., dp/dt) alters the magnitude of the adaptation (A vs. B). Upper trace = receptor discharge frequency (Hz); middle trace = recording of action potentials; lower trace = transpulmonary pressure (Ptp). (From Schweitzer and Fisher, unpublished.)

may help to alleviate the response by removing vagal smooth muscle tone. Furthermore, pharmaceutical targeting of airway afferents may also provide a useful therapeutic target in ameliorating dyspnea or counterproductive efforts during mechanical ventilation.

Rapidly Adapting Receptors

RARs are thought to contribute to cough, reflex bronchoconstriction, and rapid shallow breathing (113–115). As their name implies, this group of receptors adapt rapidly to maintained inflation of the lung (Fig. 15). RARs are less frequently

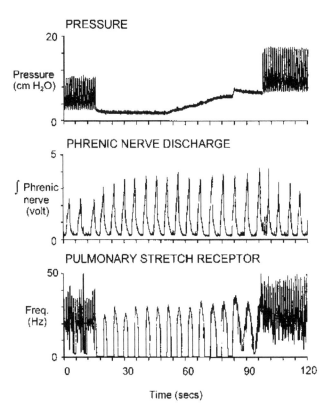

Figure 14 SAR discharge in response to efferent contraction of airway smooth muscle (ASM) in phase with phrenic discharge. Note the continued presence of a phasic discharge of the SAR in phase with the phrenic nerve discharge despite the withdrawal of ventilation of the lung and a constant airway pressure. The maintained modulation of SAR activity reflects a parallel respiratory medullary outflow to airway smooth muscle via vagal efferents. Upper trace = airway pressure; middle trace = recording of integrated phrenic nerve discharge; lower trace = discharge frequency of a SAR. Transpulmonary pressure (Ptp). (From Ref. 106.)

encountered in receptor recordings in the adult and newborn (99,101), representing some 15–18% of receptor recordings in the adult, but this may reflect both a dissection and an audio discrimination bias for smaller diameter fibers with modest discharge frequencies. RAR recordings are even more rarely encountered in the newborn, representing some 4–5% of receptors recorded from canine and opossum airways (99,101). RARs are concentrated at airway branch points in the

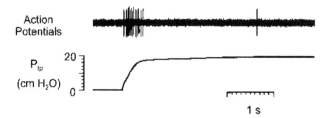

Figure 15 Adaptation of a RAR to maintained inflation: typical rapid adaptation of discharge frequency in a RAR from a newborn dog. Upper trace = recording of action potentials; lower trace = transpulmonary pressure (Ptp). (From Schweitzer and Fisher, unpublished.)

adult, but little is known of their location within neonatal airways on a morphological or neurophysiological basis. Nevertheless, RARs are thought to exert powerful effects through cough and pattern of breathing. The reduced cough reflex of the newborn is consistent with reduced RAR activity (68).

In the adult, RARs have a chemical sensitivity to compounds such as phenylbiguanide (PBG), which is a 5-hydroxytryptamine-3 receptor agonist. The potential physiologic role of G-protein-coupled receptor (GPCR) mechanisms on RAR discharge is not clear, and the impact of such mechanisms have yet to be examined in the newborn. At least some RARs respond to capsaicin, the pungent ingredient of hot peppers (116). Capsaicin is typically assumed to stimulate unmyelinated C-fiber afferents, although the coincidence of RAR activation challenges this assumption and raises the question of the apparent physiologic role of capsaicin responsiveness in RARs (116). Riccio et al. (117) reported that the phenotypic response of airway afferent cell bodies was differentiated on the basis of their location in the nodose or jugular ganglion (see Table 1). They reported that the nodose ganglion contained a predominance of cell bodies from $A\delta$ fibers, whereas the jugular ganglion was composed of almost equal populations of cell bodies of $A\delta$ and C-fiber afferents. There were also differential responses to capsaicin and hypertonic saline depending on the ganglionic location of the cell bodies. Pulmonary edema and lymphatic obstruction also activate RARs (118). Recent studies have also clearly shown that the activity of afferent nerves can be increased by allergic inflammation of the airways (119,120).

Neurotransmitters such as dopamine reduce the discharge of RARs (121), potentially through D_2 receptors (122). The GPCR-related sensitivity of RARs suggests that mechanical afferent feedback from the lung has the potential to be a highly controlled variable. It also reveals the potential to alter RAR activity pharmaceutically in order to modify respiratory sensation which may be highly beneficial in inflammatory lung disease or during mechanical ventilation. None of the responses related to RAR activity have been studied in the newborn.

C-Fiber Afferents

C-fiber or unmyelinated afferents represent >90% of the respiratory afferents from the lung (93), and they are thought to play an important role in inflammatory lung disease of infancy and adulthood (115,119,123–127). Undem's group has provided significant insight into the functional behavior and ganglionic segregation of specific sensory modalities between the nodose and jugular ganglia of the vagus nerve (117,119,125). As mentioned above, respiratory afferents in the jugular and nodose ganglion display differences in their mechanical or capsaicin sensitivity (117). Studies of the in vivo respiratory discharge and reflex effects of C-fibers show that these fibers respond not only to capsaicin but also to inflammatory mediators such as major basic protein or eosinophilic cationic protein (120,126–130).

Virtually nothing is known of either the behavior or the morphology of C-fiber (or Aδ) afferents in the neonatal lung. At the same time, knowledge of the molecular mechanisms affecting C-fibers has advanced rapidly due to the identification and cloning of the vanilloid receptor-1 (VR1) (131) and subsequent production of a VR1 knockout mouse lacking the VR1 protein (92). VR1 is a nonselective cation channel that increases its conductance in response to capsaicin and heat (92). Loss of VR1 causes a severe reduction in the response to both capsaicin and heat in $VR1^{-/-}$ mice and, as expected, results in a loss of dorsal root ganglion cell responsiveness to these stimuli (92).

Lung C-fiber afferents were initially implicated as a possible afferent mechanism in the newborn lung on the basis of the bronchomotor and cardiac effects (bronchoconstriction and bradycardia) to right heart injections of capsaicin (132). C-fiber afferents have also been suggested to be responsible for the laryngeal and pattern of breathing response of newborn lambs to capsaicin or pulmonary edema (133–135). The recent observation that the VR1 antagonist capsaizepine blocks the reflex bronchoconstrictor effects of capsaicin provides more definitive evidence that C-fiber afferents are indeed responsible (136). Figure 16 illustrates the response of a neonatal canine C-fiber afferent recording to right heart injection of capsaicin (Schweitzer and Fisher, unpublished observation). Note the brisk short latency response of the multifiber recording. Since there are no reported studies of the behavior of C-fiber afferents in the newborn, a high priority should be associated with studies of their neurophysiological cellular behavior. C-fibers are polymodal afferents that are thought to be activated by H^+, inflammatory mediators, such as lactic acid, and prostaglandins

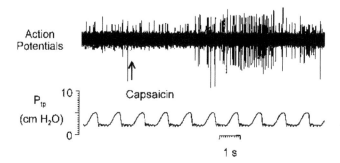

Figure 16 Response of a C-fiber afferent to capsaicin. A multifibre recording of a C-fiber afferent in a newborn dog and the response to right heart injection of capsaicin (at arrow). Note the short latency onset of activity in response to capsaicin injection.

(90,120,127,130,137). In the newborn, lactic acid causes a reflex bronchoconstriction that is at least partially mediated by C-fiber afferents, since perineural capsaicin reduces the magnitude of the bronchomotor response (138).

The morphological and neurophysiological aspects of lower-airway afferents remain an area in need of further investigation. Recent insight into the molecular mechanisms involved in the mechanical and chemical signaling of afferent receptors (92,131,139) provides unparalleled opportunities to test novel hypotheses with respect to the ontogeny of airway afferents.

Acknowledgments

Research from our laboratories is supported by the Australian National Health and Medical Research Council (M.P.S.), the Canadian Institutes of Health Research (J.T.F.), and the Ontario Thoracic Society (J.T.F.). C.S. was supported by a postdoctoral fellowship from Société des eaux minérales d'Evian. The authors wish to thank Ms. Sandra Vincent (Kingston) for her assistance in preparing the manuscript.

References

1. Spooner BS, Wessells NK. Mammalian lung development: interactions in primordium formation and bronchial morphogenesis. J Exp Zool 1970; 175:445–454.
2. Dey RD, Hung K-S. Development of innervation in the lung. In: McDonald JA, ed. Lung Growth and Development, Vol 100. New York: Marcel Dekker, 1997:244–265.

3. Tollet J, Everett AW, Sparrow MP. Spatial and temporal distribution of nerves, ganglia, and smooth muscle during the early pseudoglandular stage of fetal mouse lung development. Dev Dyn 2001; 221:48–60.

4. Pattyn A, Morin X, Cremer H, Goridis C, Brunet JF. The homeobox gene Phox2b is essential for the development of autonomic neural crest derivatives. Nature 1999; 399:366–370.

5. Young HM, Ciampoli D, Hsuan J, Canty AJ. Expression of ret-, p75(NTR)-, phox2a-, phox2b-, and tyrosine hydroxylase-immunoreactivity by undifferentiated neural crest–derived cells and different classes of enteric neurons in the embryonic mouse gut. Dev Dyn 1999; 216:137–152.

6. Chalazonitis A, Rothman TP, Chen J, Gershon MD. Age-dependent differences in the effects of GDNF and NT-3 on the development of neurons and glia from neural crest–derived precursors immunoselected from the fetal rat gut: expression of GFRα-1 in vitro and in vivo. Dev Biol 1998; 204:385–406.

7. Thompson RJ, Doran JF, Jackson P, Dhillon AP, Rode J. PGP 9.5—a new marker for vertebrate neurons and neuroendocrine cells. Brain Res 1983; 278:224–228.

8. Tharakan T, Kirchgessner AL, Baxi LV, Gershon MD. Appearance of neuropeptides and NADPH-diaphorase during development of the enteropancreatic innervation. Brain Res Dev Brain Res 1995; 84:26–38.

9. Guembe L, Villaro AC. Histochemical demonstration of neuronal nitric oxide synthase during development of mouse respiratory tract. Am J Respir Cell Mol Biol 1999; 20:342–351.

10. Young HM, Hearn CJ, Farlie PG, Canty AJ, Thomas PQ, Newgreen DF. GDNF is a chemoattractant for enteric neural cells. Dev Biol 2001; 229:503–516.

11. Durbec P, Marcos-Gutierrez CV, Kilkenny C, et al. GDNF signalling through the Ret receptor tyrosine kinase [see comments]. Nature 1996; 381:789–793.

12. Tollet J, Everett AW, Sparrow MP. A confocal microscopy study of the development of the fetal muose lung. In: Autonomic Neuroscience: Basic & Clinical, Autonomic Neruoscience: Basic & Clinical. London: Elsevier, 2000, Vol 82.

13. Tollet J. Development of neural tissue and airway smooth muscle in fetal mouse lung explants: a role for GDNF in lung innervation. Am J Respir Cell Mol Biol 2002; 26:420–429.

14. Towers PR, Woolf AS, Hardman P. Glial cell line-derived neurotrophic factor stimulates ureteric bud outgrowth and enhances survival of ureteric bud cells in vitro. Exp Nephrol 1998; 6:337–351.

15. Weichselbaum M, Sparrow MP. A confocal microscopic study of the formation of ganglia in the airways of fetal pig lung. Am J Respir Cell Mol Biol 1999; 21:607–620.

16. Burri PH. Structural aspects of prenatal and postnatal development and growth of the lung. In: McDonald JA, ed. Lung Growth and Development. New York: Marcel Dekker, 1997:1–35.

17. Weichselbaum M, Everett AW, Sparrow MP. Mapping the innervation of the bronchial tree in fetal and postnatal pig lung using antibodies to PGP 9.5 and SV2. Am J Respir Cell Mol Biol 1996; 15:703–710.

18. Sparrow MP, Weichselbaum M, McCray PB. Development of the innervation and airway smooth muscle in human fetal lung. Am J Respir Cell Mol Biol 1999; 20:550–560.

19. Weichselbaum M. The structure and distribution of the innervation of the developing lung: confocal microscope study. Department of Physiology. Nedlands: University of Western Australia, 2001.

20. Lamb JP, Sparrow MP. Sensory Innervation in the bronchial mucossa of the pig. International Tachykinin 2000, La Grande Motte, France, Oct. 17–20, 2000.

21. Weichselbaum M. Lung development and pulmonary neuroendocrine cells (PNEC), obtained by confocal laser scanning microscopy. www.neuroendocrine-cell.com 2002.

22. Sparrow MP, Warwick SP, Everett AW. Innervation and function of the distal airways in the developing bronchial tree of fetal pig lung. Am J Respir Cell Mol Biol 1995; 13:518–525.

23. Ten Have-Opbroek AA. The development of the lung in mammals: an analysis of concepts and findings. Am J Anat 1981; 162:201–219.

24. Cadieux A, Springall DR, Mulderry PK, et al. Occurrence, distribution and ontogeny of CGRP immunoreactivity in the rat lower respiratory tract: effect of capsaicin treatment and surgical denervations. Neuroscience 1986; 19:605–627.

25. Butcher L. Acetylcholinesterase histochemistry. In: Hoekfeld ABT, ed. Handbook of Chemical Neuroanatomy, Vol 1. Amsterdam: Elsevier, 1983:1–49.

26. Schemann M, Sann H, Schaaf C, Mader M. Identification of cholinergic neurons in enteric nervous system by antibodies against choline acetyltransferase. Am J Physiol 1993; 265:G1005–G1009.

27. Lee LY, Pisarri TE. Afferent properties and reflex functions of bronchopulmonary C-fibers. Respir Physiol 2001; 125:47–65.

28. Sparrow MP, Weichselbaum M. Structure and function of the adventitial and mucosal nerve plexuses of the bronchial tree in the developing lung. Clin Exp Pharmacol Physiol 1997; 24:261–268.

29. Undem BJ, Myers AC. Autonomic ganglia. In: Barnes PJ, ed. Autonomic Control of the Respiratory System. Reading, U.K.: Harwood Academic Publications, 1997:87–118.

30. Warburton D, Zhao J, Berberich MA, Bernfield M. Molecular embryology of the lung: then, now, and in the future. Am J Physiol 1999; 276:L697–L704.

31. Sparrow MP, Warwick SP, Mitchell HW. Foetal airway motor tone in prenatal lung development of the pig. Eur Respir J 1994; 7:1416–1424.

32. McCray PB Jr. Spontaneous contractility of human fetal airway smooth muscle. Am J Respir Cell Mol Biol 1993; 8:573–580.

33. Schittny JC, Miserocchi G, Sparrow MP. Spontaneous peristaltic airway contractions propel lung liquid through the bronchial tree of intact and fetal lung explants [see comments]. Am J Respir Cell Mol Biol 2000; 23:11–18.

34. Baluk P, Nadel JA, McDonald DM. Substance P–immunoreactive sensory axons in the rat respiratory tract: a quantitative study of their distribution and role in neurogenic inflammation. J Comp Neurol 1992; 319:586–598.

35. Larsell O. The ganglia, plexus and nerve-terminations of the mammalian lung and pleura pulmonis. J Comp Neurol 1922; 35:97–132.

36. Larsell O, Dow RS. The innervation of the human lung. Am J Anat 1933; 52:125–146.

37. Ploschko A. Nervenendigungen und den Ganglien der Respirations-organe. Anat Anz 1897; 13:S.12–S.22.

38. Li ZS, Fox-Threlkeld JE, Furness JB. Innervation of intestinal arteries by axons with immunoreactivity for the vesicular acetylcholine transporter (VAChT). J Anat 1998; 192:107–117.

39. Black JL. Innervation of airway smooth muscle. In: Barnes PJ, ed. Autonomic Control of the Respiratory System. Reading, U.K.: Harwood Academic Publications, 1997:185–200.

40. Rogers DF. Motor control of airway goblet cells and glands. Respir Physiol 2001; 125:129–144.

41. Uddman R, Hakanson R, Luts A, Sundler F. Distribution of neuropeptides in airways. In: Barnes PJ, ed. Autonomic Control of the Respiratory System. Reading, U.K.: Harwood Academic Publications, 1997:21–38.

42. Undem BJ, Myers AC. Neural regulation of the immune response. In: Busse WM, Holgate ST, eds. Asthma and Rhinitis. Oxford: Blackwell Scientific, 2000:927–944.

43. Rogers DF, Barnes PJ. Neural control of the airway vasculature. In: Barnes PJ, ed. Autonomic Control of the Respiratory System. Reading, U.K.: Harwood Academic Publications, 1997:229–248.

44. Barnes PJ. Neuromodulation in airways. In: Barnes PJ, ed. Autonomic Control of the Respiratory System. Reading, U.K.: Harwood Academic Publications, 1997:139–184.

45. Barnes PJ. Airway neuropeptides. In: Busse WM, Holgate ST, eds. Asthma and Rhinitis. Oxford: Blackwell Scientific, 2000:891–908.

46. Honjin R. On the ganglia and nerves of the lower respiratory tract of the mouse. J Morphol 1954; 95:263–287.

47. Honjin R. On the nerve supply of the mouse with special reference to the structure of the peripheral vegetative system. J Comp Neurol 1956; 105:587–625.

48. Ebina M, Yaegashi H, Takashi T, Motomiya M, Tanemura M. Distribution of smooth muscles along the bronchial tree: a morphometric study of ordinary autopsy lungs. Am Rev Respir Dis 1990; 141:1322–1326.

49. Schelegle ES, Green JF. An overview of the anatomy and physiology of slowly adapting pulmonary stretch receptors. Respir Physiol 2001; 125:17–31.

50. Sorokin SP, Hoyt RFJ. Neuroepithelial bodies and solitary small granule-cells. In: Massaro D, ed. Lung Cell Biology. New York: Marcel Dekker, 1989:191–344.

51. Scheuermann DW. Comparative histology of pulmonary neuroendocrine cell system in mammalian lungs. Microsc Res Tech 1997; 37:31–42.

52. Adriaensen D, Scheuermann DW. Neuroendocrine cells and nerves of the lung. Anat Rec 1993; 236:70–85; discussion 85–86.

53. Johnson EW, Eller PM, Jafek BW. Protein gene product 9.5-like and calbindin-like immunoreactivity in the nasal respiratory mucosa of perinatal humans. Anat Rec 1997; 247:38–45.

54. Luts A, Uddman R, Absood A, Hakanson R, Sundler F. Chemical coding of endocrine cells of the airways: presence of helodermin-like peptides. Cell Tissue Res 1991; 265:425–433.
55. Stahlman MT, Gray ME. Ontogeny of neuroendocrine cells in human fetal lung. I. An electron microscopic study. Lab Invest 1984; 51:449–463.
56. Stahlman MT, Gray ME. Immunogold EM localization of neurochemicals in human pulmonary neuroendocrine cells. Microsc Res Tech 1997; 37:77–91.
57. Polak JM, Becker KL, Cutz E, et al. Lung endocrine cell markers, peptides, and amines. Anat Rec 1993; 236:169–171.
58. Lauweryns JM, Cokelaere M, Deleersynder M, Liebens M. Intrapulmonary neuro-epithelial bodies in newborn rabbits. Influence of hypoxia, hyperoxia, hypercapnia, nicotine, reserpine, L-DOPA and 5-HTP. Cell Tissue Res 1977; 182:425–440.
59. Youngson C, Nurse C, Yeger H, Cutz E. Oxygen sensing in airway chemoreceptors. Nature 1993; 365:153–155.
60. Reynolds SD, Giangreco A, Power JH, Stripp BR. Neuroepithelial bodies of pulmonary airways serve as a reservoir of progenitor cells capable of epithelial regeneration. Am J Pathol 2000; 156:269–278.
61. Lauweryns JM, Peuskens JC, Cokelaere M. Argyrophil, fluorescent and granulated (peptide and amine producing?) AFG cells in human infant bronchial epithelium. Light and electron microscopic studies. Life Sci I 1970; 9:1417–1429.
62. Van Lommel A, Lauweryns JM. Neuroepithelial bodies in the Fawn Hooded rat lung: morphological and neuroanatomical evidence for a sensory innervation. J Anat 1993; 183:553–566.
63. Adriaensen D, Timmermans JP, Brouns I, Berthoud HR, Neuhuber WL, Scheuer-mann DW. Pulmonary intraepithelial vagal nodose afferent nerve terminals are confined to neuroepithelial bodies: an anterograde tracing and confocal microscopy study in adult rats. Cell Tissue Res 1998; 293:395–405.
64. Gosney JR. Neuroendocrine cell populations in postnatal human lungs: minimal variation from childhood to old age. Anat Rec 1993; 236:177–180.
65. Skogvall S, Korsgren M, Grampp W. Evidence that neuroepithelial endocrine cells control the spontaneous tone in guinea pig tracheal preparations. J Appl Physiol 1999; 86:789–798.
66. Coleridge HM, Coleridge JCC. Reflexes evoked from the tracheobronchial tree and lungs. In: Cherniack NS, Widdicombe JG, eds. Handbook of Physiology, Section 3: The Respiratory System, Vol II: Control of Breathing, Part 1. Washington: American Physiological Society, 1986:395–429.
67. Agostoni E, Chinnock M, Daly MB, Murray JG. Functional and histological studies of the vagus nerve and its branches to the heart, lungs and abdominal nerve viscera in the cat. J Physiol (Lond) 1957; 135:182–205.
68. Mortola JP, Fisher JT. Upper airway reflexes in newborns. In: Mathew OP, Sant'Ambrogio G, ed. Respiratory Function of the Upper Airway. New York: Marcel Dekker, 1988:303–357.
69. Mathew OP, Sant'Ambrogio FB. Laryngeal reflexes. In: Mathew OP, Sant'Ambrogio G, ed. Respiratory Function of the Upper Airway. New York: Marcel Dekker, 1988: 259–302.

70. Bartlett D Jr. Upper airway motor systems. In: Cherniack NS, Widdicombe JG, eds. Handbook of Physiology, Section 3, Respiratory System II. Washington: American Physiological Society, 1986:223–245.

71. Sessle BJ, Greenwood LF, Lund JP, Lucier GE. Effects of upper respiratory stimuli on respiration and single repiratory neurons in the adult cat. Exp Neurol 1978; 61:245–259.

72. Lucier GE, Storey AT, Sessle BJ. Effects of upper respiratory tract stimuli on neonatal respiration: reflex and single neuron analyses in the kitten. Biol Neonate 1979; 35:82–89.

73. Boggs DF, Bartlett D Jr. Chemical specificity of a laryngeal apneic reflex in puppies. J Appl Physiol 1982; 53:455–462.

74. Fisher JT, Mathew OP, Sant'Ambrogio G. Morphological and neurophysiological aspects of airway and pulmonary receptors. In: Haddad GG, Farber JP, eds. Developmental Neurobiology of Breathing. New York: Marcel Dekker, 1991: 219–244.

75. Sant'Ambrogio G, Sant'Ambrogio FB. Role of laryngeal afferents in cough. Pulm Pharmacol 1996; 9:309–314.

76. Mathew OP, Abu-Osba YK, Thach BT. Influence of upper airway pressure changes on genioglossus muscle respiratory activity. J Appl Physiol 1982; 52:438–444.

77. Mathew OP, Abu-Osba YK, Thach BT. Genioglossus muscle responses to upper airway pressure changes: afferent pathway. J Appl Physiol 1982; 52:445–450.

78. Mathew OP, Abu-Osba YK, Thach BT. Influence of upper airway pressure changes on respiratory frequency. Respir Physiol 1982; 49:223–233.

79. Sant'Ambrogio G, Mathew OP, Fisher JT, Sant'Ambrogio FB. Laryngeal receptors responding to transmural pressure, airflow and local muscle activity. Respir Physiol 1983; 54:317–330.

80. Sant'Ambrogio G, Mathew OP, Sant'Ambrogio FB, Fisher JT. Laryngeal cold receptors. Respir Physiol 1985; 59:35–44.

81. Sant'Ambrogio G, Mathew OP, Sant'Ambrogio FB. Characteristics of laryngeal cold receptors. Respir Physiol 1988; 71:287–298.

82. Anderson JW, Sant'Ambrogio FB, Mathew OP, Sant'Ambrogio G. Water-responsive laryngeal receptors in the dog are not specialized endings. Respir Physiol 1990; 79:33–44.

83. Anderson JW, Washburn DL, Ferguson AV. Intrinsic osmosensitivity of subfornical organ neurons. Neuroscience 2000; 100:539–547.

84. Fox AJ, Barnes PJ, Urban L, Dray A. An in vitro study of the properties of single vagal afferents innervating guinea-pig airways. J Physiol (Lond) 1993; 469:21–35.

85. Fisher JT, Mathew OP, Sant'Ambrogio G, Sant'Ambrogio FB. Reflex effects and receptor responses to upper airway pressure and flow stimuli in developing puppies. J Appl Physiol 1985; 58:258–264.

86. Al-Shway SF, Mortola JP. Respiratory effects of airflow through the upper airways in newborn kittens and puppies. J Appl Physiol 1982; 53:805–814.

87. Sant'Ambrogio FB, Anderson JW, Sant'Ambrogio G. Menthol in the upper airway depresses ventilation in newborn dogs. Respir Physiol 1992; 89:299–307.

88. Mathew OP, Anderson JW, Orani GP, Sant'Ambrogio FB, Sant'Ambrogio G. Cooling mediates the ventilatory depression associated with airflow through the larynx. Respir Physiol 1990; 82:359–368.

89. Stockwell M, Lang S, Yip R, Zintel T, White C, Gallagher CG. Lack of importance of the superior laryngeal nerves in citric acid cough in humans. J Appl Physiol 1993; 75(2):613–617.

90. Holzer P. Capsaicin: cellular targets, mechanisms of action, and selectivity for thin sensory neurons. Pharmacol Rev 1991; 43:143–201.

91. Caterina MJ, Schumacher MA, Tominaga M, Rosen TA, Levine JD, Julius D. The capsaicin receptor: a heat-activated ion channel in the pain pathway [see comments]. Nature 1997; 389(6653):816–824.

92. Caterina MJ, Leffler A, Malmberg AB, et al. Impaired nociception and pain sensation in mice lacking the capsaicin receptor. Science 2000; 288:306–313.

93. Jammes Y, Fornaris E, Mei N, Barrat E. Afferent and efferent components of the bronchial vagal branches in cats. J Auton Nerv Syst 1982; 5:165–176.

94. Sant'Ambrogio G. Information arising from the tracheobronchial tree in mammals. Physiol Rev 1982; 62:531–539.

95. Ricco MM, Kummer W, Biglari B, Myers AC, Undem BJ. Interganglionic segregation of distinct vagal afferent fibre phenotypes in guinea-pig airways. J Physiol (Lond) 1996; 496(Pt 2):521–530.

96. Krauhs JM. Morphology of presumptive slowly adapting receptors in dog trachea. Anat Rec 1984; 210:73–85.

97. McGilliard KL, Jones SE, Robertson GE, Olsen GD. Altered respiratory control in newborn puppies after chronic prenatal exposure to alpha-l-acetylmethadol (LAAM). Respir Physiol 1982; 47:299–311.

98. Schwieler GH. Respiratory regulation during postnatal development in cats and rabbits and some of its morphological substrates. Acta Physiol Scand 1968; suppl 304:1–123.

99. Fisher JT, Sant'Ambrogio G. Location and discharge properties of respiratory vagal afferents in the newborn dog. Respir Physiol 1982; 50:209–220.

100. Marlot D, Mortola JP, Duron B. Functional localization of pulmonary stretch receptors in the tracheobronchial tree of the kitten. Can J Physiol Pharmacol 1982; 60:1073–1077.

101. Farber JP, Fisher JT, Sant'Ambrogio G. Airway receptor activity in the developing opossum. Am J Physiol 1984; 246:R753-R758.

102. Sant'Ambrogio FB, Fisher JT, Sant'Ambrogio G. Adaptation of airway stretch receptors in newborn and adult dogs. Respir Physiol 1983; 52:361–369.

103. Pack AI, Ogilvie MD, Davies RO, Galante RJ. Responses of pulmonary stretch receptors during ramp inflations of the lung. J Appl Physiol 1986; 61:344–352.

104. Fisher JT, Sant'Ambrogio G. Effects of inhaled CO_2 on airway stretch receptors in the newborn dog. J Appl Physiol 1982; 53:1461–1465.

105. Fisher JT, Sant'Ambrogio FB, Sant'Ambrogio G. Stimulation of tracheal slowly adapting stretch receptors by hypercapnia and hypoxia. Respir Physiol 1983; 53:325–339.

106. Richardson CA, Herbert DA, Mitchell RA. Modulation of pulmonary stretch receptors and airway resistance by parasympathetic efferents. J Appl Physiol 1984; 57(6):1842–1849.

107. Waldron MA, Fisher JT. Neural control of airway smooth muscle in the newborn. In: Haddad G, Farber JP, eds. Developmental Neurobiology of Breathing. New York: Marcel Dekker, 1991:483–518.

108. Greenough A, Morley C, Davis J. Interaction of spontaneous respiration with artificial ventilation in preterm babies. J Pediatr 1983; 103:769–773.

109. Greenough A. The premature infant's respiratory response to mechanical ventilation. Early Hum Dev 1988; 17(1):1–5.

110. Hird MF, Greenough A. Spontaneous respiratory effort during mechanical ventilation in infants with and without acute respiratory distress. Early Hum Dev 1991; 25(2):69–73.

111. Dyke MP, Kohan R, Evans S. Morphine increases synchronous ventilation in preterm infants. J Paediatr Child Health 1995; 31(3):176–179.

112. Jarreau PH, Moriette G, Mussat P, et al. Patient-triggered ventilation decreases the work of breathing in neonates. Am J Respir Crit Care Med 1996; 153(3):1176–1181.

113. Sant'Ambrogio G, Widdicombe JG. Reflexes from airway rapidly adapting receptors. Respir Physiol 2001; 125:33–45.

114. Widdicombe JG. Afferent receptors in the airway and cough. Respir Physiol 1998; 114:5–15.

115. Widdicombe J, Lee LY. Airway reflexes, autonomic function, and cardiovascular responses. Environ Health Perspect 2001; 109(suppl 4):579–584.

116. Mohammed SP, Higenbottam TW, Adcock JJ. Effects of aerosol-applied capsaicin, histamine and prostaglandin E2 on airway sensory receptors of anaesthetized cats. J Physiol (Lond) 1993; 469:51–66.

117. Riccio MM, Kummer W, Biglari B, Myers AC, Undem BJ. Interganglionic segregation of distinct vagal afferent fibre phenotypes in guinea-pig airways. J Physiol (Lond) 1996; 496(Pt 2):521–530.

118. Ravi K, Bonham AC, Kappagoda CT. Effect of pulmonary lymphatic obstruction on respiratory rate and airway rapidly adapting receptor activity in rabbits. J Physiol (Lond) 1994; 480(Pt 1):163–170.

119. Riccio MM, Proud D, Undem BJ. Enhancement of afferent nerve excitability in the airways by allergic inflammation [review]. Pulm Pharmacol 1995; 8(4–5):181–185.

120. Lee LY, Widdicombe JG. Modulation of airway sensitivity to inhaled irritants: role of inflammatory mediators. Environ Health Perspect 2001; 109(suppl 4):585–589.

121. Jackson DM, Simpson WT. The effect of dopamine on the rapidly adapting receptors in the dog lung. Pulm Pharmacol Ther 2000; 13:39–42.

122. Lawrence AJ, Krstew E, Jarrott B. Functional dopamine D_2 receptors on rat vagal afferent neurones. Br J Pharmacol 1995; 114:1329–1334.

123. Coleridge HM, Coleridge JCG, Schultz HD. Afferent pathways involved in reflex regulation of airway smooth muscle. Pharmacol Ther 1989; 42:1–63.

124. Coleridge HM, Coleridge JCG. Pulmonary reflexes: neural mechanisms of pulmonary defense. Annu Rev Physiol 1994; 56:69–91.

125. Undem BJ, McAlexander M, Hunter DD. Neurobiology of the upper and lower airways. Allergy 1999; 54(suppl 57):81–93.
126. Ho CY, Gu Q, Lin YS, Lee LY. Sensitivity of vagal afferent endings to chemical irritants in the rat lung. Respir Physiol 2001; 127(2–3):113–124.
127. Lee LY, Pisarri TE. Afferent properties and reflex functions of bronchopulmonary C-fibers. Respir Physiol 2001; 125(1–2):47–65.
128. Lee LY, Gu Q, Gleich GJ. Effects of human eosinophil granule-derived cationic proteins on C-fiber afferents in the rat lung. J Appl Physiol 2001; 91(3):1318–1326.
129. Gu Q, Lee LY. Hypersensitivity of pulmonary C fibre afferents induced by cationic proteins in the rat. J Physiol 2001; 537(Pt 3):887–897.
130. Ho CY, Gu Q, Hong JL, Lee LY. Prostaglandin E(2) enhances chemical and mechanical sensitivities of pulmonary C fibers in the rat. Am J Respir Crit Care Med 2000; 162(2 Pt 1):528–533.
131. Caterina MJ, Schumacher MA, Tominaga M, Rosen TA, Levine JD, Julius D. The capsaicin receptor: a heat-activated ion channel in the pain pathway. Nature 1997; 389(23):816–824.
132. Anderson JW, Fisher JT. Capsaicin-induced reflex bronchoconstriction in the newborn. Respir Physiol 1993; 93:13–27.
133. Diaz V, Dorion D, Kianicka I, Letourneau P, Praud JP. Vagal afferents and active upper airway closure during pulmonary edema in lambs. J Appl Physiol 1999; 86(5):1561–1569.
134. Diaz V, Dorion D, Kianicka I, Letourneau P, Praud JP. Vagal afferents and active upper airway closure during pulmonary edema in lambs. J Appl Physiol 1999; 86(5):1561–1569.
135. Diaz V, Dorion D, Renolleau S, Letourneau P, Kianicka I, Praud JP. Effects of capsaicin pretreatment on expiratory laryngeal closure during pulmonary edema in lambs. J Appl Physiol 1999; 86(5):1570–1577.
136. Nault MA, Vincent SG, Fisher JT. Mechanisms of capsaicin- and lactic acid–induced bronchoconstriction in the newborn dog. J Physiol (Lond) 1999; 515:567–578.
137. Sasamura T, Kuraishi Y. Peripheral and central actions of capsaicin and VR1 receptor. Jpn J Pharmacol 2000; 80:275–280.
138. Marantz MJ, Vincent SG, Fisher JT. Role of vagal C-fiber afferents in the bronchomotor response to lactic acid in the newborn dog. J Appl Physiol 2001; 90:2311–2318.
139. Price MP, Lewin GR, McIlwrath SL, et al. The mammalian sodium channel BNC1 is required for normal touch sensation. Nature 2000; 407:1007–1011.

4

Chemical Control of Breathing from Fetal Through Newborn Life

**MARTHA JANE MILLER and
RICHARD J. MARTIN**

Case Western Reserve University
Cleveland, Ohio, U.S.A.

MUSA A. HAXHIU

Howard University College of Medicine
Washington, D.C., U.S.A.

I. Introduction

The mammalian newborn is perfectly adapted to transition at birth from a fetal state, totally dependent on the mother, to independent air-breathing life. This chapter will first consider how chemoreceptive neural systems develop in utero in anticipation of the need for the newborn to match metabolic needs with exchange of oxygen and carbon dioxide. Then we will consider postnatal adaptation of chemoreceptor systems to the air breathing state, as well as postnatal insults which can interrupt this orderly process of maturation.

II. Development of Chemoreception

A. Fetal Life

Rhythmic contractions of the diaphragm, intercostals, and laryngeal adductors are present in most mammals by the beginning of the second third of gestation (1–3). These spontaneous breathing movements (FBM) occur during periods of low-voltage, high-frequency sleep similar to REM sleep in the adult (4). The frequency of FBM increases with advancing gestation, occurring ~30% of the time near term in the sheep (5). In the human, there is evidence for sensitivity of fetal breathing to a number of stimuli, including maternal smoking, use of alcohol, maternal glucose, and even the time of day (6) (Fig. 1).

The level of carbon dioxide in the blood may be the primary drive for FBM, upon which sleep state acts as a powerful modulating influence. The relative suppression of fetal breathing (as compared to the adult) appears to reflect a balance of inhibitory and stimulatory influences acting on central respiratory drive. The central chemoreceptors necessary for response to changes in arterial CO_2 develop early in fetal life. For example, the sheep fetus responds to hypercapnia and hypothermia with an increase in FBM, even during high-voltage, slow-wave sleep, when breathing movements are normally absent (7). In addition, the sheep fetus is capable of responding to acute hypoxia with a reduction in FBM, and to asphyxia with powerful gasps (8–10).

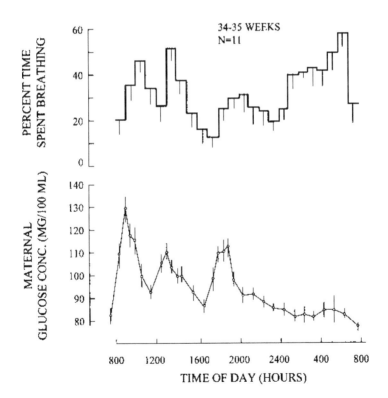

Figure 1   Percentage of time spent breathing by 11 fetuses at 34–35 weeks each hour of the day. Mothers were given meals at 8 AM, 12 noon, and 5 PM. Fetuses made breathing movements a greater percentage of the time during the second and third hours following breakfast, lunch, and dinner. (From Ref. 6.)

Pontine structures may play a critical role in suppression of hypercapnic and hypoxic chemosensory response in the fetus. As noted above, FBM are not ordinarily present during high-voltage, slow-wave sleep. Johnson and Gluckman (11) found that lesioning of the lateral pons permitted hypercapnic stimulation of FBM. These authors also noted that bilateral lesioning of the upper pons in lamb fetuses reversed depression of FBM by hypoxia (12). Thus, pontine descending inhibition is a critical influence on the pattern of FBM, and may act to conserve energy in utero, at a time when FBM are not necessary for control of CO_2 and O_2 exchange.

B. Transition to Postnatal Life

At birth, however, the fetus must convert within a few short minutes from dependence on the placenta for gas exchange, to a fully respiring organism. The rapidity and fidelity of this remarkable transition reflect the state of maturation of the entire cardiorespiratory system at birth: lungs, diaphragm and accessory muscles, circulation, and neural control of breathing.

To survive, the newborn must convert the irregular fetal pattern of breathing to the sustained, adaptive pattern of the adult. A number of influences act acutely at birth to support breathing, including cold stimulus (thermoreceptors), the arousal mechanism, the CO_2 chemoreceptors (2,13,14), oxygenation (15–17), and the postnatal increase in metabolic rate that has been demonstrated in experimental studies of mammalian newborns (18,19). In an elegant series of studies Kuipers et al. (20–22) considered the role of hypercapnic chemoresponse in initiation of postnatal breathing. When fetal lambs were placed on extra-corporeal membrane oxygenation and maintained at constant PaO_2 and temperature, onset of breathing at birth was dependent on an increase in CO_2 (20–22). Cord occlusion, long thought to be critical for onset of breathing, did not stimulate breathing in this model. These studies support the concept that CO_2 chemosensation is a critical element in the normal transition to postnatal life.

III. Maturation of Chemoreceptor Responses to CO_2/H^+

A. Developmental Changes in Ventilatory Responses

The ventilatory response to CO_2 has been clearly shown to increase with advancing postnatal and gestational age (23,24) in preterm human infants. Therefore, the breathing response to CO_2 in preterm infants is relatively impaired when compared to term neonates or adults, and it appears that this difference is both quantitative and qualitative. Whereas term neonates and adults increase their ventilation through an increase in both tidal volume and frequency, preterm infants do not appear to increase frequency in response to CO_2 (25–27). This somewhat unique response of respiratory timing during hypercapnic exposure is associated with prolongation of expiratory duration (see below).

For many years it was unclear whether this reduced ventilatory response to CO_2 in small preterm infants was the result of mechanical limitations in respiratory mechanics or decreased respiratory neural output, possibly associated with diminished chemosensitivity. Krauss et al. (28) simultaneously measured work of breathing and ventilatory response in premature infants and concluded that both mechanical and neurological factors limited the response to CO_2. Frantz et al. (23) confirmed that ventilatory responses to CO_2 are decreased in premature infants, and by measuring end-expiratory occlusion pressures suggested that decreased respiratory center sensitivity or output contributed to this phenomenon. Zhou et al. (29) have reported that phasic phrenic nerve response to hypercapnia changes from irregular to regular between 7 and 10 days of age in unanesthetized decerebrate newborn rats.

We have shown, in both unrestrained rat pups as well as in vagotomized, intubated, and ventilated rat pups, that hypercapnic ventilatory responses are impaired in newborn rats relative to adult rats, signifying a central origin for such response (30). The failure of respiratory rate to increase during hypercapnia, accompanied by a prolongation of expiratory time in this model, is analogous to the response observed by Noble et al. (25) in preterm infants. A similar response has been observed by Dreshaj in decerebrate, vagotomized, paralysed, and mechanically ventilated piglets (31). On the basis of these observations we hypothesized that an inhibitory neurotransmitter implicated in control of breathing, such as γ-aminobutyric acid (GABA), might be implicated in CO_2-induced prolongation of expiratory time. Administration of the $GABA_A$ receptor blocker, bicuculline, significantly reduced or eliminated this phenomenon in both the rat pup and piglet models (30,31), implicating brainstem GABA-ergic mechanisms in the CO_2-induced prolongation of expiratory time and the resultant diminution of ventilatory response during early development. These observations are consistent with the earlier data of Xia and Haddad (32) that the newborn rat brainstem has a much higher $GABA_A$ receptor density than the adult brainstem. Inhibitory neurotransmitters such as GABA may play an important role in the predisposition to respiratory inhibition due to diverse stimuli in early postnatal life in mammalian species (33) (Fig. 2).

As discussed later, a coordinated response of various respiratory muscle groups during both inspiration and expiration is key to maintenance of ventilatory stability. Dreshaj et al. have recently observed that hypercapnia-induced prolongation of expiratory time in decerebrate, vagotomized, spontaneously breathing piglets is associated with an increase in thyroarytenoid (laryngeal adductor) activation and an accompanying increase in laryngeal resistance (34), as seen in Figure 3. This phenomenon appears to contrast with the decrease in laryngeal resistance induced by hypercapnia in mature animals (35). We speculate that

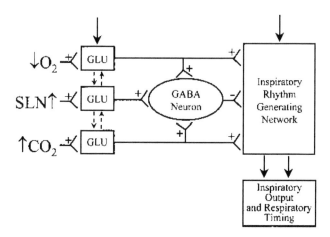

Figure 2 Schematic presentation of neuronal pathways that may be involved in chemical regulation of inspiratory output and respiratory timing during development. Oxygen deprivation or increase in CO_2 leads to activation of secondary glutamergic neurons that project to the inspiratory generating network as well as to GABA-containing neurons. Excitation of inhibitory cells decreases inspiratory activity and prolongs expiratory duration. Laryngeal stimulation, mechanical or chemical, activates second-order neurons that mainly project to GABA interneurons, which in turn inhibit activity of the inspiratory rhythm generating network, causing a decrease in tidal volume and a prolongation of expiratory time.

laryngeal braking in the neonate serves to optimize gas exchange and prevent large fluctuations in functional residual capacity when infants are exposed to hypercapnia. This pattern is primarily central in origin, and does not appear to be due to volume sensitive vagal or laryngeal sensory feedback.

B. Central Chemosensitive Sites and Postnatal Maturation

Over many years, intensive research has focused on the localization of chemo-sensory sites. These studies showed that the chemosensitive neural elements of the ventrolateral surface of the medulla play a pivotal role in the regulation of respiratory activity and ventilatory responses to CO_2 (36,37). Although more recent physiological data demonstrated the presence of chemosensitive sites in regions outside of the ventrolateral aspect of the medulla oblongata, physiological studies have established primary importance for the ventral medullary chemo-sensitive regions.

Few detailed maturational studies have focused on changes in distribution of medullary chemosensory structures that might explain the observed differences in hypercapnic ventilatory responses during development. These issues have been

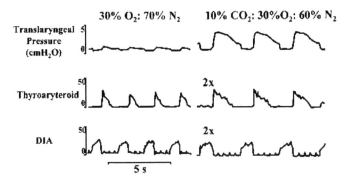

Figure 3 An example of the effects of hypercapnic loading on translaryngeal pressure (TLP) and on the EMG activity of the thyroarytenoid muscle and the diaphragm (D). Steady-state hypercapnia caused a decrease in breathing rate, entirely due to prolongation of expiratory time. Changes in respiratory activity induced by hypercapnic loading increased translaryngeal pressure and the electrical activity in all three muscles. (From Ref. 34.)

difficult to address owing to the lack of definition of a clearly structured organization of the chemosensory system at the single-cell level. Methods used to identify chemosensory neurons, such as the single-cell recording technique, do not allow the sampling of a large number of functionally active cells under awake, nonsedated experimental conditions. One way to circumvent these difficulties is to examine hypercapnia-induced expression of encoding transcription factors such as the c-fos gene, a member of the immediate early genes, and its product Fos protein (Fos). This technique has been used as a cellular marker to identify activated neurons within the CNS, as during CO_2/H^+ exposure (38,39).

Belegu et al. employed this technique during hypercapnic loading of rat pups at various postnatal days (39). Fos-positive cells were observed as expected in the ventrolateral medulla. No postnatal age-related differences were observed in the number of neurons exhibiting CO_2-induced Fos expression. Fos-positive cells were additionally observed in the lateral paragigantocellular reticular nuclei, in the medullary midline complex, and in the raphe pallidus and raphe obscurus. The number of activated cells in the midline neurons was actually higher at 5 than at 40 days of age. These findings indicate that neurons activated by increases in CO_2/H^+ concentrations are well developed from the first days of postnatal life in maturing rat pups. Therefore, deficiency in the neuronal network for sensing increases in CO_2/H^+ does not appear to play a major role in the decreased CO_2 responses observed during early maturation.

It is still possible that postnatal maturation may influence the relative importance of discrete chemosensitive sites beyond the ventrolateral medulla, such as the medullary caudal raphe nucleus (40,41). We therefore inhibited or destroyed midline chemosensitive neuronal activity employing the piglet model (42). These experiments demonstrated that the medullary midline neurons are required for full expression of both phrenic and hypoglossal responses to CO_2 (see later). These data therefore raise the possibility that dysfunction of these midline brainstem neurons may contribute to respiratory instability in early postnatal life.

There is little available information on the role of second-messenger systems in modulating ventilatory patterns and CO_2 responses during early development. Protein kinase C (PKC) appears to be involved in CO_2-induced cfos mRNA expression in the central nervous system (43). Recent data suggest that PKC modulates respiratory timing mechanisms in rats, and that the neural substrate mediating respiratory output may be more critically dependent on PKC activity in the immature animal (44). Future studies should clarify the role of this and other second-messenger systems during normal and abnormal respiratory patterning and their roles in modulating the neurotransmitter mediated pathways described earlier.

C. Central Neural Pathways for Chemosensation and Arousal

In recent years, considerable progress has been made in understanding development of central chemosensitivity at the cellular and functional levels by combining molecular biological techniques (e.g., c-fos expression) (39) and neurotransmitter immunohistochemistry. Since physiologic responses are highly coordinated and coherently assembled, a number of different neurochemicals may participate in transmission of chemical information, and in dynamic control of final motor and behavioral responses. In support of this concept, CO_2 exposure and O_2 deprivation have been shown to lead to activation of discrete cell groups along the neuraxis, including subsets of cells outside the ventrolateral medulla including monoaminergic neurons (e.g., noradrenalinergic, serotoninergic, and histaminergic cell groups). Activation of monoaminergic neurons by an increase in the concentration of CO_2 and/or H^+ will facilitate respiratory related motor activity, particularly of upper-airway dilating muscles. In addition, these neurons coordinate sympathetic and parasympathetic tone to visceral organs, and participate in adjustments of blood flow with the level of motor activity. Any deficit in CO_2 chemosensitivity of a network of monoaminergic nuclei might lead to failure of homeostatic responses to life-threatening challenges during sleep—for example, during sleep apnea or nocturnal asthma.

In the mammalian central nervous system monoaminergic neurons are well developed and provide widespread projections throughout the entire brain (45,46). Monoaminergic pathways represent key components of the reticular activating system and are implicated in diverse physiological functions, including behavioral state control (47,48). It has recently been shown that a subpopulation of these neurons that belong to dissociable neurotransmitter-specific monoamine-containing cell groups could sense changes in concentrations of CO_2 or H^+ and use their transmitter content to relay information that modulates responses to hypercapnia in a concentration-dependent manner (49). A majority of these neurons are also activated by oxygen deprivation (38).

Catecholaminergic Neuronal Groups, Arousal, and Chemoreception

Studies from our laboratory have demonstrated that noradrenaline containing neurons are part of the neural network that senses changes in arterial CO_2. In these experiments (49,50), we examined c-fos expression in catecholaminergic neurons following exposure of unanesthetized rats to hypercapnic stress. Breathing a gas mixture with elevated CO_2 induced activation of the c-fos gene in widespread regions of the CNS, as shown by the expression of Fos-like immunoreactive protein. Colocalization studies of tyrosine hydroxylase and c-fos revealed that in the brainstem 73–85% of noradrenaline containing cells expressed Fos immunoreactivity. Double-labeled cells were found in the ventrolateral medullary reticular formation (A1 noradrenaline cells), in the dorsal aspect of the medula oblongata (A2 noradrenaline cells), in the pons (A5, A6, groups), and ventrolaterally to the locus coeruleus (A7 group). Activation of these neuronal groups by hypercapnia may overcome sleep-related inhibitory inputs and send parallel signals to the medullary respiratory network for adjustment of ventilatory drive, and to CNS structures responsible for arousal.

The coerulocortical and cholinergic systems are implicated in different forms of behavioral arousal. Recently, it was shown that the number of brainstem adrenaline and noradrenaline neurons is decreased in sudden infant death syndrome (SIDS); this decrease is closely correlated with brainstem gliosis (51). Furthermore, in SIDS victims there is a deficit in catecholaminergic innervation of the diencephalon and basal ganglia, suggesting impairment of the development of the neuronal connection from the brainstem (52). Hence, catecholaminergic changes may underlie sleep-related alterations in respiratory and cardiovascular control, and failure to arouse during prolonged sleep apnea. This concept is supported by findings in infants of substance-abusing mothers. Substances such as cocaine affect the development of monoaminergic pathways (53). These infants have an increased risk of SIDS, manifest abnormal sleeping ventilatory patterns, and require a significantly longer exposure to hypercapnia before arousal (54). Furthermore, Hunt et al. (55) suggested that an arousal response deficit may be critical in the pathophysiology of SIDS. In support of this concept, Kinney et al. (56) described decreased muscarinic binding in the arcuate nucleus, which might contribute to a failure of responses to cardiopulmonary changes during sleep.

Hypercapnic arousal responses are altered in a variety of respiratory disorders, including Prader-Willi syndrome (PWS), a disease characterized by a number of abnormalities of hypothalamic function, such as hyperphagia, short stature, temperature instability, hypogonadotrophic hypogonadism, and neurosecretory growth hormone deficiency. Compared with normal controls, patients with PWS are reported to have sleep-disordered breathing, a blunted hypercapnic ventilatory response, and a significantly higher arousal threshold to hypercapnia, which may contribute to sleep-disordered breathing in this disease (57). Structural alterations in the hypothalamic paraventricular nucleus are observed in these patients (58), suggesting that a deficit in noradrenaline containing neuronal pathways may contribute to an arousal deficit and CO_2 retention.

Congenital central hypoventilation syndrome (CCHS; "Ondine's curse") is believed to be due to insensitivity of the central chemoreceptors to CO_2. Children with CCHS may present in the newborn period with absent ventilatory responses to both hypercapnia and hypoxia, suggesting either abnormal central and peripheral chemoreceptor function or abnormal central integration of chemoreceptor input. Children or adults with CCHS who have little or no arousal sensitivity to hypercapnic stress may have an altered catecholaminergic system, but subjects with CCHS who are aroused by hypercapnia may possess some central nonrespiratory-related chemoreceptor functions (59). Anatomical or functional alterations in noradrenaline-containing cells could exist in these individuals, but have yet to be demonstrated.

A part from the role of catecholaminergic neurons in chemosensation and arousal, there is increasing evidence that serotonergic midline neurons play a role in the ventilatory response to hypercapnia (60), and are involved in diverse physiologic functions. Axonal projections and terminal arborizations from these cells invade almost the entire neuraxis, from the most caudal segments of the spinal cord to the frontal cortex (61). In studies from our laboratory, we found that hypercapnic loading activated a subpopulation of serotonin-containing cells within the caudal midline nuclei (62).

It has been shown that the activity of serotonin-containing neurons is decreased during sleep. Entering slow-wave sleep (non-REM), neuronal activity slows to ~50% of the quiet waking level and loses its regularity. Finally, during REM sleep, most serotonin neurons become nearly quiescent, via activation of GABA-ergic inputs (61).

During sleep, diminished activity of serotonin neurons may lead to a decrease in airway patency. Entering sleep and in non-REM or REM sleep, respiratory drive to upper-airway dilating muscles preferentially is decreased (for review see 63). In humans, this may lead to obstructive sleep apnea, hypopnea, and autonomic stress (63,64). Furthermore, alterations in serotonergic pathways may cause failure of homeostatic responses to life-threatening challenges (e.g., asphyxia, hypercapnia) during sleep (65). In children, altered serotonergic pathways could contribute to the severity of obstructive sleep apnea; however, this hypothesis remains to be confirmed by studies focused on development of this neuronal pathway.

Histaminergic Neurons and Response to Hypercapnia

The third group of monoaminergic neurons in the CNS, histaminergic neurons, may play an important role in chemosensation and arousal, in parallel with the serotonergic and catecholaminergic neuronal groups. These histaminergic neurons are confined to the posterior hypothalamic area. Scattered groups of these neurons are referred to as the tuberomammillary nucleus. These cells give rise to widespread projections extending via the basal forebrain to the cerebral cortex, as well as to the thalamus and pontomesencephalic tegmentum. The histaminergic system may act as a regulatory network for whole-brain activity, including hormonal functions, sleep, food intake, thermoregulation, locomotor changes, and arousal (66).

Recently we observed that a subset of histamine-containing cells are activated by hypercapnic loading (49). Activation of histamine-containing cells by an increase in CO_2 or H^+ may affect central respiratory drive, via activation of NTS neurons which are heavily innervated by histaminergic fibers (67,68).

The link between sleep-related respiratory disorders in infants and maternal smoking during pregnancy (69,70) could be partly due to interference of nicotine with the development of the histaminergic CNS system. Nicotine inhibits histamine-N-methyltransferase (71), leading to altered histaminergic transmission and arousal deficit.

D. Neonatal Apnea

The incidence of apnea of prematurity is inversely related to gestational age, and probably approaches 100% in the most immature preterm infants, depending on the diagnostic criteria employed (72). Such cessation of breathing is usually accompanied by ventilatory and cardiovascular consequences, namely hypoxemia, hypercapnia, and bradycardia.

Apnea of prematurity is thought to be secondary to immaturity of brainstem centers that regulate breathing. This immaturity in regulation of breathing is also manifested by immaturity in the respiratory responses to hypercapnia, hypoxia, and an exaggerated inhibitory response to stimulation of airway receptors. Although a cause-and-effect relationship has not been documented for disturbed control of breathing and the occurrence of apnea in preterm infants, strong associations are very well established. Histologically, immaturity of the preterm brain is manifested by a decreased number of synaptic connections, dendritic arborizations, and poor myelination. Functionally, Henderson-Smart and co-workers reported that auditory-evoked responses are longer in infants with apnea than in matched preterm controls, indicating delay in brainstem conduction time (73). Furthermore, multiple inhibitory neurotransmitters and neuromodulators have been implicated in the pathogenesis of disturbances of breathing at both the peripheral and central chemoreceptors, including dopamine, adenosine, endorphins, GABA, and prostaglandins, and these may be upregulated in early life (33).

When compared to nonapneic controls, there is even greater impairment of the hypercapnic breathing response in preterm infants with apnea (74,75). Gerhardt and Bancalari (74) and others documented that the CO_2 response in preterm infants with apnea was shifted to the right and had a lower slope than in infants without apnea. In other words, at the same level of CO_2, minute ventilation in babies with apnea was lower. Pulmonary mechanics, respiratory frequency, and dead-space volume were similar in the two groups. These data strongly suggest that a central immaturity of respiratory neural output may account for the attenuated CO_2 response in preterm babies, in particular those with apnea. However, a cause-and-effect relationship between apnea of prematurity and the attenuated response to CO_2 has not been clearly established, and both might simply represent facets of a decreased respiratory drive.

Apnea is traditionally classified into three categories based on the presence or absence of obstruction of the upper airways. These are central, obstructive, and mixed apneas. Central apnea is characterized by total cessation of inspiratory efforts with no evidence of obstruction. In obstructed apnea, the infant tries to breathe against an obstructed upper airway, resulting in chest wall motion without nasal airflow throughout the entire apnea. Mixed apnea consists of obstructed respiratory efforts usually following the central pauses, and is probably the most common type of apnea. The contribution of obstruction to apnea was first described by Thach and Stark, who observed that the frequency of apnea increased when the premature infant's neck was flexed (76). Subsequently, upper-airway obstruction was found to accompany apnea even in the absence of neck flexion (77). The site of obstruction in the upper airways is mostly in the pharynx; however, it may also occur at the larynx, and possibly both sites. Mixed apneas are the most common in small premature infants and account for more than half of all apneas, followed in decreasing frequency by central and obstructive apnea (78).

The prominence of mixed apnea has led to comparative analysis of upper-airway versus chest wall muscle responses to chemoreceptor stimulation. Upper airway muscles, such as the alae nasi, genioglossus, and posterior cricoarytenoid (laryngeal abductor), typically have their onset and peak of phasic activity prior to corresponding events in the diaphragm (79). This presumably serves to ensure upper-airway patency at peak inspiratory flow. In response to hypercapnic exposure in piglets, there was a relatively linear increase in diaphragm activation (79). In contrast, genioglossus and alae nasi exhibited a higher threshold, and activities only began to increase at a significantly higher level of CO_2 (80). It is possible that during hypercapnia, as during apnea, an initial increase in diaphragm, but not upper-airway activation, superimposed upon collapsed pharyngeal or laryngeal structures, might predispose to the obstructed inspiratory efforts that characterize mixed apnea. Furthermore, decreasing central chemosensitivity by cooling at chemosensitive sites preferentially inhibits neural output to upper-airway muscles (81). In premature infants, noninvasive measurements have demonstrated that the diaphragm EMG is low during obstructed inspiratory efforts (82). However, at resolution of apnea, both diaphragm and upper-airway activities are increased. Therefore, it appears that decrease in diaphragm activity is common to both central and mixed apnea, although collapse or closure of the upper airway, and delayed upper airway muscle activation, may prolong the episode and its consequences.

Decreased central chemosensitivity may also contribute to apnea by modulation of inhibitory reflexes arising from laryngeal afferents. Laryngeal stimulation is a well-documented trigger for reflex apnea, which serves to protect the lungs from aspiration. This response is most prominent during the neonatal period (83), and while it is assumed to be an essential protective reflex, an exaggerated response has been suggested to be a cause for apnea of prematurity or SIDS. The mechanism responsible for the greater sensitivity of the respiratory system to the inhibitory effects of laryngeal stimulation early in development is not clear, although maturational changes in central chemosensitivity might contribute to postnatal alterations in the strength of this potent inhibitory reflex. We have documented in the piglet model that withdrawal of central chemosensitivity by cooling the ventral medullary surface significantly decreases the threshold current of superior laryngeal nerve stimulation needed to inhibit diaphragm activity (84). Thus, decreased CO_2/H^+ central chemosensitivity may partially explain the vulnerability of preterm infants to stimulation of laryngeal afferents, thus further accentuating respiratory instability in this population.

IV. Chemoreceptors for Oxygen and Their Role in Breathing

A. Structure and Pathways

The carotid bodies are the principal sites at which changes in arterial PO_2 are sensed. These small glomus structures are located at the bifurcation of the common carotid arteries in the neck. Each carotid body consists of clusters of type 1 (glomus) cells, which are considered to be the essential chemosensory elements. Type 1 cells are surrounded by glialike type II cells, and the entire structure is in close contact with a network of capillaries (Fig. 4). The carotid bodies sense hypoxia resulting from a decrease in partial pressure of oxygen;

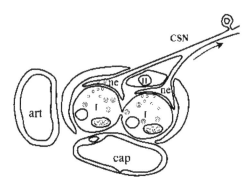

Figure 4 Diagram of the cellular components of the carotid body. The vesicle containing type 1 cells (I) are in close apposition to afferent carotid sinus nerve (CSN) endings and encapsulated by type II cells (II). The carotid body has a rich blood supply (cap, capillary; art, arteriole). (From Ref. 175.)

interestingly, they do not respond to a decrease in oxygen content alone, such as in carbon monoxide inhalation or anemia. An important modulation of the sensory activity of the carotid chemoreceptors is provided by the level of CO_2/H^+. For example, Carroll et al. (85) have shown that the carotid sinus nerve output in the kitten becomes increasingly sensitive to $PaCO_2$ with advancing age (Fig. 5).

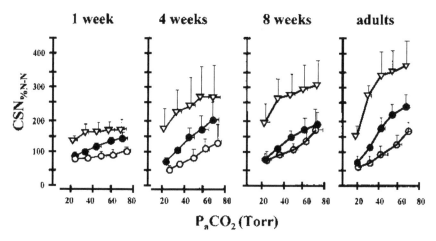

Figure 5 $CSN_{\%N-N}$ CO_2 responses in four age groups; $\bigcirc$, hyperoxia; $\bullet$, normoxia; $\triangle$, hypoxia. (From Ref. 85.)

The carotid bodies transduce a change in partial pressure of oxygen by activating sensory nerve endings of the carotid sinus nerve, a branch of the glossopharyngeal nerve. Afferent fibers traveling in the carotid sinus and vagus nerves terminate almost entirely in the *nucleus tractus solitarius* (NTS) (for review see 86; 87–90). There is evidence from studies of both adult and some newborn animal species that N-methyl-D-aspartate (NMDA) glutamate receptors in the NTS play a pivotal role in peripheral chemoreceptor-mediated hypoxic ventilatory responses. Systemic administration of the NMDA glutamate receptor antagonist MK-801 has been shown to attenuate the hypoxic ventilatory response and the peripheral chemoreceptor response to sodium cyanide in developing piglets, anesthetized dogs, and adult rats (91–93). Direct application of NK-801 to the NTS reduces the Ve response to hypoxia (94). Furthermore, NMDA glutamate receptors in the brainstem have been shown to increase with advancing postnatal age in the rat pup (95). Thus, an increase in NMDA glutamate receptors parallels the acquisition of a sustained increase in ventilation, which characterizes maturation of the hypoxic ventilatory response in the rat. From the NTS, chemoreceptor reflex pathways project to diverse sites in the lower brainstem and spinal cord (96).

B.   Mechanisms of Oxygen Chemoreception in the Carotid Body

A neural structure which controls respiration for the whole organism must be acutely sensitive to changes in partial pressure of oxygen in the arterial circulation (oxygen sensor function), and must be capable of rapid and sustained response to new challenges (modulation of sensor function and neurotransmission). In the type I cells of the carotid body, a number of biochemical changes occur during hypoxia; however, the exact molecular oxygen sensor is unknown. Chemoreceptor cells of rabbit and cat release dopamine in proportion to hypoxic stimulus, and in parallel to carotid sinus nerve output (97–99). This release of dopamine is dependent on the intracellular calcium. Neurotransmitter release (e.g., dopamine) can be triggered by depolarization involving activation of voltage dependent Ca^{2+} channels (100). Furthermore, Lopez-Barneo et al. (using isolated patches of plasma membrane) demonstrated that chemoreceptor cells possess an outward K^+ current sensitive to low PO_2 (101). Thus, this O_2-sensitive K^+ channel is a candidate for the O_2 sensor coupling arterial PO_2 to activation of the type I cell. The molecular site for oxygen sensing in the membrane could be a hemoprotein that senses low PO_2 (102,103). An alternative site for oxygen chemoreception may exist within the mitochondria of the type I cells. Biscoe and coworkers have studied these mitochondria, and found that their redox state and electrochemical potential are dependent on a PO_2 in bathing solutions, which is in the physiologic range (104). Therefore, the mitochondrion could internally signal that a change in arterial oxygen content has occurred.

For carotid sinus nerve output to increase in response to hypoxia, neurotransmitter release at the synapse between the carotid sinus nerve and the type I cell must be coupled to change in PaO_2. Many neurotransmitters and receptors have been identified in the carotid body and in the carotid sinus nerve including dopamine and D2 receptors, acetyl choline, serotonin, adenosine, substance P, and nitric oxide (for reviews see 105, 106). Endogenous dopamine is the most abundant transmitter in the carotid body , and its content appears to be highest soon after birth, thereafter decreasing over the next 7 days in the rat pup (107). Endogenous D2 dopamine receptors may act to inhibit the response of the type I cells to hypoxia, and could contribute to the low sensitivity to hypoxia of the carotid body in the immediate postnatal period. The neuromodulator adenosine is also synthesized in the carotid body, and could modulate dopamine synthesis through binding to A2a receptors (108). The current rapid advances in understanding fostered by direct recording from isolated carotid type I cells may soon clarify further details of the complex chemotransduction pathways in the carotid body.

C. Physiologic Effects of the Carotid Bodies on Breathing in Postnatal life

The carotid chemoreceptors are the primary mediators of increase in breathing during acute hypoxia. In addition, they undergo tonic activity that supports minute ventilation (109). Their sensory neural output has been studied in a variety of ways, including direct recording from the carotid sinus nerve, as well as experimental studies of the alterations in breathing evoked by carotid body denervation in experimental animals. In the fetal sheep, the carotid chemoreceptors are spontaneously active, in utero, beginning at about 90 days' gestation (110). The PaO_2 of the fetus is normally $\sim$25 mm Hg in late gestation. At this level of O_2, chemoreceptor discharge is low, and increases steeply when PaO_2 is reduced below $\sim$15 mm Hg. As noted above, stimulation of fetal carotid chemoreceptors does not significantly increase fetal breathing movements. This appears to be due to pontine descending inhibition which effectively blocks neural input from the carotid bodies to the CNS.

After birth, the acute rise in PaO_2 perfusing the carotid body has been shown to silence the chemoreceptors. Then, over the first weeks of life, arterial chemoreceptor sensitivity is reset, moving the stimulus response curve to the right, so that the carotid bodies can sense changes in PO_2 in the physiologic range (111–114) (see also Fig. 5). This chemoreceptor resetting results in an increase in the ventilatory response to hypoxia, as shown in experimental animals and in human infants over the first week of life (115–119).

The role of the carotid body in postnatal breathing has also been inferred from studies of the acute and chronic effects of carotid body denervation on respiration in animal subjects. In carotid body–denervated newborn lambs, Purves noted a decrease in Ve and rise in $PaCO_2$ with some periods of irregular breathing (120,121). The pattern of breathing is also abnormal in newborn cats and rats after carotid body denervation (122,123). Thus, these observations support the contribution of the carotid bodies to ventilation during normoxic breathing.

Some caution is warranted, however, in interpretation of these studies. Carotid body denervation requires extensive surgical dissection which can alter adjacent structures, such as baroreceptor afferents. Indeed, postsurgical sudden death of carotid-denervated animals led several groups (124–127) to propose that carotid body dysfunction could be a cause of SIDS. More recently, Forster et al. (128) reported that outcome of chemodenervation in the piglet was related to the surgical technique utilized, including route of dissection. Furthermore, carotid body denervation in goats at 1 to 4 days did not produce sudden death, or long-term effects on control of breathing (129). At this time, further evidence appears to be needed to support the hypothesis that carotid body dysfunction can contribute to the pathologic state which culminates in SIDS.

D. Carotid Chemoreceptor Involvement in Late Hypoxic Ventilatory Depression

The ventilatory response of the neonatal mammal to hypoxia exhibits a "biphasic" pattern consisting of an initial increase in minute ventilation, followed by a decline, in some cases to a level below prehypoxic levels (for review see 130). The adult mammal, in contrast, exhibits a more sustained increase in ventilation in response to prolonged hypoxia, with a more delayed hypoxic depression, or "rolloff." The initial increase in ventilation in the first few minutes of hypoxia has been attributed to the carotid chemoreceptor response. The later hypoxic ventilatory depression during the rolloff has been a subject of considerable experimental study. Theoretically, this later depression of ventilatory output could be due to a decline in chemosensory input from the carotid bodies to the CNS, or an alteration (gating) of chemosensory input within the CNS. Blanco et al. (131) addressed this question in the anesthetized newborn kitten model. In this study, minute ventilation and carotid sinus nerve (CSN) activity were simultaneously recorded prior to and during hypoxia. These authors found that CSN activity was sustained during hypoxia in the kitten, despite the onset of respiratory depression. These results support the concept that the late phase of hypoxic ventilatory depression is predominantly due to central neural inhibition. However, several groups have subsequently recorded CSN activity in response to hypoxia in the kitten and noted a biphasic pattern of output (85,132). Thus, further work is needed to fully resolve the question of the contribution of the carotid bodies to the characteristic biphasic ventilatory response in the newborn period.

E. Accessory Sites for Oxygen Chemoreception

The carotid bodies are not the only hypoxia-sensitive chemosensory tissue in the body. There are other islands of glomus tissue along the aorta and subclavian arteries, and within the abdomen (133). The aortic chemoreceptors, examples of such accessory structures, are activated by hypoxia and hypercapnia, but exert significantly less effect on breathing than carotid chemoreceptors (134,135). The role these accessory glomus tissues play in hypoxic chemosensation and control of breathing may depend on the age of the mammal and on the degree of function of the carotid bodies. After carotid body denervation in adult ponies, peripheral chemosensitivity was eliminated for several months; thereafter, chemosensitivity returned to 30–40% of normal, and sectioning of the aortic nerves almost completely eliminated peripheral chemosensitivity (136,137). Thus, accessory chemoreceptor sites in the carotid-denervated ponies may have assumed the role of the carotid bodies.

Several groups of investigators have found that activity of combined carotid body and aortic chemoreceptors may be important in the immediate neonatal period. Donnelly and Haddad found that carotid body and aortic body denervation, compared to carotid body denervation alone, resulted in significantly more apnea per hour in 3- to 9-day-old piglets (138). The time of carotid body denervation may be critical. Lowry et al. (139) found that piglets carotid body denervated at 5 days of age did not hypoventilate as compared to controls. However, animals denervated at 15 or 25 days exhibited greater hypoventilation. Lowry et al. speculated that greater plasticity of chemoreceptor function occurs in the first week of life, allowing accessory glomus tissue to assume the roles of the carotid chemoreceptors. This concept of plasticity of chemoreceptor structures is important when we consider the consequences of injury or disease which may impair carotid body chemoreception.

F. Prenatal and Postnatal Influences That Can Alter Hypoxic Chemosensitivity

Chronic Hypoxia

The carotid chemoreceptors are quite vulnerable to functional and structural change if exposed to prolonged PaO_2 outside the normal range of oxygenation. In postnatal life, long-term hypoxic exposure has been associated in humans as well as in animal models with attenuation of ventilatory responsiveness to hypoxia (140–143). In experimental animals, exposure to severe hypoxia for several weeks after birth has been shown to result in attenuation of hypoxic ventilatory response in cats (141,144), rats (145–147), and lambs (148,149,). In the rat exposed to 0.13–0.15% FiO_2 for 5–10 weeks postbirth, the normal emergence of the biphasic response to hypoxia (day 5) and the adult sustained response (day 14) was significantly delayed (Fig. 6) (150). At 5–10 weeks of age, pups exposed to chronic hypoxia still had an immature biphasic response to hypoxia, unlike the expected adult sustained response. Furthermore, chemoafferent output from the carotid sinus nerve in response to isocapnic hypoxia did not differ in chronically hypoxic and normoxic rats at 5–10 weeks. Thus, in this study, the central neural pathways which contribute to hypoxic ventilatory depression remained immature when the normal transition to postnatal air breathing was not permitted to occur.

However, there is evidence from other investigators that chronic hypoxia can also alter peripheral chemoreceptor function. Chronic hypoxia induces significant morphologic changes in the carotid body of humans and animals (151) and increases the dopamine content (152,153). Hanson et al. (154) noted in a later paper that the ventilatory response to peripheral chemoreceptor input, tested by two-breath alterations of fractional inspired oxygen, was blunted in kittens born and reared in 0.13–0.15% O_2 (tested at days 4–8 and at days 9–14). In rats, Wach (149) demonstrated that 2–3 weeks of 10% O_2 inhalation attenuated hypoxic ventilatory response. This alteration was partially reversed by a peripheral D2 receptor blocker, domperidone, suggesting that suppression of peripheral

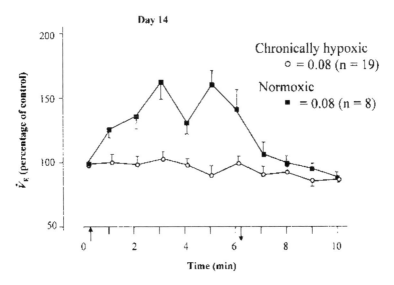

Figure 6   Respiratory responses of chronically hypoxic (○, n = 19) and normoxic (■, n = 8) rat pups to 8% O_2 on postnatal day 14. (From Ref. 150.)

chemoreceptor response contributed to the blunted hypoxic ventilatory response. Hertzberg et al. (155) also noted that newborn rats born and raised in hypoxia (0.12–0.14%) for 2 postnatal days exhibited a blunted response to hypoxia as compared to normally reared controls. Furthermore, increased carotid body dopamine turnover was detected in those pups reared in hypoxia. As noted previously, dopamine is the most abundant neurotransmitter in the carotid body, and may inhibit carotid sinus response to hypoxia through binding to postsynaptic D2 receptors (156). Theoretically, increased dopamine turnover may have reflected an increase in inhibitory neurotransmitter activity in the carotid body of chronically hypoxic animals, which could contribute to the blunted ventilatory response to hypoxia. In support of this concept, Tatsumi et al. (157) noted that adult cats exposed to hypobaric hypoxia for 3 weeks exhibited a decreased CSN response to hypoxia, which was augmented by domperidone (a peripheral dopamine D2 antagonist). Taken together, these studies suggest that chronic hypoxia may also act by increasing dopamininergic inhibition of carotid body chemosensation. At the cellular level, chronic hypoxia may also alter the O_2-sensitive K^+ channels which augment depolarization of the type I cell in response to hypoxemia (158). These findings may be pertinent to the human newborn exposed to prolonged postnatal hypoxia. For example, Sorensen and Severinghaus (140) reported that human subjects with cyanotic heart disease (TOF) exhibited a considerably decreased ventilatory response to inhalation of 40% O_2 1 year after surgical correction of their heart disease. It is not known whether this depressed hypoxic response was due to failure of postnatal resetting of the chemoreceptors, or persistence of central inhibitory gating of chemoreceptor input.

In the search for the cause of SIDS, several investigators (159–161) have examined the ultrastructure and neurotransmitter content of carotid bodies in infants who have died of SIDS compared to controls dying of defined causes. Perrin reported that the ultrastructure of the carotid body was normal in SIDS, but that dopamine and noradrenaline content were increased. At present, it is not known whether these changes could be causative or, for example, secondary to repeated hypoxic events prior to death from SIDS.

Chronic Hyperoxia

Hyperoxia may also result in significant blunting of peripheral chemoreceptor response. Two weeks of hyperoxia decreased peripheral chemoreceptor response in neonatal rats and in kittens (162,163). Ling et al. (164,165) showed that rat pups treated with 60% O_2 for the first month of life exhibited attenuated awake ventilatory responses and phrenic nerve responses to hypoxia several months later (Fig. 7). Full recovery of the hypoxic response occurred slowly in the chronically hyperoxic rats over the first 15 months of life (166). Interestingly, exposure of the

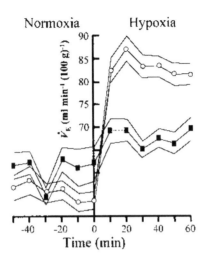

Figure 7 Hypoxic ventilatory responses in rats are depressed by exposure to chronic hyperoxia in the perinatal period (0.6 O_2). Minute ventilation (Ve) increased substantially during hypoxia in untreated control rats, and significantly less in perinatal-treated rats. Data are mans ±SEM. (O, normoxic rats; ■, perinatal exposure to hyperoxia). (From Ref. 164.)

adult rat to chronic hyperoxia did not alter the hypoxic response (164). Thus, peripheral chemoreceptors may be most vulnerable to hyperoxic injury in the newborn period.

Ericson et al. (167) have provided evidence for the cellular sites at which chronic hyperoxia alters peripheral chemoreceptor response. Four weeks of chronic hyperoxia (60% O_2) resulted in a 41% decrease in the number of unmyelinated axons in the carotid sinus nerve, compared with age-matched normoxic controls. Furthermore, chemoafferent neurons located in the petrosal ganglion exhibited degenerative changes, following 1 week of hyperoxia from birth. Marked hypoplasia of the carotid body accompanied these degenerative changes. Whether advancing age allows recovery of cellular structure or accessory chemoreceptor function in these animals is not known.

Altered Hypoxic Ventilatory Response in Premature Infants

Human infants born prematurely may have serious lung disease (RDS) requiring mechanical ventilatory support which may progress to chronic lung disease (BPD) over the first weeks of life. Such infants may exhibit repeated hypoxemic events while on mechanical ventilation and repeated apneas thereafter (168,169).

Hyperoxic exposure may also occur while the infant is in the process of recovering and still undergoing mechanical ventilation. In light of the serious perturbations in peripheral chemoreceptor function reported in animal studies after prolonged hypoxia or hyperoxia, it is not surprising to find that Calder et al. (170) and Katz-Salamon et al. (171,172) have reported blunted peripheral chemoreceptor responses in premature infants with BPD. The decrease in chemoreceptor response in infants with BPD was directly correlated with length of time on the ventilator and severity of BPD (172). At present, confirmation of peripheral chemoreceptor structural abnormalities has yet to be obtained in such infants. Furthermore, it is not known whether this defect in chemoreception in these children persists into adulthood. Theoretically, this blunting of peripheral chemoreceptor response could render the child unable to recover effectively from sleep apnea, or to increase ventilation appropriately during a serious respiratory illness. In support of this concept, studies by the Collaborative Home Infant Monitoring Evaluation Group (CHIME) , as well as independent work from our laboratory, have shown that dysfunctional respiratory control persists in some premature infants long after the need for supplemental oxygen or mechanical ventilation has passed (173,174). It is possible that a combination of repeated hypoxia and/or hyperoxia can lead to long-standing peripheral chemoreceptor dysfunction. Further advances in our understanding of the molecular basis for normal postnatal maturation of the carotid bodies may help the neonatal intensivist avoid extremes of oxygenation and create optimal conditions for postnatal development of these important structures in high-risk newborns.

References

1. Jansen AH, Chernick V. Development of respiratory control. Physiol Rev 1983; 63:437–483.
2. Jansen H, Chernick V. Fetal breathing and development of control of breathing. J Appl Physiol 1991; 70:1431–1446.
3. Harding R. State-related developmental changes in laryngeal function. Sleep 1980; 3:307–322.
4. Dawes GS, Fox HE, Leduc BM, Liggins GC, Richards RT. Respiratory movements and rapid eye movement sleep in the fetal lamb. J Physiol (Lond)1972; 220:119–143.
5. Berger PJ, Walker AM, Horne R, Brodecky V, Wilkinson MH, Wilson F, Maloney JE. Phasic respiratory activity in the fetal lamb during late gestation and labour. Respir Physiol 1986; 65:55–68.
6. Patrick J, Fetherston W, Vick H, Voegelin R. Human fetal breathing movements and gross fetal body movements at weeks 34 to 35 of gestation. Am J Obstet Gynecol 1978; 130:693–699.

7. Kuipers IM, Maertzdorf WJ, De Jong DS, Hanson MA, Blanco CE. The effect of hypercapnia and hypercapnia associated with central cooling on breathing in unanesthetized fetal lamb. Pediatr Res 1997; 41:90–95.

8. Bocking AD, Gagnon R, Milne KM, White SE. Behavioral activity during prolonged hypoxemia in fetal sheep. J Appl Physiol 1988; 65:2420–2426.

9. Hooper SB, Harding R. Changes in lung liquid dynamics induced by prolonged fetal hypoxemia. J Appl Physiol 1990; 69:127–135.

10. Koos BJ, Kianaka T, Matsuda K, Gilbert RD, Longo LD. Fetal breathing adaptation to prolonged hypoxaemia in sheep. J Develop Physiol 1988; 10:161–166.

11. Johnston BM, Gluckman PD. Lateral pontine lesions affect central chemosensitivity in unanesthetized fetal lambs. J Appl Physiol 1989; 67:1113–1118.

12. Gluckman PD, Johnston BM. Lesions in the upper lateral pons abolish the hypoxic depression of breathing in unanesthetized fetal lambs in utero. J Physiol 1987; 382:373–383.

13. Harned HS Jr, Herrington RT, Ferreiro JI. The effects of immersion and temperature on respiration in newborn lambs. Pediatrics 1970; 45:598–605.

14. Gluckman PD, Gunn TR, Johnston BM. The effect of cooling on breathing and shivering in unanaesthetized fetal lambs in utero. J Physiol 1983; 343:495–506.

15. Baier RJ, Hasan SU, Cates DB, Hooper D, Nowaczyk B, Rigatto H. Effects of various concentrations of O2 and umbilical cord occlusion on fetal breathing and behavior. J Appl Physiol 1990; 68:1597–1604.

16. Hasan SU, Rigaux A. The effects of lung distention, oxygenation and gestational age on fetal behavior and breathing movements in sheep. Pediatr Res 1991; 30:193–201.

17. Hasan SU, Rigaux A. Arterial oxygen tension threshold range for the onset of arousal and breathing in fetal sheep. Pediatr Res 1992; 32:342–349.

18. Dawes GS, Mott JC. The increase in oxygen consumption of the lamb after birth. J Physiol 1959; 146:295–315.

19. Mortola JP, Gautier H. Interaction between metabolism and ventilation: effects of respiratory gases and temperature. In: Dempsey JA, Pack AI, eds. Regulation of Breathing, 2nd ed. New York: Marcel Dekker, 1995:1011–1064.

20. Kuipers IM, Maertzdorf WJ, Keunen H, De Jong DS, Hanson MA, Blanco CE. Fetal breathing is not initiated after cord occlusion in the unanaesthetized fetal lamb in utero. J Dev Physiol 1992; 17:233–240.

21. Kuipers IM, Maertzdorf WJ, De Jong DS, Hanson MA, Blanco CE. Effect of mild hypocapnia on fetal breathing and behavior in unanesthetized normoxic fetal lambs. J Appl Physiol 1994; 76:1476–1480.

22. Kuipers IM, Maertzdorf WJ, De Jong DS, Hanson MA, Blanco CE. Initiation and maintenance of continuous breathing at birth. Pediatr Res 1997; 42:63–168.

23. Frantz ID III, Adler SM, Thach BT, Taeusch HW Jr. Maturational effects on respiratory responses to carbon dioxide in premature infants. J Appl Physiol 1976; 41:41–45.

24. Rigatto H, Brady JP, De la Torre Verduzco RT. Chemoreceptor reflexes in preterm infants. II. The effects of gestational and postnatal age on the ventilatory response to inhaled carbon dioxide. Pediatrics 1975; 55:614–620.

25. Noble LM, Carlo WA, Miller MJ, DiFiore JM, Martin RJ. Transient changes in expiratory time during hypercapnia in premature infants. J Appl Physiol 1984; l62:1010–1013.

26. Eichenwald EC, Ungarelli RA, Stork AN. Hypercapnia increases expiratory braking in preterm infants. J Appl Physiol 1993; 75:2665–2670.

27. Martin RJ, Carlo WA, Robertson SS, Day WR, Bruce EN. Biphasic response of respiratory frequency to hypercapnia in preterm infants. Pediatr Res 1985; 19:791–796.

28. Krauss AN, Klain DB, Waldman S, Auld PAM. Ventilatory response to carbon dioxide in newborn infants. Pediatr Res 1965; 9:46–50.

29. Zhou D, Huang Q, Fung ML, Li A, Darnall RA, Nattie EE, St. John WM. Phrenic response to hypercapnia in the unanesthetized, decerebrate, newborn rat. Respir Physiol 1996; 104:11–22.

30. Abu-Shaweesh JM, Dreshaj IA, Thomas AJ, Haxhiu MA, Strohl KP, Martin RJ. Changes in respiratory timing induced by hypercapnia in maturing rats. J Appl Physiol 1999; 87:484–490.

31. Dreshaj IA, Haxhiu MA, Abu-Shaweesh J, Carey RE, Martin RJ. CO_2-induced prolongation of expiratory time during early development. Respir Physiol 1999; 116:125–132.

32. Xia Y, Haddad GG. Ontogeny and distribution of $GABA_A$ receptors in rat brainstem and rostral brain regions. Neuroscience 1992; 49:973–979.

33. Moss IR, Inman JG. Neurochemicals and respiratory control during development. J Appl Physiol 1989; 67:1–13.

34. Dreshaj IA, Haxhiu MA, Miller MJ, Abu-Shaweesh J, Martin RJ. Differential effects of hypercapnia on expiratory phases of respiration in the piglet. Respir Physiol 2001; 126:43–51.

35. England SJ, Harding R, Stradling JR, Phillipson EA. Laryngeal muscle activities during progressive hypercapnia and hypoxia in awake and sleeping dogs. Respir Physiol 1986; 66:327–339.

36. Schläfke ME. Central chemosensitivity: a respiratory drive. Rev Physiol Biochem Pharmacol 1981; 90:171–249.

37. Nattie EE, Li A, Lee E, Coates EL. Central chemoreceptor location and the ventrolateral medulla. Lung Biol Health Dis 1995; 82:131–150.

38. Erickson JT, Millhorn DE. Fos-like protein is induced in neurons of the carotid sinus nerve in awake and anaesthetized rats. Brain Res 1991; 567:11–24.

39. Belegu R, Hadžiefendić S, Dreshaj IA, Haxhiu MA, Martin RJ. CO_2-induced c-fos expression in medullary neurons during early development. Respir Physiol 1999; 117:13–28.

40. Bernard DG, Li A., Nattie EE. Evidence for central chemoreception in the midline raphe. J Appl Physiol 11996; 80:108–115.

41. Li A, Randall M, Nattie EE. CO_2 microdialysis in retrotrapezoid nucleus of the rat increases breathing in wakefulness but not in sleep. J Appl Physiol 1999; 87:910–919.

42. Dreshaj IA, Haxhiu MA, Martin RJ. Role of the medullary raphé nuclei in the respiratory response to CO_2. Respir Physiol 1998; 111:15–23.

43. Kuo NT, Agani FH, Haxhiu MA, Chang CH. A possible role for protein kinase C in CO_2/H^+ induced c-fos mRNA expression in PC12 cells. Respir Physiol 1998; 111:127–135.
44. Bandla HPR, Simakajornboon N, Graff GR, Gozal D. Protein kinase C modulates ventilatory patterning in the developing rat. Am J Respir Crit Care Med 1999; 159:968–973.
45. Jacobs BL, Fornal CA. An integrative role for serotonin in the central nervous system. In: Lydic R, Babhodyan HA, eds. Behavioral and State Control: Cellular and Molecular Mechanisms. Boca Raton, FL: CRC Press, 1995:181–194.
46. Smeets WJ, Gonzalez A. Catecholamine systems in the brain of vertebrates: new perspectives through a comparative approach. Brain Res Rev 2000; 33:308–379.
47. Aston-Jones G, Bloom F. Activity of norepinephrine-containing locus coeruleus neurons in behaving rats anticipates fluctuations in the sleep-waking cycle. J Neurosci 1981;1:876–886.
48. McGinty DJ, Harper RM. Dorsal raphe neurons: depression of firing during sleep in cats. Brain Res 1976; 101:569–575.
49. Haxhiu MA, Tolentimo-Silva F, Pete G, Kc P, Mack SO. Monoaminergic neurons, chemosensation and arousal. Respir Physiol 2001; 129:191–209.
50. Haxhiu MA, Yung K, Erokwu BE, Cherniak NS. CO_2 induced c-fos expression in the CNS catecholaminergic neurons. Respir Physiol 1996; 105:35–45.
51. Obonai T, Yasuhara M, Nakamura T, Takashima S. Catecholamine neurons alteration in the brainstem of sudden infant death syndrome victims. Pediatrics 1998; 101:285–288.
52. Ozawa Y, Obonai T, Itoh M, Aoki Y, Funayama M, Takashima S. Catecholaminergic neurons in the diencephalons and basal ganglia of SIDS. Pediatr Neurol 1999; 21:471–475.
53. Mayes LC. Developing brain and in utero cocaine exposure: effects on neural ontogeny. Dev Psychopathol 1999; 11:685–714.
54. Ward SL, Bautista DB, Woo MS, Chang M, Schuetz S, Wachsman L, Sehgal S, Bean X. Responses to hypoxia and hypercapnia in infants of substance abusing mothers. J Pediatr 1992; 121:704–709.
55. Hunt CE. Impaired arousal from sleep: relationship to sudden infant death syndrome. J Perinatol 1989; 9:184–187.
56. Kinney HC, Filiano JJ, Sleeper LA, Mandell F, Valdes-Dapena M, White WF. Decreased muscarinic receptor binding in the arcuate nucleus in sudden infant death syndrome. Science 1995; 269:1446–1450.
57. Livingston FR, Arens R, Baileys SL, Keens TG, Ward SL. Hypercapnic arousal responses in Prader-Willi syndrome. Chest 1995; 108:1627–1631.
58. Swaab DF, Purba JS, Hoffman MA. Alterations in the hypothalamic paraventricular nucleus and its oxytocin neurons (putative satiety cells) in Prader-Willi syndrome: a study of five cases. J Clin Endocrinol Metab 1995; 80:573–579.
59. Marcus CL, Bautista DB, Amihyia A, Ward SL, Keens TG. Hypercapneic arousal responses in children with congenital central hypoventilation syndrome. Pediatrics 1991; 88:993–998.

60. Mason P. Physiological identification of pontomedullary serotonergic neurons in the rat. J Neurophysiol 1997; 77:1087–1098.
61. Jacobs BL, Fornal CA. An integrative role for serotonin in the central nervous system. In: Lydic R, Babhdoyan HA, eds. Behavioral State Control: Cellular and Molecular Mechanisms. Boca Raton, FL: CRC Press, 1995:181–194.
62. Haxhiu MA, Tolentimo-Silva F, Pete G, Kc P, Mack SO. Monoaminergic neurons, chemosensation and arousal. Respir Physiol 2001; 129:191–209.
63. Dempsey JA, Smith CA, Harms CA, Chow CM, Saupe KW. Sleep-induced breathing instability. Sleep 1996; 19:236–247.
64. Cherniack NS. Respiratory dysrhythmias during sleep. N Engl J Med 1981; 305: 325–330.
65. Panigrahy A, Filiano J, Sleeper LA, Mandell F, Valdes-Depena M, Krous HF, Rava LA, Foley E, White WF, Kinney HC. Decreased serotonergic receptor binding in rhombic lip–derived regions of the medulla oblongata in the sudden infant death syndrome. J Neuropathol Exp Neurol 2000; 59:377–384.
66. Panula P, Karlstedt K, Sallmen T, Peitsaro N, Kaslin J, Michelsen KA, Anichtchik O, Kukko-Lukjanov T, Lintunen M. The histaminergic system in the brain: structural characteristics and changes in hibernation. J Chem Neuroanat 2000; 18:65–74.
67. Airaksinen MS, Panula P. The histaminergic system in the guinea pig central nervous system: an immunocytochemical mapping study using an antiserum against histamine. J Comp Neurol 1988; 273:163–168.
68. Panula P, Pirvola U, Auvinen S, Airaksinen MS. Histamine-immunoreactive nerve fibers in the rat brain. Neuroscience 1989; 28:585–610.
69. Rintahaka PJ, Hirvonen J. The epidemiology of sudden death syndrome in Finland in 1969–1980. Forensic Sci Int 1986; 30:219–233.
70. Kraus N, McGee T, Comperatore C. MLRs in children are consistently present during wakefulness, stage 1 and REM sleep. Eye Hear 1989; 10:339–345.
71. Gairola C, Godin CS, Houdi AA, Crooka PA. Inhibition of histamine N-methyl-transferase activity in guinea-pig pulmonary alveolar macrophages by nicotine. J Pharm Pharmacol 1988; 40:724–726.
72. Abu-Shaweesh JM, Baird TM, Martin RJ. Apnea and bradycardia of prematurity. In: Greenough A, Milner AD, eds. Basic Mechanisms of Pediatric Respiratory Disorders, 2nd ed. London: Arnold Heath Science, 2002.
73. Henderson-Smart DJ, Pettigrew AG, Campbell DJ. Clinical apnea and brainstem neural function in preterm infants. N Engl J Med 1983; 308:353.
74. Gerhardt T, Bancalari E. Apnea of prematurity: 1. Lung function and regulation of breathing. Pediatrics 1984; 74:58–62.
75. Durand M, Cabal LA, Gonzalez F, Georgie S, Barberis C, Hoppenbrouwers T, Hodgman JE. Ventilatory control and carbon dioxide response in preterm infants with idiopathic apnea. Am J Dis Child 1985; 139:717–720.
76. Thach BT, Stark AR. Spontaneous neck flexation and airway obstruction during apneic spells in preterm infants. J Pediatr 1974; 94:275.
77. Milner AD, Boon AW, Saunders RA, Hopkins IE. Upper airway obstruction and apnea in preterm infants. Arch Dis Child 1980; 55:22–25.

78. Miller MJ, Martin RJ. Pathophysiology of apnea of prematurity. In: Polin RA, Fox WW, eds. Fetal and Neonatal Physiology, 2nd ed. Orlando, FL: W.B. Saunders, 1998.

79. Carlo WA, Martin RJ, Abboud EL, Bruce EN, Strohl KP. Effect of sleep state and hypercapnia on alae nasi and diaphragm EMGs in preterm infants. J Appl Physiol Respir Environ Exercise Physiol 1983; 54:1590–1596.

80. Carlo WA, Martin RJ, DiFiore JM. Differences in CO_2 threshold of respiratory muscles in preterm infants. J Appl Physiol 1988; 65:2434–2439.

81. Martin RJ, Dreshaj I, Miller MJ, Haxhiu MA. Role of the ventral medullary surface in modulating respiratory responses to reflex stimulation in piglets. In: Trouth CO, Millis RM, Kiwull-Schone H, Schlafke ME, eds. Ventral Brainstem Mechanisms and Control of Respiration and Blood Pressure. New York: Marcel Dekker, 1995.

82. Gauda EB, Miller MJ, Carlo WA, DiFiore JM, Martin RJ. Genioglossus and diaphragm activity during obstructive apnea and airway occlusion in infants. Pediatr Res 1989; 26:583–587.

83. Davies AM, Koening JS, Thach BT. Upper airway chemo-reflex responses to saline and water in preterm infants. J Appl Physiol 1988; 64:1412–1420.

84. Litmanovitz I, Dreshaj I, Miller MJ, Haxhiu MA, Martin RJ. Central chemosensitivity affects respiratory muscle responses to laryngeal stimulation in the piglet. J Appl Physiol 1994; 76:403–408.

85. Carroll JL, Bamford OS, Fitzgerald RS. Postnatal maturation of carotid chemoreceptor responses to O_2 and CO_2 in the cat. J Appl Physiol 1993; 75:2383–2391.

86. Jordan D. Central integration of chemoreceptor afferent activity in arterial chemoreceptors. In: O'Regan R. et al., eds. Cell to System. New York: Plenum Press, 1994:87–97.

87. Cottle MK. Degeneration studies of primary afferents of IXth and Xth cranial nerves in the cat. J Comp Neurol 1964; 122:329–343.

88. Ciriello J, Hrycyshyn AW, Calaresu FR. Glossopharyngeal and vagal afferent projections to the brainstem of the cat: a horseradish peroxidase study. J Autonom Nerv Syst 1981; 4:64–79.

89. Panneton WM, Loewy AD. Projections of carotid sinus nerve to the nucleus of the solitary tract in the cat. Brain Res 1980; 191:239–244.

90. Finley JCW, Katz DM. The central organization of carotid body afferent projections to the brainstem of the rat. Brain Res 1992; 572:108–116.

91. Ohtake PJ, Torres JE, Gozal YM, Graff GR, Gozal D. NMDA receptors mediate peripheral chemoreceptor afferent input in the conscious rat. J Appl Physiol 1998; 84:853–861.

92. Ang RC, Hoop B, Kazemi H. Role of glutamate as the central neurotransmitter in the hypoxic ventilatory response. J. Appl Physiol 1992; 72:1480–1487.

93. Lin J, Sugihara C, Huang J, Here D, Devia C, Bancalari E. Effect of N-methyl-D aspartate receptor blockade on hypoxic ventilatory response in unanaesthetized piglets. J Appl Physiol 1996; 80:1759–1763.

94. Ogawa H, Mizusawa A, Kikuchi Y, Hida W, Miki H, Shirato K. Nitric oxide as a retrograde messenger in the nucleus tractus solitarius of the rat during hypoxia. J Physiol (Lond) 1995; 486:495–504.

95. Ohtake PJ, Simakajornboon N, Fehniger MD, Xue Y-D, Gozal D. N-methyl-D-aspartate receptor expression in the nucleus tractus solitarii and maturation of hypoxic ventilatory response in the rat. Am J Respir Crit Care Med 2000;162:1140–1147.

96. Loewy AD, Burton H. Nuclei of the solitary tract: efferent projections to the lower brainstem and spinal cord of the cat. J Comp Neurol 1978; 181:421–450.

97. Fidone S, González C, Yoshizaki K. Effects of low oxygen on the release of dopamine from the rabbit carotid body in vitro. J Physiol 1982; 333:93–110.

98. González C, Almaraz L, Obeso A, Rigual R. Carotid body chemoreceptors: from natural stimuli to sensory discharges. Physiol Rev 1994; 74:829–898.

99. González C, Almaraz L, Obeso A, Rigual R. Oxygen and acid chemoreception in the carotid body chemoreceptors. Trends Neurosci 1992; 15:136–153.

100. Almaraz L, González C, Obeso A. Effects of high potassium on the release of [^{3}H]dopamine from the cat carotid body in vitro. J Physiol 1986; 379:293–307.

101. López-Barneo J, López-López JR, Ureña J, González C. Chemotransduction in the carotid body: K^+ current modulated by P_{O2} in type I chemoreceptor cells. Science 1988; 241:580–582.

102. López-López JR, González C. Time course of K^+ current inhibition by low oxygen in chemoreceptor cells of adult rabbit carotid body: effects of carbon monoxide. FEBS Lett 1992; 299:251–254.

103. Lahiri S, Iturriaga R, Mokashi A, Ray DK, Chugh D. CO reveals dual mechanisms of O2 chemoreception in the cat carotid body. Respir Physiol 1993; 94:227–240.

104. Biscoe TJ, Duchen MR. Monitoring P_{O2} by the carotid chemoreceptor. News Physiol Sci 1990; 5:229–233.

105. Fidone SJ, González C. Initiation and control of chemoreceptor activity in the carotid body. In: Fishman AP, ed. Handbook of Physiology. Bethesda, MD: American Physiological Society, 1986:247–312.

106. González C, López-López JR, Obeso A, Pérez-Garcia M, Rocher A. Cellular mechanisms of oxygen chemoreception in the carotid body. Resp Physiol 1995; 102:137–147.

107. Hertzberg T, Hellstrom S, Lagercrantz H, Pequignot JM. Development of the arterial chemoreflex and the turnover of carotid body catecholamines in the newborn rat. J Physiol 1990; 425:211–225.

108. Gauda EB, Lawson EE. Developmental influences on carotid body responses to hypoxia. Respir Physiol 2000; 121:188–208.

109. Forster HV, Pan LG, Lowry TF, Serra A, Wenninger J, Martino P. Important role of carotid chemoreceptor afferents in control of breathing of adult and neonatal mammals. Respir Physiol 2000; 119:199–208.

110. Blanco CE, Dawes GS, Hanson MA, McCooke HB. The arterial chemoreceptors in fetal sheep and newborn lambs. J Physiol 1982; 330:38P.

111. Blanco CE, Dawes GS, Hanson MA, McCooke HB. The response to hypoxia of arterial chemoreceptors in fetal sheep and new-born lambs. J Physiol 1984; 351:25–37.

112. Hanson MA, Kumar P, McCooke HB. Post-natal re-setting of carotid chemoreceptor sensitivity in the lamb. J Physiol 1986; 382:57P.

113. Kumar P, Hanson MA. Re-setting of the hypoxic sensitivity of aortic chemoreceptors in the newborn lamb. J Dev Physiol 1989; 11:199–206.

114. Mulligan EM. Discharge properties of carotid bodies. Developmental aspects. In: Haddad GG, Farber JP, eds. Developmental Neurobiology of Breathing. New York: Marcel Dekker, 1991:321–340.

115. Hanson MA, Eden GJ, Nijhuis JG, Moore PJ. Peripheral chemoreceptors and other O$_2$ sensors in the fetus and newborn. In: Pack AI, ed. Chemoreceptors and Reflexes in Breathing. New York: Oxford University Press, 1989:113–120.

116. Williams BA, Hanson MA. Role of the carotid chemoreceptors in the respiratory response of newborn lambs to alternate pairs of breaths of air and a hypoxic gas. J Dev Physiol 1990; 13:157–164.

117. Williams BA, Smyth J, Boon AW, Hanson MA, Kumar P, Blanco CE. Development of respiratory chemoreflexes in response to alternations of fractional inspired oxygen in the newborn infant. J Physiol 1991; 442:81–90.

118. Calder NA, Williams BA, Kumar P, Hanson MA. The respiratory response of healthy term infants to breath-by-breath alternations in inspired oxygen at two postnatal ages. Pediatr Res 1994; 35: 321–324.

119. Jansen AH, Chernick V. Fetal breathing and development of control of breathing. J Appl Physiol 1991; 70:1431–1446.

120. Purves MJ. The effects of hypoxia in the new-born lamb before and after denervation of the carotid chemoreceptors. J Physiol 1966; 185:60–77.

121. Purves MJ. Respiratory and circulatory effects of breathing 100% oxygen in the new-born lamb before and after denervation of the carotid chemoreceptors. J Physiol 1966; 185:42–59.

122. Schweieler GH. Respiratory regulation during postnatal development in cats and rabbits and some of its morphological substrate. Acta Physiol Scand Suppl 1968; 304:3–123.

123. Hofer MA. Lethal respiratory disturbance in neonatal rats after arterial chemoreceptor denervation. Life Sci 1984; 34:489–496.

124. Bureau MA, Lamarche J, Foulon P, Dalle D. Postnatal maturation of respiration in intact and carotid body–chemodenervated lambs. J Appl Physiol 1985; 59:869–874.

125. Carroll JL, Bureau MA. Peripheral chemoreceptor CO$_2$ response during hyperoxia in the 14-day-old awake lamb. Respir Physiol 1988; 73:339–350.

126. Donnelly DF, Haddad GG. Prolonged apnea and impaired survival in piglets after sinus and aortic nerve section. J Appl Physiol 1990; 68:1048–1052.

127. Cote A, Porras H, Meehan B. Age-dependent vulnerability to carotid chemodenervation in piglets. J Appl Physiol 1996; 80:323–331.

128. Forster HV, Pan LG, Lowry TF, Serra A, Wenninger J. Martino P. Important role of carotid chemoreceptor afferents in control of breathing of adult and neonatal mammals. Respir Physiol 2000; 119:189–208.

129. Lowry TF, Forster HV, Pan LG, Korducki MA, Probst J, Franciosi RA, Forster MM. The effect on breathing of carotid body denervation in neonatal goats. J Appl Physiol 1999; 87:1026–1034.

130. Neubauer JA, Melton JE, Edelman NH. Regulation of respiration during brain hypoxia. J Appl Physiol 1990; 68:441–451.

131. Blanco CE, Hanson MA, Johnson P, Rigatto H. Breathing pattern of kittens during hypoxia. J Appl Physiol 1984; 56:12–17.
132. Marchal F, Bairam A, Haouzi P, Crance JP, Di Giulio C, Vert P, Lahiri S. Carotid chemoreceptor response to natural stimuli in the newborn kitten. Respir Physiol 1992; 87:183–193.
133. Martin-Body RL, Robson GJ, Sinclair JD. Restoration of hypoxic responses in the awake rat after carotid body denervation by sinus nerve section. J Physiol 1986; 380:61–73.
134. Daly M, Ungar A. Comparison of the reflex responses elicited by stimulation of the separately perfused carotid and aortic body chemoreceptors in the dog. J Physiol 1966; 182:379–403.
135. Lahiri S, Mokaski A, Mulligan E, Nishino T. Comparison of aortic and carotid chemoreceptor responses to hypercapnia and hypoxia. J Appl Physiol 1981; 51:55–61.
136. Bisgard GE, Buss DD, Forster HV, Orr JA, Rasmussen B, Rawlings CA. Hypoventilation in ponies after carotid body denervation. J Appl Physiol 1976; 40:184–190.
137. Bisgard GE, Forster HV, Klein JP. Recovery of peripheral chemoreceptor function following denervation in ponies. J Appl Physiol 1980; 49:964–970.
138. Donnelly DF, Haddad GG. Prolonged apnea and impaired survival in piglets after sinus and aortic nerve section. J Appl Physiol 1990; 68:1048–1052.
139. Lowry TF, Forster HV, Pan LG, Serra A, Wenninger J, Nash R, Sheridan D, Franciosi RA. The effects on breathing of carotid body denervation in neonatal piglets. J Appl Physiol 1996; 87:2128–2135.
140. Sorensen SC, Severinghaus JW. Respiratory insensitivity to acute hypoxia persisting after correction of Tetralogy of Fallot. J Appl Physiol 1968; 25:221–223.
141. Hanson MA, Kumar P, Williams BA. The effect of chronic hypoxia upon the development of respiratory chemoreflexes in the newborn kitten. J Physiol 1989; 411:563–574.
142. Severinghaus JW. Hypoxic respiratory drive and its loss during chronic hypoxia. Clin Physiol 1972; 2:57–79.
143. Eden GJ, Hanson MA. Effects of chronic hypoxia from birth on the ventilatory response to acute hypoxia in the newborn rat. J Physiol 1987; 392:11–19.
144. Tenney SM, Ou LC. Hypoxic ventilatory response of cats at high altitude: an interpretation of 'blunting.' Respir Physiol 1977; 30:185–199.
145. Ling L, Olsen, EB Jr, Vidnik EH, Mitchell GS. Attenuation of the hypoxic ventilatory response in adult rats following one month of perinatal hyperoxia. J Physiol (Lond) 1996; 495:561–571.
146. Okubu S, Mortola JP. Long term respiratory effects of neonatal hypoxia in the rat. J Appl Physiol 1988; 64:952–958.
147. Matsuoka T, Yoda T, Ushikubo S, Matsusawa S, Sasano J, Komiyama A. Repeated acute hypoxia temporarily attenuates the ventilatory response to hypoxia in conscious newborn rats. Pediatr Res 1999; 46:120–125.
148. Sladek M, Parker RA, Grogaard JB, Sundell HW. Long-lasting effect of prolonged hypoxemia after birth on the immediate ventilatory response to changes in arterial partial pressure of oxygen in young lambs. Pediatr Res 1993; 34:821–828.

149. Wach RA, Bee D, Barer GR. Dopamine and ventilatory effects of hypoxia and almitrine in chronically hypoxic rats. J Appl Physiol 1989; 67:186–192.
150. Eden GJ, Hanson MA. Effects of chronic hypoxia from birth on the ventilatory response to acute hypoxia in the newborn rat. J Physiol 1987; 392:11–19.
151. Edwards C, Heath D, Harris P, Castillo Y, Kruger H, Ares-Stella J. The carotid body in animals at high altitude. J Pathol 1971; 104:231–238.
152. Pequignot JM, Cattet-Emard JM, Dalmaz Y, Peyrier L. Dopamine and norepinephrine dynamics in rats carotid body during long-term hypoxia. J Auton Nerv Syst 1987; 21:9–14.
153. Olson EB, Vidnik EH, McCrimmon DR, Dempsey JA. Monoamine neurotransmitter metabolism during acclimatization to hypoxia in rats. Respir Physiol 1983; 54:79–96.
154. Hanson MA, Kumar P, Williams BA. The effect of chronic hypoxia upon the development of respiratory chemoreflexes in the newborn kitten. J Physiol 1989; 411:563–574.
155. Hertzberg T, Hellstrom S, Holgert H, Lagercrantz H, Pequignot JM. Ventilatory response to hyperoxia in newborn rats born in hypoxia—possible relationship to carotid body dopamine. J Physiol 1992; 456:645–654.
156. Iturriaga R, Larrain C, Zapata P. Effects of dopaminergic blockade upon carotid chemosensory activity and its hypoxia induced excitation. Brain Res 1994; 663:145–154.
157. Tatsumi K, Pickett C, Weil JV. Decreased carotid body sensitivity in chronic hypoxia: role of dopamine. Respir Physiol 1995; 101:47–57.
158. Wyatt CN, Wright C, Bee D, Peers C. O_2 sensitive K^+ currents in carotid body chemoreceptor cells from normoxic and chronically hypoxic rats and their roles in hypoxic chemotransduction. Proc Natl Acad Sci USA 1995; 92:295–299.
159. Perrin DG, Cutz E, Becker LE, Bryan AC. Ultrastructure of carotid bodies in sudden infant death syndrome. Pediatrics 1984; 73:646–651.
160. Perrin DG, Becker LE, Madapallimatum A, Cutz E, Bryan AC, Sola MJ. Sudden infant death syndrome: increased carotid-body dopamine and nonadrenaline content. Lancet 1984; 2(8402):535–537.
161. Lick EE, Pérez-Atayde AR, Young JB. Carotid body in the sudden infant death syndrome: a combined light microscopic, ultrastructural and biochemical study. Pediatr Pathol 1986; 6:335–350.
162. Eden GJ, Hanson MA. Effects of hypoxia from birth on the carotid chemoreceptor and ventilatory responses of rats to acute hypoxia. J Physiol 1986; 374:24–35.
163. Hanson MA, Eden GJ, Nijhuis JG, Moore PJ. Peripheral chemoreceptors and other oxygen sensors in the fetus and newborn. In: Lahiri S, Forster RE, Davies RO, Pack AI, eds. Chemoreceptors and Reflexes in Breathing: Cellular and Molecular Aspects. New York: Oxford University Press, 1989:113–120.
164. Ling L, Olson EB, Vidnik EH, Mitchell GS. Attenuation of the hypoxic ventilatory response in adult rats following one month of perinatal hyperoxia. J Physiol 1996; 495:561–571.
165. Ling L, Olson EB, Vidnik EH, Mitchell GS. Integrated phrenic responses to carotid afferent stimulation in adult rats following perinatal hyperoxia. J Physiol 1997; 500:787–796.

166. Ling L, Olson EB, Vidnik EH, Mitchell GS. Slow recovery of impaired phrenic responses to hypoxia following perinatal hyperoxia in rats. J Physiol 1998; 511:599–603.

167. Erickson JT, Mauzer C, Jana A, Ling L, Olson EB, Vidnik EH, Mitchell GS, Katz DM. Chemoafferent degeneration and carotid body hypoplasia following chronic hyperoxia in newborn rats. J Physiol 1998; 509:519–526.

168. Dimaguila MAVT, DiFiore JM, Martin RJ, Miller MJ. Characteristics of hypoxemic episodes in very low birthweight infants on ventilatory support. J Pediatr 1997; 130:577–583.

169. Bolivar JM, Gerhardt T, González A. Mechanisms for episodes of hypoxemia in preterm infants undergoing mechanical ventilation. J Pediatr 1995; 127:767–773.

170. Calder NA, Williams BA, Smyth J, Boon AW, Kumar P, Hanson MA. Absence of ventilatory responses to alternating breaths of mild hypoxia and air in infants who have had bronchopulmonary dysplasia: implications for the risk of sudden infant death. Pediatr Res 1995; 35:677–681.

171. Katz-Salamon M, Lagercrantz H. Hypoxic ventilatory defense in very preterm infants: attenuation after long term oxygen treatment. Arch Dis Child 1994; 70:F90-F95.

172. Katz-Salamon M, Johnsson B, Lagercrantz H. Blunted peripheral chemoreceptor response to hyperoxia in a group of infants with bronchopulmonary dysplasia. Pediatr Pulmonol 1995; 20:101–106.

173. Ramanathan R, Corwin MJ, Hunt CE, Lister G, Tinsley LR, Baird T, Silvestri JM, Crowell DH, Martin RJ, Neuman MR, Weese-Mayer DE, Cupples LA, Peucker M, Willinger M, Keens TG. Cardiorespiratory events recorded on home monitors; comparison of healthy infants with those at increased risk for SIDS. JAMA 2001; 2199–2207.

174. DiFiore JM, Arko M, Miller MJ, Krauss A, Betkerur A, Zadell A, Kenney S, Martin RJ. Cardiorespiratory events in preterm infants referred for apnea monitoring studies. Pediatrics 1991; 108:1304–1308.

175. Peers C, Buckler KJ. Transduction of chemostimuli by the type I carotid body cell. J Membr Biol 1995; 144:1–9.

5

Upper-Airway Muscle Control During Development

Application to Clinical Disorders That Occur in Premature Infants

ESTELLE B. GAUDA

The Johns Hopkins University
Baltimore, Maryland, U.S.A.

I. Introduction

The challenges of the newborn infant are to breast or bottle feed, breathe, protect the lower airway, and cry. However, to effectively accomplish these goals, coordination among upper-airway muscles and coordination between upper-airway muscles and the diaphragm and chest wall muscles must occur. One critical function of the upper-airway muscles is to dilate or stiffen the upper airway when the greatest negative pressure is generated by contraction of the diaphragm and chest wall muscles during inspiration. This coordinated function between upper-airway muscles and chest wall muscles allows unobstructed breathing to occur.

The upper airway includes the nose, pharynx, larynx, and extrathoracic trachea. Approximately 30 pairs of muscles are involved in modulation of the diameter and function of the upper airway. Some of these muscles are listed in Table 1. The activity of these muscles is modulated by cortical inputs, state (sleep or wakefulness), and mechanoreceptor and chemoreceptor influences. Upper-airway closure during sleep is the hallmark of obstructive sleep apnea that occurs in infants, children, and adults, which can lead to respiratory and cardiovascular

Table 1 Regions of the Upper Airway and Corresponding
Muscles

Upper airway region	Muscles
Nose	Alae Nasi
Pharynx	
Nasopharynx	Palatoglossus
	Palatopharyngeal
	Tensor veli palatini
	Levator veli palatini
Oropharynx	Genioglossus
Hypopharynx	Suprahyoid
	Geniohyoid
	Mylohyoid
	Infrahyoid
	Sternohyoid
	Thyrohyoid
	Omohyoid
Larynx	Intrinsic
	PCA
	TA
	Lateral CA
	Interarytenoid
	Extrinsic
	Stylohyoid
	Geniohyoid
	Digastric (anterior and posterior)
	Mylohyoid

morbidities (1,2). However, discoordinate control of upper airway muscles is
frequent during early postnatal development. Premature infants have decreased
respiratory drive resulting in central, mixed, and obstructive apnea (3). They are
also at increased risk for aspiration during feeding (4). However, breathing and
feeding disorders both improve with postnatal maturation. There are multiple
intrinsic and extrinsic factors that modulate upper-airway function, that change
during development. The influences of these factors on upper-airway function
during maturation can account for improved coordination of upper-airway
muscles, resulting in unobstructed breathing, phonation, adequate feeding, and
normal growth and development. This chapter will review the intrinsic and
extrinsic factors that are most responsible for the developmental improvement in

function of the upper airway during postnatal maturation, with an emphasis on neural control mechanisms.

This review will be weighted heavily toward regulation of pharyngeal and laryngeal muscles during postnatal development for three reasons: [1] obstruction of the upper airway most frequently occurs at the pharynx and larynx; [2] dysfunction of the upper airway usually involves neural mechanisms that modulate the activity of pharyngeal and laryngeal muscles; and [3] regulation of the nerves and muscles that control the patency of these upper-airway structures has been studied in great detail. Because the ability to breathe and feed improves naturally with postnatal maturation in human infants, the premature infant is the natural subject in which to study maturation of mechanisms that regulate upper-airway function. Thus, clinical entities that are known to occur in premature infants related to dysfunction of the upper airway will be described followed by evidence from studies in human infants and neonatal animals that reveal possible mechanisms responsible for the clinical finding. Studies performed in adult humans and mature animals will be presented when appropriate for comparison.

II. Apnea in Premature Infants: Incidence and Characterization

Irregular respiration is common and is the hallmark of breathing in premature infants (3,5). This respiratory pattern is characterized by short and long periods of apnea, defined as cessation of airflow. While short apneas are quite common and may occur without clinical consequence, more prolonged apnea with duration of > 20 sec may be associated with bradycardia and oxygen desaturation, requiring intervention (6). Apneic and bradycardic events can be associated with cyclic changes in cerebral perfusion as measured by Doppler flow velocities in premature infants (7), and cerebral desaturation with subsequent reoxygenation measured by near infrared spectroscopy in term infants (8). Thus, prolonged apneic events may place the infant at increased risk for hypoxic ischemic reperfusion injury of the central nervous system. Prolonged apnea occurs in virtually all premature infants < 28 weeks postconceptional age, in 50% of infants at 30–32 weeks, and in < 7% of infants at 34–35 weeks (5). The postnatal age at which the last apneic episode may be detected decreases exponentially with increasing postconceptional age (9). While apnea of prematurity usually resolves by 34–37 weeks postconceptional age, apnea frequently persists beyond term in the most immature infants, those born at 24–28 weeks (10).

Three types of prolonged apnea have been described: central, obstructive, and mixed. Central apnea is characterized by the absence of diaphragmatic activity; obstructive apnea is characterized by upper-airway obstruction with persistent diaphragmatic activity; mixed apnea has features of both central and obstructive apneas. Central and mixed are the most common types of apnea that occur in premature infants (6). While it was commonly believed that central apnea was not associated with upper-airway obstruction, newer techniques (amplified cardiac oscillation method) has shown that 13% of central apneas that occur in premature infants are associated with airway closure, as described by Idiong et al. (11). Furthermore, 87% of mixed apneas were associated with a patent airway at the onset of the apnea with subsequent closure (11). Lastly, during the apneic phase of periodic breathing, pharyngeal obstruction occurs in premature infants (12). While the negative pressure generated by the chest wall muscles and diaphragmatic activity during inspiration may place the upper airway at increased risk for collapse (13,14), inspiratory effort is not necessary for upper airway obstruction to occur in individuals with disordered breathing during sleep. There is considerable evidence that upper-airway closure occurs in premature infants (outlined above) and adults during central apnea (15), suggesting that sustained central drive to both the upper-airway muscles and chest wall muscles is key for stable respiration to occur. Central drive to both these groups of muscles is significantly depressed during sleep accounting for the increased frequency of apnea during sleep (16,17).

All types of apnea and periodic breathing occur during sleep. Apnea with upper-airway obstruction occurs more often during active, REM, or indeterminate sleep (18–21). Premature infants are asleep 80% of the time, and 70% of their sleep time is in active or indeterminate sleep (22,23). Thus, airway obstruction is a common event that occurs during apnea in premature infants. With increasing maturation, the duration of the apneic events becomes shorter and the events are less likely to be associated with upper-airway obstruction (24).

III. Pharynx: A Site of Upper-Airway Obstruction and the Role of Pharyngeal Dilator Muscles in Apnea

The pharynx is a collapsible tube in a rigid chamber and has characteristics similar to a Starling resistor, as described by Smith et al. (25). The balance of upstream resistance (nasal pressure), downstream pressure (thoracic pressure), and transmural pressure determines whether the pharynx is patent, narrowed, or collapsed. Transmural pressure is determined by the difference between intraluminal and tissue pressure. Intraluminal pressure is the lateral wall pressure that acts on the luminal surface of the tube, while tissue pressure acts on the outside of the collapsible tube. Surface-adhesive factors contribute significantly to intraluminal pressure while activity of the upper-airway muscles contributes significantly to tissue pressure. The pharyngeal muscles are divided into dilators and constrictors, as listed in Table 1. The most commonly studied pharyngeal muscle is the genioglossus muscle. This muscle is located beneath the tongue and functions to protrude the tongue. Activation of the genioglossus muscle increases the pharyngeal diameter in infants, children, and adults. In addition, this muscle has phasic activity that is coincident with inspiration. Since the genioglossus is easily accessible and modulates upper-airway patency, this muscle has become the representative pharyngeal dilator muscle of the upper airway. Because of its location, the activity of genioglossus muscle has been measured noninvasively with submental (26) and sublingual (27,28) surface electromyograms (EMG) in infants. Thus, studies determining how this muscle is controlled have contributed considerably to our understanding of control of upper-airway dilator muscles during development.

IV. Brainstem Neuronal Network Responsible for Respiratory Rhythmogenesis

Respiratory rhythmogenesis has been the focus of several excellent recent reviews (29,30). A brief discussion and a schematic of the network responsible for rhythmic respiration are presented, followed by how this network is involved in controlling major upper-airway muscles during development. In addition, factors such as sleep state and afferent inputs from activation of peripheral receptors that are important modulators of respiratory rhythm and thus activity of upper airway muscles during respiration will be discussed.

As outlined in the schematic (Fig. 1), respiratory rhythm is generated by a network of neurons in the brainstem. A group of cells in the rostral ventral lateral medulla form the pre-Bötzinger complex and are essential to the network. These cells exhibit bursting pacemaker properties and are believed to be the "kernel" responsible for the generation of respiratory rhythm (29–33). Experiments show that lesioning and blocking the activity of this group of cells abolishes respiratory rhythm and gives strong support to this model of respiratory rhythm generation (34–36). In the cat, pre-Bötzinger neurons synapse on two main groups of respiratory-related neurons that form the ventral respiratory group (VRG) and the dorsal respiratory group (DRG) located in the ventrolateral medulla and the nucleus tractus solatari (nTS), respectively (37). Neurons from the VRG and DRG form synapses with the phrenic motoneuron pool that innervates the diaphragm (38). In the newborn rat, only the VRG, in contrast to both the VRG and DRG, appears to be essential for respiratory rhythmogenesis (39). A small percentage of respiratory-related neurons in the VRG send axonal projections to hypoglossal motoneurons (40). Although the pre-Bötzinger complex drives the activity of the respiratory-related neurons that innervate the muscles of respiration, activity of the neurons in the pre-Bötzinger complex can also be modulated by synaptic inputs from the nTS (37) (Fig. 1).

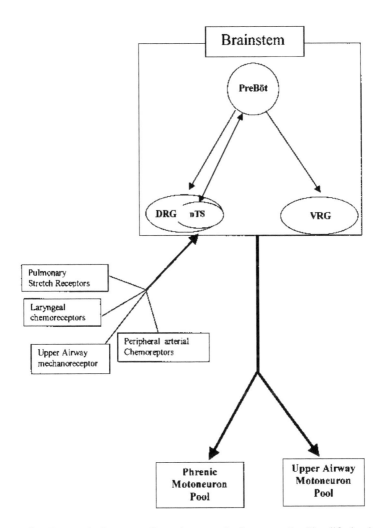

Figure 1 Neuronal elements of respiratory rhythmogenesis. Simplified schematic outlining the elements of the network in the brainstem that are essential for respiratory rhythmogenesis and the peripheral afferent inputs (integrated in the nTS) that modulate the output to the motoneuron pools that control upper airway muscles and diaphragm activity. See text for discussion. PreBöt, pre-Bötzinger complex; nTS, nucleus tractus solitari; DRG, dorsal respiratory group; VRG, ventral respiratory group.

Integration of peripheral inputs is a key feature responsible for modulating the respiratory network; information from activation or inhibition of sensory fibers in the upper airway, the lung, and peripheral arterial chemoreceptors (to be described below) is integrated and processed in the nTS (Fig. 1). Thus, the nTS is commonly known as a relay station for afferent influences that modulate respiration (41–43). Axons from key neuronal groups that regulate sleep and wakefulness also synapse directly onto motoneurons that control the activity of upper-airway muscles (44) and the diaphragm (45). Central and peripheral influences may indirectly modulate upper-airway muscles and the diaphragm via axonal projections from the nTS that synapse on to hypoglossal and phrenic motoneuron pools (44,45) (Fig. 1). Other, additional neuronal groups regulating hypoglossal and motoneuron pools are those that control sleep and wakefulness. Two major neuronal groups that control sleep and wakefulness that will be discussed are the dorsal caudal raphe in the medulla (46,47) and the locus coeruleus in the pons (48,49).

In review, the key neuronal circuits that control activity of the muscles of respiration include [1] the pre-Bötzinger complex (kernel of respiratory rhythm); [2] the nTS (relay station for peripheral inputs); [3] motoneuron pools for neurons that innervate the upper-airway muscles (specifically, hypoglossal) and diaphragm (phrenic motoneuron pool); [4] nonrespiratory, central neuronal groups (caudal raphe and locus coeruleus) that tonically excite hypoglossal motoneurons during wakefulness; and [5] peripheral circuits that send sensory information to the nTS. It should be apparent from this simplified sketch of a complex system that development can affect many parts of the network. The focus of the subsequent discussion will be on features of neurons that make up the motoneuron pools that control the upper-airway muscles, and how sleep and afferent input from the periphery affects the activity of these muscles during early postnatal development.

V. Hypoglossal Motoneurons During Postnatal Development

A. Changes in Intrinsic Properties

Motoneuron activity patterns are frequently matched to the muscle fibers they innervate. Thus, understanding the effect of development on firing properties of the hypoglossal motoneurons is directly relevant to genioglossal muscle function. With postnatal development in the newborn rat, the cell bodies of hypoglossal motoneurons undergo extensive remodeling, and change their electrophysiological properties. Specifically, remodeling of dendritic arborization of the hypoglossal motoneuron and proliferation and distribution of K^+ channels across the entire membrane of the motoneuron occurs with postnatal maturation

(50–52). As a result of these changes, the intrinsic electrical properties of hypoglossal motoneurons and the effect of synaptic inputs on the firing properties of these neurons change. Contrary to what might be expected, patch-clamp studies in isolated hypoglossal motoneurons from neonatal and adult rats show a decrease in cell excitability to depolarizing stimuli with maturation (53). Another important feature of these hypoglossal motoneurons is the ability to hyperpolarize after depolarizing stimuli—known as "after-hyperpolarization potential" (AHP).

Classic studies performed on other motoneurons and other cells have shown that the AHP following the action potential is an important determinant of repetitive firing behavior of the neuron (54). The duration of the AHP decreases and the amplitude of the AHP are smaller in hypoglossal motoneurons from adults than the AHP amplitude of the neonatal animals (53). A reduction in AHP amplitude allows faster firing and thereby contributes to enhanced excitability of the hypoglossal motoneurons from adult animals and less excitability in hypoglossal motoneurons from immature animals. The intrinsic electrical properties of the hypoglossal motoneurons are further modulated by neurotransmitters binding to excitatory neurotransmitter receptors on these neurons.

B. Changes in Neurotransmitter Receptor Expression

Similar to most other central neuronal circuits, glutamate is the major excitatory neurotransmitter that mediates the inspiratory activity of hypoglossal motoneurons by binding to N-methyl-D-aspartate (NMDA) and non-NMDA receptors (55,56). Thyrotropin-releasing hormone (TRH), serotonin (5HT), and norepinephrine (NE) are three other neuromodulators that significantly augment hypoglossal activity (for review see 57). The level of these neuromodulators in specific brainstem regions (caudal raphe and locus coeruleus nucleus) determines sleep-wake cycles (46–49). Furthermore, the level of these excitatory neuromodulators at the upper-airway motoneuron synapse determines the level of tone of the upper-airway muscles. As outlined above and shown in Figure 2, axons from the caudal raphe (the source of TRH and 5HT) and the locus coeruleus (the source of NE) synapse on hypoglossal motoneurons. TRH, 5HT, and NE all excite hypoglossal motoneurons in rats and mice during wakefulness (for review see 57, 58). However, this excitatory response is developmentally regulated (59).

TRH and NE Effects on Hypoglossal Motoneurons During Development

Absence of TRH receptor and TRH receptor binding on hypoglossal motoneurons in neonatal animals during the first week of postnatal life may account for the difference in hypoglossal motoneuron excitability to TRH during postnatal development (60,61). TRH protein binding significantly increases, reaching adult levels by 2 weeks postnatal age (60). Concurrent with these findings,

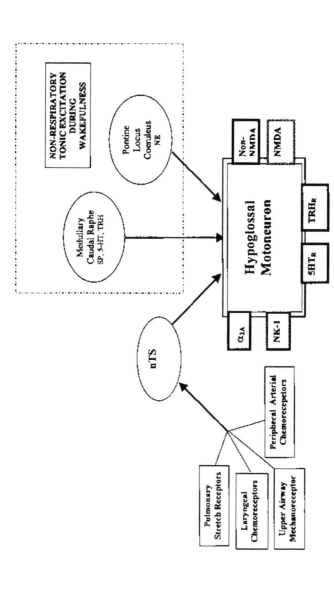

Figure 2 **Modulation of hypoglossal motoneurons during wakefulness.** Simplified schematic depicting pontine-medullary nuclei that activate hypoglossal motoneurons during wakefulness, releasing specific neuromodulators that bind to corresponding receptors on hypoglossal motoneurons. Reduction in SP, 5HT, and TRH and NE from these pontine-medullary nuclei occurs during active REM sleep, resulting in decreased activation of hypoglossal motoneurons. Peripheral afferent inputs are integrated in the nTS, and axonal projections from the nTS synapse onto hypoglossal neurons during wakefulness and sleep. SP, substance P; 5HT, serotonin; TRH, thyrotropin releasing hormone; NE, norepinephrine. The small boxes surrounding the hypoglossal motoneuron represent neuromodulator and neurotransmitter receptors: (α_{2A})-adrenergic receptor for NE, non-NMDA, and NMDA receptors for glutamate; $5HT_R$ for serotonin receptors and NK-1; neurokinin receptor for SP; TRH_R for TRH receptor.

depolarization of hypoglossal motoneurons to exogenously applied TRH achieves an adult response (for review see 62). In contrast, NE depolarizes hypoglossal motoneurons and potentiates inspiratory related hypoglossal nerve activity in brain slices from animals at birth (61). This potentiating effect of NE on inspiratory activity of hypoglossal nerve continues to increase during the first 2 weeks of postnatal life in newborn mice and at birth in rats (59,61). The responsible α_1-adrenergic receptor subtype is most likely α_{1B} as suggested by Volgin et al. (63).

5HT Effects on Hypoglossal Motoneurons During Development

Although intrinsic properties of the neonatal hypoglossal motoneurons cause an increase in AHP resulting in less capacity of the motoneurons for repetitive firing, application of 5HT significantly inhibits AHP (64). By inhibiting AHP, repetitive firing capacity of neonatal hypoglossal motoneuron increases (62,64). This effect on AHP is unique to neonatal hypoglossal motoneurons secondary to the presence of $5HT_{1A}$ receptor on these motoneurons (62,64). $5HT_{1A}$ receptors expression and receptor binding in hypoglossal motoneurons significantly decreases with postnatal maturation (62). $5HT_{1B}$, $-_{2A}$ and $-_{2C}$ are the predominant serotonin receptors detected in the adult hypoglossal motoneurons (65). Binding of 5HT to these receptors does not change AHP in adult neurons (64). Since neonatal hypoglossal motoneurons appear to be dependent on 5HT for repetitive firing capacity, any reduction of 5HT makes the infant's upper airway more susceptible to collapse—events that occur most often during sleep.

VI. Upper-Airway Muscle Atonia During Sleep: Role of TRH, NE, and 5HT

Apnea associated with upper-airway obstruction occurs during sleep with most apneic events occurring during active sleep or REM sleep (18–21). As outlined above, TRH, NE, 5HT, and substance P (SP) are neuromodulators that sustain the activity of upper-airway dilating muscles during wakefulness (57) (Fig. 2). While the caudal raphe is the source of TRH, 5HT, and SP, axonal projections from the locus coeruleus and surrounding pontine tegmentum are the sources of NE which synapse on respiratory-related DRG and VRG neurons, and hypoglossal moto-neurons (66). Although these NE axonal projections to hypoglossal motoneurons are present early in life, there is a substantial increase in NE innervation during the first 180 days of postnatal life in the rat (66). Thus, even during wakefulness, the newborn has less excitatory NE innervation to the hypoglossal motoneurons than adults.

In review, active and REM sleep is associated with a complete suppression of muscle tone in the postural muscles and a reduction of muscle tone in the respiratory related muscles such as the genioglossus and other muscles modulating upper-airway diameter. This muscle hypotonia is secondary to reduced TRH, 5HT, and NE levels in the region of the upper-airway motoneurons. Since in immature animals there are [1] reduced excitatory NE innervation to hypoglossal motoneurons, [2] presence of $5HT_{1A}$ receptors on neonatal hypoglossal motoneurons which improve the repetitive firing capabilities of the motoneuron, and [3] absence of excitatory TRH receptors, reduction in 5HT, TRH, and NE that occurs naturally during active sleep makes the newborn infant particularly vulnerable to upper-airway obstruction during sleep. Thus, it is no surprise that the premature infant should have increased incidence of apnea associated with upper-airway obstruction, which improves with maturation.

However, there are a subset of premature and term infants that have a greater incidence of apnea with and without upper-airway obstruction that persists longer than it does in other infants at the same postconceptual ages (10). These infants are at increased risk for morbidity and mortality from sudden death (67). Advances in neonatal care have allowed infants born at little more than 1/2 of gestation (23–25 weeks) to survive. Ex utero exposure to therapeutic agents may modify the development of peripheral sensory inputs that modulate respiratory rhythm and upper-airway control during sleep.

VII. Infants with BPD Have Increased Frequency of Apnea: Possible Mechanisms

Several intriguing observations related to upper-airway obstruction and apnea in premature infants have been reported. Infants born at the lowest gestation (< 26 weeks) gestation have a greater incidence of apnea that persists after term gestation (10), and infants with chronic lung disease are more likely to have apnea associated with upper-airway obstruction than control premature infants (68). Alterations in two important peripheral inputs modulating upper-airway function might help explain these clinical observations. Peripheral inputs that are integral to upper-airway muscle control, mechanoreceptor and peripheral arterial chemoreceptors, are likely to be altered in premature infants and infants with chronic lung disease.

A. Effects and Alterations in Upper-Airway Mechanoreceptors on Upper-Airway Muscle Activation

As represented in the schematics in Figures 1 and 2, mechanical and sensory stimuli in the nose and upper airway modulate upper-airway muscle activity. These sensory fibers are contained in the pharyngeal branch of the glossopharyngeal nerve (69); mechanical stimulation with negative and positive pressure in the pharynx increases and decreases genioglossus EMG activity, respectively, in adult animals (70) and young cats (71). Similarly, sensory fibers of the ethmoidal nerve that innervates the nose are involved in pressure sensation (72), and negative pressure applied to the nose also activates the genioglossus muscle (73,74) and modulates respiratory-related neurons in the nTS (75). As shown in Figure 1, nTS axonal projections synapse on hypoglossal and phrenic motoneurons (44,45).

Application of negative pressure to the nose is frequently done in humans to characterize afferent inputs that modify upper-airway muscle activation (76). In adult humans, negative pressure applied at the nose causes reflex activation of the genioglossus muscle, and topical anesthesia to the nasopharynx abolishes this response (76). Furthermore, sleep has an inhibitory influence on the reflex response of the genioglossus EMG to upper-airway negative pressure in normal adults (77).

Instead of negative pressure applied to the nose, nasal occlusion at end expiration is the preferred technique to determine the effect of upper-airway negative pressure on upper-airway muscle responses in unsedated human infants (26–28,76–79). The effects of nasal occlusion at end expiration on subsequent occluded inspiratory efforts are [1] removal of inhibitory influence of increased lung volume (pulmonary stretch receptors) on activity of upper airway muscles and nerves (80,81), [2] activation of negative pressure receptors in the upper airway, and [3] activation of peripheral arterial chemoreceptors as hypercapnia and hypoxemia develop during the occlusion (71,82). Thus, nasal occlusion does not separate the influence of lung volume, upper-airway negative pressure, and increasing chemoreceptor drive on the reflex response of the upper-airway muscles associated with each occluded effort. Nevertheless, assessing the effect of nasal airway occlusion at end expiration on the activity of the genioglossus EMG associated with the first occluded breath is generally believed to be mediated by upper-airway and pulmonary stretch mechanoreceptors. Zhang et al. also found peak genioglossus EMG activity to be greater in response to upper-airway negative pressure after blockade of pulmonary stretch receptors from the lung (81). Thus, end-expiratory occlusion is performed to remove the influence of lung volume on the response of upper-airway muscles to upper-airway negative pressure.

Nasal occlusion has been shown to significantly increase genioglossus EMG activity with the first occluded effort in micrognathic infants during sleep (14). We determined that in premature infants, genioglossus EMG activity is frequently absent during normal breathing; however, it could be induced by experimentally induced nasal occlusion (27,28). The percent of experimentally induced occlusions associated with genioglossus EMG, however, was significantly less in premature infants with apnea than in infants without apnea (28). We attributed this finding to a decrease in central respiratory drive in infants with apnea associated with upper-airway obstruction. A similar finding has also been described by Wulbrand et al., who described a concurrent decrease in submental (representing genioglossus EMG) and diaphragmatic EMG associated with apnea in premature infants (83).

It is difficult to separate the multiple effects of mechanoreceptor and chemoreceptor activity on respiratory muscle responses when upper-airway negative pressure is applied or end-expiratory airway occlusion is performed. However, separation of these multiple afferent inputs on the output of upper-airway dilating muscles can be done in experimental animals by isolating the upper airways from the lungs. We measured the response of the genioglossus and diaphragmatic EMG to [1] negative pressure applied to the isolated upper airway during normoxia and hypercapnia, [2] end-expiratory tracheal occlusion, and [3] the application of upper-airway negative pressure combined with tracheal occlusion in spontaneously breathing tracheotomized, anesthetized cats (71). We found that feedback from phasic pulmonary stretch receptors was a potent inhibitor of reflex activation of the genioglossus muscle in response to negative pressure applied to the upper airway, which can be overridden by an increase in chemoreceptor drive (hypercapnia) (71). A similar finding has recently been described in adult rats. Bailey et al. reported that hypercapnia can override lung volume–mediated inhibition on activation of genioglossus muscles in the adult rat (84). Thus, activation of the upper airway dilating muscles during obstructive sleep apnea is predicated on the activation of sensory receptors within the upper airway and concurrent increase in chemoreceptor drive.

Alterations in the sensitivity of receptors within the upper airway or decreased hypoxic or hypercapnic sensitivity may prolong apneic events. Frequent and prolonged apneic events occur in infants who are born at the youngest gestation and those who develop chronic lung disease. The most immature premature infants are intubated for extended periods of time during early postnatal development. Chronic intubation may have local effects on sensory innervation to the upper airway. Mechanical compression of the sensory fibers innervating the upper airway as a result of chronic intubation during critical stages of development may, in part, contribute the clinical observation that increased upper-airway obstruction during apnea occurs in infants with bronchopulmonary dysplasia (BPD).

B. Reduced Sensitivity of Upper-Airway Receptors

The effects of chronic intubation on subsequent activation of upper-airway and genioglossus responses have not been studied. However, the effect of chronic tracheostomy on upper-airway reflexes has been described in adult animals (85). Chronic tracheostomy bypasses important receptors in the upper airway that modulate laryngeal function (for review see 86). As a result of chronic tracheostomy, alterations in central threshold and transneuronal conduction times of the superior laryngeal nerve (SLN) occur (85). These alterations may account for the increased episodes of aspiration known to occur in adult humans with tracheostomies. The SLN is the afferent limb of many of the airway protective reflexes (described below), and when stimulated causes reflex activation of upper-airway dilating muscles (described above). Chronic intubation in newborn infants may affect development of upper-airway reflexes by bypassing important upper-airway sensory receptors similar to chronic tracheotomy in adult humans and animals.

Additionally, mechanical compression of the sensory fibers in the mucosa of the upper airway may change the developmental pattern of myelination of the SLN. In the newborn kitten, 75% of the fibers of the SLN are unmyelinated during the first postnatal month and myelinated fibers increase by 50% at 6 weeks postnatal age (87). This change in myelination as a result of development is associated with differences in response to electrical stimulation of the SLN. Electrical stimulation of the SLN evoked apnea in the younger animals and evoked swallowing in the older animals (87). It would be of considerable interest to know if chronic intubation in immature animals affects the pattern of myelination and/or threshold activation of the SLN during postnatal development.

C. Effect and Alterations in Peripheral and Central Chemoreceptor Influences on Upper-Airway Muscle Activity

As previously mentioned, upper-airway motoneurons are modulated by afferent activity from peripheral and central chemoreceptors. Peripheral arterial chemoreceptors in the carotid body respond to changes in O_2 and CO_2 tension and pH, while central chemoreceptors in the medulla respond to changes in CO_2 tension and H^+ concentration. Hypoxia, hypercapnia, and acidosis increase activity, while hyperoxia, hypocapnia, and alkalosis decrease activity from peripheral arterial chemoreceptors (88). An increase in chemoreceptor drive augments the activity of upper-airway dilating muscles during wakefulness and sleep, and in response to upper-airway negative pressure. Changes in peripheral chemoreceptor drive also affects diaphragmatic and chest wall muscle activity (89,90). Of interest, though, upper-airway dilating muscles and the nerves that innervate upper-airway muscles are preferentially modulated by peripheral chemoreceptor activity in comparison to that of the diaphragm and its innervation, the phrenic nerve (89–91). Exposure to both hyperoxia and dopamine infusion silences peripheral chemoreceptor activity (88), and abolishes the phasic electrical activity from nerves that innervate upper-airway muscles (92). The sensitivity of peripheral arterial chemoreceptors and central chemoreceptors to changes in gas tension and pH increases with maturation in animals and infants (for review see 93). Thus, a diminution in chemoreceptor drive as function of immaturity places the premature infant at increased risk for apnea with and without upper-airway obstruction.

D. Reduced Hypoxic Chemosensitivity

Reduced hypoxic chemosensitivity of peripheral arterial chemoreceptors may contribute to the increase in upper airway obstruction during apnea in infants with BPD, as observed by Fajardo et al. (68). A common technique used to test chemoreceptor function in unanesthetized animals or human infant is to assess immediate changes in ventilation in response to a hypoxic or hyperoxic challenge. Since metabolism, and thus ventilation, decreases in young animals and newborn infants during exposure to hypoxia (94), exposure to hyperoxia, known as the Dejours test, is more commonly used in this population (95–98). Acute exposure to hyperoxia silences the electrical activity of the peripheral arterial chemo-receptors (88). The reduction in ventilation, in response a single breath of 100% O_2, is proportional to the contribution of peripheral arterial chemoreceptors to breathing (95). Using the Dejours test, peripheral chemoreceptor function has been tested in infants with BPD (99). In response to a hyperoxic challenge, infants with BPD had a smaller reduction in ventilation than control infants at the same postconceptional age (99), suggesting that the peripheral arterial chemo-receptors are less responsive in infants with BPD.

Further evidence that peripheral arterial chemoreceptors are important in modulating upper airway activity in premature infants is that [1] hyperoxic exposure increases apneic events associated with upper-airway obstruction (100), [2] low-flow CO_2 decreases the frequency of apnea (101), and [3] progressive hypercapnia increases the activity of upper-airway dilating muscles (102) in premature infants. In addition to activating peripheral arterial chemoreceptors, hypercapnia also stimulates central chemoreceptors and neurons in the nTS (103–106). Thus, both peripheral and central chemoreceptors modulate activity of upper-airway dilating muscles in premature infants.

In addition to the increased frequency of apnea with upper-airway obstruction found in infants with BPD, these infants also have reduced hypoxic arousal responses (107). Reduced hypoxic arousal responses also suggests that peripheral chemoreceptor function may be altered in infants with BPD. Activation of peripheral arterial chemoreceptors is key to promoting arousal mechanisms during upper-airway obstruction (108) and during rapidly developing hypoxemia in newborn lambs (109).

The mechanisms responsible for the reduction in chemoreceptor activity in infants with BPD is unknown. However, several clues may be deduced from studies done in newborn animals. Premature infants who develop BPD are exposed to high concentrations of oxygen tension at an early developmental stage (110). Exposure to increased O_2 tension during the first month of postnatal life in newborn rats abolishes peripheral arterial chemoreceptor-mediated hypoxic chemosensitivity (111,112). This deficit persists through adulthood (111,112). In addition, hyperoxic exposure in these animals reduces the number of cell bodies of chemoafferent neurons within peripheral arterial chemoreceptors that are essential for transmitting electrical signals from the peripheral arterial chemoreceptors to the brain (113). The cellular mechanisms for this reduction in chemoafferents has not been elucidated, but the finding that hypoxic chemosensitivity is abolished after perinatal hyperoxic exposure is striking, and these results have been replicated. Mitchell and coworkers have further determined that the critical window of hyperoxic exposure to abolish hypoxic chemosensitivity is within the first 2 weeks of postnatal life in the newborn rat (113a). Perhaps, then, hyperoxic exposure during maturation of hypoxic chemosensitivity in newborn infants could, theoretically, result in the persistently diminuted peripheral arterial chemoreceptor responses, thereby contributing to prolonged apnea (68) and reduced arousal responses during asphyxial apnea as reported in infants with BPD (107).

VIII.   The Larynx: A Site of Upper-Airway Obstruction During Apnea in Premature Infants

In addition to pharyngeal muscles, intrinsic laryngeal muscles have respiratory-related activity (91,114), and the larynx is a frequent site of upper-airway closure during apnea that occurs in premature infants (115,116). The position and aperture of the larynx is controlled by extrinsic and intrinsic laryngeal muscles listed in Table 1. The mechanisms modulating the respiratory-related activity of laryngeal muscles has been characterized for the intrinsic muscles of the larynx, which include the posterior cricoarytenoid (PCA), the only dilator of the vocal cords; the thyroarytenoid (TA), powerful constrictor of the vocal cords; and the lateral cricoarytenoid and interarytenoid muscles (vocal cord constrictors). PCA muscle activity is more frequently concurrent with diaphragmatic or phrenic nerve inspiratory activity than pharyngeal or alae nasi (nasal dilator) muscle activity during unstimulated breathing in animals and infants (102,117). TA constrictor activity causes glottic closure. TA muscle activity is frequently seen during phase I expiration, and it contributes to maintaining lung volume in infants (118). TA expiratory activity is an important component of airway protective reflexes, which will be discussed below.

IX.   Role of Laryngeal Receptors in Modulation of Upper-Airway Muscle Responses

A.   Laryngeal Pressure Receptors

Inspiratory and expiratory activity of the intrinsic laryngeal muscles are modulated by inputs from mechanoreceptors and chemoreceptors (central and peripheral) via the nTS. The larynx contains several types of sensory receptors that respond to mechanical and sensory changes in the upper airway (119). These mechanical stimuli can be pressure or flow in the upper airway, or contraction of upper-airway muscles (120,121). Activation of these mechanoreceptors will reflexly activate laryngeal muscles (74,121). Specifically, negative pressure in the larynx activates pharyngeal and laryngeal dilating muscles but inhibits diaphragmatic activity (74). The afferent limb of this reflex is contained within the sensory fibers of the SLN, a branch of the vagus nerve which projects to the nTS, caudal to the dorsal cochlear nucleus (122). The efferent limb of the reflex is the recurrent laryngeal and phrenic nerves with motoneuron pools in the nucleus ambiguus (NA) and spinal cord, respectively. Mechanoreceptors regulate the activity of the pharyngeal and laryngeal muscles during breathing and contribute to upper-airway function, swallowing, and feeding.

A recent study employing pseudorabies viruses to retrogradely label connected sets of neurons in a hierarchical manner showed that neurons that project to PCA arise from neurons in the ventral medulla that are extensively involved in regulation of respiratory and cardiovascular function (123). In addition, there appeared to be direct connections from the respiratory pacemaker cells (pre-Bötzinger complex) with PCA motoneurons (123). Therefore, the anatomical interconnections between laryngeal motoneurons and respiratory neurons in the brainstem support the physiological findings of significant respiratory modulation of intrinsic laryngeal muscles.

B. Laryngeal Chemoreceptors

Sensory fibers in the larynx, which innervate "taste buds" on the epiglottis, are activated by fluids with low chloride content (124,125). In response to water in the larynx, a potent airway protective reflex, laryngeal chemoreflex (LCR), is elicited to prevent inadvertent aspiration (126,127). The physiological components of the laryngeal chemoreflex include swallowing, central reflex apnea or hypoventilation, bradycardia, and hypertension. The laryngeal chemoreflex is strongest during early postnatal development in mammalian species, and has been associated with life-threatening apnea and bradycardia in the youngest animals (128–131).

Anatomical Circuitry: Bradycardia Associated with LCR

Similar to the reflex arc of mechanoreceptor stimulation in the upper airway, the afferent limb of the laryngeal chemoreflex is contained in the sensory fibers of the SLN, which synapses in the nTS and nucleus ambiguus (NA). Axonal projections from the nTS synapse onto recurrent laryngeal motoneurons (RLN) in the NA and phrenic neuron pool in the spinal cord. Sensory fibers from the SLN also synapse onto preganglionic cardiac vagal nerves in the NA, as shown in Figure 3. Identification of SLN and cardiac vagal neurons with fluorescent dyes has

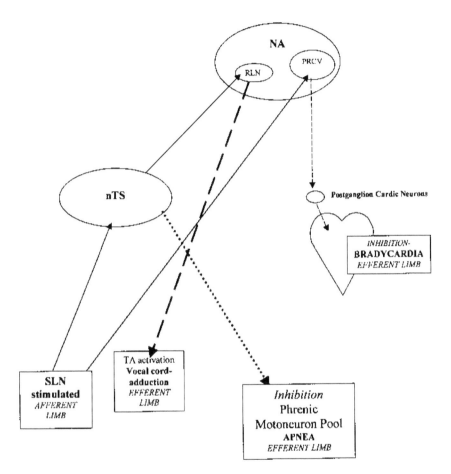

Figure 3 Neural circuitry for the laryngeal chemoreflex. The LCR occurs when
sensory fibers are stimulated in the SLN. These afferent fibers synapse on cell bodies in the
nTS which send axonal projections to the cell bodies of the recurrent laryngeal nerve
(RLN) in the nucleus ambiguus (NA) and phrenic motoneuron pool in the spinal cord.
SLN fibers also synapse on preganglionic cardiac vagal with cell bodies in the NA. Axonal
projections from the preganglionic vagal afferents synapse on preganglionic cardiac
neurons with cell bodies in the right atrium and vena cava. Stimulation of sensory fibers
of the SLN involved in the LCR results in apnea with and without vocal cord closure (TA
activation), apnea, and bradycardia. PRCV, preganglionic cardiac vagal cell bodies; RLN,
recurrent laryngeal nerve motoneurons; NA, nucleus ambiguus; TA, thyroarytenoid
muscle.

allowed for more complete characterization of synaptic inputs between these neuronal groups. Mendelowitz has demonstrated, using a patch-clamp technique in brain slices from newborn rats, that depolarization of SLN neurons directly excite cardiac vagal neurons within the NA (132,133). The result of this excitation of cardiac vagal neurons is a decrease in heart rate. Thus, some SLN fibers monosynaptically synapse upon cardiac vagal neurons accounting for the bradycardia associated with activation of the LCR. Whether the properties of the synapses change with development accounting for less significant reduction in heart rate associated with the laryngeal chemoreflex with maturation, has not been determined.

C. LCR Possible Mechanisms Explaining Apnea and Bradycardia Associated with Oral Feeding and Gastroesophageal Reflux in Premature Infants

Apnea and bradycardic events occur during bottle feeding (134,135) and gastroesophageal reflux (GER) in preterm and term infants (136–138). These apneic and bradycardic events are likely secondary to activation of the LCR during feeding and GER (for review, see 138–141). Similar to unobstructed sustained respiration, coordinated sucking and swallowing with breathing is a skill that improves with maturation (142). Discoordination of pharyngeal and palatal muscles during bottle feeding places the immature infant at increased risk for undercoating of the epiglottis (location of receptors for LCR) or penetration of liquids into the larynx. In addition, in the infant who has residual lung disease who has increased work of breathing, tachypnea, and difficulty in coordination sucking, swallowing, and breathing, bottle feeding is more likely to result in inadvertent stimulation of the LCR and direct aspiration (4). Similarly, GER, to the level of the pharynx associated with discoordinated swallow, may also stimulate laryngeal receptors and activate the LCR (141).

Reflux of acidic fluid is a potent stimulus for inducing the LCR in young animals (131) and is likely to be operative in premature and term infants (137,139). The coordinate, mature response to fluid in the larynx is to swallow, to arouse, and to cough. However, when factors associated with depressed arousal are operative, life-threatening apnea with O_2 desaturations and bradycardia may occur in response to GER to the level of pharynx in newborn animals (143). As mentioned earlier, infants with BPD have depressed arousal responses (107). Since these infants have reduced functional residual capacity (reduced O_2 storage), they are at risk for repetitive hypoxic episodes during apnea (144). Repetitive hypoxic episodes results in decreased ability to arouse in response to an acute hypoxic stimulus in newborn animals (145), placing infants with BPD at increased risk for prolonged apnea with hypoxemia associated with GER (146).

With maturation, coordination of upper-airway muscles improves, and the physiological response to stimulation of the laryngeal chemoreflex decreases (142,147). Specifically, the duration and severity of the apneic and bradycardic events decrease (148). With postnatal maturation, inhibitory afferent inputs are counterbalanced by increases in excitability of respiratory-related neurons within the respiratory network (149). Differential expression of ion channels and neurotransmitter receptor profiles that occur in hypoglossal motoneurons accounts for some of the maturational effects on hypoglossal motoneuron excitability (outlined above). Less has been reported on the effect of development on the intrinsic properties of laryngeal motoneurons. Although the percent of myelinated fibers in the SLN significantly increases with postnatal maturation (87), the mechanisms accounting for the developmental change in the physiological response to laryngeal stimulation is most likely a more sustained respiratory drive from maturation of central components of the respiratory network. Elaborate anatomical and cellular interactions between pacemaker cells in the pre-Bötzinger complex and the respiratory network in the brainstem occur with maturation and are associated with more stable respiratory patterns. Several excellent monographs have recently reviewed the studies describing cellular and anatomical factors that contribute to stable respiratory pattern during late fetal and early postnatal development (30,150). Changes in neurotransmitter profiles within the brainstem network from predominantly inhibitory to excitatory profiles contribute to the sustained rhythmic respiration that occurs with maturation (150). Thus, pharmacological therapeutic interventions to stabilize respiration and decrease the frequency of apnea, with and without upper-airway obstruction, in premature infants have frequently targeted inhibitory neurotransmitter systems.

X. Why Therapies Are Effective in Treating Apnea in Premature Infants

A. NCPAP

Multiple therapeutic interventions including pharmacological and nonpharmacological methods have been used for the treatment of apnea with upper-airway obstruction in premature infants. These interventions have previously been reviewed (151). The most commonly used nonpharmacological therapy is nasal continuous positive airway pressure (NCPAP). NCPAP decreases the frequency of mixed, central, and obstructive apnea in premature infants (152). Several factors account for this effect: NCPAP [1] splints the upper airway open, making it less collapsible (153), and [2] increases functional residual capacity, stabilizing O_2 levels (153). A stable O_2 level results in less variation between high and low respiratory drive. Increased variability in respiratory drive destabilizes breathing and precipitates apnea (154).

B. Methylxanthines: Theophylline, Caffeine, and Aminophylline

Adenosine Receptor Blockers: Adenosine Depresses Respiratory Drive

Theophylline and caffeine are the most commonly used pharmacological agents for the treatment of apnea in premature infants (151,155). The most likely mechanism responsible for the reduction in all types of apnea attributed to these methylxanthines is that xanthines are potent adenosine receptor blockers (156,157). Adenosine, a ubiquitous neuromodulator, is a breakdown product of adenosine triphosphate (ATP), and is involved in modulating many neuronal and cellular properties. In response to hypoxia, adenosine levels increase significantly (158,159). Hypoxia is associated with ventilatory depression in mature animals (160), adults (161), immature animals (162), and infants (163). Although several neuromodulators may mediate hypoxic ventilatory depression, adenosine is the major neuromodulator involved in hypoxic ventilatory depression (162), especially in immature animals. The fetus (162) and newborn are particularly sensitive to the depressive effects of adenosine on respiration. This respiratory depression results in apnea in the most immature animals (164,165). Adenosine receptor antagonists (caffeine, theophylline, and aminophylline) either abolish or attenuate the respiratory depression associated with hypoxic exposure in mature (160) and immature models (164,165). The therapeutic benefits of caffeine and theophylline in the treatment of apnea that occurs in premature infants are also well known (151,155).

Endogenous adenosine produced during hypoxia will bind to all adenosine receptors, some of which are linked to excitatory and inhibitory second-messenger systems, resulting in depolarization or hyperpolarization of the cell or neuron (166). There are four classes of adenosine receptors—A_1, A_{2A}, A_{2B}, and A_3. All four receptor subclasses have been cloned. The cellular and physiological affects of ligand binding to these receptors have been best characterized for the A_1 and A_2 subclasses of receptors (167). A_1 and A_2 receptors are coupled to G_i and G_s protein, respectively (166). Caffeine and theophylline block both A_1 and A_2 adenosine receptors (156,157). Caffeine and theophylline increase central respiratory drive by blocking the effects of adenosine on brainstem respiratory-related neurons (168,169). These respiratory depressant effects are mediated through the A_1-adenosine receptor. A_1-adenosine receptor binding has been found in key respiratory-related areas in the fetal sheep brainstem: rostral ventrolateral medulla, nTS, and NA (170). The A_1-adenosine receptors are inhibitory and are present on glutamatergic neurons that send axonal projections to phrenic motoneurons (171) and hypoglossal motoneurons (172). Adenosine binding to presynaptic A_1-adenosine receptors on glutamate containing neurons blocks the release of glutamate (173). Since glutamate is a major excitatory neurotransmitter regulating respiratory-related neurons and upper-airway motoneurons, blocking A_1-adenosine receptors with caffeine and theophylline theoretically should result in increased activity of respiratory-related and hypoglossal motoneurons, thereby stabilizing ventilation and decreasing the frequency of apnea.

$GABA_A$ Receptor Blockers: GABA Depresses Respiratory Drive

Theophylline and caffeine may also increase excitatory activity of respiratory-related neurons involved in GABA transmission. GABA, similar to glycine, has a dual role in neurotransmission during fetal and postnatal development: during early development, GABA and glycine depolarize neurons; during late development, GABA and glycine hyperpolarize neurons (174,175). During postnatal development, GABA and glycine are the two major neurotransmitters that depress respiratory drive (176). Similar to adenosine levels, GABA levels significantly increase in response to hypoxia and contribute to the ventilatory depression resulting from hypoxic exposure (177,178). Inhibitory actions of GABA are mediated through the $GABA_A$ receptor, an inotropic receptor that gates chloride channels (179). Theophylline blocks the inhibiting effects of GABA in cells transfected with recombinant $GABA_A$ receptor (180). Pharmacological experiments suggest that $GABA_A$ receptors exist on phrenic motoneurons (181). GABA binding to these receptors [1] inhibits excitatory glutamergic inputs to phrenic motoneurons in a newborn rat brainstem preparation (181), [2] inhibits respiratory drive in response to hypercapnia in premature rabbits (182), and [3] increases apnea frequency in response to repetitive hypoxic exposure in newborn piglets (183). Thus, in addition to blocking adenosine receptors, methylxanthines may also increase respiratory drive and reduce the frequency of apnea by competitive blocking of $GABA_A$ receptors on phrenic motoneurons.

XI. Conclusions

In conclusion, maturation of intrinsic and extrinsic factors influences the control of upper-airway muscles during development in premature infants with and without coexisting lung disease. By describing the events that occur in the premature infant, a natural model of respiratory system immaturity, I have discussed the effect of development on changes in key central and peripheral components of the respiratory system that ultimately leads to stable breathing patterns with maturation. Several clinical conditions naturally occur in premature infants: [1] prolonged apnea associated with upper-airway obstruction; [2] significant apnea and bradycardia associated with hypoxemia; and [3] apnea and bradycardia associated with oral feedings and GER. In this chapter, I have presented evidence from recent scientific publications that explains the changes in cellular and neuronal properties of central and peripheral neurons involved in respiratory control of upper-airway muscles which may account for these physiological events that occur in premature infants. In addition, I have discussed how some ex utero therapies used to sustain the smallest premature infants may in fact predispose these infants to chronic lung disease, more apneic events with upper-airway obstruction that persist past term gestation, and to weaken arousal responses during apnea and hypoxic exposure. Understanding the key elements responsible for maturation of the central and peripheral components responsible for stable respiration is important, since infants who have persistent apnea with upper-airway obstruction are at increased risk for sudden death (67). Lastly, I have briefly presented probable mechanisms to explain how two widely used therapies, NCPAP and methylxanthines, are effective in stabilizing breathing and thereby decreasing the frequency of apnea.

I have taken the liberty of being selective, in order to provide clarity to an extremely complex system that is constantly changing, not only during development, but also moment to moment. I encourage the reader to peruse recent reviews that I have included in the bibliography that discuss other aspects of changes that occur in the respiratory network during postnatal development.

Acknowledgments

I thank my family for the time they gave me to complete this chapter, Dr. Musa Haxhiu for his helpful suggestions, and my colleagues, Drs. Elizabeth Cristofalo and Frances Northington, for reading and editing the document.

References

1. Guilleminault C, Pelayo R. Sleep-disordered breathing in children. Ann Med 1998; 30(4):350–356.
2. Roux F, D'Ambrosio C, Mohsenin V. Sleep-related breathing disorders and cardiovascular disease. Am J Med 2000; 108(5):396–402.
3. Gabriel M, Albani M, Schulte FJ. Apneic spells and sleep states in preterm infants. Pediatrics 1976; 57(1):142–147.
4. Mercado-Deane MG, Burton EM, Harlow SA, Glover AS, Deane DA, Guill MF. Swallowing dysfunction in infants less than 1 year of age. Pediatr Radiol 2001; 31(6):423–428.
5. Henderson-Smart DJ. The effect of gestational age on the incidence and duration of recurrent apnoea in newborn babies. Aust Paediatr J 1981; 17(4):273–276.
6. Dransfield DA, Spitzer AR, Fox WW. Episodic airway obstruction in premature infants. Am J Dis Child 1983; 137(5):441–443.
7. Ramaekers VT, Casaer P, Daniels H. Cerebral hyperperfusion following episodes of bradycardia in the preterm infant. Early Hum Dev 1993; 34(3):199–208.

8. Urlesberger B, Pichler G, Gradnitzer E, Reiterer F, Zobel G, Muller W. Changes in cerebral blood volume and cerebral oxygenation during periodic breathing in term infants. Neuropediatrics 2000; 31(2):75–81.

9. Henderson-Smart DJ, Butcher-Puech MC, Edwards DA. Incidence and mechanism of bradycardia during apnoea in preterm infants. Arch Dis Child 1986; 61(3):227–232.

10. Eichenwald EC, Aina A, Stark AR. Apnea frequently persists beyond term gestation in infants delivered at 24 to 28 weeks. Pediatrics 1997; 100(3 Pt 1):354–359.

11. Idiong N, Lemke RP, Lin YJ, Kwiatkowski K, Cates DB, Rigatto H. Airway closure during mixed apneas in preterm infants: is respiratory effort necessary? J Pediatr 1998; 133(4):509–512.

12. Miller MJ, Carlo WA, DiFiore JM, Martin RJ. Airway obstruction during periodic breathing in premature infants. J Appl Physiol 1988; 64(6):2496–2500.

13. Reed WR, Roberts JL, Thach BT. Factors influencing regional patency and configuration of the human infant upper airway. J Appl Physiol 1985; 58(2):635–644.

14. Roberts JL, Reed WR, Mathew OP, Thach BT. Control of respiratory activity of the genioglossus muscle in micrognathic infants. J Appl Physiol 1986; 61(4):1523–1533.

15. Badr MS, Toiber F, Skatrud JB, Dempsey J. Pharyngeal narrowing/occlusion during central sleep apnea. J Appl Physiol 1995; 78(5):1806–1815.

16. Reis FJ, Cates DB, Landriault LV, Rigatto H. Diaphragmatic activity and ventilation in preterm infants. I. The effects of sleep state. Biol Neonate 1994; 65(1):16–24.

17. Worsnop C, Kay A, Kim Y, Trinder J, Pierce R. Effect of age on sleep onset-related changes in respiratory pump and upper airway muscle function. J Appl Physiol 2000; 88(5):1831–1839.

18. Albani M, Bentele KH, Budde C, Schulte FJ. Infant sleep apnea profile: preterm vs. term infants. Eur J Pediatr 1985; 143(4):261–268.

19. Flores-Guevara R, Plouin P, Curzi-Dascalova L, Radvanyi MF, Guidasci S, Pajot N. Sleep apneas in normal neonates and infants during the first 3 months of life. Neuropediatrics 1982; 13(suppl):21–28.

20. Hoppenbrouwers T, Hodgman JE, Harper RM, Hofmann E, Sterman MB, McGinty DJ. Polygraphic studies of normal infants during the first six months of life. III. Incidence of apnea and periodic breathing. Pediatrics 1977; 60(4):418–425.

21. Rigatto H. Control of ventilation in the newborn. Annu Rev Physiol 1984; 46:661–674.

22. Curzi-Dascalova L, Peirano P, Morel-Kahn F. Development of sleep states in normal premature and full-term newborns. Dev Psychobiol 1988; 21(5):431–444.

23. Curzi-Dascalova L, Figueroa JM, Eiselt M, Christova E, Virassamy A, d'Allest AM. Sleep state organization in premature infants of less than 35 weeks' gestational age. Pediatr Res 1993; 34(5):624–628.

24. Lee D, Caces R, Kwiatkowski K, Cates D, Rigatto H. A developmental study on types and frequency distribution of short apneas (3 to 15 seconds) in term and preterm infants. Pediatr Res 1987; 22(3):344–349.

25. Smith PL, Wise RA, Gold AR, Schwartz AR, Permutt S. Upper airway pressure-flow relationships in obstructive sleep apnea. J Appl Physiol 1988; 64(2):789–795.

26. Carlo WA, Miller MJ, Martin RJ. Differential response of respiratory muscles to airway occlusion in infants. J Appl Physiol 1985; 59(3):847–852.

27. Gauda EB, Miller MJ, Carlo WA, DiFiore JM, Johnsen DC, Martin RJ. Genioglossus response to airway occlusion in apneic versus nonapneic infants. Pediatr Res 1987; 22(6):683–687.

28. Gauda EB, Miller MJ, Carlo WA, DiFiore JM, Martin RJ. Genioglossus and diaphragm activity during obstructive apnea and airway occlusion in infants. Pediatr Res 1989; 26(6):583–587.

29. Rekling JC, Feldman JL. PreBotzinger complex and pacemaker neurons: hypothesized site and kernel for respiratory rhythm generation. Annu Rev Physiol 1998; 60:385–405.

30. Smith JC, Butera RJ, Koshiya N, Del Negro C, Wilson CG, Johnson SM. Respiratory rhythm generation in neonatal and adult mammals: the hybrid pacemaker-network model. Respir Physiol 2000; 122(2–3):131–147.

31. Johnson SM, Koshiya N, Smith JC. Isolation of the kernel for respiratory rhythm generation in a novel preparation: the pre-Botzinger complex "island." J Neurophysiol 2001; 85(4):1772–1776.

32. Koshiya N, Smith JC. Neuronal pacemaker for breathing visualized in vitro. Nature 1999; 400(6742):360–363.

33. Smith JC, Ellenberger HH, Ballanyi K, Richter DW, Feldman JL. Pre-Botzinger complex: a brainstem region that may generate respiratory rhythm in mammals. Science 1991; 254(5032):726–729.

34. Koshiya N, Guyenet PG. Tonic sympathetic chemoreflex after blockade of respiratory rhythmogenesis in the rat. J Physiol 1996; 491(Pt 3):859–869.

35. Ramirez JM, Schwarzacher SW, Pierrefiche O, Olivera BM, Richter DW. Selective lesioning of the cat pre-Botzinger complex in vivo eliminates breathing but not gasping. J Physiol 1998; 507(Pt 3):895–907.

36. St Jacques R, St John WM. Transient, reversible apnoea following ablation of the pre-Botzinger complex in rats. J Physiol 1999; 520(Pt 1):303–314.

37. Bongianni F, Corda M, Fontana GA, Pantaleo T. Reciprocal connections between rostral ventrolateral medulla and inspiration-related medullary areas in the cat. Brain Res 1991; 565(1):171–174.

38. Rikard-Bell GC, Bystrzycka EK, Nail BS. Brainstem projections to the phrenic nucleus: a HRP study in the cat. Brain Res Bull 1984; 12(5):469–477.

39. Hilaire G, Monteau R, Gauthier P, Rega P, Morin D. Functional significance of the dorsal respiratory group in adult and newborn rats: in vivo and in vitro studies. Neurosci Lett 1990; 111(1–2):133–138.

40. Woch G, Ogawa H, Davies RO, Kubin L. Behavior of hypoglossal inspiratory premotor neurons during the carbachol-induced, REM sleep-like suppression of upper airway motoneurons. Exp Brain Res 2000; 130(4):508–520.

41. Davies RO, Kalia M. Carotid sinus nerve projections to the brain stem in the cat. Brain Res Bull 1981; 6(6):531–541.

42. Furusawa K, Yasuda K, Okuda D, Tanaka M, Yamaoka M. Central distribution and peripheral functional properties of afferent and efferent components of the superior

laryngeal nerve: morphological and electrophysiological studies in the rat. J Comp Neurol 1996; 375(1):147–156.

43. Torrealba F, Claps A. The carotid sinus connections: a WGA-HRP study in the cat. Brain Res 1988; 455(1):134–143.

44. Fay RA, Norgren R. Identification of rat brainstem multisynaptic connections to the oral motor nuclei using pseudorabies virus. III. Lingual muscle motor systems. Brain Res Brain Res Rev 1997; 25(3):291–311.

45. Dobbins EG, Feldman JL. Brainstem network controlling descending drive to phrenic motoneurons in rat. J Comp Neurol 1994; 347(1):64–86.

46. Lydic R, McCarley RW, Hobson JA. Serotonin neurons and sleep. II. Time course of dorsal raphe discharge, PGO waves, and behavioral states. Arch Ital Biol 1987; 126(1):1–28.

47. Lydic R, McCarley RW, Hobson JA. Serotonin neurons and sleep. I. Long term recordings of dorsal raphe discharge frequency and PGO waves. Arch Ital Biol 1987; 125(4):317–343.

48. Kayama Y, Koyama Y. Brainstem neural mechanisms of sleep and wakefulness. Eur Urol 1998; 33(suppl 3):12–15.

49. Osaka T, Matsumura H. Noradrenergic inputs to sleep-related neurons in the preoptic area from the locus coeruleus and the ventrolateral medulla in the rat. Neurosci Res 1994; 19(1):39–50.

50. Nunez-Abades PA, Cameron WE. Morphology of developing rat genioglossal motoneurons studied in vitro: relative changes in diameter and surface area of somata and dendrites. J Comp Neurol 1995; 353(1):129–142.

51. Nunez-Abades PA, He F, Barrionuevo G, Cameron WE. Morphology of developing rat genioglossal motoneurons studied in vitro: changes in length, branching pattern, and spatial distribution of dendrites. J Comp Neurol 1994; 339(3):401–420.

52. Cameron WE, Nunez-Abades PA. Physiological changes accompanying anatomical remodeling of mammalian motoneurons during postnatal development. Brain Res Bull 2000; 53(5):523–527.

53. Berger AJ, Bayliss DA, Viana F. Development of hypoglossal motoneurons. J Appl Physiol 1996; 81(3):1039–1048.

54. Gardiner PF, Kernell D. The "fastness" of rat motoneurones: time-course of afterhyperpolarization in relation to axonal conduction velocity and muscle unit contractile speed. Pflugers Arch 1990; 415(6):762–766.

55. Funk GD, Smith JC, Feldman JL. Generation and transmission of respiratory oscillations in medullary slices: role of excitatory amino acids. J Neurophysiol 1993; 70(4):1497–1515.

56. O'Brien JA, Isaacson JS, Berger AJ. NMDA and non-NMDA receptors are co-localized at excitatory synapses of rat hypoglossal motoneurons. Neurosci Lett 1997; 227(1):5–8.

57. Kubin L, Davies RO, Pack AI. Control of upper airway motoneurons during REM sleep. News Physiol Sci 1998; 13:91–97.

58. Horner RL. Impact of brainstem sleep mechanisms on pharyngeal motor control. Respir Physiol 2000; 119(2–3):113–121.

59. Funk GD, Parkis MA, Selvaratnam SR, Walsh C. Developmental modulation of glutamatergic inspiratory drive to hypoglossal motoneurons. Respir Physiol 1997; 110(2–3):125–137.

60. Bayliss DA, Viana F, Kanter RK, Szymeczek-Seay CL, Berger AJ, Millhorn DE. Early postnatal development of thyrotropin-releasing hormone (TRH) expression, TRH receptor binding, and TRH responses in neurons of rat brainstem. J Neurosci 1994; 14(2):821–833.

61. Funk GD, Smith JC, Feldman JL. Development of thyrotropin-releasing hormone and norepinephrine potentiation of inspiratory-related hypoglossal motoneuron discharge in neonatal and juvenile mice in vitro. J Neurophysiol 1994; 72(5):2538–2541.

62. Bayliss DA, Viana F, Talley EM, Berger AJ. Neuromodulation of hypoglossal motoneurons: cellular and developmental mechanisms. Respir Physiol 1997; 110(2–3):139–150.

63. Volgin DV, Mackiewicz M, Kubin L. Alpha(1B) receptors are the main postsynaptic mediators of adrenergic excitation in brainstem motoneurons, a single-cell RT-PCR study. J Chem Neuroanat 2001; 22(3):157–166.

64. Talley EM, Sadr NN, Bayliss DA. Postnatal development of serotonergic innervation, 5-HT1A receptor expression, and 5-HT responses in rat motoneurons. J Neurosci 1997; 17(11):4473–4485.

65. Okabe S, Mackiewicz M, Kubin L. Serotonin receptor mRNA expression in the hypoglossal motor nucleus. Respir Physiol 1997; 110(2–3):151–160.

66. Aldes LD, Bartley K, Royal K, Dixon A, Chronister RB. Pre- and postnatal development of the catecholamine innervation of the hypoglossal nucleus in the rat: an immunocytochemical study. Brain Res Dev Brain Res 1996; 91(1):83–92.

67. Kato I, Groswasser J, Franco P, Scaillet S, Kelmanson I, Togari H. Developmental characteristics of apnea in infants who succumb to sudden infant death syndrome. Am J Respir Crit Care Med 2001; 164(8):1464–1469.

68. Fajardo C, Alvarez J, Wong A, Kwiatkowski K, Rigatto H. The incidence of obstructive apneas in preterm infants with and without bronchopulmonary dysplasia. Early Hum Dev 1993; 32(2–3):197–206.

69. Yoshida Y, Tanaka Y, Hirano M, Nakashima T. Sensory innervation of the pharynx and larynx. Am J Med 2000; 108(suppl 4a):51S–61S.

70. Mathew OP, Abu-Osba YK, Thach BT. Influence of upper airway pressure changes on genioglossus muscle respiratory activity. J Appl Physiol 1982; 52(2):438–444.

71. Gauda EB, Carroll TP, Schwartz AR, Smith PL, Fitzgerald RS. Mechano- and chemoreceptor modulation of respiratory muscles in response to upper airway negative pressure. J Appl Physiol 1994; 76(6):2656–2662.

72. Tsubone H. Nasal "pressure" receptors. Nippon Juigaku Zasshi 1990; 52(2):225–232.

73. Mathew OP, Abu-Osba YK, Thach BT. Genioglossus muscle responses to upper airway pressure changes: afferent pathways. J Appl Physiol 1982; 52(2):445–450.

74. Van Lunteren E, Van de Graaff WB, Parker DM, Mitra J, Haxhiu MA, Strohl KP. Nasal and laryngeal reflex responses to negative upper airway pressure. J Appl Physiol 1984; 56(3):746–752.

75. Boissonade FM, Lucier GE. Effects of ethmoidal nerve stimulation on respiration-related neurones in the dorsal medulla of the cat. Brain Res 1993; 605(2):345–348.

76. Horner RL, Innes JA, Holden HB, Guz A. Afferent pathway(s) for pharyngeal dilator reflex to negative pressure in man: a study using upper airway anaesthesia. J Physiol 1991; 436:31–44.

77. Horner RL, Innes JA, Morrell MJ, Shea SA, Guz A. The effect of sleep on reflex genioglossus muscle activation by stimuli of negative airway pressure in humans. J Physiol 1994; 476(1):141–151.

78. Cohen G, Henderson-Smart DJ. Upper airway muscle activity during nasal occlusion in newborn babies. J Appl Physiol 1989; 66(3):1328–1335.

79. Thach BT, Schefft GL, Pickens DL, Menon AP. Influence of upper airway negative pressure reflex on response to airway occlusion in sleeping infants. J Appl Physiol 1989; 67(2):749–755.

80. St John WM, Zhou D. Reductions of neural activities to upper airway muscles after elevations in static lung volume. J Appl Physiol 1992; 73(2):701–707.

81. Zhang S, Mathew OP. Decrease in lung volume-related feedback enhances laryngeal reflexes to negative pressure. J Appl Physiol 1992; 73(3):832–836.

82. Matsumoto S, Kanno T, Yamasaki M, Nagayama T, Shimizu T. Influences of lung mechanoreceptors and carotid chemoreceptors on the response of respiratory muscle activity to tracheal occlusion. Jpn J Physiol 1991; 41(1):101–115.

83. Wulbrand H, Von Zezschwitz G, Bentele KH. Submental and diaphragmatic muscle activity during and at resolution of mixed and obstructive apneas and cardiorespiratory arousal in preterm infants. Pediatr Res 1995; 38(3):298–305.

84. Bailey EF, Jones CL, Reeder JC, Fuller DD, Fregosi RF. Effect of pulmonary stretch receptor feedback and CO(2) on upper airway and respiratory pump muscle activity in the rat. J Physiol 2001; 532(Pt 2):525–534.

85. Sasaki CT, Suzuki M, Horiuchi M, Kirchner JA. The effect of tracheostomy on the laryngeal closure reflex. Laryngoscope 1977; 87(9 Pt 1):1428–1433.

86. Petcu LG, Sasaki CT. Laryngeal anatomy and physiology. Clin Chest Med 1991; 12(3):415–423.

87. Miller AJ. Characterization of the postnatal development of superior laryngeal nerve fibers in the postnatal kitten. J Neurobiol 1976; 7(6):483–494.

88. Gonzalez C, Almaraz L, Obeso A, Rigual R. Carotid body chemoreceptors: from natural stimuli to sensory discharges. Physiol Rev 1994; 74(4):829–898.

89. Haxhiu MA, Mitra J, Van Lunteren E, Prabhakar N, Bruce EN, Cherniack NS. Responses of hypoglossal and phrenic nerves to decreased respiratory drive in cats. Respiration 1986; 50(2):130–138.

90. Haxhiu MA, Van Lunteren E, Mitra J, Cherniack NS. Comparison of the response of diaphragm and upper airway dilating muscle activity in sleeping cats. Respir Physiol 1987; 70(2):183–193.

91. Haxhiu MA, Van Lunteren E, Mitra J, Cherniack NS. Responses to chemical stimulation of upper airway muscles diaphragm in awake cats. J Appl Physiol 1984; 56(2):397–403.

92. Van Lunteren E, Haxhiu MA, Mitra J, Cherniack NS. Effects of dopamine, isoproterenol, and lobeline on cranial and phrenic motoneurons. J Appl Physiol 1984; 56(3):737–745.

93. Gauda EB, Lawson EE. Developmental influences on carotid body responses to hypoxia. Respir Physiol 2000; 121(2–3):199–208.

94. Mortola JP, Rezzonico R. Metabolic and ventilatory rates in newborn kittens during acute hypoxia. Respir Physiol 1988; 73(1):55–67.

95. Alvaro RE, Weintraub Z, Kwiatkowski K, Cates DB, Rigatto H. Speed and profile of the arterial peripheral chemoreceptors as measured by ventilatory changes in preterm infants. Pediatr Res 1992; 32(2):226–229.

96. Bamford OS, Carroll JL. Dynamic ventilatory responses in rats: normal development and effects of prenatal nicotine exposure. Respir Physiol 1999; 117(1):29–40.

97. Hertzberg T, Lagercrantz H. Postnatal sensitivity of the peripheral chemoreceptors in newborn infants. Arch Dis Child 1987; 62(12):1238–1241.

98. Hertzberg T, Hellstrom S, Holgert H, Lagercrantz H, Pequignot JM. Ventilatory response to hyperoxia in newborn rats born in hypoxia—possible relationship to carotid body dopamine. J Physiol 1992; 456:645–654.

99. Katz-Salamon M, Jonsson B, Lagercrantz H. Blunted peripheral chemoreceptor response to hyperoxia in a group of infants with bronchopulmonary dysplasia. Pediatr Pulmonol 1995; 20(2):101–106.

100. Alvaro R, Alvarez J, Kwiatkowski K, Cates D, Rigatto H. Induction of mixed apneas by inhalation of 100% oxygen in preterm infants. J Appl Physiol 1994; 77(4):1666–1670.

101. Al Aif S, Alvaro R, Manfreda J, Kwiatkowski K, Cates D, Rigatto H. Inhalation of low (0.5%–1.5%) CO_2 as a potential treatment for apnea of prematurity. Semin Perinatol 2001; 25(2):100–106.

102. Carlo WA, Martin RJ, DiFiore JM. Differences in CO_2 threshold of respiratory muscles in preterm infants. J Appl Physiol 1988; 65(6):2434–2439.

103. Belegu R, Hadziefendic S, Dreshaj IA, Haxhiu MA, Martin RJ. CO_2-induced c-fos expression in medullary neurons during early development. Respir Physiol 1999; 117(1):13–28.

104. Dean JB, Lawing WL, Millhorn DE. CO_2 decreases membrane conductance and depolarizes neurons in the nucleus tractus solitarii. Exp Brain Res 1989; 76(3):656–661.

105. Jansen AH, Liu P, Weisman H, Chernick V, Nance DM. Effect of sinus denervation and vagotomy on c-fos expression in the nucleus tractus solitarius after exposure to CO_2. Pflugers Arch 1996; 431(6):876–881.

106. Sica AL, Gootman PM, Ruggiero DA. CO(2)-induced expression of c-fos in the nucleus of the solitary tract and the area postrema of developing swine. Brain Res 1999; 837(1–2):106–116.

107. Garg M, Kurzner SI, Bautista D, Keens TG. Hypoxic arousal responses in infants with bronchopulmonary dysplasia. Pediatrics 1988; 82(1):59–63.

108. Fewell JE, Taylor BJ, Kondo CS, Dascalu V, Filyk SC. Influence of carotid denervation on the arousal and cardiopulmonary responses to upper airway obstruction in lambs. Pediatr Res 1990; 28(4):374–378.

109. Fewell JE, Kondo CS, Dascalu V, Filyk SC. Influence of carotid denervation on the arousal and cardiopulmonary response to rapidly developing hypoxemia in lambs. Pediatr Res 1989; 25(5):473–477.
110. Jobe AH, Ikegami M. Prevention of bronchopulmonary dysplasia. Curr Opin Pediatr 2001; 13(2):124–129.
111. Ling L, Olson EB Jr, Vidruk EH, Mitchell GS. Phrenic responses to isocapnic hypoxia in adult rats following perinatal hyperoxia. Respir Physiol 1997; 109(2):107–116.
112. Ling L, Olson EB Jr, Vidruk EH, Mitchell GS. Integrated phrenic responses to carotid afferent stimulation in adult rats following perinatal hyperoxia. J Physiol 1997; 500(Pt 3):787–796.
113. Erickson JT, Mayer C, Jawa A, Ling L, Olson EB Jr, Vidruk EH. Chemoafferent degeneration and carotid body hypoplasia following chronic hyperoxia in newborn rats. J Physiol 1998; 509(Pt 2):519–526.
113a. Bavis RW, Olson EB Jr, Mitchell GS. Critical developmental period for hyperoxia-induced blunting of hypoxic phrenic responses in rats. J Appl Physiol 2002; 92(3):1013–1018.
114. Berkowitz RG, Sun QJ, Chalmers J, Pilowsky PM. Respiratory activity of the rat posterior cricoarytenoid muscle. Ann Otol Rhinol Laryngol 1997; 106(11):897–901.
115. Ruggins NR, Milner AD. Site of upper airway obstruction in preterm infants with problematical apnoea. Arch Dis Child 1991; 66(7 Spec No):787–792.
116. Ruggins NR, Milner AD. Site of upper airway obstruction in infants following an acute life-threatening event. Pediatrics 1993; 91(3):595–601.
117. Eichenwald EC, Howell RG III, Kosch PC, Ungarelli RA, Lindsey J, Stark R. Developmental changes in sequential activation of laryngeal abductor muscle and diaphragm in infants. J Appl Physiol 1992; 73(4):1425–1431.
118. Hutchison AA, Wozniak JA, Choi HG, Conlon M, Otto RA, Abrams RM. Laryngeal and diaphragmatic muscle activities and airflow patterns after birth in premature lambs. J Appl Physiol 1993; 75(1):121–131.
119. Widdicombe J. Airway receptors. Respir Physiol 2001; 125(1–2):3–15.
120. Fisher JT, Mathew OP, Sant'Ambrogio FB, Sant'Ambrogio G. Reflex effects and receptor responses to upper airway pressure and flow stimuli in developing puppies. J Appl Physiol 1985; 58(1):258–264.
121. Sant'Ambrogio FB, Mathew OP, Clark WD, Sant'Ambrogio G. Laryngeal influences on breathing pattern and posterior cricoarytenoid muscle activity. J Appl Physiol 1985; 58(4):1298–1304.
122. Hanamori T, Smith DV. Central projections of the hamster superior laryngeal nerve. Brain Res Bull 1986; 16(2):271–279.
123. Waldbaum S, Hadziefendic S, Erokwu B, Zaidi SI, Haxhiu MA. CNS innervation of posterior cricoarytenoid muscles: a transneuronal labeling study. Respir Physiol 2001; 126(2):113–125.
124. Nishino T. Physiological and pathophysiological implications of upper airway reflexes in humans. Jpn J Physiol 2000; 50(1):3–14.

125. Bradley RM. Sensory receptors of the larynx. Am J Med 2000; 108(suppl 4a):47S–50S.
126. Boggs DF, Bartlett D Jr. Chemical specificity of a laryngeal apneic reflex in puppies. J Appl Physiol 1982; 53(2):455–462.
127. Harding R, Johnson P, McClelland ME. Liquid-sensitive laryngeal receptors in the developing sheep, cat and monkey. J Physiol 1978; 277:409–422.
128. Downing SE, Lee JC. Laryngeal chemosensitivity: a possible mechanism for sudden infant death. Pediatrics 1975; 55(5):640–649.
129. Park HQ, Kim KM, Kim YH, Hong WP, Kim MS, Kim DY. Age dependence of laryngeal chemoreflex in puppies. Ann Otol Rhinol Laryngol 2001; 110(10):956–963.
130. Sasaki CT. Development of laryngeal function: etiologic significance in the sudden infant death syndrome. Laryngoscope 1979; 89(12):1964–1982.
131. Wetmore RF. Effects of acid on the larynx of the maturing rabbit and their possible significance to the sudden infant death syndrome. Laryngoscope 1993; 103(11 Pt 1):1242–1254.
132. Mendelowitz D. Advances in parasympathetic control of heart rate and cardiac function. News Physiol Sci 1999; 14:155–161.
133. Mendelowitz D. Superior laryngeal neurons directly excite cardiac vagal neurons within the nucleus ambiguus. Brain Res Bull 2000; 51(2):135–138.
134. Garg M, Kurzner SI, Bautista DB, Lew CD, Ramos AD, Platzker AC. Pulmonary sequelae at six months following extracorporeal membrane oxygenation. Chest 1992; 101(4):1086–1090.
135. Poets CF, Langner MU, Bohnhorst B. Effects of bottle feeding and two different methods of gavage feeding on oxygenation and breathing patterns in preterm infants. Acta Paediatr 1997; 86(4):419–423.
136. Ferlauto JJ, Walker MW, Martin MS. Clinically significant gastroesophageal reflux in the at-risk premature neonate: relation to cognitive scores, days in the NICU, and total hospital charges. J Perinatol 1998; 18(6 Pt 1):455–459.
137. Menon AP, Schefft GL, Thach BT. Airway protective and abdominal expulsive mechanisms in infantile regurgitation. J Appl Physiol 1985; 59(3):716–721.
138. Menon AP, Schefft GL, Thach BT. Apnea associated with regurgitation in infants. J Pediatr 1985; 106(4):625–629.
139. Page M, Jeffery H. The role of gastro-oesophageal reflux in the aetiology of SIDS. Early Hum Dev 2000; 59(2):127–149.
140. Thach BT, Davies AM, Koenig JS, Menon A, Pickens DL. Reflex induced apneas. Prog Clin Biol Res 1990; 345:77–84.
141. Thach BT. Reflux associated apnea in infants: evidence for a laryngeal chemoreflex. Am J Med 1997; 103(5A):120S–124S.
142. Gewolb IH, Vice FL, Schwietzer-Kenney EL, Taciak VL, Bosma JF. Developmental patterns of rhythmic suck and swallow in preterm infants. Dev Med Child Neurol 2001; 43(1):22–27.
143. Jeffery HE, Page M, Post EJ, Wood AK. Physiological studies of gastro-oesophageal reflux and airway protective responses in the young animal and human infant. Clin Exp Pharmacol Physiol 1995; 22(8):544–549.

144. Garg M, Kurzner SI, Bautista DB, Keens TG. Clinically unsuspected hypoxia during sleep and feeding in infants with bronchopulmonary dysplasia. Pediatrics 1988; 81(5):635–642.
145. Johnston RV, Grant DA, Wilkinson MH, Walker AM. Repetitive hypoxia rapidly depresses arousal from active sleep in newborn lambs. J Physiol 1998; 510(Pt 2):651–659.
146. Hrabovsky EE, Mullett MD. Gastroesophageal reflux and the premature infant. J Pediatr Surg 1986; 21(7):583–587.
147. Lanier B, Richardson MA, Cummings C. Effect of hypoxia on laryngeal reflex apnea—implications for sudden infant death. Otolaryngol Head Neck Surg 1983; 91(6):597–604.
148. Harding R, Johnson P, Johnston BE, McClelland MF, Wilkinson AR. Proceedings: cardiovascular changes in new-born lambs during apnoea induced by stimulation of laryngeal receptors with water. J Physiol 1976; 256(1):35P–36P.
149. Kurth CD, Hutchison AA, Caton DC, Davenport PW. Maturational and anesthetic effects on apneic thresholds in lambs. J Appl Physiol 1989; 67(2):643–647.
150. Hilaire G, Duron B. Maturation of the mammalian respiratory system. Physiol Rev 1999; 79(2):325–360.
151. Hascoet JM, Hamon I, Boutroy MJ. Risks and benefits of therapies for apnoea in premature infants. Drug Saf 2000; 23(5):363–379.
152. Miller MJ, Carlo WA, Martin RJ. Continuous positive airway pressure selectively reduces obstructive apnea in preterm infants. J Pediatr 1985; 106(1):91–94.
153. Duncan AW, Oh TE, Hillman DR. PEEP and CPAP. Anaesth Intensive Care 1986; 14(3):236–250.
154. Weintraub Z, Alvaro R, Kwiatkowski K, Cates D, Rigatto H. Effects of inhaled oxygen (up to 40%) on periodic breathing and apnea in preterm infants. J Appl Physiol 1992; 72(1):116–120.
155. Bhatia J. Current options in the management of apnea of prematurity. Clin Pediatr (Phila) 2000; 39(6):327–336.
156. Daly JW. Alkylxanthines as research tools. J Auton Nerv Syst 2000; 81(1–3):44–52.
157. Jacobson KA, Von Lubitz DK, Daly JW, Fredholm BB. Adenosine receptor ligands: differences with acute versus chronic treatment. Trends Pharmacol Sci 1996; 17(3):108–113.
158. Winn HR, Rubio R, Berne RM. Brain adenosine concentration during hypoxia in rats. Am J Physiol 1981; 241(2):H235–H242.
159. Yan S, Laferriere A, Zhang C, Moss IR. Microdialyzed adenosine in nucleus tractus solitarii and ventilatory response to hypoxia in piglets. J Appl Physiol 1995; 79(2):405–410.
160. Gershan WM, Forster HV, Lowry TF, Garber AK. Effect of theophylline on ventilatory roll-off during hypoxia in goats. Respir Physiol 1996; 103(2):157–164.
161. Georgopoulos D, Holtby SG, Berezanski D, Anthonisen NR. Aminophylline effects on ventilatory response to hypoxia and hyperoxia in normal adults. J Appl Physiol 1989; 67(3):1150–1156.

162. Bissonnette JM. Mechanisms regulating hypoxic respiratory depression during fetal and postnatal life. Am J Physiol Regul Integr Comp Physiol 2000; 278(6):R1391–R1400.
163. Rigatto H, Brady JP, de la Torre Verduzco R. Chemoreceptor reflexes in preterm infants. I. The effect of gestational and postnatal age on the ventilatory response to inhalation of 100% and 15% oxygen. Pediatrics 1975; 55(5):604–613.
164. Runold M, Lagercrantz H, Fredholm BB. Ventilatory effect of an adenosine analogue in unanesthetized rabbits during development. J Appl Physiol 1986; 61(1):255–259.
165. Runold M, Lagercrantz H, Prabhakar NR, Fredholm BB. Role of adenosine in hypoxic ventilatory depression. J Appl Physiol 1989; 67(2):541–546.
166. Fredholm BB, IJzerman AP, Jacobson KA, Klotz KN, Linden J. International Union of Pharmacology. XXV. Nomenclature and Classification of Adenosine Receptors. Pharmacol Rev 2001; 53(4):527–552.
167. Fredholm BB, Arslan G, Halldner L, Kull B, Schulte G, Wasserman W. Structure and function of adenosine receptors and their genes. Naunyn Schmiedebergs Arch Pharmacol 2000; 362(4–5):364–374.
168. Kawai A, Okada Y, Muckenhoff K, Scheid P. Theophylline and hypoxic ventilatory response in the rat isolated brainstem-spinal cord. Respir Physiol 1995; 100(1):25–32.
169. Schmidt C, Bellingham MC, Richter DW. Adenosinergic modulation of respiratory neurones and hypoxic responses in the anaesthetized cat. J Physiol 1995; 483(Pt 3):769–781.
170. Bissonnette JM, Reddington M. Autoradiographic localization of adenosine A1 receptors in brainstem of fetal sheep. Brain Res Dev Brain Res 1991; 61(1):111–115.
171. Dong XW, Feldman JL. Modulation of inspiratory drive to phrenic motoneurons by presynaptic adenosine A1 receptors. J Neurosci 1995; 15(5 Pt 1):3458–3467.
172. Bellingham MC. Driving respiration: the respiratory central pattern generator. Clin Exp Pharmacol Physiol 1998; 25(10):847–856.
173. Heron A, Lekieffre D, Le Peillet E, Lasbennes F, Seylaz J, Plotkine M. Effects of an A1 adenosine receptor agonist on the neurochemical, behavioral and histological consequences of ischemia. Brain Res 1994; 641(2):217–224.
174. Miles R. Neurobiology. A homeostatic switch. Nature 1999; 397(6716):215–216.
175. Singer JH, Berger AJ. Development of inhibitory synaptic transmission to motoneurons. Brain Res Bull 2000; 53(5):553–560.
176. Bonham AC. Neurotransmitters in the CNS control of breathing. Respir Physiol 1995; 101(3):219–230.
177. Hoop B, Beagle JL, Maher TJ, Kazemi H. Brainstem amino acid neurotransmitters and hypoxic ventilatory response. Respir Physiol 1999; 118(2–3):117–129.
178. Soto-Arape I, Burton MD, Kazemi H. Central amino acid neurotransmitters and the hypoxic ventilatory response. Am J Respir Crit Care Med 1995; 151(4):1113–1120.
179. Hevers W, Luddens H. The diversity of GABAA receptors. Pharmacological and electrophysiological properties of GABAA channel subtypes. Mol Neurobiol 1998; 18(1):35–86.

180. Sugimoto T, Sugimoto M, Uchida I, Mashimo T, Okada S. Inhibitory effect of theophylline on recombinant GABA(A) receptor. Neuroreport 2001; 12(3):489–493.

181. Su CK, Chai CY. GABAergic inhibition of neonatal rat phrenic motoneurons. Neurosci Lett 1998; 248(3):191–194.

182. Hedner T, Hedner J, Bergman B, Iversen K, Jonason J. Effects of GABA and some GABA analogues on respiratory regulation in the preterm rabbit. Biol Neonate 1983; 43(3–4):134–145.

183. Miller MJ, Haxhiu MA, Haxhiu-Poskurica B, Dreshaj IA, DiFiore JM, Martin RJ. Recurrent hypoxic exposure and reflex responses during development in the piglet. Respir Physiol 2000; 123(1–2):51–61.

6

Developmental Trend of Sleep Characteristics in Premature and Full-Term Newborns

LILIA CURZI-DASCALOVA

INSERM, Hôpital Robert Debré
Paris, France

I. Introduction

Behavioral states (e.g., sleep and wakefulness) are constellations of physiological and behavioral variables that are stable over time and repeat themselves (1). The concept of behavioral states has made it possible to group movements and physiological parameters in definable entities whose graduate organisation during nervous system maturation can be studied (2). The emergence of behavioral sleep and wake states in infants is one of the remarkable achievements of the central nervous system and a good indicator of normal or abnormal development (3). Sleep can be considered as a window on the developing brain (4). Changes in state are accompanied by changes in many key physiological measurements. Thus, even when state is not of direct interest, its links with cardiorespiratory, neurophysiological, and behavioral functions mandate that state be monitored and taken into account as an essential covariate when investigating these functions (5,6).

The main three behavioral states: wakefulness; slow-wave sleep (SWS), or non-rapid eye movement sleep (NREM); and paradoxical or rapid eye movement (REM) sleep are produced by the activity of excitatory and inhibitory neurons located in several brainstem and forebrain centers organized into "systems" or "networks," each of which is responsible for controlling a given state. General principles of sleep-wake control and the development of brain structures involved (and related references) have been reviewed recently (3).

The degree of differentiation at birth and the rate of age-related modifications in states depend on the maturation of involved brain structures. In general, REM sleep appears first, followed by NREM and wakefulness. Because of some differences, especially in electroencephalographic (EEG) and motor patterns, REM sleep in young animals and in infants during the first months of age is usually named active sleep (AS), and NREM sleep is usually named quiet sleep (QS).

II. Development of Behavioral States in Animals

Distinct behavioral states have been described in chronically implanted fetuses of animal species whose brains are relatively mature at birth. In a study using rest-activity and heart rate (HR) evaluation, Belich et al. (7) documented cyclic occurrence of three states in rabbit fetuses beyond 25 days of gestation. REM and NREM states were found in lambs between 120 and 140 days of gestation (normal length of gestation, 150 days), while SWS increased. The timing of the fetal sleep cycle was not correlated with that of the maternal sleep cycle (8,9). In guinea pig fetuses, Astic et al. (10) recorded REM sleep beyond 41 days of gestation, with a peak at 50 days of gestation, i.e., at the time of first appearance of SWS. REM sleep then decreased until birth (normal length of gestation, 65 days), while SWS increased (Fig. 1A). Two distinct EEG states have been described in baboon fetuses recorded at 143–153 days of gestation (normal length of gestation, 175–185 days). State 1 (QS) was distinguishable from state 2 (AS) based on the presence of *tracé alternant*. A smaller percentage of time was spent in state 1 than in state 2 (11).

In guinea pigs and sheep, whose brain is relatively mature at birth, the characteristics of the three main states, including EEG patterns, were similar during the first few days of life and adulthood (12,13) (Fig. 1B). AS and QS, definition based on concordance of the electrocorticogram, electro-oculogram (EOG), and nuchal electromyogram (EMG), were found in preterm lambs born at 133–135 days of gestation. Compared to full-term lambs (147 days of gestation), the preterm lambs spent more time in AS (14).

Behavioral observations and polysomnographic recordings in chronically implanted kittens and rat pups showed that three main behavioral states were recognizable during the first few days of life (15). These states were designated as [1] wakefulness (defined by moving and eating behavior), [2] QS (short periods of quiescence), and [3] AS, or paradoxical, "sismic" REM sleep characterized by neck muscle atony, rapid eye movements, and generalized sismic movements. In these species characterized by marked immaturity at birth, AS prevailed (Fig. 1B),

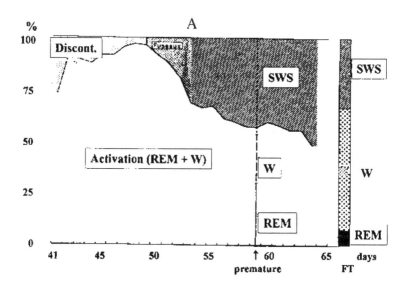

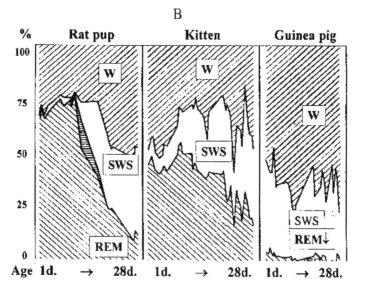

Figure 1 Fetal and neonatal behavioral states. (A) Fetal behavioral states in guinea pig (chronic polygraphic study) (From Ref. 10.) (B) Behavioral states during the first month of life in guinea pig (mature brain at birth), rat pups, and kittens (immature brain in at birth) (chronic polygraphic study) (From Ref. 13.) Discont: discontinuous EEG; SWS: slow-wave sleep; W: wakefulness; REM: rapid-eye-movements sleep. FT: full-term newborn; d: age in days.

but EEG findings were similar in all three states (13,16,17). Based on data obtained by electrolytic lesions of anterior raphe nuclei and on analyses of monoaminergic brain system in rats and cats (with immature brain at birth), some authors suggest that AS and QS during the first few weeks of life may not be the exact counterparts of REM and NREM sleep (18,19; other references in 3).

REM sleep occupies a larger proportion of time in newborns than in adult animals (3,13) (Fig. 1).

III. Behavioral States in Early Human Ontogenesis

A. Fetal Studies

Advances in real-time ultrasonography made it possible to demonstrate that during the last trimester of pregnancy, human fetuses exhibit behavioral states similar to those observed in newborns with similar postconceptional age (PCA). Estimates of the time of first appearance of behavioral states in utero have varied. Prechtl and coworkers (20) defined four fetal behavioral states: state F1, characterized by a slower regular HR, with startles but no eye movements; state 2F, with an irregular HR, eye movements, and occasional gross body movements; state 3F, with a fast regular HR and eye movements but no body movements; and state 4F, with a fast irregular HR, eye movements, and continual body movements. Based on the above criteria and state scoring, utilizing a 3-min moving window, the first studies by Prechtl and coworkers found evidence of behavioral state development in human fetuses between 36 and 38 weeks gestational age (21). However, using a similar scoring system, Visser et al. (22) reported correlations among HR, eye movement, and gross body movement patterns in normal fetuses at 30 to 32 weeks' gestation. Okai et al. (23) documented stable periods of REM and NREM of more than 3 min duration between 28 and 31 weeks gestational age; they also found a strong correlation between the occurrence of rapid eye movements and breathing movements after 27 weeks' gestation. Interestingly, thoracic and abdominal fetal respiratory movements usually occur out of phase during state 2F, a characteristic also found during AS in newborns (5,24).

Fetal states are independent of maternal behavioral states (25).

Monitoring of fetal EEG activity and heart rate variability in healthy fetuses during normal labor demonstrated two alternating sleep states identical to AS and QS observed in newborns (26,27).

Based on the HR pattern and the presence or absence of eye and gross body movements, behavioral states were assigned similarly in low-risk babies recorded during the last weeks of pregnancy and during the first 2 weeks of postnatal life. The proportions of AS, QS, and indeterminate sleep (IS) were virtually identical in fetuses and neonates (28).

B. Behavioral States in Premature and Full-Term Newborns

Behavioral states should be considered not only as a basis for descriptive behavioral classification but also as distinct modes of brain activity. Scoring of behavioral states should never be based on a single variable. In the definition of states there is no limit to the number of variables that can be included in the analysis. However, only relevant variables should be taken into account (1). Also, the results obtained depend on the variables taken into account and on the resolution of the time unit chosen for their classification (29).

Nonsleep States

Definition of nonsleep states is based mainly on behavioral criteria. Carefully recorded information obtained by continuous direct or video monitoring observation is the only way to define crying, quiet wakefulness, and active wakefulness. Charge-sensitive mattress recording can be useful for studying nonsleep states. To our knowledge, systematic polygraphic investigations and quantification of nonsleep states in premature infants have not been conducted to date.

Quiet Wakefulness

This is rare before 35 weeks PCA. It is defined by wide-open eyes with or without exploratory eye movements. Body movements are absent or scarce (30). Beyond 35 weeks, low-voltage theta EEG, characteristic of wakefulness, can be distinguished from the active sleep EEG pattern (29,31). Chin EMG reveals high-voltage activity on which is superimposed phasic activity related to facial movements. Respiration is usually regular (29). Quiet wakefulness corresponds to Prechtl state 3 (1), for which one of the criteria is a stable HR.

Active Wakefulness

This is defined by open eyes, eye movements, repetitive eye openings and closings, frequent gross body movements, and irregular respiration (29). Active wakefulness corresponds to Prechtl state 4 (1), for which one of the criteria is a variable HR with accelerations.

Crying (Prechtl's State 5)

This is accompanied by gross body movements and crying vocalization. The eyes may remain open or closed. Polygraphic parameters are usually uninterpretable because of the presence of artifacts. Although some authors include crying in the waking period (30), crying may be classified as a separate state because of its specific behavioral characteristics (1).

Even when most of the feeding time (breast or bottle) is spent in wakefulness, progressive transition to other behavioral states, characterized by changes in EEG patterns, can be observed despite persistent nutritive sucking. Continuous gavage feeding usually does not disturb sleep states (29).

Sleep States

The first description of sleep states was based on observation of simultaneous cyclic modification of respiratory rate and body and eye movements in young babies (32,33). Whereas the classification of sleep states was developed mainly on the EEG patterns in adults (34), polygraphic recording became the gold standard for state classification and developmental physiology in newborns. Because of EEG and some quantitative behavioral characteristics differ in neonates as compared with adults, the pioneers of sleep studies of newborns argued that specific terms were needed to design sleep states in neonates (35–41). They used combinations of several parameters to define states. Two major sleep states are usually distinguished in early human ontogenesis: active and quiet sleep, to which subsequently has been added an indeterminate sleep (IS) state. Based mainly on behavioral "gestalt" evaluation of patterns, Prechtl and coworkers, who do not use EEG pattern as a state criterion, classified QS-like periods as state 1, and AS-like periods as state 2; this classification does not allow distinction of IS (1,38). Attempts at state classification based on a single parameter (movement or HR) have also been made (42–44).

Polysomnography is easy to perform in newborns, if some technical requirements are taken into account (29):

1. The person in charge of the recording must have some training in neonatal care.
2. The data should be interpreted by a person conversant with age-related EEG characteristics in premature and full-term newborns (29,45–47).
3. Piezoelectric transducers rather than EOG should be used for eye movement detection because of the very low amplitude of retino-corneal electrical potential differences in neonates (Fig. 2) (29).
4. Chin EMG recording may be unsuccessful because of the possibility of low-amplitude activity at this level.
5. Extremely lightweight transducers should be used for leg movement detection.

Use of recording methods that are not suited to newborns causes errors in sleep state identification. When the technician is experienced in neonatal polysomnography, the baby usually falls asleep before the end of electrode placement.

State scoring data depend on the answer to a number of questions:

1. What are the variables chosen for state definition (state-specific criteria; Table 1, Fig. 3)?
2. What is the minimum duration of the state?
3. What is the tolerated duration of parameter discrepancies without interruption of the ongoing state (state smoothing)?

A.R., healthy 33 week preterm infant

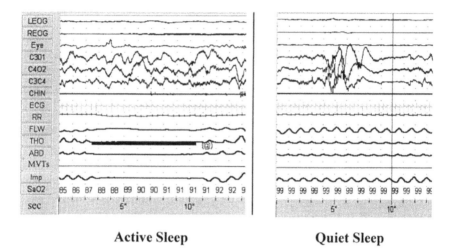

Active Sleep   Quiet Sleep

Figure 2 Example of digitized polysomnographic recordings in a healthy preterm infant at a postconceptional age (PCA) of 33 weeks. Active sleep (left panel) is characterized by a continuous EEG pattern and rapid eye movements (observed and detected only by piezotransducer recording). Quiet sleep (right panel) is characterized by both a discontinuous EEG pattern and the absence of eye movements. (From Ref. 29.) LEOG, REOG: left and right electro-oculogram; eye: eye movements recorded using a piezotransducer (Sleep Watch transducer, Respironics); C3O1 and C4O2: EEG recordings; RR: cardiotachography based on instantaneous heart rate measurement; FLW: nasobuccal airflow detected by thermistors; tho and abd: thoracic and abdominal respiratory movements detected by strain gauges; MVTs: sum of right hand and left leg movements, detected by actimeters; sec: time in seconds; Imp: respiratory movements detected by impedance technique.

4.   When does a given state start?
5.   When does a given state end?

Briefly, a major state begins with the establishment of a typical stable constellation of several state-specific criteria (> 1, 3 min, etc.), is not interrupted by brief incidents (< 60 sec), and ends with a longer-lasting discrepancy (> 60 sec) between parameters or a new constellation specific for another state (29).

In daily practice, sleep states in newborns are recognized by the minimum requirement of two concordant criteria: the EEG patterns (visually classified as continuous versus discontinuous), and the presence or absence of REMs. According to Pan and Ogawa (48), automatic analysis of EEG criteria

Table 1 Summary of the Major Variables (A) and Ancillary Variables (B) Used for Sleep State Scoring at Various Conceptional Ages

(A) Major variables for sleep state scoring

| | CA in weeks | | | | | |
| | 27–34 | | 35–36 | | 37–41 | |
State	AS	QS	AS	QS	AS	QS
EEG	cont: Δ + Θ, or Δ, or semidiscont.	discontinuous	cont: Δ + Θ, or Δ	discontinuous or semidiscont.	continuous: Θ, or, Δ + Θ, or Δ	tracé alternant
Eye movements	+	–	++	–	+++	–

(B) Other variables

| | CA in weeks | | | | | | | |
| | 31–34[a] | | 35–36 | | 37–38 | | 39–41 | |
State	AS	QS	AS	QS	AS	QS	AS	QS
Respiratory rate[a]	irregular	regular or irregular	irregular	regular or irregular	irregular	regular or irregular	irregular	regular or irregular
Tonic chin EMG[b]	–	+ or – (20%)	–	+ or – (20%)	–	+ or – (20%)	–	+ or – (20%)
Body movements[b]	+++ (20%)	++ (5.2%)	+++ (22%)	++ (7%)	+++ (22%)	++ (10%)	++ (14%)	+ (3%)

[a] No quantitative data available for infants younger than 31 weeks PCA.
[b] In parentheses: % of time spent with this parameter.
CA, conceptional age; cont, continuous EEG trace; discont, discontinuous EEG trace; Δ, delta EEG activity; Θ, theta EEG activity. The number of pluses is a relative indication of eye or body movement density. Note that ~20% of quiet sleep is spent with inhibited tonic chin EMG. Body movements decrease in amount with age. For irregular respiration definition and amount, see Ref. 29 and text.

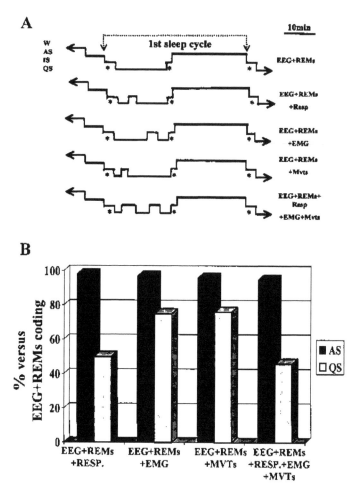

Figure 3 Sleep state determination based on differing state criteria. AS: active sleep; QS: quiet sleep. (A) Hypnograms in a normal full-term newborn (39 weeks PCA, healthy). The amount of AS (defined on the basis of EEG and eye movement criteria only) was virtually unchanged when additional criteria were used (regular or irregular respiration; presence or absence of chin EMG; presence or absence of body movements; and concordance of all five criteria). In contrast, use of additional criteria resulted in a reduction in quiet sleep in favor of indeterminate sleep (IS), which was especially striking when concordance of all five criteria was required. (B) Mean values of AS and QS, expressed as percent of EEG + REM–defined values, in a group of 10 full-term (39–41 weeks) appropriate-for-gestational-age (AGA) infants. Addition of tonic chin EMG as a criterion, for example, decreased the mean QS amount to 75% of that defined by EEG + REMs. AS amount remained nearly the same when different criteria were required for state coding. (From Refs. 61, 70.)

(power, discontinuity, etc.) may predict sleep state changes in preterm infants of > 30 weeks PCA. Scher et al. (49) found that increasing values of spectral theta predicted state changing in a cohort of asymptomatic 28–36 weeks PCA infants. Despite advances in automatic sleep analysis, especially in adults, there is no computerized method for state scoring in newborns (49–53). For instance, state scoring based on heart rate variability (HRV) is not reliable; 11% of the AS and 40% of QS epochs are misclassified in normal full-term newborns when only HRV measures are used; such a classification is even less accurate in premature infants (29,54). State scoring in premature and full-term newborns therefore continues to be done manually on a computer screen or on paper.

Two main sleep states can be distinguished in neurologically normal newborns.

Active Sleep (Figs. 2–4, Table 1)

AS is characterized by the concordance of more continuous EEG and presence of REMs. In very premature babies, REMs are few and isolated, but their presence in successive 20- or 30-sec epochs are necessary for the definition of AS. Their number increases with increasing PCA. Near full term, bursts of REMs become more frequent. In term infants, REMs are usually of lower density at the beginning of given AS, increasing over time before decreasing toward the end of the state (29).

EEG during AS in newborns is characterized by more continuous delta and theta waves than QS. Delta waves amount and amplitude progressively decrease with age, mostly beyond 34 weeks PCA. Concordance between continuous EEG and REMs during stable (> 3 min) periods has been described at about 27 weeks PCA. In < 34 weeks PCA, AS with REMs can be associated with semi-continuous EEG pattern composed of short EEG depressions and continuous delta activity during at least 70% of a given 20- or 30-sec scoring period (29,47). Beyond 37 weeks PCA, two types of AS can be distinguished: the EEG of AS following wakefulness contains a larger amount of slow waves, while AS following the QS state is characterized by faster, lower-amplitude, predominantly theta activity (6,29,45,47,55).

Tonic chin EMG is inhibited during most of the AS time. The remainder ($\sim 10\%$) of AS time is characterized by chin activation following phasic EMG bursts related to body and facial movements (56,57). Active REM sleep is also concomitant to inhibition of postural midline muscles, involved in paradoxical thoracoabdominal respiratory movements and obstructive sleep apnea observed in newborns (24,58,59).

AS is characterized by irregular respiration and more body movements than QS (see below, motor activity).

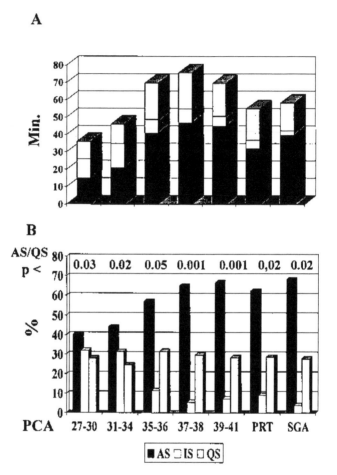

Figure 4 Sleep states and sleep cycle duration in preterm and term infants. Neurologically normal preterm AGA infants at various ages (PCA in weeks), preterm infants at term (PRT), and full-term, small-for-gestational-age (SGA) neonates are shown. (A) Sleep states and sleep cycle duration are given in minutes. (B) Sleep states as percentage of total sleep time. In A, sleep cycle duration at a given age is given by the sum of AS, IS, and QS duration. (Abbreviations as in Fig. 3.)

Quiet Sleep (Figs. 2–4, Table 1)

QS is defined by the absence of REMs and more discontinuous EEG than in AS. EEG patterns for QS definition at different ages are as follows: [1] Up to 36 weeks PCA: discontinuous EEG; however, at 35–36 weeks PCA, QS may include periods with more continuous delta activity (semidiscontinuous tracing); [2]

Beyond 37 weeks PCA: "trace alternant" or continuous delta activity. In near term infants, QS EEG may be more continuous at the beginning of the state, before the appearance of typical "trace alternant" (6,29,31,45,52,60).

Tonic chin EMG is present in $\sim 80\%$ of QS between 31 and 41 weeks PCA (no data for younger premature infants). Normal, full-term newborns spend on average 22% of their QS with absent tonic chin EMG; similar percentages have been observed in NREM sleep in older infants and adults (56,57,61–63) (Fig. 3).

Respiratory rate can be regular or irregular. The amount of irregular respiration described depends on the method of evaluation. We are scoring respiratory rate as irregular when in given (20 or 30 sec) epoch the duration of the longest respiratory cycle is 50% longer than the shortest one. Based on such quantified evaluation, we found that the mean amount of QS epochs with irregular respiration was between 45% and 70% (50% in normal, full-term newborns; Fig. 3). However, in all PCA groups studied, the amount of irregular respiration was significantly higher in AS than in QS (5,61). As a generalization (gestalt pattern), respiratory rate is described as regular in QS (38).

Body and facial movements are fewer in QS than in AS (see below, motor activity).

Indeterminate Sleep

IS exhibits characteristics of both AS and QS. It is also called undifferentiated sleep, coincidence sleep, ambiguous sleep, or no-state (29,40,64,65). IS periods are mainly characterized by absence of REMs during continuous EEG tracing. IS can interrupt an ongoing state or be related to a between-state transition (66) (Fig. 3A). IS occupies $\sim 30\%$ of total sleep time from 27 to 34 weeks PCA and decrease to $< 10\%$ starting at 35 weeks PCA. This decrease of IS favors AS amount (61) (Fig. 4).

Between-State Transitions

Although sleep during transitions between QS and AS exhibits features of both states, it is described as an independent, individualized mode of central nervous system functioning. The order of disappearance of AS sleep parameters during the switch from AS to QS sleep, and their order of appearance during the switch from QS to AS sleep, may help to determine which brain structures control these sleep states (67).

A stable, well-organized pattern of between-sleep-states transitions has been described in healthy 30–41 weeks PCA newborn infants. Duration of AS to QS transitions was significantly longer than duration of QS to AS transitions and was independent of PCA. The sequence of changes in parameters (REM and EEG) was invariable: REM cessation was the first change in AS to QS transitions, and REM appearance was the last change in the QS to AS transitions (64,66). Theses findings are in keeping with studies in human fetuses (21,69,70). They are in agreement with observations of well-defined sleep states very early in human ontogenesis (3,53).

Sleep Cycling

The time pattern of sleep states in neonates is fairly stereotyped. In contrast with older infants and adults who are normally falling asleep in NREM sleep, wakefulness in newborns is followed by a brief episode of AS (shorter than those between two QS episodes). Then, a short period of transitional sleep can precede the onset of QS, which is followed by a longer episode of AS (either directly or with intervening transitional sleep; Fig. 3A). Each sleep cycle includes one complete AS and one complete QS state. Sleep cycle duration is measured from the end (or the beginning) of a given state to the end (or the beginning) of the next state of the same type (Fig. 3A).

Sleep cycle duration is variable across infants and across successive cycles in a given infant. Nevertheless, mean sleep cycle duration increases with age, from 40 min at 27–30 weeks PCA to 45 min at 31–34 weeks PCA and 50–70 min between 35 and 41 weeks PCA (3,29) (Fig. 4A).

Sleep state duration and percentages of different states in the sleep cycle are age dependent. In healthy infants, IS occupies $\sim 30\%$ of the total sleep time from 27 to 34 weeks PCA, and decreases to $< 10\%$ starting at 35 weeks PCA. This decrease in IS favors AS, which becomes the predominant state, occupying $> 60\%$ of the sleep time between 35 weeks PCA and term (3,6,29,70) (Fig. 4B). To our knowledge, the balance between AS and wakefulness, described in older infants (3,71), has never been studied in newborn babies.

Using time-lapse video recordings, Ingersol and Thoman (72) found that very low birth (born < 1500 g) preterm infants showed marked stability and developmental changes in the organization of sleep-wake states from a very early age, and that their states were related to demographic variables as well as temporal measures of care giving.

Normal sleep cycling is observed in neurologically normal premature reaching term and small-for-gestational-age neonates, as well as in artificially ventilated premature infants (70,73) (Fig. 4). Disturbance of sleep cycling may be observed during the first days of life in newborns with mild CNS abnormalities. At this ontogenetic moment, the presence of sleep states organization has a good prognostic value, as far as neurological future of the infant is considered (74). Later sleep cycling may appear in babies with more severe CNS damage. Holdish-Davis (75) found that, despite illness, high-risk preterm babies between 29 and 39 weeks continued to achieve appropriate developmental sleep organization.

Studies in human infancy have shown little or no evidence of circadian sleep-wake rhythmicity at birth (76–78).

C. Influence of Environmental Factors on Sleep Organization in Neonates

Quantified studies on environment and behavioral state organization in neonates mainly included infants evaluated before discharge from neonatal care departments.

Sleep architecture is sensitive to *environmental temperature*. In both premature and full-term newborns cool exposure decreases total sleep time as a consequence of an earlier awakening, whereas AS duration increases at the expense of QS (79–81). Tirosh et al. (82) found that moderate heating provokes a significant decrease in the proportion of AS and an increase in QS. The modification of sleep structure by a warm environment was not confirmed in other studies (80). Discrepancy between these studies is probably related to differences in the amplitude and the trend of temperature changes. Augmented humidity does not change sleep structure if the incubator air temperature remains constant (83). In contrast to adults, active thermoregulation occurs in the premature infant during REM sleep (81,84). Mean rectal temperature has been found lower in AS than in QS in only term, not premature, infants (81,85).

Prone sleeping position is frequent, especially in sick premature babies. Keene et al. (86) did not find significant differences in cardiorespiratory stability between supine and prone positions in preterm infants. However, many epidemiological investigations suggested that, in older infants, prone sleeping increases risk of sudden infant death syndrome (87). This augmented risk has been related to arousal thresholds that increase when sleeping prone (88). There are few reports on the effect of body position on behavioral states organization in neonates. In healthy full-term newborns, Amemiya et al. (89) and Myers et al. (90) observed more awake time in the supine than in the prone position; wakefulness occurred at the expense of state 1 (QS) and/or state 2 (AS). Newborn infants slept more in the prone position than in the supine, and QS was significantly more in the prone position (90,91). In 36 weeks PCA asymptomatic preterm infants, Goto et al. (92) described more awakenings during all sleep states in supine than in prone position. After each feeding, the first QS was significantly shorter when sleeping supine, but overall, the total sleep and percent sleep state were not affected by sleep position.

Bosque et al. (93) found slightly lower total sleep and percentage sleep time in neonates who experienced *kangaroo care* as compared with those sleeping in incubators.

Ariagno et al. (94) did not demonstrate significant difference between sleep parameters (sleep time, AS, QS, sleep transitions) in asymptomatic 36 weeks PCA infants receiving neonatal individualized developmental care program (NIDCAP) as compared with those receiving routine care. In < 32 weeks PCA infants, Bertelle and Sizun (95) found significantly higher total sleep time

(P < .02), QS duration (P < .02), and shorter sleep latency (P < .006) in NIDCAP than in routine, non-NIDCAP caring conditions.

In general, both in the literature and in our own experience, sleep state differentiation was documented earlier during ontogenesis in studies performed after the 1980s than in those done previously (3). This is probably ascribable to improvements made in neonatal care in industrialized countries during recent decades.

D. Sleep and Methylxanthines

Methylxanthine derivatives are currently used to prevent or decrease apneas in premature neonates. They cross the blood brain barrier (96,97), and their antiapnea effect has been ascribed to respiratory center stimulation (98–100). Available data on the effects of methylxanthine derivatives on sleep are hetero-geneous and partly conflicting. Most of them were obtained with theophylline because this was the first drug used to control apnea in premature neonates. Drug effects probably depend on the drug used, animal species investigated, dosage, whether use is acute or chronic, and age.

In premature babies treated by theophylline because of apnea, Demarquez et al. (96) described an increase of awakening and a decrease of QS and IS. Dietrich et al. (101) found a decreased amount of AS, while Gabriel et al. (102) described that AS amount remained unaffected. Thoman et al. (103) found that 2 to 5-week-old postterm babies treated by theophylline when born premature presented more wakening and AS, but noted that the clinical history of treated babies was not similar to control groups. Theophylline is partially converted to caffeine in preterm population (104).

In many neonatal departments, caffeine is preferred to theophylline because of lower side effects on heart rate, urinary sodium excretion, gastrointestinal intolerance, and behavior (105,106). Emory et al. (107) found correlations between salivary caffeine levels and the number of state changes and startles observed during administration of the Brazelton Neonatal Assessment Scale. Preliminary data from Hayes et al. (108) suggested a dose-related effect of caffeine in premature infants with a decrease in QS and increase in AS and drowsiness as defined by the method of Thoman et al. (42) for state-scoring in newborns, which relies mainly on motor behavior criteria.

To assess the potential effect on sleep organization of caffeine in standard maintenance dosages, we recently performed 10-h polysomnographic recordings in 15 neurologically normal and clinically stabilized 33–34 weeks PCA neonates, of whom 10 had been treated for > 3 days with once-a-day oral caffeine citrate, 5 mg/kg, given around 2 PM. We analyzed [1] the usual sleep-wake parameters, including wakefulness, AS, QS, and IS expressed as the number of episodes, duration, and percentage of total sleep time; [2] the duration and order of

Table 2 Wakefulness and Sleep Parameters in Caffeine-Treated and Non-Caffeine-Treated Infants

Criteria	Caffeine	No Caffeine	*P* value
W: number	14.9 ± 8.9	20.4 ± 11.3	0.3
AS: number	26.7 ± 6.8	33.6 ± 9.8	0.2
QS: number	9.7 ± 3	9 ± 3.5	0.9
IS: number	30.7 ± 6.9	28.2 ± 8	0.6
W: % of recording	6.1 ± 4.3	7.6 ± 4.3	0.5
AS: % of TST	64.3 ± 9.7	63 ± 15.2	0.8
QS: % of TST	14.8 ± 3.4	14.9 ± 5.4	1
IS: % of TST	20.9 ± 8.2	22.1 ± 10.5	0.8
State transitions: number	81.6 ± 22.9	91.2 ± 15.1	0.4
AS ⇒ QS transition in min	6.4 ± 3.1	6.1 ± 3.7 (5.8)	0.7
QS ⇒ AS transition in min	1.7 ± 1.8	1.5 ± 1.8	0.7

Means ± SD.
W, wakefulness; AS, active, REM sleep; QS, quiet, NREM sleep; IS, indeterminate sleep; TST, total sleep time; min, between-state transition duration in minutes.
None of the comparisons showed significant differences (*P* at least > .3).
Source: Ref. 109.

parameter modifications during transitions between the main AS and QS states; and [3] the characteristics of morning data (before caffeine) compared to evening data (after caffeine). We found no significant differences between the controls and the infants on maintenance caffeine (Table 2). We conclude that caffeine in a standard maintenance dosage does not modify sleep organization in neurologically normal and clinically stable 33–34 weeks PCA infants (109).

IV. Neurophysiological Correlates of Sleep States in Premature and Full-Term Newborns

A. Sleep, Motor Activity, and Reflexes

Amount of Motor Activity

The amount of motor activity was one of the first criteria for behavioral states description (32,33). Indeed, Dreyfus-Brisac, Monod, and Samson-Dolfus, the pioneers of sleep ontogenesis studies in France (110), first designed the principal two states in newborns by the terms "sommeil calme" and "sommeil agité," which were later equated with the English terms quiet sleep and active sleep. Behavioral states classification based on motor activity recording alone has been advocated (42).

In both AS and QS, in newborns ≥31 weeks PCA (lower age limit of the study), the initiation of spontaneous trunk and limb movements, under pyramidal control, is inhibited during diaphragmatic contraction. This inhibition is seen neither with movements accompanying sighs nor with movements mediated by cranial nerves (111). Groom et al. (28) described stable individual differences in motor activity level: infants who moved at a certain rate as fetuses generally moved at the same rate as neonates.

When motor activity of the upper and lower limbs is recorded continuously, periods with total quietness are nearly absent in normal premature and full-term newborns (112,113). However, from 31 weeks PCA (the youngest PCA studied), the amount of time spent moving is significantly greater during AS than during QS (Fig. 5). The amount of movement in both sleep states remains stable until 38 weeks PCA and decreases significantly in full-term (39–41 weeks PCA) newborns (112). Thus, 39 weeks PCA is a turning point characterized by a significant decrease in motor activity during both AS and QS. The prevalence of body movements in AS as compared with QS in premature infants reaching the normal term and in small-for-gestational-age newborns is similar to that observed in AGA newborns of the same PCA (70,114) (Fig. 5).

In parallel with between-state differences in quantified motor activity, state-segregated motor patterns have been described by observation of neonatal behavior (115,116). It is well established that rhythmic chin movements (about 3/sec) appear only (but not always) in QS; they usually occur in bursts (29). Startles are highly characteristic of QS, while sigh frequency is lower in QS than in AS (114,117). REMs, and small face and limb movements, mainly occur in AS; their appearance allows detection of the onset of AS by visual observation.

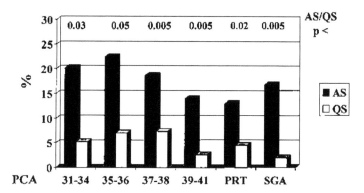

Figure 5 Percentage of time spent with body movements in different sleep states. (From Refs. 29, 112, 114). (Abbreviations as in Fig. 4.)

Following some historical description of motor development in neonates (38,91,115), the detailed study of Hayes et al. (116) demonstrated that state-segregated behaviors were more likely to exhibit co-occurrence in infants 30 weeks PCA and older.

Motor Reflex Responses

The amplitude of the motor **reflex** responses to various stimuli depends on the level of CNS structures (spinal/brain stem/cortical) involved and on the degree of alpha and gama motoneurons' inhibition/facilitation according to sleep states. Most of the proprioceptive reflexes are of higher amplitude in QS than in AS, in contrast with exteroceptive skin reflexes which are usually of higher amplitude in AS than in QS. Table 3 summarizes some of the scarce data on between-state differences of responses to sensory stimulations observed in neonates.

It is of highest importance to check behavioral state when evaluating neurological status in newborns (51) using posture, muscle tone, motor, and reflex parameters. Indeed, all these parameters are state dependent. Some of the historical misunderstanding in evaluation of neurological maturation in neonates seems to be partially related to the fact that some authors did the examination in wakefulness after stimulating the baby (126), while others observed what was happening during sleep (127,128).

B. Developmental Regulation of Sleep and Autonomic Functions

"Emotional" Sweating

Phasic modifications of electrical skin properties measured at the palms and soles are related to emotions and mental activity during wakefulness, and sponta-neously appear during sleep, prevailing during NREM sleep as compared with REM sleep in adults (129,130). It has been reported that they reflect sweat gland activity and are principally under sympathetic ANS control (131). The earliest age at which spontaneous skin potential responses (SPRs) have been found in sleeping newborns is 28 weeks PCA, which is the age at which sweat glands become functionally mature (132). SPRs increase gradually with PCA, more rapidly during AS than during QS (Fig. 6). The transition to an adultlike prevalence of SPRs during QS is due to a steady increase in SPRs in QS during the first 5 months of postterm life (oldest age studied), whereas the SPR increase during AS stops earlier (133).

Storm (134) found that beyond 29 weeks gestational age and at > 10 days of postnatal age (lower age limit of the study), skin conductance changes in connection with heel prick were lowest in sleep and highest during crying

Table 3 Effect of States on the Intensity of Nonrespiratory Reflexes in Normal Newborn Infants

Reflex group	Reflexes—details	PCA	AS/QS	Wake/sleep	Notes
Proprioceptive (118)	Knee, biceps and lip jerks, Moro	FT	QS > AS	QS > W > AS	
Proprioceptive (118)	Vestibuloocular, tonic myotatic	FT	AS > QS	W > AS > QS	
Exteroceptive skin, tactile (118)	Palmar and plantar graspingfinger	FT	AS > QS	W > AS > QS	Inhibition in QS
Exteroceptive skin, tactile (118)	lip protrusion, toe, tibial, fibular, axilary	FT	AS > QS	W = AS > QS	
Exteroceptive skin, pressure (118)	Babkin	FT	AS > QS	W = AS > QS	
Exteroceptive skin, pressure (118)	Palmo-mental	FT	AS > QS	W = AS > QS	
Exteroceptive skin, nociceptive (118)	Babinski, abdominal, thigh, pubic	FT	AS > QS	W = AS > QS	
Spinal monosynaptic (119)	H reflex	FT, Prem	QS > AS		FT > Prem
Spinal monosynaptic (120)	H reflex	FT		Wake > Sleep	Depression in sleep
Skin polysynaptic (121)	Tibialis ant. and biceps contraction	FT	AS > QS		Depression in QS
Brainstem (122)	Blink reflex	FT, Prem		Wake = QS	
Proprioceptive (123)	Achiles'			Wake > Sleep	Depression in sleep
Baroreceptor (124)	Tilting, cardiovascular	FT	AS = QS		
Vagal (125)	Occular compression, longest R-R interval	Near-term	AS > QS	W > AS > QS	Vagal escape?

PCA, postconceptional age; AS, active, REM sleep; QS, quiet, NREM sleep; FT, full-term infants; prem, premature infants.

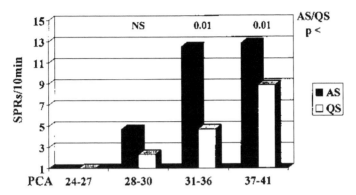

Figure 6 Spontaneous skin potential responses (SPRs) in active (AS) and quiet (QS) sleep. SPRs were first detected at a PCA of 28 weeks. (From Ref. 132.)

($P < .05$). The mean skin conductance level mirrored the behavioral state from 34 weeks gestational age ($P < .05$).

Respiratory Patterns

The first descriptions of sleep states in infants were based on observed differences in respiratory rate: breathing was more irregular during AS and more regular during QS (32,33,55). Striking state-related changes in respiratory pattern have been documented from the time of appearance of differentiated sleep states (5). Sleep-related respiratory characteristics in newborns are described in other chapters in this book. Breathing parameters usually taken into account to evaluate sleep states or respiratory control normality/abnormality are central respiratory pauses, breathing regularity/irregularity, breathing frequency, and percentage of time with out-of-phase (paradoxical) occurring between thoracic and abdominal breathing movements. These parameters present large between-subject differences and fluctuations between one moment to the next in a given subject. Data from the literature usually concern clinically and neurologically normal AGA newborns older than 30 weeks PCA, because younger premature infants usually have neonatal respiratory distress syndrome and are not appropriate for normal respiratory development evaluation. Four parameters investigated showed significant between-state characteristics.

Central respiratory pauses of short duration are a normal phenomenon in newborns. They have been documented during wakefulness following body movements (135). However, they mainly occur during sleep. The apnea index, defined as the percentage of nonbreathing time, is significantly higher during AS than during QS. It remains at a high level until 38 weeks PCA and decreases significantly during both AS and QS at 39–41 weeks PCA (136). Premature infants at term and SGA newborns have significantly more respiratory pause than AGA infants of the same PCA (136,137) (Fig. 7).

Beyond 35 weeks PCA, *respiratory frequency* is significantly higher during AS than during QS. During both AS and QS, respiratory frequency increases significantly at 39–41 weeks PCA (Fig. 7), and continues to increase during the first 2 months of life decreasing progressively thereafter (138).

Phase shift between thoracic and abdominal breathing, a normal phenomenon during the first months of life (24,58,139–142), is closely related to selective intercostal muscle inhibition in AS and to high chest wall compliance (24). From 31 to 41 weeks PCA, the time spent with a 180° thoracoabdominal phase shift remains unchanged and is significantly greater during AS compared with QS.

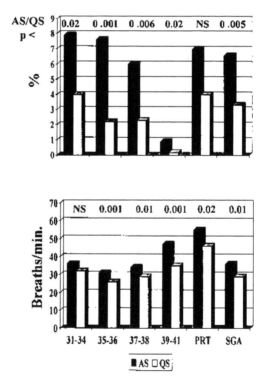

Figure 7 Apnea index (percentage of nonbreathing time) and breathing frequency in the two sleep states are shown. (From Refs. 29, 70, 136–138.) (For abbreviations, see Fig. 3.)

In premature and full-term newborns, *irregular breathing* prevails significantly during AS, covering > 90% of the time spent in this state. However, 20–50% of QS is also accompanied with irregular breathing, with no differences between the youngest premature and full-term newborns (29,61).

Artificially ventilated (18–54/min intermittent positive pressure ventilation) but neurologically normal infants are more dependent on the machine for ventilation in QS than in AS (143).

Heart Rate (HR) and Heart Rate Variability (HRV)

HR and HRV give valuable information on sympathetic and parasympathetic tone during different sleep states in early ontogenesis (144,145). It is now well established that sympathetic tone prevails in AS, while parasympathetic tone prevails in QS (54,145,146). Because of methodological differences in frequency band definition, it is difficult to compare published data on age-related modifications. HR and high-frequency HRV (related to the respiratory cycle and principally under parasympathetic control) are the only parameters that are comparable when different ages are considered.

Beyond 35 weeks PCA, HR is significantly faster and high-frequency HRV significantly lower during AS than during QS. Although HR and high-frequency HRV do not exhibit significant interdependence (54), they exhibit parallel trend of age-related modifications. From 31 to 41 weeks PCA, HR decreases and high-frequency HRV increases during both AS and QS (54,70) (Fig. 8).

In general, HR and HRV levels are modified in "at-risk" (but neurologically normal) premature infants at term and small-for-gestational-age infants (70,147–151) (Fig. 8).

Sleep states in term neonates are also related to changes in cerebral hemodynamic (152,153).

V.   Comments and Summary

Sleep or wake onset and sleep state changes are coordinated processes involving simultaneous or quasisimultaneous changes in sensory, motor, autonomic, hormonal, and cerebral processes. The neural structures underlying each of these processes must reach a certain degree of development before the corresponding state can appear. Differentiated behavioral states are present in humans *in utero* during the third trimester of gestation.

Polysomnography, the gold standard for state definition, is easy to perform in newborns if the persons in charge of the recording are conversant with age-related EEG and REM characteristics and if they have some training in neonatal care.

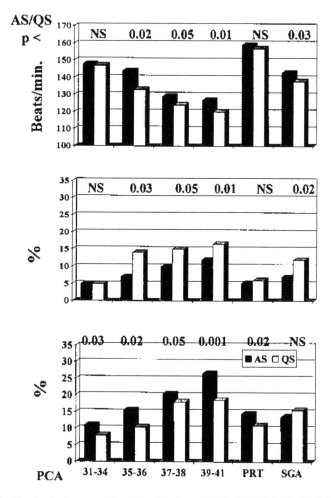

Figure 8 Heart rate (top panel) and heart rate variability (HRV) in the high-frequency (middle panel) and low-frequency (bottom panel) spectra in the two sleep states. (From Refs. 29, 54, 148, 149.) (For abbreviations, see Fig. 3.)

Scoring of behavioral states should never be based on single variable. The quantified results obtained depend on the variables taken into account. As early as 27 weeks PCA, stable AS and QS states can be distinguished, based on concordance between the EEG and REM characteristics of a given state. Additional criteria, such as respiratory rate, HR, tonic chin EMG, and body movement have virtually no effect on the amount of AS (which is maturing earlier in the ontogenesis). In contrast to AS, up to the normal term, QS can be reduced in duration in favor of IS by the presence of irregular respiration, inhibited tonic chin EMG, and body movements.

Between 27 and 34 weeks PCA, IS state is 30% of the sleep time (definition based on EEG + REM criteria). Its amount significantly decreases beyond 35–36 weeks PCA in favor of AS. Up to the normal term in humans, sleep is characterized by stable periods ($\sim$20–22%) of QS (NREM) and a very high (up to 70%) percentage of AS (as opposed to 20% in adults).

Knowledge of early state differentiation is important because a number of physiological parameters are correlated to sleep states and a number of abnormalities occur primarily in one or the other of the main sleep states. Most of state-dependent differences in cardiorespiratory changes or disturbances are related to the physiological specificity of the given state (Fig. 9).

AS is considered a more "dangerous" state in regard to cardiorespiratory disturbances. It is normally characterized by postural muscle hypotonia, sensitivity of brainstem respiratory centres to behaviorallike (environmental or endogenous) stimuli, and prevalence of sympathetic ANS tone. These AS characteristics are not only involved in out-of-phase thoracoabdominal respiratory movements and prevalence of obstructive respiratory events, but also in the persistence of more autonomous respiratory movements in artificially ventilated infants and in some cases of mild central alveolar hypoventilation (Ondine syndrome). These state-dependent respiratory abnormalities will be discussed in other chapters. The prevalence of sympathetic tone explains the higher amplitude of low-frequency HRV in this state.

QS is normally characterized by the presence of postural muscle tone, high dependence of brainstem respiratory centers functioning to "chemical" (mainly CO_2) stimuli, and prevalence of parasympathetic, vagal ANS tone. These QS characteristics may explain the higher dependence on the ventilator in artificially

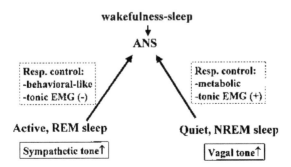

Figure 9 Schema of physiological interactions of active and quiet sleep on the control of respiration, heart rate, and heart rate variability. ANS: autonomic nervous system.

ventilated infants and the dramatic respiratory arrest in case of central alveolar hypoventilation. The higher parasympathetic tone explains the higher amplitude of HF HRV in this state. In addition, EEG abnormalities are more readily detected during QS than during AS.

Finally, sleep cycling seems to be one of the basal functions of the central nervous system, established early during human ontogenesis and resistant to some deviations from the norm as prematurity, intrauterine growth retardation, and artificial ventilation if the neurological and the biological status are not affected.

References

1. Prechtl HFR. The behavioral states of the newborn infant (a review). Brain Res 1974; 76:183–212.
2. Parmelee AH, Garbanati JA. Clinical neurobehavioral aspects of state organisation in newborn infants. In: Yabuuchi H, Watanabe K, Okada S, eds. Neonatal Brain and Behavior. Nagoya: University of Nagoya Press, 1987:131–144.
3. Curzi-Dascalova L, Challamel MJ. Neurophysiological basis of sleep development. In: Loughlin GM, Carroll JL, Marcus CL, eds. Sleep and Breathing in Children: A Developmental Approach. New York: Marcel Dekker, 2000:3–37.
4. Kohyama J. Sleep as a window on the developing brain. Curr Prob Pediatr 1998; 28:69–100.
5. Curzi-Dascalova L. Physiological correlates of sleep development in premature and full-term newborns. Clin Neurophysiol 1992; 22:151–166.
6. Sahni R, Schulze KF, Stefanski M, Myers MM, Fifer WP. Methodological issues in coding sleep states in immature infants. Dev Psychobiol 1995; 28:85–101.
7. Belich AI, Nazarova LA. The development of the rest-activity cycle in rabbit fetus. J Evol Biochem Physiol 1988; 24:217–222.
8. Ruckebush Y, Gaujoux M, Eghbali B. Sleep cycles and kinesis in the foetal lamb. Electroenceph Clin Neurophysiol 1977; 42:226–237.
9. Gauwerky J, Wernicke K, Boos R, Kubli F. Heart rate variability, breathing and body movements in normoxic fetal lambs. J Perinat Med 1982; 10(suppl 2):111–112.
10. Astic L, Sastre JP, Brandon AM. Polygraphic study of vigilance states in the guinea-pig fetus. Physiol Behav 1973; 11:647–654.
11. Stark RI, Haiken J, Nordli D, Myers MM. Characterization of electroencephalographic state in fetal baboons. Am J Physiol 1991; 26:R496–500.
12. Jouvet D, Valatx JL. Etude polygraphique du sommeil chez l'agneau. C R Soc Biol 1962; 156:1411–1414.
13. Jouvet-Mounier D. Etude comparée de l'ontogenèse des états de vigilance chez le chat, le rat et le cobay au cours du premier mois post-natal. Bordeaux Med 1969; 4:895–903.
14. Walker AM, De Preu ND. Preterm birth in lambs: sleep patterns and cardiorespiratory changes. J Dev Physiol 1991; 16:139–145.

15. Vogel GM, Feng P, Kinney GG. Ontogeny of REM sleep in rats: possible implication for endogenous depression. Physiol Behav 2000; 68:453–461.

16. Valatx JL, Jouvet D, Jouvet M. Evolution électroencéphalographique des différents états de sommeil chez le chaton. Electroenceph Clin Neurophysiol 1964; 7:218–233.

17. Garma L, Verley R. Ontogenèse des états de veille et de sommeil chez les mammifères. Rev Neuropsyciatr Infant 1969; 17:487–504.

18. Adrien J, Bourgoin S, Hamon M. Midbrain raphe lesion in the newborn rat. I. Neurophysiological aspect of sleep. Brain Res 1977; 127:99–110.

19. Franc M, Page J, Heller HC. The effect of REM sleep-inhibiting drugs in neonatal rats: evidence for a distinction between neonatal active sleep and REM sleep. Brain Res 1997; 778:64–72.

20. Prechtl HFR. Assessment of fetal neurological function and development. In: Levene MI, Bennett MJ, Jonathan P, eds. Fetal and Neonatal Neurology and Neurosurgery. London: Churchill Livingstone, 1988:35–40.

21. Nijhuis JG, Van de Pas M, Jongsma HW. State transitions in uncomplicated pregnancy after term. Early Hum Dev 1998; 2:152–132.

22. Visser GHA, Poelmann-Weesies G, Cohen TMN, Bekedam DJ. Fetal behavior at 30–32 weeks of gestation. Pediatr Res 1987; 22:655–658.

23. Okai T, Kozuma S, Shinozuka N, Kuwabara Y, Mizuno M. A study on the development of sleep-wakefulness cycle in the human foetus. Early Hum Dev 1992; 29:391–396.

24. Curzi-Dascalova L. Phase relationships between thoracic and abdominal respiratory movements during sleep in 31–38 weeks CA normal infants. Comparison with full-term (39–41 weeks) newborns. Neuropediatrics 1982; 13(suppl):15–20.

25. Hoppenbrouwers T, Ugartechea JC, Combs D, Hodgman JE, Harper RM, Sterman MB. Studies of maternal-fetal interaction during the last trimester of pregnancy: ontogenesis of the basic rest-activity cycle. Exp Neurol 1978; 61:136–153.

26. Challamel MJ, Revol M, Bremond A, Fargier P. Electroencéphalogramme foetal au cours du travail. Modifications physiologiques des états de vigilance. Rev Fr Gynecol 1975; 70:235–239

27. Rosen MG, Dierker LJ, Hertz RH, Sorokin Y, Timortritdch IE. Fetal behavioral states and fetal evaluation. Clin Obstet Gynecol 1979; 22:605–611.

28. Groom LJ, Swiber MJ, Atterbury JL, Bentz LS, Holland SB. Similarity and differences in behavioral state organization during sleep periods in perinatal infant before and after birth. Child Dev 1997; 68:1–11.

29. Curzi-Dascalova L, Mirmiran M. Manual of Methods for Recording and Analysing Sleep-Wakefulness States in Preterm and Full-Term Infants. Paris: INSERM, 1996.

30. Curzi-Dascalova L, Monod N, Guidasci S, Korn G. Transition veille-sommeil chez les nouveau-nés et les nourrissons avant l'âge de 3 mois. Rev EEG Neurophysiol 1981; 11:1–10.

31. Dreyfus-Brisac C. Ontogenesis of brain bioelectrical activity and sleep organisation in neonates and infants. In: Falkner F, Tanner JM, eds. Human Growth, Vol 3. New York: Plenum, 1979:157–182.

32. Denissova MP, Figurin NL. Periodic phenomena during sleep in infants. News in nervous system reflexology and physiology. (In Russian.) 1926; 2:338–345.
33. Aserinsky E, Kleitman N. A motility cycle in sleeping infants as manifested by ocular and gross bodily activity. J Appl Physiol 1955; 8:11–18.
34. Rechtschaffen A, Kales A, eds. A Manual of Standardized Terminology, Techniques and Scoring System for Sleep Stages of Human Subjects. Washington: U.S. Public Health Service, Government Printing Office, 1968.
35. Monod N, Dreyfus-Brisac C, Morel-Kahn F, Pajot N. Les premières étapes de l'organisation du sommeil chez le prématuré et le nouveau-né à terme. Rev Neurol 1964; 110:304–305.
36. Roffwarg HP, Muzio JN, Dement WC. Ontogenetic development of human sleep-dream cycle. Science 1966; 152:604–619.
37. Parmelee AH, Wenner WH, Akiyama Y, Schultz M, Stern E. Sleep states in premature infants. Dev Med Child Neurol 1967; 9:70–77.
38. Prechtl HFR, Akiyama Y, Zinkin P, Grant DK. Polygraphic studies in the full-term newborns. I. Tehnical aspects and qualitative analysis. Clin Dev Med 1968; 27:1–21.
39. Dreyfus-Brisac C. Ontogenesis of sleep in human prematures after 32 weeks of conceptional age. Dev Psychobiol 1970; 3:91–121.
40. Anders T, Emde R, Parmelee A, eds. A Manual of Standardized Terminology, Techniques and Criteria for Scoring of States of Sleep and Wakefulness in Newborn Infants. Los Angeles: UCLA Brain Information Service, MINDS Neurological Information Network, 1971.
41. Wolff P, Ferber R. The development of behavior in human infants, premature and newborn. Annu Rev Neurosci 1979; 2:291–307.
42. Thoman EB, McDowell K. Sleep cycling in infants during the earliest postnatal weeks. Physiol Behav 1989; 45:217–522.
43. Erkenjunti M, Kero P, Halonen JP, Mikola H, Sainio K. SCSB method compared to EEG-based polygraphy in sleep state scoring of newborn infants. Acta Pediatr Scand 1990; 79:274–279.
44. Schechtman VL, Harper RK, Harper RM. Development of heart rate dynamics during sleep-wake states in normal infants. Pediatr Res 1993; 34:618–623.
45. Dreyfus-Brisac C. Neonatal electroencephalography. In: Scarpelli EM, Cosmi EV, eds. Rev Perinatol Med, Vol 3. New York: Raven Press, 1979:397–472.
46. Stockard-Pope JE, Werner SS, Bickford RG. Atlas of Neonatal Electroencephalography, 2d ed. New York: Raven Press, 1992.
47. Lamblin MD, André M, Challamel MJ, Curzi-Dascalova L, d'Allest AM, De Giovanni E, Moussali-Salefranque F, Navelet Y, Plouin P, Radvany-Bouvet MF, Samson-Dolfus D, Vecchierini-Blineau MF. EEG in premature and full-term infants: developmental features and glossary. Neurophysiol Clin 1999; 29:123–219.
48. Pan XL, Ogawa T. Microstructure of longitudinal 24 hour electroencephalograms in healthy preterm infants. Pediatr Int 1999; 41:18–27.
49. Scher MS, Dokianakis SG, Steppe DA, Banks DL, Sclabassi RJ. Computer classification of state in healthy preterm neonates. Sleep 1997; 20:132–141.

50. Giaquinto S, Marciano F, Monod N, Nolfe G. Application of statistical equivalence to newborn EEG recordings. Electroenceph Clin Neurophysiol 1977; 42:406–413.

51. Scher MS. Understanding sleep ontogeny to assess brain dysfunction in neonates and infants. J Child Neurol 1998; 13:467–474.

52. Myers MM, Fifer WP, Grose-Fifer J, Sahni R, Stark RI, Schulze KF. A novel quantitative measure of trace-alternant EEG activity and its association with sleep states in preterm infants. Dev Psychobiol 1997; 31:167–174.

53. Kuhle S, Klebermass K, Olischar M, Hulek M, Prusa AR, Kohlhauser C, Birnbacher R, Weninger M. Sleep-wake cycles in preterm infants below 30 weeks of gestational age. Preliminary results of a prospective amplitude-integrated EEG study. Wien Klin Wochenschr 2001; 113:219–223.

54. Clairambault J, Curzi-Dascalova L, Kauffmann F, Médigue C, Leffler C. Heart rate variability in normal sleeping full-term and preterm neonates. Early Human Dev 1992; 28:169–183.

55. Monod N, Pajot N. Le sommeil du nouveau-né et du prématuré. I. Analyse des études polygraphiques (mouvements oculaires, respiration et EEG) chez le nouveau-né à terme. Biol Neonat 1965; 8:281–307.

56. Curzi-Dascalova L, Plassart E. Activité tonique du muscle mentonnier pendant le sommeil du nouveau-né à terme et du nourrisson. J Physiol (Paris) 1976; 72:5A.

57. Schloon H, O'Brien MJ, Scholten CA, Prechtl HFR. Muscle activity and postural behavior in newborn infants. Neuropaediatrie 1976; 7:384–415.

58. Curzi-Dascalova, L. Thoracico-abdominal respiratory correlations in infants: constancy and variability in different sleep states. Early Hum Dev 1978, 2:25–38.

59. Gaultier C. Le contrôle de la ventilation. In: Dehan M, Micheli JL, eds. Le poumon du nouveau-né. Progrès en pédiatrie, périnatologie. Paris: Doin, 2000:53–60.

60. Eiselt M, Schendel M, Dorschel J, Curzi-Dascalova L, D'Allest AM, Zwiener U. Quantitative analysis of discontinuous EEG in premature and full-term newborns during quiet sleep. Electroenceph Clin Neurophysiol 1997; 103:528–534.

61. Curzi-Dascalova L, Peirano P, Morel-Kahn F. Development of sleep states in normal premature and full-term newborns. Dev Psychobiol 1988; 21:431–444.

62. Salzarulo P. L'atonie musculaire pendant le sommeil chez l'homme. Riv Psicol 1968; Suppl:201–220.

63. Liefting B, Bes F, Faglioli I, Salzarulo P. Electromyographic activity and sleep states in infants. Sleep 1994; 17:718–722.

64. Monod N, Curzi-Dascalova, L. Transitional sleep states in full-term newborns. Rev EEG Neurophysiol (Paris) 1973; 3:87–96.

65. Salzarulo P, Fagioli I. Changes of sleep states and physiological activities across the first year of life. In: Kalverboer A, Genta ML, Hopkins B, eds. Current Issues in Developmental Psychology. Biopsychological Perspectives. Dordrecht: Kluwer, 1999:3–74.

66. Curzi-Dascalova L. Between-sleep states transition in premature babies. J Sleep Res 2001; 10:153–158.

67. Gottesmann C. The transition from slow-wave sleep to paradoxical sleep: evolving facts and concepts of the neurophysiological processes underlying the intermediate stage of sleep. Neurosci Behav Rev 1996; 20:367–387.

68. Arduini D, Rizzo G, Caforio L, Boccolini MR, Romanini C, Mancuso S. Behavioural state transitions in healthy and growth retarded fetuses. Early Hum Dev 1989; 19:155–165.
69. Groom LJ, Benanti JM, Bentz LS, Singh KP. Morphology of active sleep-quiet sleep transitions in normal human term fetuses. J Perinat Med, 1996; 24:171–176.
70. Curzi-Dascalova L. Développement du sommeil et des fonctions sous contrôle du système nerveux autonome chez les nouveau-nés prématurés et à terme. Arch Pediatr 1995; 2:255–262.
71. Louis J, Cannard C, Bastuji H, Challamel MJ. Sleep ontogenesis revisited: a longitudinal 24-h home polygraphic study on 15 normal infants during the first two years of life. Sleep 1997; 20:323–333.
72. Ingersoll EW, Thoman EB. Sleep/wake states of preterm infants: stability, developmental changes, diurnal variation, and relation with caregiving activity. Child Dev 1999; 70:1–10.
73. Curzi-Dascalova L, Figueroa JM, Eiselt M, Christova E, Virassami A, D'Allest AM, Guimaraes H, Gaultier C, Dehan M. Sleep state organization in premature infants of less than 35 weeks' gestational age. Pediatr Res 1993; 34:624–628.
74. Pezzani C, Radvanyi-Bouvet MF, Relier JP, Monod N. Neonatal electroencephalography during the first twenty-four hours of life in full-term newborn infants. Neuropediatrics 1986; 17:11–18.
75. Holditch-Davis D. The development of sleeping and waking states in high-risk preterm infants. Infant Behav Dev 1990; 13:513–531.
76. Parmelee AH Jr, Stern E. Development of states in infants. In: Clements CD, Purpura DD, Mayer F, eds. Sleep and the Maturating Nervous System. New York: Academic Press, 1972:199–215.
77. McGraw K, Hoffmann R, Harker C, Herman JH. The development of circadian rhythms in human infants. Sleep 1999; 22:303–310.
78. Mirmiran M, Ariagno RL. Influence of light in the NICU on the development of circadian rhythms in preterm infants. Semin Perinatol 2000; 4:247–257.
79. Azas Y, Fleming PJ, Levine M, McCabe R, Stewart A, Johnson P. The relationship between environmental temperature, metabolic rate, sleep state, and evaporate water loss in infants from birth to three months. Pediatr Res 1992; 32:417–423.
80. Bach V, Telliez F, Zoccoli G, Lenzi P, Leke A, Libert JP. Interindividual differences in the thermoregulatory response to cool exposure in sleeping neonates. Eur J Appl Physiol 2000; 81:455–462.
81. Bach V, Telliez F, Lenzi P, Chardon K, Leke A, Libert JP. Awakenings, sleep-wake cycle and thermal environment in neonates. In: Salzarulo P, Ficca G, eds. Awakening and Sleep-Wake Cycle Across Development. Amsterdam: Benjamins, 2002:131–148.
82. Tirosh E, Bader D, Hodgins H, Cohen A. Sleep architecture as related to temperature changes in neonates at term. Clin Physiol 1996; 16:603–608.
83. Telliez F, Bach V, Delanaud S, M'Baye H, Leke A, Apédoh A, Abdiche M. Influence du niveau d'humidité de l'air sur le sommeil du nouveau-né en incubateur. RBM 1999; 21:171–176.

84. Darnall RA Jr, Ariagno RL. The effect of sleep state on active thermoregulation in the premature infant. Pediatr Res 1982; 16:512–514.
85. Scher MS, Dokianakis SG, Sun M, Steppe DA, Guthrie RD, Sclabassi RJ. Rectal temperature changes during sleep state transitions in term and preterm neonates at postconceptional term age. Pediatr Neurol 1994; 10:191–194.
86. Keene DJ, Wimmer JR Jr, Mathew OP. Does supine positioning increase apnea, bradycardia, and desaturation in preterm infants? J Perinatol 2000; 1:17–20.
87. Mitchel EA, Brunt JM, Everard C. Reduction in mortality from sudden infant death syndrome in New Zealand. Arch Dis Child 1994; 70:291–294.
88. Kahn A, Grosswasser J, Franco P, Scaillet S, Sawaguchi T, Kelmanson I, de Broca A, Dan B, Servais L. Factors influencing the determination of arousal thresholds in infants—a review. Sleep Med 2000; 1:273–278.
89. Amemiya F, Vos JE, Prechtl HF. Effects of prone and supine position on heart rate, respiratory rate and motor activity in fullterm newborn infants. Brain Dev 1991; 13:148–154.
90. Myers MM, Fifer WP, Schaeffer L, Sahni R, Ohira-Kist K, Stark RI, Schulze KF. Effect of sleeping position and time after feeding on the organization of sleep/wake states in prematurely born infants. Sleep 1998; 21:343–349.
91. Hashimoto T, Hiura K, Endo S, Fukuda K, Mori A, Tayama M, Miyao M. Postural effects on behavioral states of newborn infants—a sleep polygraphic study. Brain Dev 1983; 5:286–291.
92. Goto K, Mirmiran M, Adams MM, Longford RV, Baldwin RB, Boeddiker MA, Ariagno RL. More awakenings and heart rate variability during supine sleep in preterm infants. Pediatrics 1999; 103:603–609.
93. Bosque EM, Brady JP, Affonso DD, Wahlberg V. Physiologic measures of kangaroo versus incubator care in terciary-level nursery. J Obstet Gynecol Neonatal Nurs 1995; 24:219–226.
94. Ariagno RL, Thoman EB, Boeddiker MA, Kugener B, Constantinou JC, Mirmiran M, Baldwin RB. Developmental care does not alter sleep and development of premature infants. Pediatrics 1997; 100:1026–1027.
95. Bertelle V, Sizun J. Analyse comparée du sommeil de l'enfant prématuré avec et sans programme de soin de développement. Mémoire, Faculté de Médecine de Brest, France, 2001.
96. Demarquez JL, Brachet-Lierman A, Paty J, Deliac MM, Philippe JC, Paix M, Babin JP, Martin C. Traitement préventif des apnées du prématuré par la théophylline: étude clinique, pharmacocinétique, neurophysiologique. Arch Fr Pediatr 1978; 35:793–805.
97. McCall AL, Millington WR, Wurtman RJ. Blood-brain barrier transport of caffeine: dose-related restriction of adenine transport. Life Sci 1982; 31:2709–2715.
98. Robert JL, Mathew OP, Thach BT. The efficacity of theophylline in premature infants with mixed and obstructive apnea and apnea associated with pulmonary and neurologic disease. J Pediatr 1982; 100:968–970.
99. Aranda JV, Turmen T, Davis J, Trippenbach T, Grondin D, Zinman R, Watters G. Effect of caffeine on control of breathing in infantile apnea. J Pediatr 1983; 103:975–983.

100. Nehlig A, Daval JL, Debry G. Caffeine and central nervous system: mechanisms of action, biochemical, metabolic and psychostimulant effects. Brain Res Rev 1992; 17:139–170.
101. Dietrich J, Krauss AN, Reidenberg M, Drayer DE, Auld PA. Alteration in state in apneic pre-term infants receiving theophylline. Clin Pharmacol Ther 1978; 24:474–478.
102. Gabriel M, Witolla C, Albani M. Sleep and aminophylline treatment of apnea in preterm infants. Eur J Pediatr 1978; 128:145–149.
103. Thoman EB, Holditch Davis D. Theophylline affected sleep-wake development in premature infants. Neuropediatrics 1985; 16:13–18.
104. Calhoun LK. Pharmacologic management of apnea of prematurity. J Perinat Neonatal Nurs 1996; 9:56–62.
105. Bairam A, Boutroy MJ, Badonnel Y, Vert P. Le choix entre théophylline et caféine dans le traitement des apnées du prématuré. Arch Fr Pediatr 1990; 47:461–465.
106. Comer AM, Perry CM, Figgit DP. Caffeine citrate: a review of its use in apnoea of prematurity. Pediatr Drugs, 2001; 3:61–79.
107. Emory EK, Konopka S, Hronsky S, Tuggey R, Dave R. Salivary caffeine and neonatal behavior: assay modification and functional significance. Psychopharmacology (Berl) 1988; 94:64–68.
108. Hayes MJ, Akilesh M, Davare AA, Parker KG. Comparison of theophylline and caffeine pharmacotherapy on behavioral state and spontaneous movement in infants between 30–35 weeks PCA. Sleep Res Online 1999; 2(suppl 1):203.
109. Curzi-Dascalova L, Aujard Y, Gaultier C, Rajguru M. Sleep organization in premature 33/34-week postmenstrual age infants treated with maintenance-dose caffeine. J Pediatr 2002; 140:766–771.
110. Dreyfus-Brisac C, Monod N, Blanc C, Samson D, Ziegler T. Veille sommeil et réactivité chez le nouveau-né à terme. EEG Clin Neurophysiol 1956; suppl 6:425–431.
111. Curzi-Dascalova L. Relationships between body movements and phase of respiratory cycle in newborns. J Dev Physiol 1991; 16:99–103.
112. Peirano P, Curzi-Dascalova L, Vicente G. Influence of states of sleep and age on body motility in normal premature and full-term neonates. Neuropediatrics 1986; 17:186–190.
113. Giganti F, Cioni G, Biagioni E, Puliti MT, Boldrini A, Salzarulo P. Activity patterns assessed throughout 24-hour recording in preterm and term infants. Dev Psychobiol 2001; 38:133–142.
114. Peirano P, Curzi-Dascalova L, Morel-Kahn F, Lebrun F. Motor activity in sleeping small-for-gestational-age full-term neonates. Brain Dysfunc 1988; 1:32–42.
115. Cioni G, Ferrari F, Prechtl HF. Posture and spontaneous motility in full-term infants. Early Hum Dev 1989; 18:247–262.
116. Hayes MJ, Plante LS, Fielding BA, Kumar SP, Delivoria-Papadopoulos M. Functional analysis of spontaneous movements in preterm infants. Dev Psychobiol 1994; 27:271–287.

117. Curzi-Dascalova L, Plassart E. Respiratory and motor events in sleeping infants: their correlation with thoracico-abdominal relationships. Early Hum Dev 1978; 2:39–50.
118. Prechtl HFR. Pattern of reflex behavior related to sleep in the human infant. In: Clemente C, Purpura D, Meyer F, eds. Sleep and Maturing Nervous System. New York: Academic Press, 1972:288–301.
119. Vakhrameeva IA, Finkel ML. Dynamics of the reflex excitability of spinal motoneurons during day sleep in newborn infants. (In Russian.) Zh Evol Biochem Physiol 1976; 12:161–168.
120. Vecchierini-Blineau MF, Guiheneuc P. Excitability of the monosynaptic reflex pathway in the child from birth to four years of age. J Neurosurg Psychiatry 1981; 44:309–314.
121. Vecchierini-Blineau MF, Guiheneuc P. Lower limb cutaneous polysynaptic reflexes in the child, according to age and state of waking and sleeping. J Neurosurg Psychiatry 1982; 45:331–338.
122. Tanaka J. Developmental changes in electrically elicited blink reflex in infancy and childhood. (In Japanese.) No Ta Hattatsu 1989; 21:271–277.
123. Vakhrameeva IA, Kamenskaya AG, Naulainen BA. Depression of the Achilles' reflex during daytime sleep in newborn infants. Hum Physiol 1980; 6:359–366.
124. Thoresen M, Cowan F, Walloe L. Cardiovascular responses to tilting in healthy newborn babies. Early Hum Dev 1991; 26:213–222.
125. Ramet J, Hauser B, Dehan M, Curzi-Dascalova L, Gaultier C. Effect of state of alterness on the heart rate response to ocular compression in human infants. Biol Neonate 1995; 68:270–275.
126. Saint-Anne Dargassis S. Neurological Development in the Full-Term and Premature Neonate. Amsterdam: Elsevier, 1977.
127. Prechtl HFR. The study of neural development as a perspective of clinical problems. In: Connolly KJ, Prechtl HFR, eds. Maturation and Development: Biological and Psychological Perspectives. Philadelphia: Lippincott, 1981; 77/78:198–215.
128. Cioni G, Prechtl HF. Preterm and early postterm motor behaviour in low-risk premature infants. Early Hum Dev 1990; 23:159–191.
129. Broughton RJ, Poiré R, Tassinari CA. The electrodermogram (Tarchanoff effect) during sleep. Electroenceph Clin Neurophysiol 1965; 18:691–708.
130. Johnson LC, Lubin A. Spontaneous electrodermal activity during waking and sleeping. Psychophysiology 1966; 3:8–17.
131. Darrow CW, Gullikson GR. The peripheral mechanisms of the galvanic skin response. Psychophysiology 1970; 6:597–600.
132. Curzi-Dascalova L, Pajot N, Dreyfus-Brisac C. Spontaneous skin potential responses in sleeping infants between 24 and 41 weeks of conceptional age. Psychophysiology 1973; 10:478–487.
133. Curzi-Dascalova L, Dreyfus-Brisac C. Distribution of skin potential responses according to states of sleep during the first months of life in human babies. Electroenceph Clin Neurophysiol, 1976; 41:399–407.
134. Storm H. Development of emotional sweating in preterms measured by skin conductance changes. Early Hum Dev 2001; 62:149–158.

135. Mathew OP, Thopil CK, Belan M. Motor activity and apnea in preterm infants. Is there a causal relationship? Am Rev Respir Dis 1991; 144:842–844.

136. Curzi-Dascalova L, Christova-Gueorguieva E. Respiratory pauses in normal prematurely born infants. A comparison with full-term infants. Biol Neonate 1983; 44:325–332.

137. Curzi-Dascalova L, Peirano P, Christova E. Respiratory characteristics during sleep in healthy small-for-gestational-age newborns. Pediatrics 1996; 97:554–559.

138. Curzi-Dascalova L, Lebrun F, Korn G. Respiratory frequency according to sleep state and age in normal premature infants. A comparison with full-term infants. Pediatr Res 1983; 27:152–156.

139. Finkel LM. The activity of respiratory muscles in newborn infants during wakefulness and sleep. (In Russian.) Zh Evol Biochem Fiziol 1975; 11:92–95.

140. Curzi-Dascalova L, Plassart E. Mouvement respiratoires au cours du sommeil du nouvea-né à terme: comparaison des enregistrements thoraciques et abdominaux. Rev EEG Neurophysiol 1976; 65:97–104.

141. Knill R, Andrews W, Bryan AC, Brayan MH. Respiratory load compensation in infants. J Appl Physiol 1976; 40:357–361.

142. Henderson-Smart DJ, Read DJC. Depression of respiratory muscles and defective responses to nasal obstruction during active sleep in the newborn. Austr Paediatr 1966; 12:261–266.

143. Curzi-Dascalova L, Relier JP, Peirano P, Castex M, Vasseur O. Degree of dependence on the ventilator according to sleep states in artificially ventilated premature infants. Am J Perinatol 1986; 3:169–173.

144. Gootman PM. Neural regulation of cardio-vascular functions in the perinatal period. In: Gootman N, Gootman PM, eds. Perinatal Cardiovascular Function. New York: Marcel Dekker, 1983:265–327.

145. Porges SW, Doussard-Roosevelt JA, Stifter CA, McClenny BD, Riniolo TC. Sleep state and vagal regulation of heart rate patterns in the human newborn: an extension of the polyvagal theory. Psychophysiology 1999; 36:14–21.

146. Goto K, Sato K, Izumi T. Sleep state transition and changes in autonomic function in newborn infants. Psychiatry Clin Neurosci 2000; 54:303–304.

147. Van Ravenswaaij-Art CMA, Hopman JCW, Kollé LAA, Van Amen JPL, Stoelinga GBA, Van Geijn HP. Influences of heart rate variability in spontaneously breathing preterm infants. Early Hum Dev 1991; 27:187–205.

148. Eiselt M, Curzi-Dascalova L, Clairambault J, Kauffmann F, Medigue C, Peirano P. Heart rate in low risk prematurely born infants reaching normal term. A comparison with full-term newborns. Early Hum Dev 1993; 32:183–195.

149. Spassov L, Curzi-Dascalova L, Clairambault J, Kauffmann F, Eiselt M, Medigue C, Peirano P. Heart rate and heart rate variability in small-for-gestational-age newborns. Pediatr Res 1994; 35:500–505.

150. Patzak A, Schlüter B, Orlow W, Mrowka R, Gerhardt D, Schubert E, Persson PB, Barschdorff D, Trowitzsch E. Linear and nonlinear properties of heart rate control in infants at risk. Am J Physiol 1997; 273:R540–R547.

151. Sahni R, Schulze KF, Kashyap S, Ohira-Kist K, Myers MM, Fifer WP. Body position, sleep states and cardiorespiratory activity in developing low birth weight infants. Early Hum Dev 1999; 54:197–206.
152. Münger DM, Bucher HU, Duc G. Sleep state changes associated with cerebral blood volume changes in healthy term newborn infants. Early Hum Dev 1998; 52:27–42.
153. Peirano P, Curzi-Dascalova L, Morel-Kahn F, Lebrun F. Motor activity in sleeping small-for-gestational-age full-term neonates. Brain Dysfunc 1988; 1:32–42.

7

Metabolic and Ventilatory Interaction in the Newborn

JACOPO P. MORTOLA

McGill University
Montreal, Quebec, Canada

I. Introduction

The expectation that pulmonary air convection must meet metabolic demands is a very likely one for organisms that depend on the lungs for gas exchange. Because pulmonary ventilation ($\dot{V}_E$) is an important determinant of alveolar ventilation ($\dot{V}_A$), and metabolic rate, in conditions of equilibrium, corresponds to oxygen consumption ($\dot{V}_{O_2}$) or carbon dioxide production ($\dot{V}_{CO_2}$), the closeness between metabolism and $\dot{V}_E$ implies stability in alveolar and blood gases.* Indeed, in adult mammals, the expectation of a close relationship between $\dot{V}_E$ (or $\dot{V}_A$) and metabolic rate has been verified on numerous circumstances. During moderate levels of exercise, the alveolar and arterial CO_2 partial pressures (respectively, $PACO_2$ and $PaCO_2$) remain nearly constant, until anaerobic metabolism provides an additional stimulus to $\dot{V}_E$. Equally, variations in ambient temperature (Ta) offer examples of changes in $\dot{V}_{O_2}$ accommodated by nearly proportional changes in $\dot{V}_E$ (1). Pharmacological interventions raising metabolic rate result in isocapnic hyperpnea, whether in normoxic or hypoxic conditions (2), and parallel changes

---

* The alveolar gas equation for CO_2 states that the alveolar partial pressure of CO_2 is proportional to the ratio between CO_2 production and alveolar ventilation [$PACO_2 = (\dot{V}_{CO_2}/\dot{V}_A) \cdot Pb$, where Pb is barometric pressure].

of $\dot{V}_{O_2}$ and $\dot{V}_E$ are observed daily, during the normal circadian patterns (3). However, some deviations from the expectation are also known, such as responses to exercise with hyperventilation* and hypocapnia (4), or cases of hypo- or hyperventilation during warm or cold exposures (5). These deviations from the expected pattern indicate that priorities other than strictly gas exchange may intervene in dictating the level of $\dot{V}_E$. For example, in the cold, the necessity of reducing the respiratory heat loss can pose a limit to the degree of hyperpnea, whereas the opposite may occur when body temperature (Tb) increases, as during muscle exercise in a warm environment.

In newborns, numerous situations could modify the relationship between $\dot{V}_E$ and metabolic needs. For example, sleep, which is the predominant state in the neonatal period, in adults is known to alter numerous control mechanisms, including the $\dot{V}_A$-$\dot{V}_{CO_2}$ balance (6). Second, the homeostatic mechanisms controlling Tb, so effective in adult mammals, are less functional in the newborn, partly because of its small size and mostly because of the incomplete thermal control. Changes in Tb can have a direct influence on the $\dot{V}_E$ level, in addition to the effect mediated by the change in metabolic rate (1). Further, because the electrochemical neutrality varies with temperature, a change in Tb could require some degree of hypo- or hyperventilation for the purpose of maintaining a constant relative alkalinity and protection of the pH-dependent protein functions (alphastat regulation) (7–9). Third, the structural characteristics of the respiratory system, which in newborns is prone to distortion and mechanical inefficiency (10), may pose a limit to the $\dot{V}_E$ levels necessary to meet large metabolic demands. Also, if the peripheral chemoreceptors were important in detecting gaseous metabolism, their low postnatal sensitivity (11–14) could reduce the ability of $\dot{V}_E$ to track changes in metabolic rate. Finally, but not of little importance, the common neonatal strategy of changing metabolic rate with changes in oxygenation (15) places additional demands on the coupling between metabolic rate and $\dot{V}_E$.

In this chapter I plan to consider conditions thought, or well known, to modify the metabolic requirements of the newborn, and examine the corresponding $\dot{V}_E$ changes. Unfortunately, the survey is limited by the paucity of studies that have specifically addressed this issue. Nevertheless, the review of the available data permits some tentative conclusions regarding the extent of the coupling between $\dot{V}_E$ and metabolic rate in newborn mammals.

II. Glossary of Terms and Definitions

a, A   arterial, alveolar

---

* *Hyperventilation* is a level of $\dot{V}_A$ exceeding that required by metabolic demands (see also Sec. II).

HVR	hypoxic ventilatory response, ml/min
O_2, CO_2	oxygen, carbon dioxide, ml_{STPD}
PO_2, PCO_2	partial pressure of O_2, CO_2, mm Hg
Ta, Tb	temperature, ambient or body, °C
$\dot{V}_E$, $\dot{V}_A$	minute, alveolar ventilation, ml_{BTPS}/min
$\dot{V}_{O_2}$, $\dot{V}_{CO_2}$	rate of O_2 consumption, CO_2 production, ml_{STPD}/min
W	body weight

Gaseous metabolism ($\dot{V}_{O_2}$ and $\dot{V}_{CO_2}$) and *metabolic rate* are used interchangeably.

Hypoxia: A decrease in O_2 availability at the tissue level.

Hyper-, *hypopnea*: Respectively, an increase and decrease in the absolute value of $\dot{V}_E$, relative to normoxia.

Hyperventilation: An increase in $\dot{V}_E$ relative to metabolic demands. More precisely, an increase in $\dot{V}_A/\dot{V}_{CO_2}$, i.e. a decrease in $PaCO_2$, irrespective of the absolute value of $\dot{V}_E$ or $\dot{V}_A$.

Hypoventilation: An increase in $PaCO_2$.

Hypometabolism: A drop in metabolic rate, relative to the normoxic value.

Thermoneutrality: The range of Ta over which, in normoxia, Tb is maintained with minimal $\dot{V}_{O_2}$.

III. Interspecies Differences in Metabolic Rate

As in adults, in newborn mammals body weight–specific oxygen consumption ($\dot{V}_{O_2}$/W) is greater in the smaller species.* Are these interspecies differences accommodated by corresponding differences in $\dot{V}_E$? An ideal approach to answer this question would be that of measuring simultaneously $\dot{V}_E$ (or $\dot{V}_A$) and $\dot{V}_{O_2}$ (or $\dot{V}_{CO_2}$) in many species under identical conditions—for example, at thermoneutrality and at similar times of the circadian cycle. This has never been done. However, after combining the results of many studies and averaging the data pertaining to any given species, the figure that emerges (Fig. 1) is that of a direct proportionality between $\dot{V}_{O_2}$ and $\dot{V}_E$ (10). The very small marsupials fall on the same line of the more precocial eutherian mammals. On average, $\dot{V}_E/\dot{V}_{O_2}$ equals 41 (ml_{BTPS}/ml_{STPD}), which corresponds to $\dot{V}_{O_2}$ being $\sim 2.5\%$ of $\dot{V}_E$.

On the assumptions that $\dot{V}_E$ is directly proportional to $\dot{V}_A$, and that the right-to-left shunts are minimal and similar among species, the proportionality between $\dot{V}_E$ and $\dot{V}_{O_2}$ implies an interspecies similarity in the pressures of alveolar and blood gases. Data of alveolar gas pressures are too few for any conclusion;

---

* However, the interspecies differences are not nearly as marked as they are in adults. In fact, in adults $\dot{V}_{O_2} \propto W^{0.75}$, whereas in newborn mammals $\dot{V}_{O_2} \propto$ to $W^{0.99}$ (eutherian mammals and marsupials, combined) or $\propto$ to $W^{0.91}$ (eutherians only) (10).

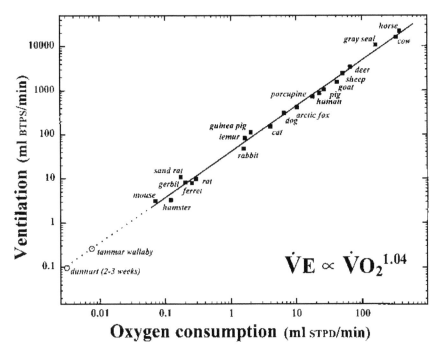

Figure 1 Average values of pulmonary ventilation and the corresponding values of oxygen consumption in newborn species. Data (represented in double log scale) of eutherian mammals (*filled symbols*) are from Ref. 10; values of the marsupials (*open symbols*) are from Ref. 64 (dunnart) and Ref. 63 (wallaby). In the dunnart at 2–3 weeks, up to one-third of total gas exchange occurs through the skin.

those of arterial blood gases, from a number of newborn species, are quite scattered, but do not show any systematic differences with the species body size (10); the overall interspecies averages are respectively, 82 and 40 mm Hg for arterial PO_2 and PCO_2, and 7.39 for pH.*

IV. Metabolic Rate During Body Growth and Aging

In the newborn, $\dot{V}_{O_2}/W$ is usually higher than in the adult, with the exception of some of the small rodents; in these species, in the first days after birth $\dot{V}_{O_2}/W$ actually increases, and only after several days does it begin the usual postnatal

---

* These values exclude those obtained on the day of birth, because of the rapid changes occurring at this time.

decline (10). Although it is known that also $\dot{V}_E/W$ is higher in newborns than in adults, whether or not $\dot{V}_E$ follows closely the postnatal changes in resting $\dot{V}_{O_2}$ has never been specifically addressed by experimental studies. A coarse perusal of published data on Sprague-Dawley rats of different postnatal ages, between a few days to 1 month, reveals a large variability in $\dot{V}_E/\dot{V}_{O_2}$, with values ranging from 25 to 45. This variability could be caused by differences in methodology and in study protocols, which can influence $\dot{V}_{O_2}$ and $\dot{V}_E$ in numerous ways. In addition, at any given age, differences in gender, Ta, Tb, time of day, and state of arousal could cause variability in $\dot{V}_E/\dot{V}_{O_2}$ by altering normoxic $\dot{V}_{O_2}$.

In Figure 2, data of $\dot{V}_E/kg$ of normoxic rats during growth have been plotted not as function of their age, but as function of their normoxic $\dot{V}_{O_2}/W$, irrespective of the factors responsible for its value. Neither in male nor in female rats was $\dot{V}_E$ directly proportional to $\dot{V}_{O_2}$, and a pattern emerged of $\dot{V}_E/\dot{V}_{O_2}$ tending to be lower in those conditions characterised by a high normoxic $\dot{V}_{O_2}/kg$. Hence, a source of variability in $\dot{V}_E/\dot{V}_{O_2}$ during growth would not be the postnatal age per se, but the metabolic condition of the animal. Whether or not this information may be of general value waits confirmatory data from other species.

V. Circadian Patterns of Metabolism

In human infants and a few other newborn mammals in which measurements have been performed, it is possible to document the existence of circadian patterns in Tb and metabolic rate, reminiscent of what is well known in adults. Studies in artificially reared animals demonstrated that the neonatal rhythm is of endogenous origin, rather than the result of maternal influences (17,18). After a couple of weeks, at least in rats, the Tb oscillations gradually decrease in amplitude, almost disappearing around weaning age, to increase again thereafter (19–21); this pattern is an intriguing phenomenon with no clear explanation.

In the rat pups, not only are $\dot{V}_{O_2}$ and Tb lower during the morning hours,* but also the thermogenic response to a cold environment is decreased, presumably because of a lowering in the set point of thermoregulation (22). One implication of this is that, for the same cold stimulus, the propensity for hypothermia is greater in the morning than in the evening hours. Rat pups respond to this situation behaviorally, by increasing in the morning their tendency to huddle (Czerwinski, Seifert, and Mortola, 1999, unpublished observations).

In adult rats, $\dot{V}_E$ and $\dot{V}_{O_2}$ oscillate throughout the day with very similar patterns, such that $\dot{V}_E/\dot{V}_{O_2}$ presents minimal variations (3). Continuous record-

---

* The rat, like most rodents, is a nocturnal animal, with higher mean levels of activity at night.

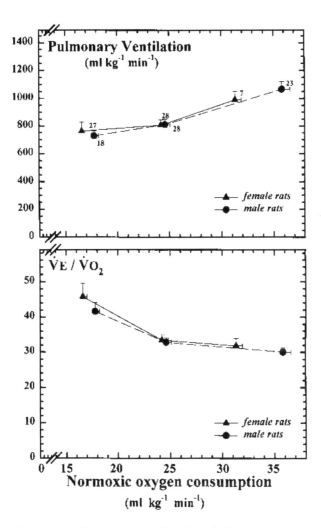

Figure 2 Pulmonary ventilation (top panel) and ventilation oxygen consumption ratio ($\dot{V}_E/\dot{V}_{O_2}$, bottom panel) in rats of different ages and at different metabolic levels. Numbers indicate the number of rats for each range of $\dot{V}_{O_2}$. Data between genders did not differ significantly, but for either gender $\dot{V}_E/\dot{V}_{O_2}$ was lower when $\dot{V}_{O_2}$/kg was higher. (From Ref. 16.)

ings are difficult to obtain in young pups, because of their frequent needs for maternal care. Nevertheless, from intermittent measurements in 6-day-old rats it was clear that both $\dot{V}_{O_2}$ and $\dot{V}_E$ were higher at 7:00 PM than at 7:00 AM, with a similar $\dot{V}_E/\dot{V}_{O_2}$ (23) (Fig. 3). It would be interesting to obtain circadian $\dot{V}_E$ data at later stages of postnatal development, when, as mentioned above, the amplitude of the circadian patterns undergoes rapid changes. If indeed $\dot{V}_E$ was following closely the circadian oscillations of metabolism, as it seems, it would mean that, as in adults, also in newborns the presence of a biological clock does not compromise the normal role of $\dot{V}_E$ in protecting blood gases. At the same time, such results would indicate that the normal AM–PM difference in Tb, of $\sim 1°C$, has no appreciable effects on the relationship between $\dot{V}_E$ and $\dot{V}_{O_2}$.

In adult rats, not only $\dot{V}_E/\dot{V}_{O_2}$ during air breathing, but also the hyperventilatory responses to hypoxia or hypercapnia (i.e., the percent increase in $\dot{V}_E/\dot{V}_{O_2}$ from normoxia) are quite similar between the AM and PM hours (24–26). In newborn rats the hypoxic effects on $\dot{V}_E$ were proportional to those on $\dot{V}_{O_2}$ in both the evening and the morning hours, such that the level of hypoxic hyperventilation remained the same (23).

VI. Changes in Temperature

A. Cold

The metabolic responses of newborn mammals to changes in Ta have been extensively investigated. The thermoneutral range is typically smaller, and at higher Ta values, than in adults. As in adults, also in newborns a reduction in Ta below thermoneutrality stimulates heat production, which in newborns is mostly nonshivering thermogenesis, and behavioral heat conservation.

In adults, the increase in metabolic rate during exposure to cold is accompanied by a proportional increase in $\dot{V}_E$ (1). In lambs also, a decrease in Ta was met by proportional increases in $\dot{V}_{O_2}$ and $\dot{V}_E$ (27), with no changes in Tb, blood gases, or pH (28). In 11-day-old dogs exposed to Ta 20°C, $\dot{V}_{O_2}$ and $\dot{V}_A$ increased proportionately from the corresponding values at 30°C, with minimal changes in $PaCO_2$, arterial O_2 content, and PaO_2 (29).

On the other hand, in newborn rats a reduction in Ta of just a few degrees reduced the ventilation metabolism ratio (Fig. 3), and at 36°C $\dot{V}_E/\dot{V}_{O_2}$ was $\sim 35–38\%$ higher than at 24°C (30,31). From a coarse review of the published data, it seems that the drop in ventilation–metabolism ratio in the cold may have some relationship with the drop in Tb, which occurs readily when small newborns like the rat are exposed to cold (Fig. 4). Because changes in Tb could influence the $\dot{V}_E$ level (32), this could explain the greater inability of the neonatal rat in maintaining $\dot{V}_E/\dot{V}_{O_2}$ in the cold in comparison to the newborn dog or sheep. Whether or not a cause-and-effect relationship between

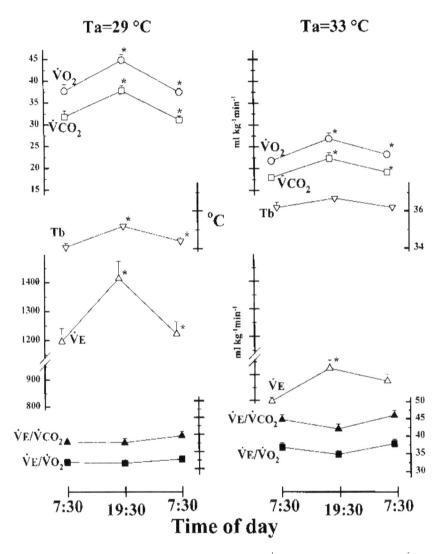

Figure 3 Mean values of pulmonary ventilation ($\dot{V}_E$), oxygen consumption ($\dot{V}_{O_2}$), carbon dioxide production ($\dot{V}_{CO_2}$), and body temperature (Tb) in 6-day-old rats, in the morning (7:30) and evening hours (19:30), at ambient temperatures (Ta) of 29 or 33°C. Gaseous metabolism and $\dot{V}_E$ increased in the evening hours, in proportion to one another. Bars indicate SEMs, which, when not represented, were within symbol size. * Significant difference from the preceding measurement. (From Ref. 23.)

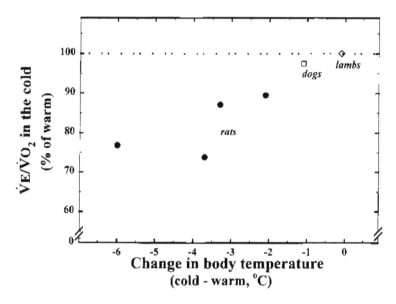

Figure 4 Ventilation oxygen consumption ratio ($\dot{V}_E/\dot{V}_{O_2}$) in cold conditions, expressed as percent of the value in warm conditions (100%, dotted horizontal line), for newborn rats, dogs, and lambs, as function of the change in body temperature between hypoxia and normoxia. In the small newborn rat, cold reduced body temperature and $\dot{V}_E/\dot{V}_{O_2}$ more than in the larger newborns. Values of $\dot{V}_E/\dot{V}_{O_2}$, when not available at the source, were calculated from the changes in $PaCO_2$. (From Refs. 23, 28–31, 33.)

Tb and $\dot{V}_E/\dot{V}_{O_2}$ really exists will require further measurements. A reduced hyperpnea in the cold limits the pulmonary heat loss, but, at the same time, this mechanism for Tb protection implies some departure from complete acid base homeostasis.

B. Heat Exposure

Most mammals live at temperatures below thermoneutrality. This probably applies also to the majority of newborns, especially those of the medium-size and large species. Over the thermoneutral range, because, by definition, $\dot{V}_{O_2}$ is at its minimum, the only possibility for maintaining Tb against a progressive increase in Ta is by mechanisms of heat loss. These latter mechanisms, typically, are very limited in newborns, and this is the main reason for their narrow range of thermoneutrality. Hence, especially in some of the smallest species, warm conditions can readily provoke an increase in Tb—i.e., hyperthermia (10).

Above thermoneutrality, $\dot{V}_{O_2}$ increases partly because of the energetic cost of the functions activated by the hyperthermia, and partly because of the Q_{10} effect.*

To these conditions of warm exposure, or overt hyperthermia, some adult mammals respond with thermal polypnea, a rapid and shallow pattern that can result in major increases of $\dot{V}_E$ with a minimal impact on $\dot{V}_A$ (5). In newborns, experimental data on the $\dot{V}_E$ response to heat stress are very few. In lambs and human infants heat exposure resulted in no or modest increases in Tb and a substantial increase in breathing rate (34,35). In these studies tidal volume was not measured, but the fact that the elimination of CO_2 increased, whereas $\dot{V}_{O_2}$ did not change, suggested that the subjects were hyperventilating. In another study, in lambs of different age groups (27), as Ta was raised $\dot{V}_E/\dot{V}_{O_2}$ clearly increased. The data in animals agree with previous observations in infants (36,37), and would indicate that in newborns, as in adults, during heat exposure the priorities of respiratory regulation are shifting from the control of blood gases to the control of heat loss. Indeed, during heat stress, the evaporative heat loss from the respiratory tract can increase by 50% (infants) to 100% (lambs) (34,35).

In lambs, infants, and newborn rats, the breathing pattern has been consistently found to be more irregular in warm than in cold conditions, and in infants, the propensity to apneic episodes in warm conditions has been considered a potentially life-threatening situation (38). Chemical stimuli, such as hypoxia or hypercapnia, usually result in a breathing pattern more regular than during air breathing, and also the cold-induced increase in metabolic rate appears to act as a stimulus, stabilizing breathing. Hence, during warm conditions in normoxia the chemical and metabolic stimuli on breathing are minimal, and this situation could favor breathing irregularities (31).

VII. Changes in Respiratory Gases

Within the aim of the present chapter it is of interest to consider the changes in oxygenation, because both hyperoxia and hypoxia alter metabolic rate in many newborn species. However, changes in inspired CO_2 (hypercapnia), at least between 1% and 5% of inspired CO_2, typically have negligible effects on neonatal $\dot{V}_{O_2}$ and Tb (33,39,40).

A. Hyperoxia

Data on the effects of hyperoxia on pulmonary convection ($\dot{V}_E$ or $\dot{V}_A$) and metabolic rate ($\dot{V}_{O_2}$ or $\dot{V}_{CO_2}$) are limited to a few species. In mice, lambs,

---

* The Q_{10} (Arrhenius) factor expresses the change in reaction velocity for a $10°C$ change in temperature, $Q_{10} = (A'/A'')^{[10/(T'-T'')]}$, where A' and A'' are the enzymatic activities, or reaction velocities, at the corresponding temperatures T' and T''.

newborn rats, and infants, hyperoxia most commonly increases $\dot{V}_{O_2}$ (10). The basis for this phenomenon is not clear. The simplest interpretation is that normoxic $\dot{V}_{O_2}$ may be limited by the availability of O_2, and that hyperoxia would resolve this limitation (1).

The time profile of the $\dot{V}_E$ response to hyperoxia has been examined in human infants. After the immediate and brief reduction in $\dot{V}_E$ presumably due to the lowering in carotid body inputs, $\dot{V}_E$ increases at or above the normoxic value (41–47). Experiments aiming to address the question of whether a proportionality exists between the ventilatory and metabolic responses have been performed in the newborn mouse and the human infant, with discordant results. In 1- to 2-day-old mice, 5 min of 100% O_2 breathing resulted in an increase in $\dot{V}_{O_2}$ and a drop in breathing rate and $\dot{V}_E$ (48). However, in the infant, after a few minutes of hyperoxia $\dot{V}_{O_2}$, $\dot{V}_E$, and $\dot{V}_A$ increased, with a drop in end-tidal CO_2, indicating that air convection increased disproportionately more than metabolic rate did (45–47).

Presumably, the lack of proportionality between metabolic rate and $\dot{V}_E$ in hyperoxia can be attributed to the numerous factors which, in addition to $\dot{V}_{O_2}$ itself, impact on the $\dot{V}_E$ level. After the sudden inhibition of the chemoreceptor inputs, the high O_2 reduces the hemoglobin capacity for CO_2 and, consequently, provokes a reduction in cerebral tissue pH, which stimulates breathing. Hyperoxia could also stimulate breathing by direct action on the brain structures (49) and, possibly, via activation of the airway receptors.

B. Hypoxia

As mentioned earlier, in first approximation in normoxia the level of $\dot{V}_E$ varies in proportion to the metabolic processes. Although this phenomenon has been noticed and documented by experiments for over a century, the mechanisms which permit $\dot{V}_E$ to track metabolism are still unknown. Similarly, the metabolic level is an important determinant of the magnitude of the ventilatory response to hypoxia (HVR, ml/min). In fact, for any given level of hypoxia, the HVR is not a fixed, predetermined value; rather, it increases when metabolic rate is elevated, and decreases in situations of low metabolism (15), as if the metabolic level, from a functional view point, was controlling the gain of the inputs from the chemoreceptors (Fig. 5, top panel). From the concept that metabolic rate is fundamental in determining the magnitude of the HVR, it also follows that a drop in metabolism during hypoxia can lower the HVR; if the metabolic drop was marked, then, the HVR can be nil or even negative (i.e., the $\dot{V}_E$ level in hypoxia is less than in normoxia; Fig. 5, B–B^4 in bottom panel). Because of these two reasons (the importance of $\dot{V}_{O_2}$ in determining $\dot{V}_E$ and the HVR, and the possibility of a change in $\dot{V}_{O_2}$ during hypoxia), it is important not to confuse the HVR as an index of the hyperventilation. In fact, a correct assessment of the

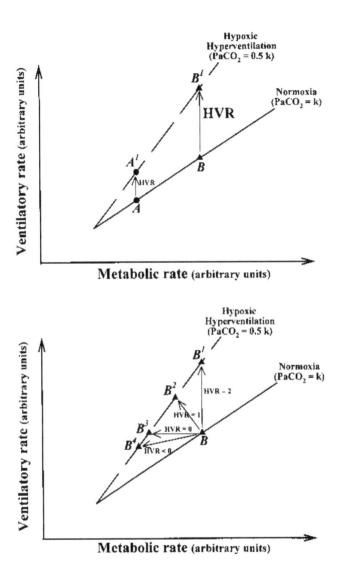

Figure 5 (*Top*) Schematic representation of the relationship between metabolic rate and pulmonary ventilation, in normoxia (continuous line), or during an hypoxic condition creating an hyperventilation = 2× the normoxic value (i.e., halving the $PaCO_2$, dashed line). Any point on the dashed line indicates the same level of hyperventilation. However, from A to A^1 the magnitude of the hyperpneic response (HVR) is half that from B to B^1. In other words, although A-A^1 and B-B^1 indicate the same hyperventilatory response, B-B^1

degree of hyperventilation is not obtained simply from the HVR; rather, it can be conveniently expressed by the increase in $\dot{V}_E/\dot{V}_{O_2}$ or the drop in $PaCO_2$. The schematic examples in Figure 5, bottom, show that the same degree of hypoxic hyperventilation (i.e., the same increase in $\dot{V}_E/\dot{V}_{O_2}$) can be achieved with qualitatively different combinations of HVR and hypometabolism (B^1 to B^4).

With this premise, we can now examine the hypoxic hyperventilation of newborn and young animals, with attention to the degree of stability of the hyperventilatory response in conditions known to change normoxic $\dot{V}_{O_2}$, such as body growth and exposure to cold, and among species with different metabolic requirements.

Hypoxic Hyperventilation: Newborns of Small and Large Species

For the same level of hypoxia, the variability in the magnitude of the hypoxic hyperventilation is very large, in both adult and newborn species. In the latter, even small differences in postnatal age, in addition to the different degree of maturity at birth, have an important impact on the function of the chemoreceptors and on the HVR (10). Nevertheless, despite the variability, several points can be made from these comparisons of newborn and adult species exposed to the same degree of hypoxia (inspired $O_2 = 10\%$; Fig. 6). First, the newborn's hyperventilation shows a scatter among species similar to, and within the range of, the responses measured in adult species. Second, there is no obvious trend for a change in the magnitude of the hyperventilatory response with normoxic $\dot{V}_{O_2}/W$. In other words, the magnitude of the normoxic $\dot{V}_{O_2}/W$ of the species does not systematically influence the degree of hypoxic hyperventilation. In many newborns hypoxia decreases Tb, and this is more marked in the smallest species which have the highest normoxic $\dot{V}_{O_2}/kg$. Hence, the fact that there is no systematic interspecies trend in the magnitude of the hyperventilation, nor a systematic difference from the adults, suggests that the drop in Tb does not have a major effect on the degree of the hypoxic hyperventilation.

Hypoxic Hyperventilation and Body Growth

In newborn rats, as in other newborn species, the HVR is almost nil, whereas the hypometabolic response to hypoxia is very pronounced. By comparison, in adult

---

requires twice as much HVR than A-A^1, because in B metabolic rate is twice than in A. (*Bottom*) From B to B^1, B^2, B^3, or B^4, the hypoxic hyperventilation is the same, namely 2× normoxia. However, the hyperventilation in B-B^1 is strictly achieved by hyperpnea, with no hypometabolism; in B-B^3 is achieved only by hypometabolism; with no HVR; and in B-B^2 there is a combination of hyperpnea and hypometabolism. Finally, B-B^4 is an example of hyperventilation achieved with a large hypometabolic response and a negative HVR.

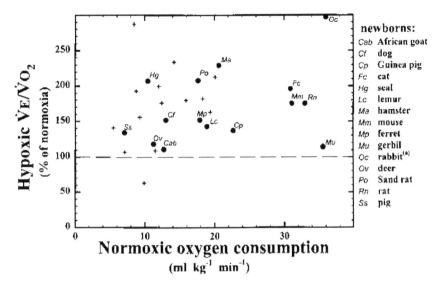

Figure 6   Ventilation–oxygen consumption ratio ($\dot{V}_E/\dot{V}_{O_2}$) in hypoxia (10% inspired O_2) expressed as percent of the normoxic value (dashed line) in various newborn species. All newborn species hyperventilated (i.e., increased $\dot{V}_E/\dot{V}_{O_2}$), but the degree of hypoxic hyperventilation was very variable. +, Response of adult species exposed to the same level of inspired oxygen as the newborns. (From Refs. 50–52.)

rats the hypoxic hypometabolism is small, whereas the HVR is marked. The combination of these two responses is what determines the hyperventilation (increase in $\dot{V}_E/\dot{V}_{O_2}$), and in newborn rats this is almost as large as in older rats of different age and body weight (53).

Similarly to what adopted above (Sec. IV; Fig. 2), it is convenient to represent the level of the hypoxic hyperventilation not as function of age or W, but as function of the normoxic $\dot{V}_{O_2}$. When analyzed in this fashion (Fig. 7), results of prepuberty rats appear to be very similar to those of older animals (16). Hence, the hyperventilatory response to hypoxia is almost the same at various levels of normoxic $\dot{V}_{O_2}$, whether it is achieved predominantly by hypometabolism, by hyperpnea, or by any combination of the two.

Figure 7, incidentally, shows a rather important difference in the degree of hypoxic hyperventilation between genders, the response being more pronounced in female than in male rats, irrespective of normoxic $\dot{V}_{O_2}$. Sex hormones are known to play a role in the control of $\dot{V}_E$ (54), but the fact that the difference is also manifest before puberty indicates that these hormones cannot be considered a major factor responsible for the gender difference in hypoxic hyperventilation.

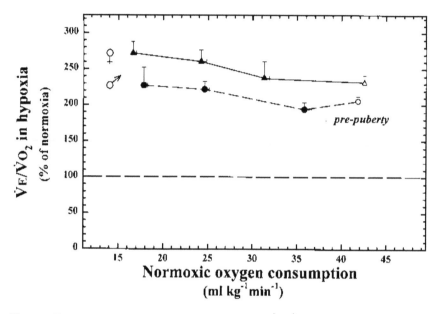

Figure 7 Ventilation–oxygen consumption ratio ($\dot{V}_E/\dot{V}_{O_2}$) during hypoxia (10% inspired O_2), expressed as percent of the normoxic value (dashed line) in prepuberty (open symbols) and postpuberty rats (filled symbols) with different metabolic levels. At all levels of oxygen consumption ($\dot{V}_{O_2}$/kg), the hyperventilatory responses were larger in females. For either gender, the values of prepuberty rats were comparable to those of older animals with high $\dot{V}_{O_2}$/kg. (From Ref. 16.)

Hypoxic Hyperventilation and Changes in Temperature

Analysis of the hypoxic hyperventilation during exposure to cold is included in this chapter because cold and hypoxia combined cause major effects on Tb and $\dot{V}_{O_2}$; hence, it is an opportunity to verify the strength of the metabolism-ventilation linkage when some of the primary variables are modified.

The experiment summarised in Figure 8 refers to 11-day-old puppies (29), studied in warm (open symbols) or cold conditions (filled symbols). In warm conditions, a progressive decrease in the inspired O_2 significantly reduced $\dot{V}_{O_2}$ when PaO_2 was ~ 40 mm Hg or less, and $\dot{V}_A$ started to rise only when the hypoxia was severe. In the cold, normoxic $\dot{V}_{O_2}$ was higher than in warm conditions, as expected because of the increased thermogenesis, and this increase was accompanied by a proportional increase in $\dot{V}_E$. With hypoxia, $\dot{V}_{O_2}$ was beginning to drop significantly at $PaO_2 \sim 50$ mm Hg, i.e., at a higher value than in warm conditions, and $\dot{V}_A$ decreased. As apparent from the $PaCO_2$ values (Fig. 8, top right), the degree of hyperventilation in the cold was identical to that

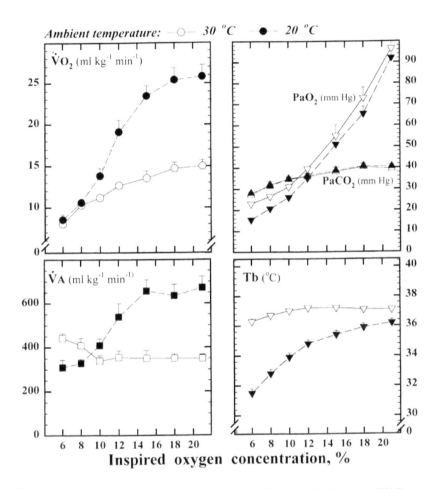

Figure 8 Eleven-day-old dogs, exposed to progressive hypoxia, in warm (30°C, open symbols) and cold conditions (20°C, filled symbols). $\dot{V}_{O_2}$, oxygen consumption; $\dot{V}_A$, alveolar ventilation; PaO_2 and $PaCO_2$, arterial pressure of, respectively, oxygen and carbon dioxide; Tb, body temperature. (From Refs. 29, 53.)

in the warm condition. Hence, this experiment illustrates the remarkable similarity in hypoxic hyperventilation despite the major differences in metabolic and ventilatory responses. In other words, gas convection responds appropriately, maintaining the adequate $\dot{V}_E/\dot{V}_{O_2}$, irrespective of what the metabolic level may be.

It is important to point out that the drop in Tb with hypoxia, which occurs both in warm and in cold conditions as the consequence of the hypometabolism (1), was substantially more marked in the cold, when the decrease in Tb was as large as 5°C (Fig. 8, bottom right). Since $\dot{V}_E$ and $\dot{V}_A$ were able to perfectly track the metabolic requirements, the conclusion should be reached that even a rather large change in Tb does not have any appreciable impact on the magnitude of the puppy's hyperventilatory response. It would be of interest to extend these observations to other species, like newborn rats, which in normoxia are unable to maintain a constant $\dot{V}_E/\dot{V}_{O_2}$ when Tb drops (Sec. VII.B).

The drop in Tb during hypoxia also occurs in the human infant, and it is not uncommon for neonatologists to artificially increase the incubator temperature in an attempt to raise the Tb of the hypoxic infant; this practice has been questioned, since it could be harmful to the infant's strategy for survival (10). In newborn cats and dogs, during hypoxia, an artificial increase in Ta until Tb is at the normoxic level increased the ventilation–metabolism ratio, possibly with a mismatch between $\dot{V}_E$ and $\dot{V}_A$ (55,56), a response that could reflect the necessity of the newborn to heat-dissipate.

VIII. Extrapulmonary Gas Exchange

Attempts to gain further insights into the relationship between pulmonary convection and metabolic rate have been made by adding to the lungs an additional gas exchanger, such as an extracorporeal membrane lung. If the level of $\dot{V}_E$ was related to tissue metabolism via neural or humoral information originated by the cellular activities, one would expect $\dot{V}_E$ to change in proportion with the changes in total metabolic rate, irrespective of how gas exchange is partitioned between the lungs and the extracorporeal gas exchanger. On the other hand, if gaseous metabolism ($\dot{V}_{O_2}$ or $\dot{V}_{CO_2}$) is the primary mechanism linking cellular activity to $\dot{V}_E$, then $\dot{V}_E$ should vary depending on pulmonary $\dot{V}_{O_2}$ or $\dot{V}_{CO_2}$, rather than on total metabolic rate.

In lamb and goat fetuses, even after disconnection from the placenta, regular breathing did not initiate as long as the membrane lung was operating, that is, as long as the metabolically produced CO_2 was not allowed to rise above normal (57–59). Earlier experiments in conscious resting adult sheep connected to an extracorporeal membrane lung indicated that $\dot{V}_E$ decreased as the rate of the artificial exchanger increased, and eventually $\dot{V}_E$ ceased when the removal of CO_2 equaled that metabolically produced (60). Hence, the eventuality that the gaseous aspect of cellular metabolism is the important variable in setting $\dot{V}_E$ is more than a mere hypothesis, and it finds support in some experimental observations.

Naturally occurring dual gas exchangers can be found among lower vertebrates, but they are rare among mammals and birds; two notable exceptions, the neonatal marsupial and the avian embryo at term, offer additional experimental opportunities to explore the relationship between pulmonary convection and metabolic rate during the early developmental processes.

Marsupial neonates are born at a very early stage of development, being the most altricial of all mammals (10). Some of them are born after < 2 weeks of gestation, with body weights 10–100 times smaller than that of a newborn mouse! In addition to the lungs, these animals rely heavily on the skin for gas exchange, while the respiratory apparatus is quite inefficient (61,62).

In the tammar wallaby (birth weight $\sim 450\,mg$), the skin accounts for $\sim 30\%$ of total $\dot{V}_{O_2}$ on the day of birth, and its contribution to total gas exchange remains significant for the first few postnatal days. During this time, $\dot{V}_E$ was found to be proportional to total $\dot{V}_{O_2}$, not to the gas exchange of the lungs or skin separately considered. This observation led to the conclusion that even at such early stages of development in mammals the mechanisms coupling $\dot{V}_E$ to the whole body metabolism were already operational, and that total $\dot{V}_{O_2}$ was the relevant parameter setting the $\dot{V}_E$ level (62,63).

A different conclusion, however, emerged from experiments in the neonatal dunnart, in which changes in whole-body metabolic rate were provoked by changes in temperature. The Julia Creek dunnart is a marsupial born with a body weight of only $\sim 15\,mg$, with the skin contributing almost the entirety of the body gaseous exchange for several days (61). In experiments performed at ~ 2–3 weeks postnatally (64), when the skin provided $\sim 1/3$ of total $\dot{V}_{O_2}$, a drop in Ta from 36 to 32°C greatly decreased both skin and lung $\dot{V}_{O_2}$, but had only a minor effect on $\dot{V}_E$. Only with more severe cooling did all parameters decline together, a result predictable from the Q_{10} effect on biological reactions.

In the chick embryo, the lungs become a functional gas exchange organ as soon as the embryo pierces into the air cell at the blunted end of the egg, and at this stage some aspects of its regulation of breathing resemble those of the neonatal mammal. Hence, during the last day of incubation the embryo has a double route for gas exchange, one provided by the chorioallantoic membrane and the other by the lungs. Over the last 24–36 h of incubation, the gas exchange function of the chorioallantoic membrane gradually declines, as that of the lungs increases its relative importance. During all this time, an experimental increase in T resulted in increases of both total gas exchange and $\dot{V}_E$. However, the increase in $\dot{V}_E$ was less than that of *total* $\dot{V}_{O_2}$; rather, it was proportional to *pulmonary* $\dot{V}_{O_2}$ (Fig. 9). Hence, in line with the majority of the observations just summarized, the observations in the chick embryo also imply that the $\dot{V}_E$ control mechanisms are linked to peripheral cellular needs not via neural or humoral information, but via the gaseous component of tissue metabolism. Yet, how the mechanisms setting $\dot{V}_E$ are sensing the level of gaseous metabolism remains mysterious. The peripheral receptors could be involved by sensing $PaCO_2$, but the close proportionality between $\dot{V}_E$ and $\dot{V}_{O_2}$ or $\dot{V}_{CO_2}$ would imply a very high gain of the $\dot{V}_E$ response to CO_2, and this is not what emerged from some experiments on the avian embryo's peripheral chemosensitivity (Menna and Mortola, unpublished measurements).

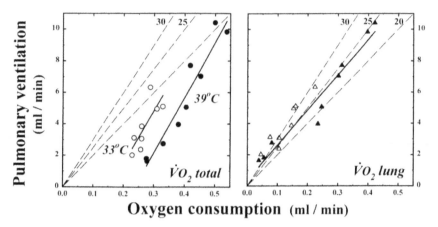

Figure 9 Chick embryos during the last 36 h of incubation. Pulmonary ventilation is plotted against oxygen consumption ($\dot{V}_{O_2}$) of the whole embryo ($\dot{V}_{O_2}$ total, left panel), or against the component of $\dot{V}_{O_2}$ exchanged through the lungs ($\dot{V}_{O_2}$ lung, right panel), at 33°C (open symbols) and at 39°C (filled symbols). Dashed lines join constant $\dot{V}_E / \dot{V}_{O_2}$, of the values indicated. Continuous lines are the linear regressions through the data points. An increase in temperature provoked an increase in $\dot{V}_{O_2}$ total disproportionately greater than the increase in $\dot{V}_E$, which, on the contrary, had a unique relationship with $\dot{V}_{O_2}$ lung. (From Ref. 65.)

IX. Summary and Concluding Remarks

Does pulmonary ventilation track the changes in metabolic rate in newborns? The question seems not to have a unique answer. In fact, from the information in our hands and summarized in the previous sections, the answer would seem to be *yes* or *no*, depending on the experimental conditions (Table 1). In reality, a closer scrutiny reveals that the $\dot{V}_E - \dot{V}_{O_2}$ relationship breaks down when Ta changes, i.e., when the respiratory system is engaged as an effector organ for thermoregulation. Because in newborns the mechanisms for the control of heat loss are less effective than in adults, as indicated by the narrow thermoneutral range, the possibility of $\dot{V}_E$ becoming a means for heat control is a more likely event than it is in adults. When this happens, the only option for a coexistent homeostasis of blood gases is left to the flexibility of the dead space, which permits a dissociation between $\dot{V}_E$ and $\dot{V}_A$. Some adult mammals are capable of varying the dead space in order to fulfill thermoregulatory tasks with the respiratory system without seriously compromising blood gas homeostasis (5); to what extent this strategy is used in the neonatal period has not been the object of specific studies.

Adult mammals, by use of all their mechanisms of thermoregulation, maintain homeothermy, and Tb changes only in extreme conditions. Newborns,

Table 1 In Newborns, Are Changes in Gas Convection Proportional to Those of Metabolic Rate?

Conditions	Answer	Section
Normoxia, among species	Yes	III
Normoxia, during growth and aging	Probably No ($\dot{V}_E/\dot{V}_{O_2}$ is lower when $\dot{V}_{O_2}$ is higher)	IV
Normoxia, during circadian oscillations	Yes	V
Normoxia, during cold exposure	Yes, when Tb is maintained No, when Tb decreases ($\dot{V}_E/\dot{V}_{O_2}$ decreases at low Ta, presumably for heat conservation)	VI.A
Normoxia, during heat exposure	No ($\dot{V}_E/\dot{V}_{O_2}$ increases with the increase in Ta, presumably for heat loss)	VI.B
Hyperoxia, compared to normoxia	Variable $\dot{V}_E/\dot{V}_{O_2}$ responses	VII.A
Hypoxia, during circadian oscillations	Yes	V
Hypoxia, among species	Yes (although, large variability)	VII.B
Hypoxia, during growth and aging	Yes	VII.B
Hypoxia, during cold exposure	Yes	VII.B
Hypoxia, during heat exposure	No ($\dot{V}_E/\dot{V}_{O_2}$ increases with the increase in Ta, presumably for heat loss)	VII.B

on the contrary, are far less capable of protecting Tb, especially in hypoxia (1). The lax homeothermy, the limited thermogenesis, and the propensity for hypometabolism of many newborn mammals represent a pattern quite reminiscent of the ectothermic behavior of lower vertebrates. In ectothermic animals, a decrease in Ta is often accompanied by an increase in $\dot{V}_E/\dot{V}_{O_2}$, while the opposite occurs when Ta increases (5). These responses are considered appropriate for the constancy of protein functions. In fact, the pH of electrochemical neutrality varies inversely with temperature, and the maintenance of the net charge of proteins requires a change in blood pH to meet electrochemical balance. Specifically, alpha-stat regulation, which refers to the control of the fractional dissociation ratio (termed alpha) of the imidazole group of the amino acid histidine (alpha-stat regulation) (7), implies changes in pH inversely with temperature; adjustments in the relationship between ventilation and metabolism (namely $\dot{V}_A/\dot{V}_{CO_2}$) are a particularly suitable means to achieve it. Therefore, one could ask whether or not also the newborn mammal, like the ectotherms, may adopt alpha-stat regulation, in place of pH stability, and adjust the ventilation metabolism ratio to accommodate the changes in Tb. The data available do not support this possibility. For example, in newborn dogs during hypoxia (Fig. 8), the hypocapnia and alkalosis were of the same magnitude in cold and warm conditions, despite the much lower Tb in the former case; hence, there was no indication of alpha-stat regulation. Also, a decrease in Tb (such as cold exposure in normoxia) can be accompanied by a decrease in $\dot{V}_E/\dot{V}_{O_2}$ (Table 1), which is the opposite of what demanded by alphastat regulation.

In conclusion, all the evidence suggests that in newborn mammals $\dot{V}_E$ tracks metabolic rate with the priority of controlling blood gases and maintaining pH stability. These priorities can find some compromise in the control of heat loss, when respiration is used as an effector organ for thermoregulation, but they are not sacrificed for alpha-stat regulation. Hence, the newborn mammal uses survival techniques, such as hypoxic hypometabolism and hypothermia, reminiscent of the ectothermic behavior of lower vertebrates, but its control of breathing is geared for pH stability and homeothermy.

References

1. Mortola JP, Gautier H. Interaction between metabolism and ventilation: effects of respiratory gases and temperature. In: Dempsey JA, Pack AI, eds. Regulation of Breathing, Lung Biology in Health and Disease Series. New York: Marcel Dekker, 1995:1011–1064.
2. Saiki C, Mortola JP. Effect of 2,4-dinitrophenol on the hypometabolic response to hypoxia of conscious adult rats. J Appl Physiol 1997; 83:537–542.
3. Seifert EL, Mortola JP. The circadian pattern of breathing in conscious adult rats. Respir Physiol 2001; 129:297–305.
4. Dempsey JA, Forster HV, Ainsworth DM. Regulation of hyperpnea, hyperventilation, and respiratory muscle recruitment during exercise. In: Dempsey JA, Pack AI, eds. Regulation of Breathing, Lung Biology in Health and Disease Series. New York: Marcel Dekker, 1995:1065–1134.
5. Mortola JP, Frappell PB. Ventilatory responses to changes in temperature in mammals and other vertebrates. Annu Rev Physiol 2000; 62:847–874.
6. Phillipson EA, Bowes G. Control of breathing during sleep. In: Cherniack NS, Widdicombe JG, eds. Handbook of Physiology. Section 3, Respiration. Vol II, Control of Breathing. Bethesda, MD: American Physiological Society, 1986:649–689.
7. Reeves RB. The interaction of body temperature and acid-base balance in ectothermic vertebrates. Annu Rev Physiol 1977; 39:559–586.
8. Nattie EE. The alphastat hypothesis in respiratory control and acid-base balance. J Appl Physiol 1990; 69:1201–1207.

9. Jennings DB. Breathing for protein function and [H^+]homeostasis. Respir Physiol 1993; 93:1–12.

10. Mortola JP. Respiratory Physiology of Newborn Mammals. A Comparative Perspective. Baltimore: Johns Hopkins University Press, 2001.

11. Blanco E, Dawes GS, Hanson MA, McCooke HB. The response to hypoxia of arterial chemoreceptors in fetal sheep and new-born lambs. J Physiol (Lond) 1984; 351:25–37.

12. Carroll JL, Bamford OS, Fitzgerald RS. Postnatal maturation of carotid chemoreceptor responses to O_2 and CO_2 in the cat. J Appl Physiol 1993; 75:2383–2391.

13. Bamford OS, Sterni LM, Wasicko MJ, Montrose MH, Carroll JL. Postnatal maturation of carotid body and type I cell chemoreception in the rat. Am J Physiol 1999; 276:L875–L884.

14. Mulligan EM. Discharge properties of the carotid bodies. Developmental aspects. In: Haddad GG, Farber JP, eds. Developmental Neurobiology of Breathing, Lung Biology in Health and Disease Series. New York: Marcel Dekker, 1991:321–340.

15. Mortola JP. Ventilatory responses to hypoxia in mammals. In: Haddad GG, Lister G, eds. Tissue Oxygen Deprivation. From Molecular to Integrated Function, Lung Biology in Health and Disease Series. New York: Marcel Dekker, 1996:433–477.

16. Mortola JP, Saiki C. Ventilatory response to hypoxia in rats: gender differences. Respir Physiol 1996; 106:21–34.

17. Mumm B, Kaul R, Heldmaier G, Schmidt I. Endogenous 24-hour cycle of core temperature and oxygen consumption in week-old Zucker rat pups. J Comp Physiol B 1989; 159:569–575.

18. Redlin U, Nuesslein B, Schmidt I. Circadian changes of brown adipose tissue thermogenesis in juvenile rats. Am J Physiol 1992; 262:R504–R508.

19. Spiers DE. Nocturnal shifts in thermal and metabolic responses of the immature rat. J Appl Physiol 1988; 64:2119–2124.

20. Kittrell EM, Satinoff E. Development of the circadian rhythm of body temperature in rats. Physiol Behav 1986; 38:99–104.

21. Nuesslein B, Schmidt I. Development of circadian cycle of core temperature in juvenile rats. Am J Physiol 1990; 259:R270–R276.

22. Seifert EL, Mortola JP. Light-dark differences in the effects of ambient temperature on gaseous metabolism in newborn rats. J Appl Physiol 2000; 88:1853–1858.

23. Saiki C, Mortola JP. Hypoxia abolishes the morning-night differences of metabolism and ventilation in 6-day-old rats. Can J Physiol Pharmacol 1995; 73:159–164.

24. Peever JH, Stephenson R. Day-night differences in the respiratory response to hypercapnia in awake adult rats. Respir Physiol 1997; 109:241–248.

25. Seifert EL, Mortola JP. Circadian pattern of ventilation during acute and chronic hypercapnia in conscious adult rats. Am J Physiol 2002; 282:R244–R251.

26. Seifert EL, Mortola JP. Ventilatory and metabolic responses to hypoxia during the light and dark phases of the day (abstract). FASEB J 2001; 15:A97.

27. Andrews DC, Symonds ME, Johnson P. Thermoregulation and the control of breathing during non-REM sleep in the developing lamb. J Dev Physiol 1991; 16:27–36.

28. Sidi D, Kuipers JRG, Heymann MA, Rudolph AM. Effects of ambient temperature on oxygen consumption and the circulation in newborn lambs at rest and during hypoxemia. Pediatr Res 1983; 17:254–258.
29. Rohlicek CV, Saiki C, Matsuoka T, Mortola JP. Oxygen transport in conscious newborn dogs during hypoxic hypometabolism. J Appl Physiol 1998; 84:763–768.
30. Merazzi D, Mortola JP. Effects of changes in ambient temperature on the Hering-Breuer reflex of the conscious newborn rat. Pediatr Res 1999; 45:370–376.
31. Cameron YL, Merazzi D, Mortola JP. Variability of the breathing pattern in newborn rats: effects of ambient temperature in normoxia or hypoxia. Pediatr Res 2000; 47:813–818.
32. Gautier H. Interactions among metabolic rate, hypoxia, and control of breathing. J Appl Physiol 1996; 81:521–527.
33. Saiki C, Mortola JP. Effect of CO_2 on the metabolic and ventilatory responses to ambient temperature in conscious adult and newborn rats. J Physiol (Lond) 1996; 491:261–269.
34. Riesenfeld T, Hammarlund K, Sedin G. Influence of radiant heat stress on respiratory water loss in newborn lambs. Biol Neonate 1988; 53:290–294.
35. Riesenfeld T, Hammarlund K, Sedin G. The effect of a warm environment on respiratory water loss in fullterm newborn infants on their first day after birth. Acta Pediatr Scand 1990; 79:893–898.
36. Sulyok E, Jequier E, Prod'hom LS. Thermal balance of the newborn infant in a heat-gaining environment. Pediatr Res 1973; 7:888–900.
37. Sulyok E, Jequier E, Prod'hom LS. Respiratory contribution to the thermal balance of the newborn infant under various ambient conditions. Pediatrics 1973; 51:641–650.
38. Bader D, Tirosh E, Hodgins H, Abend M, Cohen A. Effect of increased environmental temperature on breathing patterns in preterm and term infants. J Perinatol 1998; 18:5–8.
39. Várnai I, Farkas M, Donhoffer S. Thermoregulatory effects of hypercapnia in the newborn rat. Comparison with the effect of hypoxia. Acta Physiol Ac Sci Hung 1970; 38:225–235.
40. Mortola JP, Lanthier C. The ventilatory and metabolic response to hypercapnia in newborn mammalian species. Respir Physiol 1996; 103:263–270.
41. Cross KW, Oppé TE. The effect of inhalation of high and low concentration of oxygen on the respiration of the premature infant. J Physiol (Lond) 1952; 117:38–55.
42. Cross KW, Warner P. The effect of inhalation of high and low oxygen concentrations on the respiration of the newborn infant. J Physiol (Lond) 1951; 114:283–295.
43. Graham BD, Reardson HS, Wilson JL, Tsao MU, Baumann ML. Physiologic and chemical response of premature infants to oxygen-enriched atmosphere. Pediatrics 1950; 6:55–71.
44. Rigatto H, Brady JP. Periodic breathing and apnea in preterm infants. II. Hypoxia as a primary event. Pediatrics 1972; 50:219–227.
45. Davi M, Sankaran K, Rigatto H. Effect of inhaling 100% O_2 on ventilation and acid-base balance in cerebrospinal fluid of neonates. Biol Neonate 1980; 38:85–89.

46. Mortola JP, Frappell PB, Dotta A, Matsuoka T, Fox G, Weeks S, Mayer D. Ventilatory and metabolic responses to acute hyperoxia in newborns. Am Rev Respir Dis 1992; 146:11–15.

47. Mortola JP, Frappell PB, Frappell DE, Villena-Cabrera N, Villena-Cabrera M, Peña F. Ventilation and gaseous metabolism in infants born at high altitude, and their responses to hyperoxia. Am Rev Respir Dis 1992; 146:1206–1209.

48. Mortola JP, Tenney SM. Effects of hyperoxia on ventilatory and metabolic rates of newborn mice. Respir Physiol 1986; 63:267–274.

49. Miller MJ, Tenney SM. Hyperoxic hyperventilation in carotid-deafferented cats. Respir Physiol 1975; 25:23–30.

50. Trippenbach T. Ventilatory and metabolic effects of repeated hypoxia in conscious newborn rabbits. Am J Physiol 1994; 266:R1584–R1590.

51. Mortola JP, Rezzonico R, Lanthier C. Ventilation and oxygen consumption during acute hypoxia in newborn mammals: a comparative analysis. Respir Physiol 1989; 78:31–43.

52. Frappell P, Lanthier C, Baudinette RV, Mortola JP. Metabolism and ventilation in acute hypoxia: a comparative analysis in small mammalian species. Am J Physiol 1992; 262:R1040–R1046.

53. Mortola JP. How newborn mammals cope with hypoxia. Respir Physiol 1999; 116:95–103.

54. Tatsumi K, Hannhart B, Moore L. Influence of sex steroids on ventilation and ventilatory control. In: Dempsey JA, Pack AI, eds. Regulation of Breathing, Lung Biology in Health and Disease Series. New York: Marcel Dekker, 1995:829–864.

55. Pedraz C, Mortola JP. CO_2 production, body temperature and ventilation in hypoxic newborn cats and dogs before and after body warming. Pediatr Res 1991; 30:165–169.

56. Rohlicek CV, Saiki C, Matsuoka T, Mortola JP. Cardiovascular and respiratory consequences of body warming during hypoxia in conscious newborn cats. Pediatr Res 1996; 40:1–5.

57. Kuipers IM, Maertzdorf WJ, Keunen H, De Jong DS, Hanson MA, Blanco CE. Fetal breathing is not initiated after cord occlusion in the unanaesthetized fetal lamb in utero. J Dev Physiol 1992; 17:233–240.

58. Kuipers IM, Maertzdorf WJ, De Jong DS, Hanson MA, Blanco CE. Initiation and maintenance of continuous breathing at birth. Pediatr Res 1997; 42:63–168.

59. Kozuma S, Hidenori N, Unno N, Kagawa H, Kikuchi A, Fujii T, Baba K, Okai T, Kuwabara Y, Taketani Y. Goat fetuses disconnected from the placenta, but reconnected to an artificial placenta, display intermittent breathing movements. Biol Neonate 1999; 75:388–397.

60. Phillipson EA, Duffin J, Cooper JD. Critical dependence of respiratory rhythmicity on metabolic CO_2 load. J Appl Physiol 1981; 50:45–54.

61. Mortola JP, Frappell PB, Woolley PA. Breathing through skin in a new-born mammal. Nature 1999; 397:660.

62. MacFarlane PM, Frappell PB, Mortola JP. Mechanics of the respiratory system in the newborn tammar wallaby. J Exp Biol 2002; 205:533–538.

63. MacFarlane PM, Frappell PB. Convection requirement is established by total metabolic rate in the newborn tammar wallaby. Respir Physiol 2001; 126:221–231.
64. Frappell PB, Mortola JP. Respiratory function in a newborn marsupial with skin gas exchange. Respir Physiol 2000; 120:35–45.
65. Menna TM, Mortola JP. Metabolic control of pulmonary ventilation in the developing chick embryo. Respir Physiol 2002; 130:43–55.

8

Respiratory Control Disorders
An Overview

OOMMEN P. MATHEW

Brody School of Medicine at East Carolina University
Greenville, North Carolina, U.S.A.

I. Introduction

Respiratory control is complex. Our current understanding of the generation and execution of this vital function, especially in the neonate, is fragmentary at best. Generation of respiratory rhythm from a developmental perspective is addressed in Chapter 1. This rhythm, generated by the central pattern generators located in the brainstem, is continuously modified by proprioceptive and chemical feedback mechanisms. In addition to these involuntary components, higher centers provide a source for voluntary control of respiration. These involuntary and voluntary feedback loops and their impacts on rhythm generation are discussed in greater detail in preceding chapters.

II. Respiratory Control Disorders

The neural signal for breathing is converted into the motor act of breathing, the final step in this sequence, by the respiratory muscles. Adequacy of this respiratory output is reflected in the arterial blood gases, which in turn are determined by alveolar ventilation and metabolism. Although global changes in the normal and diseased lungs can be assessed by blood gas, it lacks the ability to assess regional variations that may be important in understanding and treating the disease process. Abnormalities can occur anywhere in this chain, resulting in respiratory failure. The causes of respiratory failure in the neonate are summarized in Table 1. Of course, most cases of respiratory failure, both acute and chronic, are not the result of primary respiratory control abnormalities. They are often caused by diseases, which can be classified as obstructive or restrictive respiratory diseases. Respiratory distress syndrome, pneumonia, pulmonary edema, and airway obstruction account for the majority of these diseases. Respiratory failure may be de novo or a complication of a chronic respiratory

Table 1   Causes of Respiratory Failure in the Newborn

Central nervous system disorders
  Immaturity
  Depression
  Infection
  Associated with malformation
    Chiari malformation
    Dandy-Walker malformation
    Möbius syndrome
  Associated with genetic syndrome
    Congenital central hypoventilation syndrome
    Joubert's syndrome
  Miscellaneous
    Respiratory flutter
Peripheral nervous system disorders
  Agenesis or injury to phrenic nerve
  Diseases or injury to spinal cord
    Birth trauma to spinal cord
    Anterior horn cell diseases
  Neuromuscular disorders
    Myasthenia gravis
    Congenital myotonic dystrophy
    Congenital myopathies
Chest wall disorders
  Skeletal dysplasia
    Asphyxiating thoracic dystrophy
  Severe kyphoscoliosis
Diseases of the lung and airways
  Obstructive respiratory diseases
  Restrictive respiratory diseases

---

disease (such as bronchopulmonary dysplasia) due to an intercurrent illness. Nevertheless, changes in respiratory control occur secondarily, and they are addressed in more detail in Chapters 20 and 21.

The most common respiratory control disorder in the neonate is apnea of prematurity. It is the focus of several chapters to follow. Other respiratory control disorders are quite rare. Central nervous system causes of apnea are listed in Table 2. Some of the respiratory control changes are very transient and usually of little clinical consequence. Yet, better understanding of these events may provide unique insights into respiratory control. For example, both sighs and hiccups are far more frequent in the neonate than in the older child or adult (1,2). Activities of both diaphragm and upper-airway muscles (genioglossus and posterior cricoary-tenoid) are increased concurrently during sighs (3), resulting in 2–3 times the normal tidal volume. On the other hand, the diaphragmatic contraction during hiccup generates an even larger negative intrapleural pressure, and yet very little air enters the lungs (2). The lack of airflow during this brief, powerful diaphragm contraction is the result of upper-airway obstruction. During a typical hiccup spell, which lasts several minutes, nonintubated newborn infants may develop hypoxia, hypercarbia, and acidosis due to hypoventilation, whereas in intubated infants hyperventilation ensues (2). Upper-airway obstruction during diaphragmatic pacing (in the absence of a tracheotomy) has a similar basis. The activation of diaphragm during gasping is similar to hiccup in some respects (e.g., duration of activation, time to peak activity); however, concurrent increased activation of upper-airway muscles keeps the airway open facilitating autoresuscitation (4).

Cry is an involuntary, reflexive modification of respiration. This is often the way respirations begin in the delivery room. Until vocalization becomes an integral part of our life, cry is one common way we express our displeasure. A disorder that illustrates this aspect of respiratory control is breath-holding spells. It is an involuntary, reflexic, nonepileptogenic paroxysmal phenomenon that is not uncommon in childhood. This stereotypical behavior is often precipitated by anger, fear, pain, or frustration, and can result in loss of consciousness. An

Table 2 CNS Causes of Apnea in the Neonatal Period

Apnea of prematurity	Malformation
Depression	Tumors
Sedatives	Seizures
Narcotics	Hemorrhage
Hypoxia	Infarction
Infection	Hydrocephalus

underlying autonomic dysregulation has been implicated in the loss of consciousness (5). A positive family history is obtained in one-third of cases. An autosomal-dominant trait with reduced penetrance has been documented in some families (6). Typical color change associated with this phenomenon is pallor or cyanosis. Significant improvement in the severity and frequency of symptoms has been noted with iron therapy, even in infants without iron deficiency (7,8). Severe bradycardia may occur during spells with pallor. This group of infants with severe bradycardia have been successfully treated with pacemakers (9). Although it is not often diagnosed during the neonatal period, breath-holding spell may have its origin in the neonatal period. One large study (193 patients) reports the origin of breath-holding spells in the first month of life in 5% and in the first 2 months in 7% of patients (10).

Another related disorder, expiratory apnea, was reported by Southall and coworkers (11). It is characterized by episodes of severe hypoxemia occurring while awake in young infants after a sudden noxious stimulus. Rapid onset of severe hypoxia in these infants with expiratory apnea has been attributed to sudden right-to-left intrapulmonary shunting. This is not a benign disorder; several infants required tracheotomy. Significant mortality was observed in this group as well. A family history of breath-holding spells was present in nearly half the infants. The relationship between expiratory apnea and breath-holding spells is not entirely clear.

III. Assessment of Respiratory Control Disorders

From a conceptual framework, respiratory output can be measured anywhere along the efferent limb from the controller downward. However, some of these measurements are not feasible in the human neonate, whereas others are not practical in routine clinical practice. In the newborn infant, respiratory output has been measured at the level of the respiratory muscles, albeit primarily for research purposes. Although invasive recordings of respiratory muscles have been accomplished, surface EMG recording is typically utilized. Surface EMG of the diaphragm has been recorded in the newborn for more than two decades (12). The raw EMG signal obtained through surface electrodes is rectified and integrated to provide a quantitative measure of the respiratory output. Since this is not a standardized measurement, it has limited value in assessing adequacy of the respiratory output. However, changes in muscle activity with progressive hypercapnia, hypoxia, and respiratory loading can be evaluated in this fashion. Relative increase or decrease in activity, especially when compared to simultaneous recordings of other respiratory muscles, such as the upper-airway muscles, may provide a better understanding of respiratory control. It can also be useful in assessing the changes in respiratory output during sleep. Furthermore, spectral analysis of the raw EMG has been utilized in documenting muscle fatigue. When muscle fatigue occurs, the low-frequency component increases with a concomitant reduction in the high-frequency component, resulting in decreased high- to low-frequency ratio (13). One drawback of surface EMG is that it is often contaminated with activity from neighboring muscles.

Pressure changes produced by the respiratory muscles have been used primarily as a research tool in the neonate. Transdiaphragmatic pressure, the difference between intrathoracic and intra-abdominal pressure, is an index of force output of the diaphragm. Typically this is measured with the aid of esophageal and gastric catheters. Airway occlusion pressure is the pressure measured at the mouth during the occluded inspiratory effort. This noninvasive test is relatively easy to perform in humans. A valve on the expiratory side of the breathing circuit is occluded at end expiration. The pressure change during the first 0.1 sec of the inspiratory effort is known as the $P_{0.1}$. This index of respiratory output, first reported by Whitelaw et al. (14), is an excellent index of neural output of the respiratory center. Since no significant changes in lung volume occur during the initial phase of the first occluded breath, $P_{0.1}$ is considered to be unaffected by elastance and resistance, and is thought to be relatively insensitive to the effects of mechanical thoracopulmonary limitation. However, it may not reflect the true neural output in cases of muscle weakness or fatigue. It may also produce low values when the diaphragm is at a mechanical disadvantage, as in hyperinflation, often seen in severe chronic lung disease. Pressure generated during airway occlusion has been used to predict successful extubation in ventilator-dependent patients. Its predictive value in neonates is limited (15); still it is one of the valuable measures of neural respiratory output.

Another useful way to assess respiratory motor output is to measure ventilation, which is the product of tidal volume and frequency. Tidal volume in turn is determined by inspiratory flow and inspiratory duration. In normal subjects the mean inspiratory flow (VT/Ti) reflects inspiratory drive. Resistive and elastic loading of the lung and chest wall can alter the breathing pattern and ventilation through airway and chest wall mechanoreceptors and chemoreceptors. Maximal inspiratory pressure, maximum voluntary ventilation, and supine and sitting vital capacities have been found useful in the evaluation of conditions such as diaphragmatic paralysis in the adult. These measurements are not feasible in neonates, but maneuvers like crying vital capacity may yield useful information.

The role of routine pulmonary function testing in the evaluation of neonatal respiratory control disorders is not established. Ventilation can be measured qualitatively with thermistors or quantitatively with a pneumotach attached to the face mask. Alternatively, ventilation can be measured using nasal flow meters. This is based on the premise that neonates are preferential nose breathers. A thermistor or CO_2 monitoring device must be incorporated into the system to detect oral breathing. Alteration of the breathing pattern by the instruments used is well documented (16). One must also be very vigilant for the occurrence of leaks. A noninvasive way to measure ventilation is to use respiratory inductive plethysmography. An expandable coil is worn around the chest and abdomen. This is particularly useful to document paradoxical movement of the chest and abdomen, which is common among preterm infants. When used quantitatively, it requires careful calibration. Changes in both frequency and tidal volume can be determined from these measurements for judging adequacy of ventilation.

Chemical control of breathing is evaluated by the ventilatory responses to hypercapnia and hypoxia. Peripheral chemoreceptors sense changes in PaO_2. The carotid body plays a predominant role in this response in humans. Changes in CO_2 are sensed by central chemoreceptors located in the rostral medulla. Changes in PCO_2 and arterial pH are also sensed by the carotid body. Ventilatory response to hypoxia is unique in the newborn. This biphasic ventilatory response to hypoxia as well as the ventilatory response to hypercapnia is discussed in more detail in Chapter 5.

Another important variable in respiratory control, especially in the human neonate, is sleep. The development of sleep states and the state-dependent changes in respiratory pattern form the background to the most common respiratory control disorder in the newborn, viz: apnea of prematurity. Various aspects of this common disorder are discussed in subsequent chapters. Sleep has important implications to respiratory control in other disorders, such as chronic lung diseases and certain neurological and neuromuscular diseases. Sleep and breathing in children are the focus of a recent monograph, and several chapters in that monograph are very relevant to neonates (17). Some respiratory control abnormalities may be masked by the volitional control system and become manifest when the infant falls asleep. Congenital central hypoventilation syndrome is a typical disorder in this category.

Finally, airway protective reflexes, elicited by the inhalation or aspiration of an offending material, reflexively modify breathing pattern. One way to protect the airway is to prevent further inspiration. Invariably, maintenance of tidal ventilation is suppressed. This can be accomplished by the apneic response. Another aspect of these protective reflexes is to expel the offending agent or foreign body by coughing and other expiratory reflex. Significant maturational changes in these reflexes occur during development. One common observation is that coughing is rarely observed during intubation and suctioning in preterm and term infants during the immediate neonatal period. These maneuvers invariably elicit cough in an older infant. Irritant or rapidly adapting vagal afferents are presumed to mediate these responses. Stimulation of these endings in the premature infant may result in apnea instead (18).

IV. Summary

Understanding of respiratory control in the normal infant is a prerequisite for the diagnosis and treatment of disorders of respiratory control. This is especially true in the newborn because several aspects of normal respiratory control are unique to these infants when compared to older children or adults. Common respiratory control disorders such as apnea of prematurity are discussed in detail in subsequent chapters; insights gained from conditions such as sigh, gasp, and breath holding are briefly discussed. Assessment of respiratory control disorders includes monitoring of respiratory output under varied conditions. These include monitoring of respiratory muscle EMG, respiratory pressure and timing changes, ventilatory changes to hypoxia and hypercapnia, and state-dependent changes. In the final analysis, adequacy of respiratory control is often determined clinically on the basis of arterial blood gases or noninvasive monitoring of gas exchange with pulse oximetry and capnometry. In suspected cases, further tests may be needed to confirm these observations.

References

1. Thach BT, Taeusch HW Jr. Sighing in newborn human infants: role of inflation-augmenting reflex. J Appl Physiol 1976; 41:502–507.
2. Brouillette RT, Thach BT, Abu-Osba YK, Wilson SL. Hiccups in infants: characteristics and effects on ventilation. J Pediatr 1980; 96:219–225.
3. Van Lunteren E, Van de Graaff WB, Parker DM, et al. Activity of upper airway muscles during augmented breaths. Respir Physiol 1983; 53:87–98.
4. Mathew OP, Thach BT, Abu-Osba YK, Brouillette RT, Roberts JL. Regulation of upper airway maintaining muscles during progressive asphyxia. Pediatr Res 1984; 18:819–822.
5. DiMario FJ Jr, Burleson JA. Autonomic nervous system function in severe breath-holding spells. Pediatr Neurol 1993; 9:268–274.
6. DiMario FJ Jr, Sarfarazi M. Family pedigree analysis of children with severe breath-holding spells. J Pediatr 1997; 130:647–651.
7. Daoud AS, Batieha A, al-Sheyyab M, Abuekteish F, Hijazi S. Effectiveness of iron therapy on breath-holding spells. J Pediatr 1997; 130:547–550.
8. Mocan H, Yildiran A, Orhan F, Erduran E. Breath holding spells in 91 children and response to treatment with iron. Arch Dis Child 1999; 81:261–262.
9. Kelly AM, Porter CJ, McGoon MD, Espinosa RE, Osborn MJ, Hayes DL. Breath-holding spells associated with significant bradycardia: successful treatment with permanent pacemaker implantation. Pediatrics 2001; 108:698–702.
10. Lombroso CT, Lerman P. Breathholding spells (cyanotic and pallid infantile syncope). Pediatrics 1967; 39:563–581.
11. Southall DP, Talbert DG, Johnson P, et al. Prolonged expiratory apnoea: a disorder resulting in episodes of severe arterial hypoxaemia in infants and young children. Lancet 1985; 2:571–577.
12. Prechtl HF, Van Eykern LA, O'Brien MJ. Respiratory muscle EMG in newborns: a non-intrusive method. Early Hum Dev 1977; 1:265–283.
13. Muller N, Gulston G, Cade D, et al. Diaphragmatic muscle fatigue in the newborn. J Appl Physiol 1979; 46:688–695.

14. Whitelaw WA, Derenne JP, Milic-Emili J. Occlusion pressure as a measure of respiratory center output in conscious man. Respir Physiol 1975; 23:181–199.
15. Barrington KJ, Finer NN. A randomized, controlled trial of aminophylline in ventilatory weaning of premature infants. Crit Care Med 1993; 21:846–850.
16. Fleming PJ, Levine MR, Goncalves A. Changes in respiratory pattern resulting from the use of a facemask to record respiration in newborn infants. Pediatr Res 1982; 16:1031–1034.
17. Loughlin GM, Carroll JL Marcus CL. Sleep and Breathing in Children: A Developmental Approach. New York: Marcel Dekker, 2000.
18. Fleming PJ, Bryan AC, Bryan MH. Functional immaturity of pulmonary irritant receptors and apnea in newborn preterm infants. Pediatrics 1978; 61:515–518.

9

Monitoring in the NICU

CHRISTIAN F. POETS

University of Tübingen
Tübingen, Germany

I. Introduction

The predominant goal of monitoring is to allow for early detection of increased cardiorespiratory instability and/or potentially dangerous pathophysiology. Cardiorespiratory monitoring in the NICU largely comprises continuous surveillance of the electrocardiogram and chest wall movements, and the noninvasive determination of blood gases. This chapter will focus on a review of techniques applied to monitor these parameters, with particular emphasis on blood gas monitoring.

II. Electrocardiography (ECG) and Heart Rate Monitoring

The ECG records electrical depolarisation of the myocardium. During continuous monitoring, only heart rate can be determined with sufficient precision; any analysis of P and T waves, axis, rythm or QT times requires a printout and/or a 12-lead ECG. Heart rate monitoring is often fraught with artifacts, which may result from poor sensor contact or motion. Artifacts can be reduced by optimal positioning of electrodes (Fig. 1) and by using pregelled electrodes with skin-friendly adhesive (1,2).

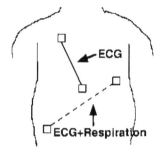

Figure 1 Schematic drawing of the optimal electrode pair location for impedance monitoring of ECG only (straight line) or both ECG and breathing movement monitoring (dashed line). (From Ref. 1.)

III. Monitoring of Chest Wall Movements

A. Impedance plethysmography

This is the technique most commonly used for monitoring chest wall movements in the NICU. It is based on the physical principle that changes in the ratio of air to fluid in the thorax, occurring during the respiratory cycle, create changes in transthoracic impedance (3). This ratio, however, is also influenced by fluctuations in blood volume occurring during the cardiac cycle and by changes in impedance at the electrode skin interface. Particularly, fluctuations in blood volume, also referred to as "cardiac artifact," may become a source of considerable interference to the breathing signal and may even result in both a failure of impedance monitors to detect apnea (4) and a misclassification of obstructive as central apneas. Artifacts can be reduced, but not completely abolished, by optimal electrode placement (Fig. 1).

B. Inductance Plethysmography

Changes in the volume of the thoracic and abdominal compartment create changes in inductance, which is registered via abdominal and thoracic bands. The sum of these changes is proportional to tidal volume, and several methods have been developed to calibrate the systems so that tidal volume can be quantified (5,6). However, this only works as long as the patient does not shift position. Thus, this technique is only of limited usefulness for tidal volume measurements in unsedated infants. Another potential advantage is that it allows for the detection of paradoxical breathing, a pattern that occurs frequently during normal infant sleep, but appears to be more prevalent in conditions associated with an increased work of breathing (e.g., upper-airway obstruction or chronic lung disease) (7).

C. Strain Gauges

These are usually made of mercury in silicon rubber and sense respiratory efforts by measuring changes in electrical resistance in response to stretching. Strain gauges are not widely used for monitoring in the NICU, and their measurements are not reproducible enough to quantitate tidal volume (8).

D. Pressure or Volume Displacement Capsules

These detect movements of an infant's diaphragm by means of an air-filled capsule that is taped to the abdomen and connected to a pressure transducer via a narrow air-filled tube. The outward movement of the abdomen during inspiration compresses the capsule to produce a positive pressure pulse that is interpreted as a breath. The technique is predominantly used in apnea monitors and trigger devices for infant ventilators, not for ICU monitoring; it is also not suitable for quantifying tidal volume (9).

In a study comparing the ability of impedance and inductance plethysmography to detect apneas, the overall reliability of both systems was good. The impedance system, however, failed in three specific situations: [1] obstructed breaths were consistently misinterpreted as breaths; [2] cardiac artifact caused false breath detection in 11 of 29 studies; and [3] the first 1–2 breaths following a sigh were often missed owing to the impedance signal going off scale (10). Another study compared the pressure capsule with an impedance monitor and found a lower specificity, but a higher sensitivity, of the capsule for the detection of apneas (11). Thus, impedance appears less reliable than inductance plethysmography and possibly also less sensitive than abdominal pressure plethysmography for apnea detection.

IV. Transcutaneous Partial Pressure of Oxygen (PTcO₂) Monitoring

A. Principle of Operation

$PTcO_2$ electrodes measure the partial pressure of oxygen through the skin. They consist of a platinum cathode and silver reference anode, encased in an electrolyte solution and separated from the skin by an O_2-permeable membrane. Electrodes are heated to improve oxygen diffusion and to arterialize the capillary blood. Oxygen is reduced at the cathode, generating an electric current proportional to the O_2 concentration in the capillary bed underneath the sensor. Sensors require a 10–15 min warmup period after application and have to be calibrated once every 4–8 hours. Probably because they are somewhat cumbersome to use (see below), most American NICUs have abandoned these devices, but they are widely used in Europe.

B. Factors Influencing Measurements

The agreement between arterial and skin surface PO_2 depends on a fragile balance between factors that increase the PO_2, namely a shift to the right of the oxygen dissociation curve and a decreased O_2 solubility in blood, both of which are caused by the heating of the skin, and factors which decrease the PO_2, namely the oxygen consumption in the heated skin and inside the electrode (12).

Sensor Temperature

There is good agreement with arterial PO_2 (PaO_2) only at 44°C, but then frequent (every 2–4 hours) resiting is necessary. At lower sensor temperatures, $PTcO_2$ will underread PaO_2, with the difference becoming larger with increasing PaO_2 (13). This is particularly important in preterm neonates, in whom high PaO_2 levels must be reliably detected to minimize the risk of retinopathy of prematurity.

Probe Placement

$PTcO_2$ will underread PaO_2 if the sensor is placed on a bony surface, if pressure is applied on the sensor, or if too much contact gel is used. With patent ductus arteriosus and right-to-left shunt, $PTcO_2$ will be higher on the upper than on the lower half of the thorax (14).

Peripheral Perfusion

$PTcO_2$ depends on skin perfusion. If the latter is reduced, e.g., owing to hypotension, anemia, acidosis (pH <7.05), hypothermia, or marked skin edema, $PTcO_2$ will be falsely low. If an underreading of PaO_2 occurs, it is advisable to check the patient for these conditions (15,16).

Skin Thickness

Close agreement with PaO_2 can only be found in neonates. This does not imply, however, that PTcO2 monitors can only be used in this age group. Studies in children and adults did in fact show that the ratio between $PTcO_2$ and PaO_2 is extremely constant in these patients (independent of age and PaO_2); it merely is 20% lower than in neonates, i.e., ~0.8 (17–19).

Response Times

In vitro response time (90% response to a sudden change in PO_2 from 19 to 0 kPa) is ~8 sec (20). The median in vivo response time (interval between oxygen saturation measured by pulse oximetry (SPO_2) falling to 60% and $PTcO_2$ reaching 2.7 kPa) was 16 sec in one study (21).

C. Detection of Hypoxemia and Hyperoxemia

Under optimal measurement conditions (sensor temperature $\geq 44°C$, hemodynamically stable preterm neonates, $PaO_2 < 13\,kPa$), $PTcO_2$ can be expected to be within $\pm 1.3–2.0\,kPa$ of PaO_2 95% of the time (22,23). Clinically, however, it seems more important to know whether the $PTcO_2$ monitor will reliably detect all situations where a patient has either too little or too much oxygen. Unfortunately, there is as yet no clear definition of what constitutes a dangerously high or low level of oxygenation. Most investigators defined hypoxemia as a $PaO_2 < 6.7\,kPa$ or as an $SaO_2 < 80\%$, and hyperoxemia as a $PaO_2 > 11–13\,kPa$ (24–28), but it should be born in mind that these thresholds were chosen rather arbitrarily. Whatever the ideal threshold, the data available suggest that $\sim15\%$ of both hypoxemic and hyperoxemic instances are missed by $PTcO_2$ monitors, whereas their specificity, particularly with regard to hypoxemia, is somewhat higher (23–31).

V. Pulse Oximetry (SPO₂)

A. Principle of Operation

Pulse oximeters, unlike $PTcO_2$ monitors, do not measure the concentration of oxygen that is dissolved in plasma, but the proportion of hemoglobin molecules in the arterial blood which are loaded with oxygen. Deoxygenated hemoglobin absorbs more light in the red band (at 600–750 nm), i.e., it looks less red, whereas oxygenated hemoglobin absorbs more light in the infrared band (850–1000 nm). The ratio of the absorbance of red and infrared light sent through a tissue correlates with the proportion of oxygenated to deoxygenated hemoglobin in the tissue. Conventional pulse oximeters determine the arterial component within this absorbance by identifying the peaks and troughs in the absorbance over time, thereby obtaining a "pulse-added" absorbance that is independent of the absorbance characteristics of the nonpulsating parts of the tissue. These pulse-added light absorbances are then associated algorithmically with empirically determined arterial oxygen saturation (SaO_2) values (12).

Next-generation instruments use additional and/or different techniques. For example, the Signal Extraction Technology (Masimo, Irvine, CA) scans through all red-to-infrared ratios (and corresponding SPO_2 values) found in the tissue, determines the intensity of these and chooses the right-most peak of these intensities, which will correspond to the absorbance by the arterial blood in the tissue. It also uses frequency analysis, time domain analysis, and adaptive filtering to establish a "noise reference" in the detected physiological signal (32), thereby improving the ability to separate between signal and noise (see below). Other next-generation instruments use differential signal amplification to achieve this goal.

B. Factors Influencing Measurements

Pulse oximeters are easier to use than $PTcO_2$ monitors: they do not require calibration or heating of the skin, and they provide immediate information about arterial oxygenation. However, it is probably because of this apparent ease of use that potentially erroneous measurements on a pulse oximeter are more at risk of being overlooked than those occurring with a $PTcO_2$ monitor. A thorough understanding of the factors potentially affecting the precision of a pulse oximeter is therefore particularly important (12).

Probe Placement

The light-receiving diode must be placed exactly opposite the emitting diode, and both must be shielded against ambient light and not be applied with too much pressure. Light bypassing the tissue can cause both falsely high and falsely low values. The sensor site must be checked every 6–8 hours. It was recently shown that 42% of nurses in a neonatal intermediate-care nursery exceeded a pressure on the skin of 50 mm Hg during fixation of a pulse oximeter sensor (33). Such high pressures may result in a reduced signal-to-noise ratio and may thus severely impair the precision of the SPO_2 measurements (33). Highly flexible sensors provide better skin contact and thus better signal-to-noise ratio.

Peripheral Perfusion

Conventional oximeters require a pulse pressure >20 mm Hg or a systolic blood pressure >30 mm Hg to operate reliably (34). Because next-generation oximeters rely less on pulse detection, they continue to operate even at lower blood pressure levels (35).

Response Times

In theory, the response time of a pulse oximeter to a sudden fall in oxygen levels, e.g., during an apnea, depends only on the time it takes for the blood to travel from the lung to the sensor site, which, if the sensor is placed around a toe, is ~4 sec in neonates (36). However, all pulse oximeters currently available average their values over periods of time varying from 2 to 15 sec or from 4 to 32 heart beats in order to level-out any erroneous measurement which may occasionally occur even under optimal conditions. This averaging, however, has unwanted consequences:

1. It delays the response to a true fall in SPO_2 values.
2. It may lead to a mixing up of true with falsely low SPO_2 readings during periods of intermittent body movements (e.g., during feeding), which can result in the erroneous impression that the patient suffers

episodes of prolonged hypoxemia. Such erroneous readings may be indistinguishable from those where the patient is truly hypoxemic, particularly if the light plethysmographic (pulse) waveforms are not available for analysis of the signal quality.

3. The use of an averaging mode can lead to erroneous conclusions in situations where a precise measurement of SPO_2 is required, e.g., during sleep studies.

4. The averaging of SPO_2 values makes it almost impossible to define normal ranges for the frequency and severity of intermittent falls in SPO_2 in infants or children, since such data would only be valid for the specific averaging mode with which they have been obtained. This is particularly true for the next-generation instruments, which use variable averaging times depending on measurement conditions, i.e., 2–4 sec averaging under optimal conditions, and up to 15 sec averaging during periods of motion.

Motion Artifact

The pulsatile (=arterial) component contributes only ~1% to the total absorbance measured by the pulse oximeter (37). Hence, at least conventional pulse oximetry is very sensitive to sudden changes in background signal, e.g., due to body movements. As already mentioned, next-generation instruments use various techniques to identify and read through periods with low signal-to-noise ratios as there are during motion. This resulted in a dramatic (>90%) decrease in false-alarm rates (38,39). However, some of these improvements in false-alarm rates were apparently achieved at the expense of not identifying true desaturation during motion (40), which is unacceptable. Thus, each next-generation pulse oximeter should be tested for its reliability in detecting desaturations during motion before recommending it for use in unsedated patients, particularly infants.

With conventional oximeters, it is important to identify whether or not a reading may have been affected by motion artifact. This can be best achieved if the light plethysmographic waveforms from which the SPO_2 measurements were derived are displayed. Whenever these waveforms are distorted, SPO_2 readings become unreliable. An alternative way is to compare the pulse rate from the oximeter with the heart rate from an ECG monitor, which should be identical (41). Without these validation measures, readings from these instruments cannot be interpreted.

For next-generation instruments, which are less reliant on a clean peak-and-trough detection and thus an undisturbed pulse waveform, there is currently no independently validated method to identify periods of poor measurement conditions and thus potentially unreliable SPO_2 readings. An interesting approach in this regard is the signal quality indicator developed by Masimo ("signal IQ"). In a preliminary evaluation of this tool, involving manual analysis of raw red-to-infrared absorption curves during 223 falls in SPO_2 to <85% in nine preterm infants, we recently found that below a signal IQ of 0.3, which is the threshold suggested by the manufacturer to indicate poor measurement conditions, the likelihood of artifactual measurements was indeed high (6/8, or 75%), whereas above this value, erroneous measurements were not observed (42).

Other Hemoglobins and Pigments

Methemoglobin (MetHb) will cause SPO_2 readings to tend toward 85%, independent of SaO_2. Carboxyhemoglobin (COHb) will cause overestimation of SaO_2 by 1% for each percent COHb in the blood (43). Fetal hemoglobin (HbF) and bilirubin do not affect pulse oximeters, but may lead to an underestimation of SaO_2 by co-oximeters (44). In patients with dark skin, SPO_2 values may be falsely high, particularly during hypoxemia (45,46).

Algorithms

Pulse oximeters, in contrast to co-oximeters, do not *measure* O_2 saturation, but derive their values from a "look-up" table which is based on empirical data from healthy adults. These may vary between brands and even between different software versions from the same manufacturer. Also, some instruments subtract a priori the typical levels of COHb, MetHb, etc. in healthy nonsmoking adults from their measurements and will thus display SPO_2 values that are some 2–3% lower than those displayed by other instruments. This approach, i.e., to display the so-called *fractional* SPO_2 instead of the usual *functional* SPO_2, has been largely abandoned in recent years, probably because it resulted in an unacceptably poor ability of instruments using this approach to detect hyperoxemia (47).

C. Detection of Hypoxemia and Hyperoxemia

In the absence of motion, pulse oximeters have both a high sensitivity and a high specificity for the detection of hypoxemia ($SaO_2 < 80\%$), although they tend to overestimate SaO_2 during extreme hypoxemia ($SaO_2 < 70\%$) (48,49). Because of the shape of the O_2 dissociation curve, however, they are less well suited for detecting hyperoxemia. The upper alarm limits that have to be chosen on individual instrument brands to avoid hyperoxemia reliably range from 88% to 95% (47,50,51). An upper alarm limit of 95% was recently confirmed for three next-generation instruments (Agilent Viridia, Böblingen, Germany; Masimo SET, Nellcor Oxismart, Pleasanton, CA) (52). The reliability in detecting PaO_2 values >80 mm Hg via noninvasive monitoring can likely be increased if both SPO_2 and $PTcO_2$ are monitored.

VI. Transcutaneous Partial Pressure of Carbon Dioxide (PTcCO$_2$) Monitoring

A. Principle of Operation

The PTcCO$_2$ sensor consists of a pH-sensing glass electrode and a silver–silver chloride reference electrode, covered by a hydrophobic CO$_2$-permeable membrane from which they are separated by a sodium bicarbonate–electrolyte solution. As CO$_2$ diffuses across the membrane, there is a pH change of the electrolyte solution (CO$_2$ + H$_2$O/HCO$_3^-$ + H$^+$), which is sensed by the glass electrode. All instruments have built-in correction factors because their uncorrected measurements will be some 50% higher than arterial PCO$_2$ (PaCO$_2$; see below). They must also be calibrated at regular intervals and require a 10–15 min run-in time following resiting.

B. Factors Influencing Measurements

Similar to PTcO$_2$ monitors, the correlation between PTcCO$_2$ and PaCO$_2$ depends on electrode temperature, probe placement, and peripheral perfusion, although not to the same extent as with the former type of monitor.

Sensor Temperature

The carbon dioxide tension measured at the skin will always be higher than that in the arterial blood. This difference between PTcCO$_2$ and PaCO$_2$ becomes larger with increasing sensor temperature (53). This inherent overestimation of PaCO$_2$ by the PTcCO$_2$ electrode is caused by [1] an increased CO$_2$ production resulting from an increased skin metabolism due to the heated sensor, [2] a higher CO$_2$ in the tissue than in the arterioles, [3] the anaerobic heating coefficient of blood for carbon dioxide, and [4] a countercurrent exchange in the dermal capillary loops (54). As diffusibility for CO$_2$ is greater than that for O$_2$, a good correlation between PaCO$_2$ and PTcCO$_2$ can already be obtained at an electrode temperature of 37°C (53). Nonetheless, the correlation can be significantly improved if the electrode is heated to 42°C. Further heating of the electrode seems to have no effect on the correlation between arterial and transcutaneous CO$_2$ values, although it will further increase the above-mentioned systematic overestimation of PaCO$_2$ by the PTcCO$_2$ electrode (53). Hence, if only PTcCO$_2$ is measured, the optimal sensor temperature with regard to skin irritation will be 42°C, whereas combined sensors, which contain both a PTcO$_2$ and a PTcCO$_2$ electrode, should be heated to 44°C (the optimal temperature for PTcCO$_2$ measurements), and this will not jeopardize the precision of the PTcCO$_2$ measurement (55).

Sensor Placement and Skin Thickness

$PTcCO_2$ measurements are relatively independent of sensor site or skin thickness, but $PTcCO_2$ may be falsely high if pressure is applied onto the sensor.

Peripheral Perfusion

$PTcCO_2$ monitors are comparatively independent of blood pressure, pH, and body temperature. In a study on 24 newborn infants with severe cardiocirculatory maladaptation and pH values ranging from 6.9 to 7.6, hematocrits between 0.28 and 0.65, body temperatures between 35.5 and 38.1°C, and systolic blood pressures between 15 and 70 mm Hg, no *systematic* influence of pH, hematocrit, body temperature, or systolic blood pressure on the relation between $PTcCO_2$ and $PaCO_2$ was observed (56). Nonetheless, $PTcCO_2$ may severely overestimate $PaCO_2$ if systolic blood pressure falls to <15 mm Hg (56) and/or under conditions of severe hemorrhagic shock (57). The *precision* of the $PTcCO_2$ measurement, however, may already start to be impaired if $PaCO_2$ is >6 kPa and/or if arterial pH is <7.30 (58,59).

Response Times

The 90% in vitro response time to a sudden change in $PaCO_2$ is between 30 and 50 sec (55,60). Data on the in vivo response time of $PTcCO_2$ monitors are not available.

C. Detection of Hypocarbia and Hypercarbia

Most investigators who validated $PTcCO_2$ monitors in infants and children reported that the instruments predicted $PaCO_2$ to within ±0.8–1.2 kPa 95% of the time (53,61,62). This precision is somewhat higher than that of $PTcO_2$ monitors (see above). Only two studies investigated the sensitivity and specificity of $PTcCO_2$ monitors to hypercarbia and hypocarbia. One found a sensitivity of 96% (21/22) for hypocarbia (defined as $PaCO_2 < 4.3$ kPa) and of 76% (31/42) for hypercarbia ($PaCO_2 > 6.1$ kPa); specificity was not analyzed (26). The other found a sensitivity of 72% (13/18) for hypocarbia ($PaCO_2 < 4.5$ kPa) and of 88% (58/66) for hypercarbia ($PaCO_2 > 5.6$ kPa). Specificity was 83% (151/183) and 88% (106/121), respectively (27). Thus, sensitivity and specificity of $PTcCO_2$ monitors are no better than those of $PTcO_2$ monitors.

VII. End-Tidal Carbon Dioxide (ETCO$_2$) Monitoring (Capnometry)

A. Principle of Operation

$ETCO_2$ analyzers usually operate via infrared capnometry; i.e., they are based on the principle that CO_2 absorbs light in the infrared band. An infrared beam is directed through a gas sample and the absorption of light caused by the CO_2 molecules in the sample measured. The amount of light absorbed by the sample is proportional to the concentration of CO_2 in the sample. Instruments must be calibrated at regular intervals to provide accurate measurements.

B. Factors Influencing Measurements

Gas Sampling Technique

Two approaches exist:

1. With mainstream capnometers, the CO_2 analyzer is built into an adapter which is placed in the breathing circuit. They have a fast response time (10 msec) and therefore are reliable even at high respiratory rates. Their disadvantage is that they can only be used in intubated patients and require 1–10 mL extra dead space.

2. Sidestream capnometers aspirate the expired air via a sample flow. They do not create extra dead space, but their precision is considerably lower than that of mainstream capnometers, particularly at high respiratory rates. This is because there are conflicting requirements with regard to the ideal sample flow. On the one hand, sample flow must be low to avoid dilution of expired gas by entrainment of ambient air at the sampling tube–patient interface. Such air entrainment will occur when the expired gas flow falls below the sample flow. Sample flow should also be low to avoid dispersion of the gas sample inside the sample tube due to nonlaminar flow conditions. On the other hand, sample flow must be high to achieve rapid filling and emptying, i.e., a short time constant, of the sample cell (63,64). Theoretical and practical analyses have shown that the ideal sample flow at which air entrainment is avoided while still keeping the time constant of the sample cell reasonably short is $\sim$150–200 mL/min (63,64). Even at this relatively high sample flow, some instruments start to systematically underread $ETCO_2$ if respiratory rate exceeds 30/min. This error, however, will remain clinically insignificant up to respiratory rates of 60–70/min (65).

Influence of V/Q Mismatch

$ETCO_2$ will only approximate $PaCO_2$ if [1] CO_2 equilibrium is achieved between end-capillary blood and alveolar gas, [2] $ETCO_2$ approximates the average alveolar CO_2 during a respiratory cycle, and [3] ventilation/perfusion relationships are uniform within the lung (66). These conditions are rarely achieved in patients with respiratory disorders. The reliability of an $ETCO_2$ measurement can be assessed from the expiratory signal: this must have a steep rise, a clear end-expiratory plateau, and no detectable CO_2 during inspiration (Fig. 2).

Influence of Sampling Site and Length of Tubing

The length of the tubing influences the total delay time of the capnograph and thereby the accuracy of the instruments: if total delay time exceeds respiratory cycle time, $ETCO_2$ measurements will become falsely low. The sampling tube should therefore be as short as possible. In addition, the sampling site should be as close as possible to the patient's airway. This is particularly important in sidestream instruments, where the error of the measurement can be significantly reduced if the sampling tube is moved from the proximal to the distal end of the endotracheal tube (67).

Response Times

While mainstream capnometers respond almost instantly to a change in $ETCO_2$, sidestream instruments require between 0.7 and 1.8 sec (or longer, if additional tubing is put between the patient and the sample cell) to transport the gas sample to the sample cell (68). As mentioned above, the response or delay time should be shorter than the patient's respiratory cycle time.

Calibration Errors

Most sidestream capnometers use water-permeable catheters to minimize the risk of tube blocking by airway secretions. This results in a dry gas being measured in the sample cell. The atmospheric barometric pressure compensation automatically performed by all capnometers when displaying $ETCO_2$ as a partial pressure

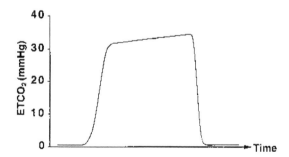

Figure 2   Normal capnogram. During initial expiration, CO_2 remains close to zero as gas from the anatomic dead space leaves the airway. CO_2 then rises sharply as alveolar gas mixes with dead space gas. The curve then levels as purely alveolar gas is exhaled (alveolar plateau). The CO_2 value at the end of this plateau represents the end-tidal PCO_2.

measurement rather than as a concentration must therefore be corrected for water vapor pressure. This is not always done by manufacturers and can lead to an overestimation of true $ETCO_2$ by 0.5–1.3 kPa (69). Users should therefore be aware whether their instrument corrects its measurements for water vapor pressure.

VIII. False Alarms in the NICU

With an increasing number of parameters being monitored, false alarms become a major burden on both patients and staff. In particular, preterm infants may respond to the noise generated by these alarms, and the subsequent interventions, with increased cardiorespiratory instability (70,71). A high rate of false alarms also carries the risk of desensitizing caregivers, potentially resulting in danger-ously long response times to true alarms (72). Thus, particular attention should be given to the question of which parameters should be monitored, which brand offers the best performance, including the lowest number of false alarms, and how alarm limits should be set.

The issue of differences in false-alarm rates between monitor brands has received surprisingly little attention, given the ubiquity of the problem. In a recent comparison of alarm rates from three widely used monitor systems (Viridia, Agilent; Kolormon, Kontron Instruments,Watford, UK [with Masimo pulse oximetry]; Solar 8000, GE Marquette, Freiburg, Germany) in a tertiary neonatal intensive care unit, there was, on average, one alarm every 9 min of monitoring (73). The median number of true alarms did not differ significantly among systems, whereas the median number of false alarms differed widely, with the Agilent system generating 32 (range 7–77) such alarms per 8 h, compared to 8 (0–19) for the Kontron and 15 (2–32) for the GE system ($P < .01$ Agilent vs. Kontron & GE; $P < .05$ Kontron vs. GE). These differences between systems were mainly due to differences in pulse oximeter and $PTcCO_2$ monitor alarm rates, each of which contributed ~40% to the total number of alarms.

Thus, there are marked differences between both parameters and manu-facturers in the frequency with which false alarms occur. Reductions in alarm rates may be sought, for example, by using improved pulse oximeter technology or by relying solely on pulse oximetry for hypoxemia and hyperoxema detection. This approach, however, must be weighed against the physiological shortcomings of measuring SPO_2 in the high range of PO_2, where small changes in the former are associated with large changes in the latter (74). Another approach is to lower hypoxemia alarms or to prolong averaging times, both of which may have marked effects on alarm rates, but again must be weighed against the risks associated with alarm delays (74). The issue of false alarms is an area that should receive more attention if noninvasive monitoring in the NICU is to improve further.

IX. Alarm Settings

A monitor should sound an alarm early enough to avoid the progression of an intermittent cardiorespiratory instability or disturbance to potentially dangerous pathophysiology, but not too early to avoid desensitization of caregivers (see above). Unfortunately, there are no systematic studies on the effects of different alarm settings on patient outcome. Thus, any recommendation on alarm limits can only be based on observational studies. For example, with regard to heart rate alarms, there is evidence that cerebral perfusion remains relatively constant during apnea/bradycardia as long as heart rate stays >80/min, but it falls sharply if heart rate drops to below this limit (75). Nevertheless, given the large interindividual differences in heart rate between infants, is may be more logical to define individual alarm limits, e.g., to alarm if heart rate falls to <2/3 of baseline (36).

With regard to apnea alarms, it can be argued that an infant can indefinately remain apneic as long as neither blood gases nor heart rate is affected; this is why, as a practical consequence, we usually disable apnea alarms on our NICU monitors (we never monitor *only* respiratory movements). With regard to hyperoxemia, an observational study found that the risk of retinopathy of prematurity increased by 50% for every 12 h PaO_2 was >80 mm Hg (10.7 kPa) (76). Hence, this threshold is now commonly used as the upper limit of the recommended range for PaO_2 (77), but it is less clear whether 40, 45, or 50 mm Hg would serve as an optimal lower alarm limit. For other parameters, e.g. CO_2, there is not even observational evidence as to what constitutes a safe range; in contrast, there are conflicting data whether hypercapnia or normocapnia is beneficial (78). Hence, it is impossible to give unequivocal recommendations on alarm limits for this parameter.

The alarm limits suggested in Table 1 are those normally used in the author's NICU in both term and preterm infants (if not stated otherwise).

Table 1 Alarm Limits for NICU Monitors

	Lower limit	Upper limit
Heart rate (1/min)	80	220
Respiratory rate/apnea duration	disabled	disabled
SPO_2 in preterm neonates receiving oxygen (%)	85	95
SPO_2 in preterms not receiving O_2 or in term infants (%)	85	disabled
$PTcO_2$ in preterm neonates receiving oxygen (kPa)	6.0	10.7[a]
$PTcCO_2$ (kPa)	6.0	7.3
$ETCO_2$ (never monitored as only parameter)	disabled	7.3

[a]Not disabled in infants *not* receiving oxygen to alarm for poor sensor-skin contact.

These alarm limits can only serve as an orientation, not as a recommendation, and may vary depending on patient condition, resting heart rate, and bicarbonate levels.

References

1. Baird TM, Goydos JM, Neuman MR. Optimal electrode location for monitoring the ECG and breathing in neonates. Pediatr Pulmonol 1992; 12:247–250.
2. Cartlidge PHT, Rutter N. Karaya gum electrocardiographic electrodes for preterm infants. Arch Dis Child 1987; 62:1281–1282.
3. Sackner MA, Krieger BP. Non-invasive respiratory monitoring. In: Scharf SM, Cassidy SS, eds. Heart-Lung Interactions in Health and Disease. Lung Biology in Health and Disease, Vol 42. New York: Marcel Dekker, 1989:663–805.
4. Southall DP, Richards JM, Lau KC, Shinebourne EA. An explanation for failure of impedance apnoea alarm systems. Arch Dis Child 1980; 55:63–65.
5. Sackner MA, Watson H, Belsito AS, Feinerman D, Suarez M, Gonzalez G, Bizousky F, Krieger B. Calibration of respiratory inductive plethysmograph during natural breathing. J Appl Physiol 1989; 66:410–420.
6. Adams JA, Zabaleta IA, Stroh D, Johnson P, Sackner MA. Tidal volume measurements in newborns using respiratory inductive plethysmography. Am Rev Respir Dis 1993; 148:585–588.
7. Sivan Y, Davidson Ward S, Deakers T, Keens TG, Newth CJL. Rib cage to abdominal asynchrony in children undergoing polygraphic sleep studies. Pediatr Pulmonol 1991; 11:141–146.
8. Adams JA, Zabaleta IA, Stroh D, Sackner MA. Measurement of breath amplitudes: comparison of three noninvasive respiratory monitors to integrated pneumotachograph. Pediatr Pulmonol 1993; 16:254–258.
9. Banovcin P, Seidenberg J, Von der Hardt H. Pressure sensor plethysmography: a method for assessment of respiratory motion in children. Eur Respir J 1995; 8:167–171.
10. Brouillette RT, Morrow AS, Weese-Mayer DE, Hunt CE. Comparison of respiratory inductive plethysmography and thoracic impedance for apnea monitoring. J Pediatr 1987; 111:377–383.
11. Railton R, Fisher J, Mitchell I, Barclay RPC. Long-term respiration monitoring in infants—a comparison of impedance and pressure capsule monitors. Clin Phys Physiol Meas 1983; 4:91–94.
12. Poets CF, Southall DP. Non-invasive oxygen monitoring in infants and children: practical considerations and areas of concern. Pediatrics 1994; 93:737–746.
13. Löfgren O, Jacobson L. The influence of different electrode temperatures on the recorded transcutaneous pO_2 level. Pediatrics 1979; 64:892–897.
14. Pearlman SA, Maisels MJ. Preductal and post-ductal transcutaneos oxygen tension measurements in premature newborns with hyaline membrane disease. Pediatrics 1989; 83:98–100.

15. Versmold HT, Linderkamp O, Holzmann M, Strohhacker I, Riegel K. Transcutaneous monitoring of pO_2 in newborn infants: where are the limits? Influence of blood pressure, blood volume, blood flow, viscosity and acid base state. Birth Defects: Original Article Series, Vol XV, No. 4. New York: Alan R. Liss, 1979:285–294.
16. Tremper KK, Waxman K, Shoemaker WC. Effects of hypoxia and shock on transcutaneous pO_2 values in dogs. Crit Care Med 1979; 7:526–531.
17. Vyas H, Helms P, Cheriyan G. Transcutaneous oxygen monitoring beyond the neonatal period. Crit Care Med 1988; 16:844–847.
18. Monaco F, Nickerson BG, McQuitty JC. Continuous transcutaneous oxygen and carbon dioxide monitoring in the pediatric ICU. Crit Care Med 1982; 10:765–766.
19. Tremper KK, Shoemaker WC. Transcutaneous oxygen monitoring of critically ill adults, with and without low flow shock. Crit Care Med 1981; 9:706–709.
20. Okken, A, Rubin, IL, Martin RJ. Intermittent bag ventilation of preterm infants on continuous positive airway pressure: the effect on transcutaneous PO_2. J Pediatr 1978; 93:279–282.
21. Poets CF, Samuels MP, Noyes JP, Jones KA, Southall DP. Home monitoring of transcutaneous oxygen tension in the early detection of hypoxaemia in infants and young children. Arch Dis Child 1991; 66:676–682.
22. Pollitzer MJ, Whitehead MD, Reynolds EOR, Delpy D. Effect of electrode temperature and in vivo calibration on accuracy of transcutaneous estimation of arterial oxygen tension in infants. Pediatrics 1980; 65:515–522.
23. Martin RJ, Robertson SS, Hopple MM. Relationship between transcutaneous and arterial oxygen tension in sick neonates during mild hyperoxemia. Crit Care Med 1982; 10:670–672.
24. Bossi E, Meister B, Pfenninger J. Comparison between transcutaneous PO_2 and pulse oximetry for monitoring O_2-treatment in newborns. Adv Exp Med Biol 1987; 220:171–176.
25. Duc G, Frei H, Klar H, Tuchschmid P. Reliability of continuous transcutaneous PO_2 in respiratory distress syndrome of the newborn. Birth Defects 1979; 15:305–313.
26. Geven WB, Nagler E, De Boo T, Lemmens W. Combined transcutaneous oxygen, carbon dioxide tensions and end-expired CO_2 levels in severely ill newborns. Adv Exp Med Biol 1987; 220:115–120.
27. Wimberley PD, Frederiksen PS, Witt-Hansen J, Melberg SG, Friis-Hansen B. Evaluation of a transcutaneous oxygen and carbon dioxide monitor in a neonatal intensive care department. Acta Paediatr Scand 1985; 74:352–359.
28. Stebbens VA, Poets CF, Alexander JA, Arrowsmith WA, Southall DP. Oxygen saturations and breathing patterns in infancy. I. Fullterm infants in the second month of life. Arch Dis Child 1991; 66:569–573.
29. Fanconi S, Doherty P, Edmonds JF, Barker GA, Bohn DJ. Pulse oximetry in pediatric intensive care: comparison with measured saturations and transcutaneous oxygen tension. J Pediatr 1985; 107:362–366.
30. Mok J, Pintar M, Benson L, McLaughlin FJ, Levison H. Evaluation of non-invasive measurements of oxygenation in stable infants. Crit Care Med 1986; 14:960–963.

31. Southall DP, Bignall S, Stebbens VA, Alexander JR, Rivers RPA, Lissauer T. Pulse oximeter and transcutaneous arterial oxygen measurements in neonatal and paediatric intensive care. Arch Dis Child 1987; 62:882–888.
32. Barker SJ, Shah NK. Effects of motion on the performance of pulse oximeters in volunteers. Anesthesiology 1997; 86:101–108.
33. Bucher HU, Keel M, Wolf M, Von Siebental K, Duc G. Artifactual pulse-oximetry estimation in neonates. Lancet 1994; 343:1135–1136.
34. Morris RW, Nairn M, Torda TA. A comparison of fifteen pulse oximeters. Part I: A clinical comparison. Part II: A test of performance under conditions of poor perfusion. Anaesth Intens Care 1989; 17:62–82.
35. ECRI. Evaluation: next-generation pulse oximetry. Health Devices 2000; 29:347–379.
36. Poets CF, Stebbens VA, Samuels MP, Southall DP. The relationship between episodes of bradycardia, apnea and hypoxemia in preterm infants. Pediatr Res 1993; 34:144–147.
37. Tremper KK, Barker SJ. Pulse oximetry. Anesthesiology 1989; 70:98–108.
38. Bohnhorst B, Poets CF. Major reduction in alarm frequency with a new pulse oximeter. Intensive Care Med 1998; 24:277–278.
39. Rheineck-Leyssius AT, Kalkman CJ. Advanced pulse oximeter technology compared to simple averaging. II. Effect on frequency of alarms in the postanesthesia care unit. J Clin Anesth 1999; 11:196–200.
40. Bohnhorst B, Peter CS, Poets CF. Pulse oximeters' reliability in detecting hypoxemia and bradycardia: comparison between a conventional and two new generation oximeters. Crit Care Med 2000; 28:1565–1568.
41. Poets CF, Stebbens VA. Detection of movement artifact in recorded pulse oximeter saturation. Eur J Pediatr 1997; 156:808–811.
42. Urschitz MS, Von Einem V, Seyfang A, Poets CF. Use of pulse oximetry in automated O_2 delivery to ventilated infants. Anesthesiology 2002; 94:537–540.
43. Zijlstra WG, Buursma A, Meeuwsen–van der Roest WP. Absorption spectra of human fetal and adult oxyhemoglobin, de-oxyhemoglobin, carboxyhemoglobin, and methemoglobin. Clin Chem 1991; 37:1633–1638.
44. Veyckemans F, Baele P, Guillaume JE, Willems E, Robert A, Clerbaux T. Hyper-bilirubinemia does not interfere with hemoglobin saturation measured by pulse oximetry. Anesthesiology 1989; 70:118–122.
45. Emery JR. Skin pigmentation as an influence on the accuracy of pulse oximetry. J Perinatol 1987; 7:329–330.
46. Zeballos RJ, Weisman IM. Reliability of noninvasive oximetry in black subjects during exercise and hypoxia. Am Rev Respir Dis 1991; 144:1240–1244.
47. Bucher HU, Fanconi S, Baeckert P, Duc G. Hyperoxemia in newborn infants: detection by pulse oximetry. Pediatrics 1989; 84:226–230.
48. Boxer RA, Gottesfeld I, Sharanjeet S, Lacorte MA, Parnel AV, Walker P. Noninvasive pulse oximetry in children with cyanotic congenital heart disease. Crit Care Med 1987; 15:1062–1064.
49. Fanconi S. Reliability of pulse oximetry in hypoxic infants. J Pediatr 1988; 112:424–427.

50. Southall DP, Bignall S, Stebbens VA, Alexander JR, Rivers RPA, Lissauer T. Pulse oximeter and transcutaneous arterial oxygen measurements in neonatal and paediatric intensive care. Arch Dis Child 1987; 62:882–888.

51. Poets CF, Wilken M, Seidenberg J, Southall DP, Von der Hardt H. The reliability of a pulse oximeter in the detection of hyperoxemia. J Pediatr 1993; 122:87–90.

52. Bohnhorst B, Peter C, Poets CF. Detection of hyperoxemia in neonates: data from 3 new pulse oximeters. Arch Dis Child Fetal Neon Ed 2002; 87:217–219.

53. Herrell N, Martin RJ, Pultusker M, Lough RRT, Fanaroff A. Optimal temperature for the measurement of transcutaneous carbon dioxide tension in the neonate. J Pediatr 1980; 97:114–117.

54. Monaco F, McQuitty JC, Nickerson BG. Calibration of a heated transcutaneous carbon dioxide electrode to reflect arterial carbon dioxide. Am Rev Respir Dis 1983; 127:322–324.

55. Wimberley PD, Pedersen KG, Olsson J, Siggaard-Andersen O. Transcutaneous carbon dioxide and oxygen tension measured at different temperatures in healthy adults. Clin Chem 1985; 31:1611–1615.

56. Brünstler I, Enders A, Versmold HT. Skin surface PO_2 monitoring in newborn infants in shock: effect of hypotension and electrode temperature. J Pediatr 1982; 100:454–457.

57. Tremper KK, Menteles RA, Shoemaker WC. Effects of hypercarbia and shock on transcutaneous carbon dioxide at different electrode temperatures. Crit Care Med 1980; 8:608–610.

58. Hand IL, Shepard EK, Krauss AN, Auld PAM. Discrepancies between transcutaneous and end-tidal carbon dioxide monitoring in the critically ill neonate with respiratory distress syndrome. Crit Care Med 1989; 17:556–559.

59. Martin RJ, Beoglos A, Miller MJ, DiFiore JM, Robertson SS, Carlo WA. Increasing arterial carbon dioxide tension: influence on transcutaneous carbon dioxide tension measurements. Pediatrics 1988; 81:684–687.

60. Merritt TA, Liyamasawad S, Boettrich C, Brooks JG. Skin-surface CO_2 measurements in sick preterm and term infants. J Pediatr 1981; 99:782–786.

61. Epstein MF, Cohen AR, Feldman HA, Raemer DB. Estimation of $PaCO_2$ by two noninvasive methods in the critically ill newborn infant. J Pediatr 1985; 106:282–286.

62. Martin RJ, Herrell N, Pultusker M. Transcutaneous measurement of carbon dioxide tension: effect of sleep state in term infants. Pediatrics 1981; 67:622–625.

63. Epstein RA, Reznik AM, Epstein MAF. Determinants of distortions in CO_2 catheter sampling systems: a mathematical model. Respir Physiol 1980; 41:127–136.

64. Gravenstein N. Capnometry in infants should not be done at lower sampling flow rates. J Clin Monit 1989; 5:63–64.

65. From RP, Scamman FL. Ventilatory frequency influences accuracy of end-tidal CO_2 measurements. Anesth Analg 1988; 67:884–886.

66. Clark JS, Votteri B, Ariagno RL, Cheung P, Eichhorn JH, Fallat RJ, Lee SE, Newth CJL, Rotman H, Sue DY. Noninvasive assessment of blood gases. Am J Respir Dis 1992; 145:220–232.

67. Schena J, Thompson J, Crone RK. Mechanical influences on the capnogram. Crit Care Med 1984; 12:672–674.

68. McEvedy BAB, McLeod ME, Kirpalani H, Volgyesi GA, Lerman J. End-tidal carbon dioxide measurements in critically ill neonates: a comparison of sidestream and mainstream capnometers. Can J Anaesth 1990; 37:322–326.

69. Severinghaus JW. Water vapour calibration errors in some capnometers: respiratory conventions misunderstood by manufacturers. Anesthesiology 1989; 70:996–998.

70. Long JG, Lucey JF, Philip AGS. Noise and hypoxemia in the intensive care nursery. Pediatrics 1980; 65:143–145.

71. Long JG, Philip AGS, Lucey JF. Excessive handling as a cause of hypoxemia. Pediatrics 1980; 65:203–207.

72. Lawless ST. Crying wolf: false alarms in a pediatric intensive care unit. Crit Care Med 1994; 22:981–985.

73. Ahlborn V, Bohnhorst B, Peter CS, Poets CF. False alarms in the neonatal intensive care unit: comparison between 3 modular monitoring systems. Acta Paediatr 2000; 89:571–576.

74. Rheineck-Leyssius AT, Kalkman CJ. Influence of pulse oximeter settings on the frequency of alarms and detection of hypoxemia: theoretical effects of artifact rejection, alarm delay, averaging, median filtering or lower setting of the alarm limit. J Clin Monit Comput 1998; 14:151–156.

75. Perlman JM, Volpe JJ. Episodes of apnea and bradycardia in the preterm infant: impact on cerebral circulation. Pediatrics 1985; 76:333–338.

76. Flynn JT, Bancalari E, Snyder ES, et al. A cohort study of transcutaneous oxygen tension and the incidence and severity of retinopathy of prematurity. N Engl J Med 1992; 326:1050–1054.

77. Amercian Academy of Pediatrics Committee on Fetus and Newborn. Guidelines for Perinatal Care. Washington: American Academy of Pediatrics, 1988:246–247.

78. Ambalavanan N, Carlo WA. Hypocapnia and hypercapnia in respiratory management of newborn infants. Clin Perinatol 2001; 28:517–532.

10

Periodic Breathing

HENRIQUE RIGATTO

University of Manitoba
Winnipeg, Manitoba, Canada

I. Introduction

Periodic breathing, a respiratory pattern in which breathing activity alternates
with breathing pauses, is common in neonates. This is particularly true in preterm
infants (1–12). Its high prevalence in preterm infants reflects immaturity of the
respiratory control system. The importance of this breathing pattern relates not
only to its association with more prolonged apneas, but also to the presence of
significant desaturations and bradycardias observed in very small infants (13,14).
When its presence is excessive in neonates at term, and is accompanied by
hypoxemia, it also reflects a predisposition for apparent life-threatening events
(ALTE) episodes in the first few weeks of life (15–18).

In this chapter, I shall discuss some of the important clinical characteristics of
periodic breathing in neonates and how these characteristics relate to Cheyne-
Stokes respiration in adults. An effort has been made to give a historical view of
how knowledge of this respiratory pattern has evolved. The physiological mechanisms that disrupt the normal control of breathing at this age will be examined.
Finally, the clinical significance of periodic breathing in neonates is discussed.

II. Concept, Morphology, and Prevalence

A. Concept

Periodic breathing is a respiratory pattern characterized by an alternation between
breathing periods and apnea (1–5,19). In the neonate, the duration of the

breathing and apneic intervals are frequently similar, each lasting about 7–10 sec. In some infants, however, the breathing will be longer or shorter than the apnea (20,21). Low ventilation/apnea ratios are associated with hypoventilation whereas high ratios are associated with hyperventilation (Fig. 1). In the early 1970s we thought the criteria for labeling an infant as having periodic breathing should be standardized, and we suggested that it should be observed for at least 2 min (1). During the following years this criterion has somewhat varied, but most authors required at least three respiratory cycles (1 cycle = 1 breathing + 1 apneic interval) to say that the infant is breathing periodically (9–11,22,23). We have also established that the apneic interval should not be less than 3 sec, to avoid mistaking a prolonged expiration for apnea.

B. Morphology

We have recently studied the morphology of periodic breathing in neonates asleep and in adult subjects falling asleep (19). We found that the crescendo/decrescendo pattern of the breathing interval predominated in the premature infant and this tended to decrease in favor of a decrescendo pattern toward adulthood (Fig. 2). We suggested that this might be related to a greater ability of the adult respiratory apparatus to translate the intense chemical stimulus, high CO_2 and low O_2 at the end of apnea, into a large tidal volume compared to the infant who is frequently incapable of doing this because of significant airway narrowing and increased airway resistance. The average duration of the respiratory cycle is $\sim$15 sec in infants and twice as long in adults, $\sim$30 sec. The number of breaths is similar in infants and adults and therefore the longer duration of the respiratory cycle in adults are due to their longer breath duration. The "duty cycle" (breathing interval/cycle duration) remains consistent with age. As reported by others also, at the beginning of the breathing interval, PCO_2 is highest and PO_2 and saturation lowest.

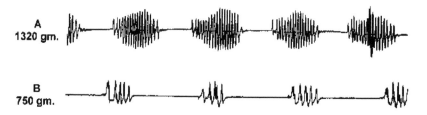

Figure 1 Respiratory flow illustrating two patterns of periodic breathing in two small preterm infants. (A) Ventilation/apnea ratio is $\sim$2, and the infant hyperventilates in relation to epochs of regular breathing. (B) Ratio is 0.4, and the infant hypoventilates.

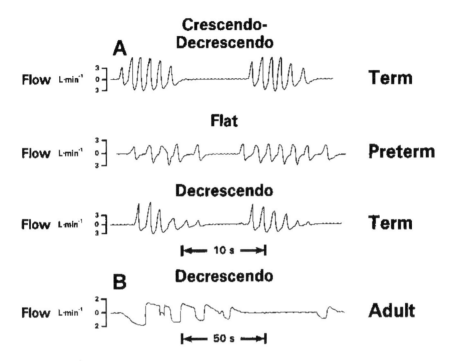

Figure 2 Illustration of periodic breathing in neonates and adult subjects. (A) Tracings show the common crescendo/decrescendo pattern in these neonates. Term neonates already show some tendency to have a decrescendo pattern. (B) Note the predominant decrescendo pattern of the adult subject. (From Ref. 19.)

C. Prevalence

The true prevalence of periodic breathing in neonates is not precisely known. Studies on the subject have examined diverse populations, and have used different criteria to define periodic breathing leading to divergent estimates (3,8–10,22,24–29). In general, the prevalence of periodic breathing is high in preterm infants and lower in term infants. In preterm infants <1000 g at birth, our data show a prevalence of 100% during the neonatal period. Others have also found a very high prevalence: Gotzbach et al. (3), 100 %; Fenner et al. (8), 72.5%; Matthews et al. (30), 91%; Hodgman et al. (26), 91%; Wilson and Howard (31), 76%; and Albani et al. (28), 75%. In term infants the prevalence reported has usually been less: Richard et al. (32), 69–80%, Kelly et al. (33), 78%; Fenner et al. (8), 41.03%; Deming and Washburn (34), 8%; Howard and Bower (35), 40%; Albani et al. (28), 36%; and Flores et al. (36), 30%. This high initial prevalence of periodic breathing decreases significantly in both preterm and term infants during the first 6–8 weeks of life. The percent of sleeping time occupied by periodic breathing in preterm infants ranged from 8% to 19% (24–26,28,37), whereas in the full-term infant it ranged from 0% to 5% (3,33,36,38,39). Using similar methodology, Kelly et al. (33) and Gotzbach et al. (3,5) found this percentage to be 12% in preterm infants and <2% in term infants. This value decreased to <1% at 12 months of age in term infants. Values at 12 months of age for preterm infants have not been reported.

III. History

Hippocrates (40), in the First Book of the Epidemics, makes reference to an unusual type of breathing. In describing the case of Philiscus, who died of an acute disease of a somewhat indefinite kind, accompanied by an enlargement of the spleen, he remarks: Τουτέῳ πνεῦμα διὰ τέλεος ὥσπες ἀνακαλουμένῳ αραιὸν, μέγα, which Galen in his work "On Difficulty of Breathing," translated as: "His respiration was rare and large, like a person who forgot for a time the need of breathing, and then suddenly remembered" (41). This appears to be the first description of periodic breathing in humans. For centuries this type of breathing did not receive much attention, and only in 1780 did Nicolas, a physician of Grenoble, described this periodic respiration in a general officer of 81 years (42). With the exception of the observation made by the Father of Medicine and by the learned physician of Grenoble, this peculiar form of respiration remained largely ignored until 1818, when Cheyne (43), in Dublin, observed it in a patient with "fatty degeneration of the heart." More descriptions followed, including that of Stokes in 1854 (44) who labeled this respiration as pathognomonic of fatty degeneration of the heart. This periodic respiration became then known as Cheyne-Stokes respiration, although other nomenclatures have been suggested over the years such as "pendulumlike breathing" (45), "brief recurrent apnea" (46), and "intermittent respiration" (47).

During the 1800s there was intense interest in this type of respiration, with reports of its occurrence under both pathological and healthy conditions (48). Observations in pathological conditions were made when patients were terminally ill, usually with involvement of the heart, brain, or both. General infections could also be associated with this pattern of breathing. Many investigators observed this respiration under experimental conditions in lower species, including frogs, tortoise, and alligators (48). This pattern was first observed in a healthy sleeping adult by Henry Kennedy in 1874 (49). Other reports confirmed this observation and suggested that sleep greatly favored the appearance of periodic respiration (50–55). Mosso (52,53) also emphasized the low O_2 of high altitude as a triggering element for this respiration.

In children, the first report appears to be that of Bjôrnström in 1870 (56), who reported periodic respiration in a 3-month-old child with "capillary" bronchitis. Other reports in children followed, including the observation that it could be observed in healthy infants during sleep (55,57–61). The first description in a neonate appears to be that of O'Connell in 1884 (62), who reported periodic breathing in a neonate 12 h old. No indication of the diagnosis was given.

From the end of the 1800s into the beginning of the 1900s efforts were made to document this type of respiration. The experiments of Douglas and Haldane (63) in the beginning of the 1900s became a landmark in the history of periodic breathing. By rebreathing inside a long thin tube the investigators became hypoxemic and developed periodic breathing; they then suggested that periodic breathing was due to "want of oxygen." The effective graphic recording of periodic breathing in newborn infants started to cluster in the second quarter of the last century (34,64,65), although description of Cheyne-Stokes breathing in preterm infants was made during the first three decades of that century (66). During this period efforts to document this breathing pattern in premature infants during sleep were also made.

In the middle of the last century, Cross (6,7,67) and Miller et al. (12,68,69) examined this respiration in many of their studies regarding control of ventilation in response to oxygen and carbon dioxide. Efforts then began to study the unstable nature of respiration in the small neonate and to search for tools to control it. Significant work followed during the second half of the last century which tried to elucidate the mechanisms underlying periodic breathing not only in small infants but also in adults (1–5,70–78).

IV. Mechanisms of Periodic Breathing

A. General

Respiratory Rhythm Generation and Its Components

Physiologists have been interested in the automaticity of respiration and its control for centuries (79). If we ignore ancient thoughts of its being dependent on vital spirits and phlogistic influences, the first scientific effort to understand respiratory control was made by LeGallois in 1812 (80), who sectioned the brain rostral to caudal and noticed that when he reached a specified level in the upper medulla, breathing would cease. He called this particular region, located near the origin of the Xth nerve in the medulla, "the principle of life." Flourens (81) expanded on LeGallois' experiments, sectioning the spinal cord, and localized the *noeud vitale* in the anterior medulla, a 2.5-mm region on both sides of the calamus scriptorius. The intellectual focus at the time was primarily to localize where breathing originated. Historically, it is of interest that Gibson in 1892 (48) stated that "after severing all the sensory stimuli to the respiratory center in the medulla, inspiratory movements of the face and larynx continued, although thoracic movements necessarily came to an end. In this observation there is clear proof that the respiratory center is in its nature thoroughly automatic."

In 1868 Hering-Bruer (82) described the role of the vagus nerve in breathing and suggested that respiration was entirely self-regulated, inspiration-inducing increase in lung volume which in turn inhibited inspiration through vagal stimulation, allowing expiration to begin. Expiration, in turn, would extinguish itself and allow inspiration to begin again. It is somewhat remarkable that such a physiological theory survived for so many years, when none of the key elements to be controlled, such as CO_2 and O_2, were incorporated. In 1908, Haldane (83) produced evidence that respiration was essentially controlled by CO_2 originating in the tissues, in a negative feedback design, in which CO_2 stimulates breathing and breathing in turn reduces CO_2. In 1930, Heymans and Heymans (84) suggested that the response to changes in O_2 in the blood was mediated through the carotid bodies, located in the bifurcation of the carotid artery. For this discovery, Corneille Jean François Heymans received the Nobel Prize for Physiology and Medicine in 1938.

Since then, most of the work related to the respiratory system has been done on the chemical responsiveness of the system and its mechanical properties. The last decade has heralded a new step forward in the paradigm, with the discovery that the *noeud vitale* region, localized just rostral to the obex in the upper medulla, contains neurons with intrinsic pacemaker properties (85–87). It is now known that most of these neuronal cells occupy a very discrete region of the anterior medulla named the pre-Bötzinger complex (88). This region appears to be a unique kernel of inspiratory pacemaker neurons, distinguishing it from the primary expiratory neurons present in the Bötzinger region itself (Fig. 3). This little "nest," not more than 300 µm in diameter, appears fundamental to the generation of inspiratory rhythm which is then modified by various other inputs, such as peripheral chemoreceptors, mechanoreceptors, behavioral inputs, and so on. Of interest is that the pre-Bötzinger complex has its dendrites adjacent to the surface of the upper ventrolateral medulla, a region that has been thought for many years to be the location for central chemosensitivity to CO_2 (89,90).

The pre-Bötzinger neuronal complex has recently been shown to be responsive to CO_2 (91,92), although the pacemakers in question were already found to be highly responsive to CO_2 a decade ago (85,87). Although much work still needs to be done, we seem to have identified all the key elements of respiratory control. The major issue still remaining is to discover how the rhythm is modulated and sustained.

Critical Role of CO_2

In parallel with efforts to discover the cellular structures that comprise the respiratory control system, new developments occurred in the area of chemical

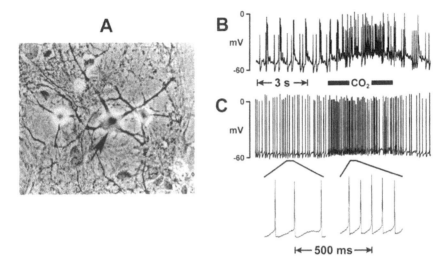

Figure 3 (A) Illustration of a pacemaker neuron in culture stained with antibodies against choline acetyltransferase. These cells are multipolar and appear uniquely responsive to CO_2. (B) A bursting pacemaker cell increases firing frequency with administration of CO_2. (C) Single beating neuron also increases frequency of firing with CO_2. Lower tracing is a computer registration with enlarged time scale of the membrane potentials. Membrane potentials are preceded by a spontaneous gradual ramp depolarization which slope increases with administration of CO_2.

control of ventilation. Experiments from various laboratories have shown that the respiratory control system needs CO_2 to function (93–97). Under normal circumstances, the CO_2 stores in the body are such that a basic level of arterial CO_2 tension, ~40 torr, is maintained. If, such as during climbing to high altitude, CO_2 decreases below a minimum level—the so-called "CO_2 apneic threshold"—breathing stops. This notion of a CO_2 apneic threshold is crucial to our understanding of periodic breathing and apnea in humans. Newborn infants, particularly preterm infants, switch spontaneously from regular to periodic breathing, and it is possible to determine the CO_2 apneic threshold under resting conditions (98). We found that the average CO_2 apneic threshold in preterm infants is only 1.5 torr lower than the actual or baseline PCO_2, whereas in adults it is ~5 torr lower (72–74,98; Fig. 4). This closeness of the CO_2 apneic threshold to the baseline CO_2 in neonates, together with other aspects of the immature respiratory feedback loop, likely contributes to the high prevalence of periodic breathing in infants compared with adults.

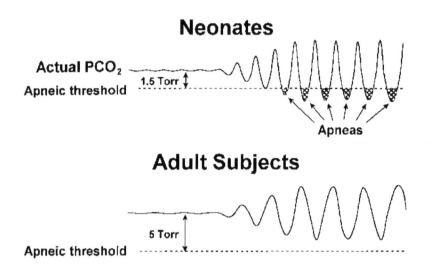

Figure 4 Diagrammatic representation of the relationship between the CO_2 apneic threshold and the baseline or actual PCO_2 levels in neonates and adults. Because of the proximity of these two levels in neonates, PCO_2 is much more likely to dive below the apneic threshold than in the adult.

B. The Neonate

The Respiratory Controller in the Neonate

The respiratory system is more unstable during the neonatal period than at any other period in life. At no other age does Douglas and Haldane's (63) assertion hold truer: "The surprising fact is not that we breathe regularly, but that we do not breathe periodically most of the time." Indeed, we have found many neonates who breathe periodically most of the time.

The fundamental requirement for apnea to occur in a given infant is that CO_2 come below the apneic threshold. This threshold, as mentioned earlier, is very close to the actual baseline PCO_2 of the infant. This means that any instability, such as that created by a brief hypoxic event, a sigh, a stretch, a leg movement, or a change in sleep state, is likely to make breathing transiently periodic. In infants, periodic respiration is not related to an increase in circulation time as it is in adults with heart or central nervous system compromise. The important elements contributing to periodicity in these infants are the systemic low O_2 levels, sleep, low functional residual capacity, and sighs. All of these may have different actions, but a common denominator is the approximation of the CO_2 apneic threshold to the actual baseline CO_2. The role of these factors are elaborated below.

Hypoxia

Premature infants are normally somewhat hypoxic. Their level of arterial O_2 tension is frequently in the 50–70 torr range. Because of this, their carotid chemoreceptor drive at rest is a significant component of the overall drive to breathe. When these infants are given an increased inspired O_2 sufficient to produce a "physiologic" denervation of the peripheral chemoreceptors, they become apneic (1,6,7,99–102). The duration of this apnea is a measure of prior baseline oxygenation, long apneas correlating well with low arterial O_2 tension (102–104). In parallel with this increased peripheral chemoreceptor drive, the low O_2 tension inhibits the respiratory center. This combination of an inhibited respiratory center in the presence of a comparatively increased peripheral chemoreceptor drive is very prone to induce respiratory instability. Because of the exponential increase in peripheral chemoreceptor activity at low levels of arterial O_2 tension, small changes in PO_2 cause large fluctuations in respiratory drive.

Hypoxia has been known to be associated with periodic breathing for centuries. In the 1800s Mosso (52,53) first documented how easily breathing of adult subjects could become periodic at high altitude. In the adult, hypoxia induces hyperventilation with a decrease in CO_2 tension below the apneic threshold level, causing apnea. In preterm infants, the hyperventilation with hypoxia is poorly sustained, and in the very small preterm infant it is entirely absent, the response being characterized by a decrease in minute ventilation (105). What happens is that hypoxia also induces a decrease in metabolism in these infants, with a decrease in CO_2 production (106,107). This allows for a low baseline CO_2 tension which is susceptible to periodic dips below threshold level. We and others have shown how easy it is to make breathing periodic in a newborn infant by decreasing the inspired O_2 concentration (2,6,31,35,69,108). On the contrary, it is very easy to change a periodic breathing pattern into a regular pattern by increasing the inhaled O_2 concentration (6,31,35,109).

Sleep

Sleep has been known to favor the appearance of periodic respiration for a long time (48,110–112). Puddicombe in 1893 (51) first reported an adult patient in whom Cheyne-Stokes respiration was induced by sleep. Mosso (52,53), in his expeditions to high altitude, reports on the profound effect of sleep in inducing periodic breathing. In newborn infants, sleep is also a very important factor. We suggested as early as 1972 that because sleep decreases ventilation with a decrease in the CO_2 response curve and a decrease in arterial O_2 tension, it may be an important factor contributing to periodic breathing (1). During sleep, the unbalancing of respiration relates to the disproportionate feedback from O_2 and CO_2 chemosensors in the presence of an inhibited respiratory center. The overall gain of the system is decreased, with a decrease slope of the ventilatory response to CO_2, but because the baseline CO_2 level increases, there is a greater change in PCO_2 per given change in ventilation. The decreased gain of the system tends to stabilize breathing, but this is counterbalanced by greater oscillations in CO_2, which may come below the apneic threshold and cause apnea. Depending on the balance of these two opposing forces, breathing may remain stable or may oscillate into periodicity during sleep. Why oscillations persist following the initial apnea remains a matter of debate. The assumption is that PCO_2, having decreased below threshold, creates the first apnea. PCO_2 then increases during the apneic pause and creates the chemical stimulus for breathing to resume. Because of the intensity of this stimulus at the end of apnea, breathing is very forceful and quickly eliminates the added CO_2, bringing it again below threshold for a new apnea. The cycle then tends to perpetuate itself until the cause for bringing the PCO_2 below threshold is eliminated.

Periodic breathing is present not only in REM sleep, as suggested originally (37,113), but also in quiet sleep. Periodic breathing is very common in infants during *tracé alternans* in quiet sleep (14,105,112). Periodic breathing in quiet sleep tends to be very "regular"—that is, with relatively consistent durations of the breathing and apneic intervals—whereas in REM sleep it is very irregular, likely owing to the various behavioral influences (Fig. 5). The regular shifts in sleep state with the associated changes in ventilation likely lead to what Douglas and Haldane (63) called "the hunting of the respiratory centre." Sleep can also contribute to periodic breathing through other mechanisms. For example, chest distortion during REM sleep may trigger a respiratory pause through the intercostal phrenic inhibitory reflex (114). The decrease in functional residual capacity during REM sleep reduces the buffering capacity of O_2, induces hypoxemia, and predisposes to instability (115).

Low Functional Residual Capacity (FRC)

The reduced outward recoil of the chest wall, which in preterm infants is close to zero, is by far the most important feature of the immature respiratory apparatus (116,117). This is mainly due to lack of mineralization of the bones of the chest wall. Gehardt and Bancalari (118) found the chest wall compliance in the preterm infant at 32 weeks of gestation to be $6.4 \, ml \cdot cmH_2O^{-1} \cdot kg^{-1}$, as opposed to $4.2 \, ml \cdot cmH_2O^{-1} \cdot kg^{-1}$ in the term infant. Because the recoil of the lung is just slightly less than that in adult subjects, the functional residual capacity of small infants is only 10% of vital capacity. This is quite near the closing volume, resulting in significant atelectasis (119–121). Together with the inactivation of intercostal muscles during REM sleep and 30% decrease in lung volume (115), the reduced outward recoil of the chest wall significantly compromises the respiratory pump, favoring instability of the control system.

The functional implications of a low FRC are various. The low volume means low O_2 stores with less buffering capacity. Additionally, atelectasis allows

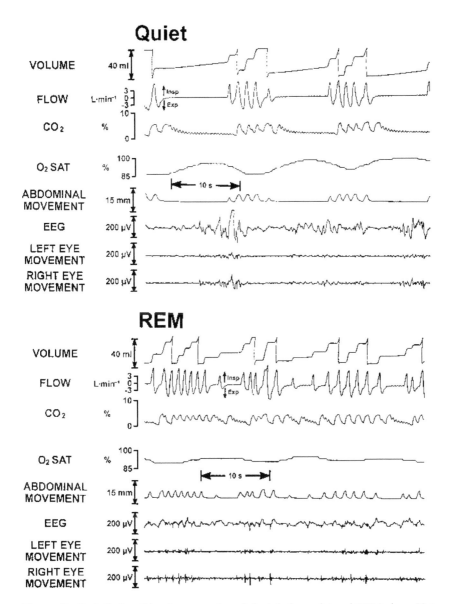

Figure 5 Periodic breathing in one preterm infant during quiet and REM sleep. Note that periodic breathing is more regular in quiet sleep; that is, the apneas and breathing intervals are nearly constant, as opposed to the irregular periodicity observed in REM sleep. Also note the presence of sighs in REM sleep. (From Ref. 14.)

for intrapulmonary right-to-left shunt, reducing O_2 tension and favoring the establishment of periodic breathing. In preterm infants, Poets et al. (122) showed that FRC was significantly lower during nonregular than during regular breathing, and this was associated with fast desaturation. Thibeault et al. (123) showed a decrease in lung volume associated with periodic breathing. Conversely, maneuvers that increase FRC tend to eliminate periodicity. In the prone position FRC increases, chest wall stabilizes with less distortion, ventilation/perfusion and saturation improve, and periodic breathing decreases (124–129). Negative pressure applied around the chest wall eliminates periodic breathing (123; Fig. 6), and continuous positive airway pressure reduces apnea of prematurity and periodic breathing (130).

Sighs

Sighs are more common during the neonatal period than at any other age in humans (131,132). They are more frequent in REM than in quiet sleep. They appear in the respiratory tracing as a "breath-on-the-top-of-a-breath," and represent one of earliest examples in physiology of positive feedback in man (133). The increased presence of sighs at this age likely relates to the increased tendency of lung volume to decrease; sighs would then restore lung volume. Sighs are twice as frequent in preterm as in term infants, which is consistent with a role in sustaining lung volume (131). The exact mechanism producing sighs is not known, but it is believed that vagal-mediated changes in pulmonary irritant reflexes and possibly chest wall reflexes, induced by a decrease in lung volume and compliance, are important (132,134,135). Asphyxia and hypoxemia also appear to be relevant in the neonate (131,136).

Are sighs important in triggering periodic breathing? In preterm infants we found that sighs were equally distributed before and after the respiratory pauses (131,137). In general, when occurring after the apnea, they occupy the first or second breath of the breathing interval, suggesting a decrease in lung volume during apnea (115,122). In term infants, however, sighs appeared to frequently trigger a run of periodic breathing (138). Our experience confirms this. The almost instantaneous changes that occur with a sigh include a decrease in PCO_2 below threshold, an increase in PO_2, and an increase in pH (139). It is likely that the most important factor is the decline in PCO_2 below threshold, thus initiating an epoch of periodic breathing.

The Airway in Periodic Breathing

During periodic breathing airway obstruction is rare (5,14,24,25). However, Miller and coworkers (140) have shown airway obstruction in their premature infants with periodic breathing. We have used the presence of a magnified cardiac oscillation signal present in the respiratory flow tracing to determine patency of

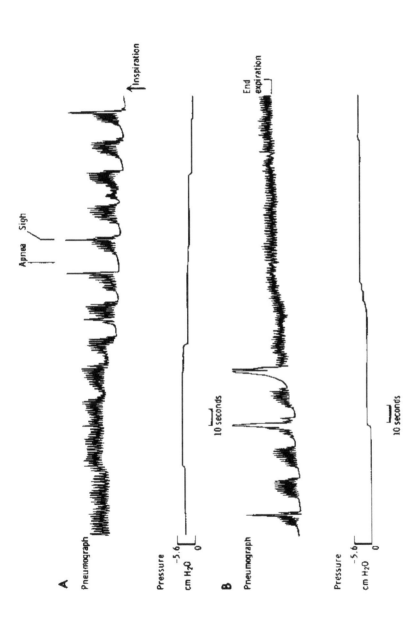

Figure 6 Pneumograph tracing with infant in the negative pressure chamber. A and B are continuous. (A) Negative pressure applied with a return to atmospheric pressure. When negative pressure is applied, the baseline is shifted upward, indicating an increase in FRC. Breathing is regular, tidal volume is smaller, and no sighs are apparent. When pressure is released, periodic breathing and sighs return. (B) Note disappearance of periodic breathing and sighs as FRC is increased again. (From Ref. 123.)

the airway and its absence to detect obstruction (141; Fig. 7). Using this method we found that the airway is almost never closed, the magnitude of the cardiac oscillation remaining relatively unchanged during apnea (Fig. 8). In a few instances where there is evidence of narrowing of the airway, it begins at ~1 sec into the respiratory pause, and is maximal at ~8 sec into the apnea (142; Fig. 9). We further investigated whether contraction of the respiratory muscles of the chest was important in causing some degree of obstruction. We found that obstruction was frequently observed in the absence of any respiratory effort (143). We therefore believe that some degree of obstruction, when it occurs, has to do with a lack of tone and flaccidity of the upper-airway smooth muscle, which occurs simultaneously with the induction of central apneas (144). Thus, obstruction is usually coincident with, rather than a cause of, apnea.

Maneuvers That Reduce Periodic Breathing in the Neonate

Periodic breathing per se does not require management in the neonate, but it is useful to recognize the various manoeuvres that are able to reduce or abolish it. *Inhaled O_2* is usually very effective (1,6,68). This effect has been known since the first half of the last century (31,35,145). In the earlier observations, 100% O_2 was used to show this effect, but lately lower concentrations of inhaled O_2 were also shown to be effective (109; Fig. 10). Even a modest increase in inhaled O_2 to 23–25% makes a significant difference. There are two reasons fundamentally for

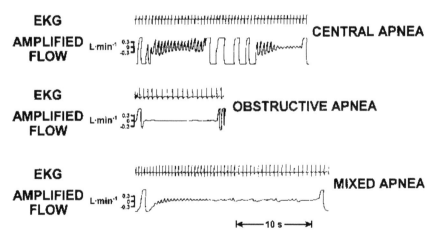

Figure 7   Classification of respiratory pauses according to the cardiac airflow oscillation method. Central apneas are those in which the cardiac airflow oscillation is present, obstructive apneas are those in which it is absent, and mixed apneas are those in which the oscillation is present during part of the apnea. (From Ref. 141.)

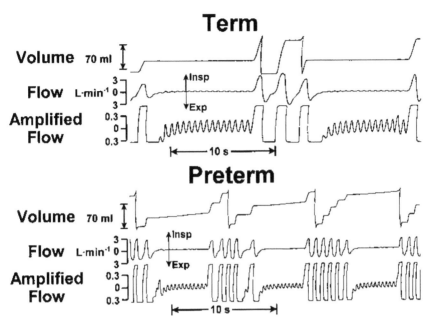

Figure 8 Periodic breathing in a preterm and a term infant to illustrate the commonly seen patency of the airway throughout the apneic period. Note the constant amplitude of the cardiac airflow oscillation, which can be better recognized when the standard flow tracing is amplified tenfold (bottom tracing).

this action of O_2. First, inhaled O_2 increases the stores of O_2 in the body, providing a buffer against hypoxemia. Second, increased O_2 facilitates breathing. It has been suggested that hypoxia acts as an anesthetic inhibiting the central neuronal network responsible for breathing (146); supplemental O_2 alleviates this. Since we do not treat periodic breathing per se, O_2 is not used for this purpose. However, periodic breathing and prolonged apnea of prematurity frequently occur together, and in the management of apnea we recommend saturations to be kept at 94% (range 92–96%) and we adjust inhaled O_2 accordingly.

Carbon dioxide is also very effective in making breathing continuous in infants with respiratory periodicity (1,31,35,67,68,108,147,148). Wilson et al. (31) were probably the first to show this in babies in the first half of the last century, although such effects had been shown earlier in adults (83). We have examined different concentrations of inhaled CO_2 in treatment of respiratory periodicity and apnea in infants, and have found that concentrations as low as 0.5% are very effective (149). CO_2, the natural stimulus to breathe, increases ventilation, making it continuous. If used in low concentration, the increase in ventilation is sufficient to keep the arterial CO_2 tension unchanged, so its action is

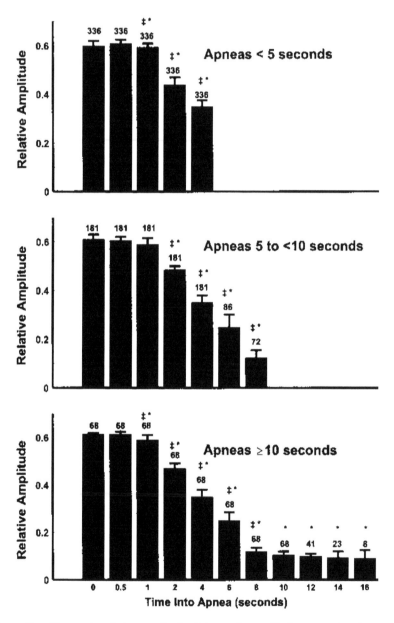

Figure 9   Changes in relative amplitude of the cardiac oscillations over time for apneas of different durations. Note that the critical period of maximum narrowing occurs at the same time despite different durations. Values are mean ±SE with number of apneas shown above each data bar. *$P \leq .05$ compared with preceding with time 0; $\pm P \leq .05$ compared with the preceding time interval. (From Ref. 142.)

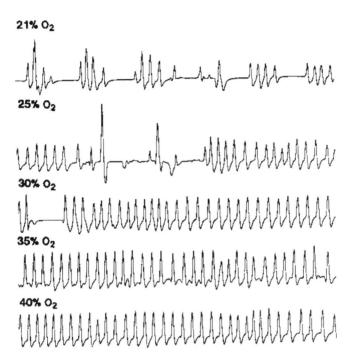

Figure 10 Illustration of the change in respiratory pattern with gradual increase in inspired O_2. Respiratory flow recorded in one preterm infant, age 16 days, 1600 g. Note regularization of breathing pattern with increased inspired O_2. (From Ref. 109.)

through an increase in respiratory drive. We have found that all respiratory pauses, not just those present in periodic breathing, are reduced or abolished by low inhaled CO_2. Because of this experimental observation we are now conducting a clinical trial using low inhaled CO_2 to treat apnea of prematurity, and comparing this effect with that obtained with theophylline (Fig. 11). The attraction of this strategy is that CO_2 is devoid of adverse side effects, unlike methylxanthines.

In the past we have suggested that anything that stimulates breathing will make respiration continuous (100,150). *Methylxanthines* do exactly that. The rationale for using methylxanthines was based on the evidence that this medication was also effective to treat Cheyne-Stokes respiration in adults. The use of aminophylline was first suggested by Shannon et al. (151) and Uauy et al. (152) in 1975 as effective in the treatment of apnea of prematurity. In the infants having apnea, periodic breathing is also present and eliminated with this medication (153). We examined the action of theophylline on breathing, both physiologically and pharmacokinetically (150,154). Theophylline increases breathing primarily by increasing tidal volume, but frequency may also increase. Methylxanthines

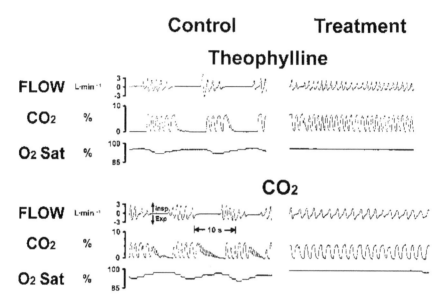

Figure 11 Illustration of the effects of theophylline and low inhaled CO_2 concentration (0.5%) on the respiratory pattern in two preterm infants. Note that CO_2 seems as effective as theophylline to regularize breathing. (From Ref. 149.)

have an additional effect on the respiratory musculature, enhancing muscular contraction. A loading dose of theophylline of 8 mg/kg and a maintenance dose of 6 mg/kg/day are currently used to treat apnea of prematurity. This regimen also eliminates periodic breathing.

Increase in FRC reduces periodic breathing (123–127). Chest wall distension, using either negative pressure around the chest or continuous positive airway pressure (CPAP), is a physiological maneuver that effectively reduces apnea of prematurity and periodic breathing. Thibeault et al. (123) elegantly showed the effect of negative pressure applied on the chest wall in correcting respiratory periodicity in preterm infants. The effect is mediated through various mechanisms including better oxygenation with increased lung volume, change in reflex feedback from the lungs, and possible inhibition of the costophrenic inhibitory reflex (114,155).

V. The Clinical Scenario

A. Preterm Infants

Periodic breathing is rare in the first few days of life (1,2). It generally becomes prominent in the second, third, and maybe fourth weeks of life, after which it tends to decrease to reach a nadir at about 6–12 weeks in small babies (1,2,5,6,8–11,14,24,25). The average length of the periodic cycle is ~15 sec, and of the apneic interval 7 sec. The absence of periodic breathing in the first few days has never been clearly explained, but it may relate to better FRC at this age, with better oxygenation (123). Perhaps an increased respiratory drive, with increased respiratory frequency due to increased pulmonary impedance, may also play a role. Increased impedance may be due to the presence of residual pulmonary fluid in the lungs as well as some minor air trapping (156). The decreased FRC after the first few days of life in preterm infants has been shown previously (123), a change which is associated with lower arterial O_2 tension and higher arterial CO_2 tension, giving the profile that Burnard et al. in 1958 (157) labeled the "respiratory insufficiency of prematurity." These physiological changes set the stage for the appearance of respiratory periodicity. In many small preterm infants who stay on the ventilator for a while this is still observed after they are extubated, although the whole scenario is shifted to a slightly more advanced postnatal age.

The sequence of events described above was very much the norm in the days prior to the use of methylxanthines and early closure of the ductus arteriosus. With these procedures, changes in PO_2 and PCO_2 are not as large as before. We have examined values for alveolar PCO_2 and PO_2 during periodic breathing and found that they may be at different levels for different babies (158; Fig. 12). It appears that each baby has a critical combination of CO_2 and O_2 tensions at which periodic breathing is observed.

Documentation of periodic breathing clinically can easily be done by observing the infant's respiration. It alternates between bursts of breathing efforts and respiratory pauses. In general, desaturations during periodic breathing are modest, there is no change in color of the infant, and there is no or minimal change in heart rate. In some very small infants, however, significant desaturations and bradycardias may be observed (13). These events can be observed through conventional monitors. In a recent work examining the factors that determine active resuscitation in the nursery, we found nursing notes quoting periodic breathing associated with significant desaturations and bradycardias (159). This seems to indicate that the periodic breathing observed in the nursery and triggering an alarm is likely associated with longer apneas than usual, meaning that periodic breathing is occurring on the edge of true "pathological" apneas.

Periodic breathing is frequently associated with prolonged apnea in preterm infants. In a study carried out in our laboratory we were able to show that a prolonged apnea ($\geq$20 s) almost never occurred in the absence of preceding short pauses such as observed in periodic breathing, and that the risk of a prolonged apnea occurring increased significantly when the preceding period contained an increased number of apneic episodes, increased duration of the longest apnea, or increased duration of the apneic time (160; Fig. 13). We believe that periodic

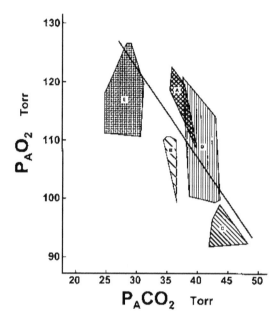

Figure 12 Illustration of various combinations of P_AO_2 and P_ACO_2 preceding apneic intervals during periodic breathing. Five infants—A, B, C, D, and E—are represented. Each vertex represents the P_AO_2, P_ACO_2 of the breath preceding apnea. Thus each vertex also represents an apnea. Note that infants may become apneic anywhere along the regression line. Each infant also chooses a combination of these values at which apnea occurs, and these are very specific for each infant. (From Ref. 158.)

breathing is a marker for apnea of prematurity, since apnea almost never occurs abruptly in infants breathing regularly, but only in infants whose respiratory pattern is characterized by significant periodicity.

B. Term Infants

The presence of periodic breathing is not unique to preterm infants, as mentioned before. It is also present in some term infants. Their presence as a percentage of sleep time is low, however, ~2% soon after birth and decreasing to <1% by 5–6 weeks of age. It then appears to remain at this low level for the first year of life. The morphology of this periodic breathing is very much the same as that of preterm infants, with an average respiratory cycle length of 14 sec and apnea length of 6 sec. In our apnea laboratory we have studied a significant number of infants at term who breathed periodically for >50% of the time, some for the entire sleep time. The striking finding was that they were invariably hypoxemic,

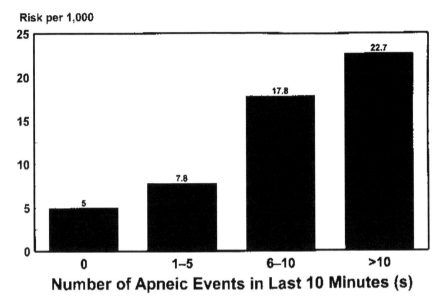

Figure 13 Likelihood of a prolonged apneic episode during the 11th minute of monitoring according to the number of apneic episodes. The risk per 1000 is plotted against the number of apneic episodes in the last 10 min. There is a significant increase in the risk between periods preceding the prolonged apnea without any apnea and periods that contain an increased number of apneic episodes. (From Ref. 160.)

with transcutaneous PO_2 in the 50–65 torr range .These infants came to us from the normal newborn area or were admitted because of an ALTE episode at home. They were polygraphically studied for 3–4 h through various behavioral states. Of interest is the fact that the healthy adult with Cheyne-Stokes respiration is also hypoxemic (161).

Because the term newborn infant is not monitored for apneic events in the nursery, the diagnosis of periodic breathing is made by observation of the infant's respiration. There is no significant decrease in heart rate or oxygen saturation.

C. Adult Subjects

Although this chapter is about periodic breathing in neonates, it would not be complete without a review of its presence in adulthood. In past centuries, periodic (Cheyne–Stokes) breathing was described mostly in adult subjects in the later years of life, usually >60, who had significant involvement of heart or central nervous system (48,77,162). This involvement was very significant from a clinical point of view, since the therapeutic tools to treat these diseases were essentially nonexistent. Today, such involvement is of much lesser degree and consequently we see less Cheyne-Stokes respiration due to pathological involvement of these systems.

The duration of the respiratory cycle in pathological conditions is very prolonged, averaging ~ 60 sec, with the breathing interval occupying slightly >50% of the cycle (162–165). Usually patients who present with this type of breathing pattern are very sick and semicomatose. There are interesting descriptions in the literature of patients being able to communicate only during the breathing period, and of instances in which a question posed during one breathing interval could only be answered in the next breathing interval, the patient being unconscious during the apneic interval (48,166). Because the respiratory pattern in these patients is generally related to increased circulation time, the priority is to correct the primary pathology. Aminophylline may help to correct the respiratory pattern in some patients.

Cheyne-Stokes respiration in situations of health, such as during climbing to high altitudes and during sleep, is made of much shorter respiratory cycles, ~ 30 sec, although they are still twice as long as those observed in neonates. Periodic breathing of high altitude is very common and triggered by low O_2 hyperventilation. This periodic respiration immediately ceases when the climber descends to low altitude. It is also much more dramatic during sleep, when the subject "rarely breathes," as described by Mosso in 1884 (52,53). Today, climbers to high altitude usually breathe from O_2 tanks to avoid the ill effects of this type of respiration, such as intense dyspnea.

Periodic breathing during sleep is rare in adults at rest. After Mosso's (52,53) first description, Fenoglio (54) tried to see whether Mosso's observations were correct and studied 100 males and 100 females of old age, during sleep (48). He found six males presenting with this type of periodic respiration during sleep but no females. It is more frequently observed when the subject falls asleep, indicating an unbalancing of the respiratory chemosensor system (165). It is also transient. We studied this breathing pattern in subjects investigated for sleep apnea and found it to be transient also (19). However, even during sleep, this periodic respiration is frequently associated with some abnormal clinical findings, such as transient partial upper-airway obstruction, hypoxemia, or both. The rarity of it in normal adult subjects is clearly reflected by the fact that when physiological measurements are needed, such as to calculate the CO_2 apneic threshold, forced ventilation is required to induce it.

VI. Clinical Significance in Neonates

The traditional view of periodic breathing has been that this is a benign respiratory pattern and we should not be too concerned about it. This view has been based on the following assumptions: [1] This respiratory pattern per se does not cause a major decrease in O_2 saturation or heart rate and therefore it is benign (3–5,9,10). [2] Some studies in the literature have not linked it to more prolonged apnea (3–5,9–11). [3] Its relationship to subsequent risk, such as ALTE or SIDS, could not be clearly established (3,5,11,26,168–175).

We have been concerned about this traditional view for the following reasons:

1. The only form of periodic breathing that seems innocent to us is that occurring very transiently when the subject falls asleep, or when there is a sharp change in sleep state with a brief disturbance of the chemical control of breathing (14,100,102,150,167). All other forms are highly pathological, including that of the climber at high altitude who feels miserable and highly dyspneic with periodic breathing, and that of term neonates with excessive periodicity. By excessive we mean breathing periodically for 50% or more of the sleeping time.
2. We have found and presented data suggesting that periodic breathing per se can be detrimental in very small preterm infants (13,176). We found that preterm infants < 1500 g had significant decrease in minute ventilation (38%) during periodic breathing, accompanied by a decrease in O_2 saturation from 92% to 80% during the apneic period (Fig. 14). Transcutaneous O_2 tension was low too. In small babies, breathing periodically for most of the sleeping time may represent a considerable exposure to low O_2.
3. I believe that periodic breathing and prolonged apnea of prematurity have the same basic physiological roots, with apnea reflecting a more severe instability (1,2,14,177–180). In a study carried out in our

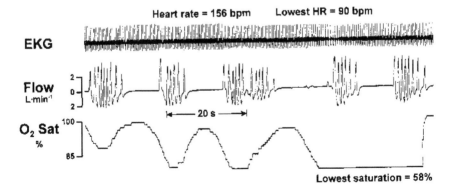

Figure 14 Illustration of a periodic breathing pattern associated with major desaturation and decrease in heart rate. It usually happens somewhere during an epoch of periodic breathing, when there is a minor delay in resuming breathing at the end of an apneic pause.

laboratory and mentioned earlier (160), we noticed that these prolonged apneas almost never occurred in the absence of preceding short apneas, and the appearance was preceded by shorter pauses. We have observed this link consistently in our polygraphic studies, the long apnea usually occurring in an ocean of small apneas such as in periodic breathing (Fig. 15).

4. We have also examined more critically the periodic breathing occurring in term infants (18). We found that this pattern of breathing occurs excessively when the transcutaneous PO_2 is low for this age group, usually 50–65 torr. These are infants who are breathing periodically for >50% of the time and frequently for the entire sleep time. Furthermore, in a group of infants with this periodicity and hypoxemia, the incidence of ALTE was much higher—55% in the periodic group and only 9% in the nonperiodic group. It is clear from our observations and those of others that ALTE is more frequent in infants who have excessive periodic breathing and are hypoxemic (17,18,23,181).

ALTE is not an innocent event and should not be ignored. It is usually associated with a significant hypoxic event and is a very alarming situation for the parents. The possibility that excessive periodic breathing may be followed by ALTE makes it important for us to be vigilant. It is relevant that previous studies failing to show a correlation between periodic breathing and future risk of

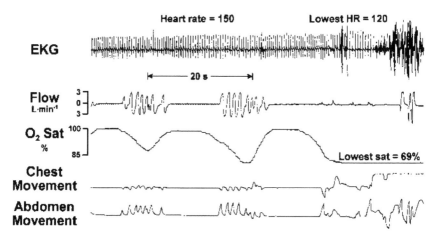

Figure 15 Illustration of a periodic breathing pattern followed by a prolonged mixed apnea, with desaturation and bradycardia. Note progressive increase in desaturation during periodic breathing preceding apnea. The prolonged apnea is mixed with a central component initially followed by airway collapse and obstruction.

prolonged apnea or ALTE included infants who breathed periodically as little as 15% of the sleeping time (3–5, 10,11,15,168,170,171,174,182,183). The overall prevalence of periodic breathing was <50% of the sleeping time. With little periodicity we do not expect an increased risk of future complications. In our experience, the risk is increased when these infants breathe at least 50% of the time periodically, and is very high when this percentage increases to 80–100% of the time.

VII. Long-Term Developmental Speculation

Preterm infants do not always come out of the perinatal period intact. One-third of small preterm infants intact at 2 years of age will show some degree of neurologic dysfunction at school age (184). The etiology and mechanisms of these late sequellae are not known, but the problem is of great concern. Many feel that much of it derives from the development of the immature brain in the unphysiological conditions of the newborn nursery (185,186). If so, these deleterious conditions will have to be identified and examined. Preterm infants are subject to a number of physiological insults, which does not affect survival but may affect the development of the immature brain. Because periodicity often coexists with prolonged apneas and significant hypoxemia, a preterm infant who breathes periodically for >50% of the time or for the entire sleep time may be subject to a more damaging insult than we have so far appreciated. As mentioned earlier, this periodicity often coexists with prolonged apneas and significant hypoxemia. Our speculation is that this exposure is not healthy and may be damaging. Unfortunately, studies trying to unravel the role of these events on late outcome have used developmental markers which do not have the discriminating power to assess the weight of these early individual insults (171). These conventional markers are affected by so many other variables that they are unable to assess accurately the effect of one single variable. New strategies are needed to assess the effects of these events on the ultimate outcome, but prevention by adjusting inspired O_2 or distending chest pressures seems a reasonable thing to do. Although we have dramatically reduced mortality, we are far from understanding the morbidity of these neonates later in life.

Acknowledgments

We are indebted to Marie T. Meunier Jackson for helping in the typing and preparation of this chapter. Also, Don Cates, Kim Kwiatkowski, Ian McIntyre, and Ruben Alvaro provided valuable comments and criticisms. Claudio Rigatto reviewed the chapter and made valuable corrections. Our research cited in this chapter was supported over the years by the Medical Research Council of

Canada, the Children's Hospital of Winnipeg Foundation, Inc., and the Manitoba Lung Association.

References

1. Rigatto H, Brady JP. Periodic breathing and apnea in preterm infants. I. Evidence for hypoventilation possibly due to central respiratory depression. Pediatrics 1972; 50:202–218.
2. Rigatto H, Brady JP. Periodic breathing and apnea in preterm infants. II. Hypoxia as a primary event. Pediatrics 1972; 50:219–228.
3. Glotzbach SF, Baldwin MA, Lederer NE, Tansey PA, Ariagno RL. Periodic breathing in preterm infants: Incidence and characteristics. Pediatrics 1989; 84:785–792.
4. Glotzbach SF, Tansey PA, Baldwin RB, Ariagno RL. Periodic breathing cycle duration in preterm infants. Pediatr Res 1989; 25:258–261.
5. Glotzbach SF, Ariagno RL. Periodic Breathing. In: Beckerman RB, Brouillette RT, Hunt CE, eds. Respiratory Control Disorders in Infants and Children. Baltimore: Williams & Wilkins, 1992:142–160.
6. Cross KW, Oppé TE. The effect of inhalation of high and low concentrations of oxygen on the respiration of the premature infant. J Physiol 1952; 117:38–55.
7. Cross KW, Warner P. The effect of inhalation of high and low oxygen concentrations on the respiration of the newborn infant. J Physiol 1951; 114:283–295.
8. Fenner A, Schalk U, Hoenicke H, Wendenburg A, Roehling T. Periodic breathing in premature and neonatal babies: Incidence, breathing pattern, respiratory gas tensions, response to changes in the composition of ambient air. Pediatr Res 1973; 7:174–183.
9. Barrington KJ, Finer NN, Wilkinson MH. Progressive shortening of the periodic breathing cycle duration in normal infants. Pediatr Res 1987; 21:247–251.
10. Barrington KJ, Finer NN. Periodic breathing and apnea in preterm infants. Pediatr Res 1990; 27:118–121.
11. Finer NN, Barrington KJ. Prolonged periodic breathing: significance in sleep studies. Pediatrics 1992; 89:450–453.
12. Miller HC, Behrle FC, Smull NW. Severe apnea and irregular respiratory rhythms among premature infants. Pediatrics 1959; 23:676–685.
13. Alvaro RE, Hussain A, Idiong, N, Lin Y-J, Kwiatkowski K, Rigatto H. Periodic breathing (PB) in small infants (≤1500 g):ventilatory correlates and significance. Pediatr Res 1997; 41:244A.
14. Rigatto H. Breathing and sleep in preterm infants. In: Loughlin GM, Carroll JL, Marcus CL, eds. Sleep and Breathing in Children. A Developmental Approach. New York: Marcel Dekker, 2000:495–515.
15. Guilleminault C, Ariagno R, Korobkin R, Nagel L, Baldwin R, Coons S, Owen M. Mixed and obstructive sleep apnea and near miss for sudden infant death syndrome. 2. Comparison of near miss and normal control infants by age. Pediatrics 1979; 64:882–891.

16. Kelly DH. Walker AM, Cahen L, Shannon DC. Periodic breathing in siblings of sudden infant death syndrome victims. Pediatrics 1980; 66:515–520.

17. Southall DP, Janczynski RE, Alexander JR, Taylor VG, Stebbens VA. Cardio-respiratory patterns in infants presenting with apparent life-threatening episodes. Biol Neonate 1990; 57:77–87.

18. Lin Y-J, Idiong N, Kwiatkowski K, Cates D, Rigatto H. Periodic breathing in term infants—Is it benign? Pediatr Res 1997; 41:161A.

19. Weintraub Z, Cates D, Kwiatkowski K, Al-Hathlol K, Hussain A, Rigatto H. The morphology of periodic breathing in infants and adults. Respir Physiol 2001; 127:173–184.

20. Chernick V, Heldrich F, Avery ME. Periodic breathing of premature infants. J Pediatr 1964; 64:330–340.

21. Chernick V, Avery ME. Response of premature infants with periodic breathing to ventilatory stimuli. J Appl Physiol 1966; 21:434–440.

22. Kelly DH, Shannon DC. Periodic breathing in infants with near-miss sudden infant death syndrome. Pediatrics 1979; 63:355–360.

23. Shannon DC, Carley DW, Kelly DH. Periodic breathing: quantitative analysis and clinical description. Pediatr Pulmonol 1988; 4:98–102.

24. Curzi-Dascalova L, Christova GL, Lebrun F, Firtion G. Respiratory pauses in very low risk prematurely born infants reaching normal term. A comparison to full term newborns. Neuropediatrics 1984; 15:13–17.

25. Curzi-Dascalova L, Christova GE. Respiratory pauses in normal prematurely born infants. A comparison with full-term newborns. Biol Neonate 1983; 44:325–332.

26. Hodgman JE, Gonzales F, Hoppenbrouwers T, Cabal LA. Apnea, transient episodes of bradycardia, and periodic breathing in preterm infants. Am J Dis Child 1990; 144:54–57.

27. Hoppenbrouwers T, Hodgman JE, Harper RM, Hofmann E, Sterman MB, McGinty DJ. Polygraphic studies of normal infants during the first six months of life. III. Incidence of apnea and periodic breathing. Pediatrics 1977; 60:418–425.

28. Albani M, Bentele KHP, Budde C, Schulte FJ. Infant sleep apnea profile: preterm vs. term infants. Eur J Pediatr 1985; 143:261–268.

29. Hageman JR, Holmes D, Suchy S, Hunt CE. Respiratory pattern at hospital discharge in asymptomatic preterm infants. Pediatr Pulmonol 1988; 4:78–83.

30. Matthews TG, Martin LT, Tulsiani S, Gill P. Periodic breathing, and sleep apnoea in normal and premature Irish infants. Ir Med J 1981; 74:83–84.

31. Wilson JL, Long SB, Howard PJ. Respiration of premature infants—response to variations of oxygen and to increased carbon dioxide in inspired air. Am J Dis Child 1942; 63:1080–1085.

32. Richards JM, Alexander JR, Shinebourne EA, deSwiet M, Wilson AJ, Southall DP. Sequential 22-hour profiles of breathing patterns and heart rate in 110 full-term infants during their first 6 months of life. Pediatrics 1984; 74:763–777.

33. Kelly DH, Stellwagen LM, Kaitz E, Shannon DC. Apnea and periodic breathing in normal full-term infants during the first twelve months. Pediatr Pulmonol 1985; 1:215–219.

34. Deming J, Washburn AH. Respiration in infancy. I. A method of studying rates, volume, and character of respiration with preliminary report of results. Am J Dis Child 1935; 49:108–124.

35. Howard PJ, Bauer AR. Irregularities of breathing in the newborn period. Am J Dis Child 1949; 77:592–609.

36. Flores R, Sternberg B, Peirano P, Guidasci S, Ddurupt N, Monod N. Respiratory pauses and periodic breathing assessed by cardio-pneumography in normal infants and in SIDS siblings. Neuropediatrics 1986; 17:59–62.

37. Parmelee AH, Stern E, Harris MA. Maturation of respiration in prematures and young infants. Neuropaediatrie 1972; 3:294–304.

38. Hunt CE, Brouillette RT, Hanson D, David RJ, Stein IM, Weissbluth M. Home pneumograms in normal infants. J Pediatr 1985:106:551–555.

39. Gordon D, Southall DP, Kelly DH, Wilson A, Akselrod S, Richards J, Kenet B, Cohen RJ, Shannon DC. Analysis of heart rate and respiratory patterns in sudden infant death syndrome victims and control infants. Pediatr Res 1986; 20:680–684.

40. Littré É. Oeuvres complètes d'Hippocrate. Paris: Ballière, 1840, ii:684.

41. Begbie JW. On the difficulty of breathing. Br Med J 1875; ii:164–171.

42. Gallois. Histoire des maladies épidemiques qui ont régné dans la province de Dauphiny depuis l'ánnée 1780. Journal de la Société de Médecine et de Pharmacie de l'Isère, 8me année, 1884:267.

43. Cheyne J. A case of apoplexy in which the fleshy part of the heart was converted into fat. Dublin Hospital Reports 1818; ii:216–223.

44. Stokes W. Symptoms of Periodic Respiration. The Diseases of the Heart and of the Aorta. Dublin: Hodges & Smith, 1854; xvi:324.

45. Brückner C. Ueber das Cheynes-Stokes'sche Respirations-Phanomen. Arch Pathol Anat Physiol Klin Med 1871; ii:155.

46. Laycock T. Notes of a clinical lecture on brief recurrent apnoea as a cause of sleeplessness in cardiac disease. Med Times Gazette 1873; i:433–435.

47. Baas JH. Ueber intermittendes Athmen. Dtsch Arch Klin Med 1874; xiv:609–612.

48. Gibson GA. Cheyne-Stokes Respiration. Edinburgh: Oliver & Boyd, 1893:1–133.

49. Kennedy H. Causes of Cheyne-Stokes respiration. Dublin J Med Sci 1874; 1(viii):521.

50. Saloz C. Cheyne-Stokes respiration. In: Contribution à l'ètude clinique et expé-mentale du phénomène respiratoire de Cheyne-Stokes. Geneva: Schuchardt, 1881; 156.

51. Puddicombe FM. On Cheyne-Stokes' respiration. Lancet 1883; i:816.

52. Mosso A. Life of man on the high Alps. London: Unwin TF, 1898; xv:45.

53. Mosso A. La respiration périodique et la respiration superflue ou de lux. Arch Ital Biol, 1886; vii:48–127.

54. Fenoglio I. Respirazione periodica nei vecchi e respiro Cheyne e Stokes. Sperimentale 1886; 1(vii):113–136.

55. Finlayson J. Observations on the state of the pupil in Cheyne-Stokes respiration. Glasgow Med J 1884; 4(xxviii):221–224.

56. Bjornström F. Om Cheyne-Stokes respirationsphaenomen. Upsala Läkareförenings Förhandlingar 1871; vi:307–312.

57. Rehn H. Zwei Beobachtungen von Cheyne-Stokes'schem Respirations—Phänomen bei Lungenaffectionen im kindlichen Alter. Jahrbuch für Kinderheilkunde und physische Erziehung 1871; iv:432.

58. Roth. Zur Casuistik des Cheyne-Stockes'schen Respiration-phänomens. Dtsch Arch Klin Med 1872; x:310–315.

59. De Cérenville EB. Thoracic-aneurism and Cheyne-Stokes respiration. Bulletin de la Société médicale de la Suisse romande, dixième année, 1876:152.

60. Hein I. Ueber die Cheyne-Stokes'sche Athmungsform. Wien Med Wochenschr 1877; xxvii:317, 341.

61. Filatow N. N Zwei Fälle von Cheyne-Stokes'schen Respiration mit glücklichem Ausgang'bei Kindern. Centralzeit Kinderkrankh 1878; ii:35–40.

62. O'Connell P. Cheyne-Stokes respiration in a newly-born child. Brit Med J 1884; i:220.

63. Douglas CG, Haldane JS. The causes of periodic breathing or Cheyne-Stokes breathing. J Physiol (Lond) 1908–1909; 38:401.

64. Deming J, Hanner JP. Respiration in infancy. II. A study of rate, volume, and character of respiration in healthy infants during the neonatal period. Am J Dis Child 1936; 51:823–831.

65. Shaw LA, Hopkins FR. The respiration of premature infants. Am J Dis Child 1931; 42:335–341.

66. Rommel O, Maschke AS. Prematurity and congenital debility. In: Pfaundler M, Schlossman A, eds. The Diseases in Children, Vol II, 2nd ed. Philadelphia: Lippincott, 1912:86–87.

67. Cross KW, Hooper JMD, Oppé TE. The effect of inhalation of carbon dioxide in air on the respiration of the full-term and premature infants. J Physiol 1953; 122:264–273.

68. Miller HC. Effect of high concentrations of carbon dioxide and oxygen on the respiration of full-term infants. Pediatrics 1954; 14:104–113.

69. Miller HC, Smull NW. Further studies on the effects of hypoxia on the respiration of newborn infants. Pediatrics 1955; 16:93–103.

70. Avery ME, Chernick V, Dutton RE, Permutt S. Ventilatory response to inspired carbon dioxide in infants and adults. J Appl Physiol 1963; 18:895–903.

71. Lahiri S, Maret KH, Sherpa MG, Peters RM Jr. Sleep and periodic breathing at high altitude: Sherpa natives versus sojourners. In: West JB, Lahiri S. eds. High Altitude and Man. Bethesda: American Physiology Society, 1984:73–90.

72. Dempsey JA. Skatrud JB. A sleep-induced apneic threshold and its consequences. Am Rev Respir Dis 1986; 133:1163–1170.

73. Skatrud JB, Dempsey JA. Interaction of sleep state and chemical stimuli in sustaining rhythmic ventilation. J Appl Physiol 1983; 55:813–822.

74. Younes M. The physiologic basis of central apnea and periodic breathing. Curr Pulmonol 1989; 10:265–365.

75. Cherniack NS, Longobardo GS, Levine OR, Mellins R, Fishman AP. Periodic breathing in dogs. J Appl Physiol 1966; 21:1847–1854.

76. Cherniack NS. Respiratory dysrhythmias during sleep. N Engl J Med 1981; 305:325–330.
77. Cherniack NS, Longobardo GS. Abnormalities in respiratory rhythm. In: Fishman AP, Cherniack NS, Widdicombe JG, Geiger SR, eds. Handbook of Physiology. The Respiratory System, Vol 2, pt 2, Ch 22. Bethesda: American Physiology Society, 1986:729–749.
78. Cherniack NS. Sleep apnea and its causes. J Clin Invest 1984; 73:1501–1506.
79. Gottlieb LS. A History of Respiration. Springfield, Il: C.C. Thomas, 1964.
80. LeGallois CJJ. Experiences sur le principe de la vie, notamment sur celui des mouvements du coeur, et sur la siege de ce principe. Paris: D'Haute, 1812:365.
81. Flourens P. Détermination du noeud vital ou point premier moteur du mécanisme respiratoire dans les vertébrés à sang froid. C R Acad Sci Paris 1862; 54:314–317.
82. Hering E. Die Selbsteuerung der Athmung durch den Nervus vagus. Sitzungsber Kaiserl Akad Wiss Vienna Math-Naturwiss Kl 1868; 57(pt 2):672–677.
83. Haldane JS, Priestley JG. The regulation of the lung-ventilation. J Physiol (Lond) 1905; 32:225–266.
84. Heymans JF, Heymans C. Sur les modifications directes et sur la régulation réflexe de l'activité du centre respiratoire de la tête isolée du chien. Arch Int Pharmacodyn Ther 1927; 33:273–372.
85. Rigatto H, Fitzgerald SF, Willis MA, Yu C. Search of the central respiratory neurons. II. Electrophysiologic studies of medullary fetal cells inherently sensitive to CO_2 and low pH. J Neurosci Res 1992; 33:590–597.
86. Smith JC, Ellenberger HH, Ballanyi K, Richter DW, Feldman JL. Pre-Bötzinger complex: a brainstem region that may generate respiratory rhythm in mammals. Science 1991; 254:726–729.
87. Fitzgerald SC, Willis MA, Rigatto H. In search of the central respiratory neurons: I. Dissociated cell cultures of respiratory areas from the upper medulla. J Neurosci Res 1992; 33:579–589.
88. Koshiya N, Smith JC. Neuronal pacemaker for breathing visualized in vitro. Nature 1999; 400:360–363.
89. Loeschke HH, Koepchen HP, Gertz KH. Über den einflub von wasserstoffi onenkonzentration und CO_2-druck im liqujor cere brospinalis auf die atmuiyg. Pflugers Arch 1958; 266:569–585.
90. Mitchell RA, Loeschcke HH, Severinghaus JW, Richardson BW, Massion WH. Regions of respiratory chemosensitivity on the surface of the medulla. Ann NY Acad Sci 1963; 109:661–681.
91. Johnson SM, Trouth CO, Smith JF. Chemosensitivity of respiratory pacemaker neurons in the pre-Bötzinger complex in vitro. Soc Neurosci 1998; 875 (abs).
92. Solomon IC, Edelman NH, O'Neal MH. CO_2/H^+ chemoreception in the cat pre-Bötzinger complex in vivo. J Appl Physiol 2000; 88:1996–2007.
93. Phillipson E, Duffin J, Cooper JD. Critical dependence of respiratory rhythmicity on metabolic CO_2 load. J Appl Physiol 1981; 50:45–54.
94. Phillipson EA, Bowes G. Control of breathing during sleep. In: Fishman AP, Cherniack NS, Widdicombe JG, Geiger SR. Handbook of Physiology, Vol II, pt 2. Bethesda: American Physiology Society, 1986:649–689.

95. Kolobow T, Gattinoni L, Tomlinson TA, Pierce JE. Control of breathing using an extracorporeal membrane lung. Anesthesiology 1977; 46:138–141.
96. Kuipers IM, Maertzdorf WJ, DeJong DS, Hanson MA, Blanco CE. Effect of mild hypocapnia on fetal breathing and behavior in unanesthetized normoxic fetal lambs. J Appl Physiol 1994; 76:1476–1480.
97. Canet E, Praud JP, Laberge JM, Blanchard PW, Bureau MA. Apnea threshold and breathing rhythmicity in newborn lambs. J Appl Physiol 1993; 74:3013–3019.
98. Khan A, Qurashi M, Kwiatkowski K, Cates D, Rigatto H. The vulnerability of the "CO_2 Apneic Threshold? in neonates. Pediatr Res 2001; 49:380A.
99. Dripps RD, Comroe JH Jr. The effect of the inhalation of high and low oxygen concentrations on respiration, pulse rate, ballistocardiogram and arterial oxygen saturation (oximeter) of normal individuals. Am J Physiol 1947; 149:277–291.
100. Rigatto H, Desai U, Leahy FAN, Kalapesi Z, Cates D. The effect of 2% CO_2, 100% O_2, theophylline and 15% O_2 on "respiratory drive" and "effective" timing in preterm infants. Early Hum Dev 1981; 5:63–70.
101. Rigatto H, Kalapesi Z, Leahy F, MacCallum M, Cates D. Ventilatory response to 100% and 15% O_2 during wakefulness and sleep in preterm infants. Early Hum Dev 1982;7:1–10.
102. Haider AZ, Rehan V, Al-Saedi S, Alvaro R, Kwiatkowski K, Cates DB, Rigatto H. Effect of baseline oxygenation on the ventilatory response to inhaled 100% oxygen in preterm infants. J Appl Physiol 1995; 79:2101–2105.
103. Haider AZ, Rehan V, Alvaro R, Al-Saedi S, Kwiatkowski K, Cates DB, Rigatto H. Low baseline oxygenation predisposes preterm infants to mixed apneas during inhalation of 100% O_2. Am J Perinatology 1996; 13:363–369.
104. Alvaro RE, Weintraub Z, Kwiatkowski K, Cates DB, Rigatto H. Speed and profile of the arterial peripheral chemoreceptors as measured by ventilatory changes in preterm infants. Pediatr Res 1992; 32:226–229.
105. Alvaro R, Alvarez J, Kwiatkowski K, Cates D, Rigatto H. Small preterm infants (≤ 1500 g) have only sustained decrease in ventilation in response to hypoxia. Pediatr Res 1992; 32:403–406.
106. Mortola JP, Rezzonico R, Lanthier C. Ventilation and oxygen consumption during acute hypoxia in newborn mammals: a comparative analysis. Respir Physiol 1989; 78:31–48.
107. Rehan V, Haider AZ, Alvaro RE, Nowaczyk B, Cates DB, Kwiatkowski K, Rigatto H. The biphasic response to hypoxia in preterm infants is not solely due to a decrease in metabolism. Pediatr Pulmonol 1996; 22:287–294.
108. Brady JP, Ceruti E. Chemoreceptor reflexes in the newborn infants: effects of varying degrees of hypoxia on heart rate and ventilation in a warm environment. J Physiol (Lond) 1966; 184:631–645.
109. Weintraub Z, Alvaro RE, Kwiatkowski K, Cates D, Rigatto H. The effects of inhaled oxygen (up to 40%) on periodic-breathing and apnea in preterm infants. J Appl Physiol 1992; 72:116–120.
110. Bülow K. Respiration and wakefulness in man. Acta Physiol Scand 1963; 59(supple 209):1–110.

111. Berssenbrugge A, Dempsey J, Skatrud, J. Hypoxic versus hypocapnic effects on periodic breathing during sleep. In: West JB, Lahiri S, eds. High Altitude in Man. Bethesda: American Physiology Society, 1984:73–90.

112. Prechtl H. The behavioural states of the newborn infant. Brain Res 1974; 76:185–212.

113. Aserinsky E. Periodic respiratory pattern occurring in conjunction with eye movement during sleep. Science 1965; 150:763–766.

114. Knill R, Bryan AC. An intercostal-phrenic inhibitory reflex in human newborn infants. J Appl Physiol 1976; 40:352–356.

115. Henderson-Smart DJ, Read DJ, Reduced lung volume during behavioral active sleep in the newborn. J Appl Physiol 1979; 46:1081–1085.

116. Agostoni E, Mead J. Statics of the respiratory system. In: Fenn WO, Rahn H, eds. Handbook of Physiology, 3. Respiration, Vol 1. Washington: American Physiology Society, 1964:387–409.

117. Agostoni E. Volume-pressure relationships of the thorax and lung in the newborn. J Appl Physiol 1959; 14:909–913.

118. Gerhardt T, Bancalari E. Chest wall compliance in full-term and premature infants. Acta Paediatr Scand 1980; 69:359–364.

119. Heldt GP, McIlroy MB. Distortion of the chest wall and work of the diaphragm in preterm infants. J Appl Physiol 1987; 62:164–169.

120. Kosch PC, Stark AR. Dynamic maintenance of end-expiratory lung volume in full-term infants. J Appl Physiol 1984; 57:1126–1133.

121. Hershenson MB. The respiratory muscles and chest wall. In Bekerman RC, Brouillette RT, Hunt CE, eds. Respiratory Control Disorders in Infants and Children. Baltimore: Williams & Wilkins, 1992:28–46.

122. Poets CF, Rau GA, Neuber K, Gappa M, Seidenberg J. Determinants of lung volume in spontaneously breathing preterm infants. Am J Respir Crit Care Med 1997; 155:649–653.

123. Thibeault DW, Wong MM, Auld PAM. Thoracic gas volume changes in premature infants. Pediatrics 1967; 40:403–411.

124. McEvoy C, Mendoza ME, Bowling S, Hewlett V, Sardesai S, Durand M. Prone positioning decreases episodes of hypoxemia in extremely low birth weight infants (1000 grams or less) with chronic lung disease. J Pediatr 1997; 130:305–309.

125. Martin RJ, Herrell N, Rubin D, Fanaroff A. Effect of supine and prone positions on arterial oxygen tension in the preterm infant. Pediatrics 1979; 63:528–531.

126. Douglas WW, Rehder K, Beynen FM, Sessler AD, Marsh HM. Improved oxygenation in patients with acute respiratory failure: the prone position. Am Rev Respir Dis 1977; 115:559–566.

127. Wagaman MJ, Shutack JG, Moomjian AS, Schwartz JG, Shaffer TH, Fox WW. Improved oxygenation and lung compliance with prone position in neonates. J Pediatr 1979; 94:787–791.

128. Lioy J, Manginello FP. A comparison of prone and supine positioning in the immediate postextubation period of neonates. J Pediatr 1988; 112:982–984.

129. Albert RK, Leasa D, Sanderson M, Robertson HT, Hlastala MP. The prone position improves arterial oxygenation and reduces shunt in olei-acid-induced acute lung injury. Am Rev Respir Dis 1987; 135:628–633.

130. Kattwinkel J, Nearman HS, Fanaroff AA, Katona PG, Klaus MH. Apnea of prematurity. 1975; 86:588–592.

131. Alvarez JE, Bodani J, Fajardo CA, Kwiatkowski K, Cates DB, Rigatto H. Sighs and their relationship to apnea in the newborn infant. Biol Neonate 1993; 63:139–146.

132. Thach BT, Tauesch HW. Sighing in human newborn infants: role of inflation-augmenting reflex. J Appl Physiol 1976; 41:502–507.

133. Comroe JH Jr. Physiology of Respiration. Chicago: Year Book, 1966:83.

134. Bendixen HH, Smith GM, Mead J. Pattern of ventilation in young adults. J Appl Physiol 1964; 19:195–198.

135. Glogowska M, Richardson PS, Widdicombe JG, Winning AJ. The role of the vagus nerves, peripheral chemoreceptors and other afferent pathways in the genesis of augmented breaths in cats and rabbits. Respir Physiol 1972; 16:179–196.

136. Bartlet Jr D. Origin and regulation of spontaneous deep breaths. Respir Physiol 1971; 12:230–238.

137. Weintraub Z, Alvaro R, Mills S, Cates D, Rigatto H. Short apneas and their relationship to body movements and sighs in preterm infants. Biol Neonate 1994; 66:188–194.

138. Ardila R, Yunis K, Bureau MA. Relationship between infantile sleep apnea and preceding hyperventilation event. Clin Invest 1986; 9:A151.

139. Fleming PJ, Goncalves AL, Levine MR, Woollard S. The development of stability of respiration in human infants: changes in ventilatory responses to spontaneous sighs. J Physiol 1984; 347:1–16.

140. Miller MJ, Carlo WA, DiFiore JM, Martin R Jr. Airway obstruction during periodic breathing in premature infants. J Appl Physiol 1988; 64:2496–2500.

141. Lemke RP, Al-Saedi SA, Alvaro RE, Wiseman NE, Cates DB, Kwiatkowski K, Rigatto H. Use of a magnified cardiac airflow oscillation to classify neonatal apnea. Am J Respir Crit Care Med 1996; 154:1537–1542.

142. Lemke RP, Idiong N, Al-Saedi S, Kwiatkowski K, Cates DB, Rigatto H. Evidence of a critical period of airway instability during central apneas in preterm infant. Am J Respir Crit Care Med 1998; 157:470–474.

143. Idiong N, Rigatto H. Airway closure during mixed apneas in preterm infants: is respiratory effort necessary? J Pediatr 1998; 133:509–512.

144. Mitchell RA, Herbert DA, Baker DG. Inspiratory rhythm and airway smooth muscle tone. J Appl Physiol 1985; 58:911–920.

145. Graham BD, Reardon HS, Wilson JL, Tsao MU, Baumann ML. Physiologic and chemical response of premature infants to oxygen-enriched atmosphere. Pediatrics 1950; 6:55–71.

146. Severinghaus JW. Effect of low oxygen tension in the central respiratory network. Personal communication to H. Rigatto, 1991.

147. Krauss AN, Klain DB, Waldman S, Auld PAM. Ventilatory response to carbon dioxide in newborn infants. Pediatr Res 1975; 9:46–50.

148. Kalapesi Z, Durand M, Leahy FAN, Cates DB, MacCallum M, Rigatto H. Effect of periodic or regular respiratory pattern on the ventilatory response to low inhaled CO_2 in preterm infants during sleep. Am Rev Respir Dis 1981; 123:8–11.

149. Al-Saif S, Alvaro R, Manfreda J, Kwiatkowski K, Cates D, Rigatto H. Inhalation of low (0.5–1.5) CO_2 as a potential treatment for apnea of prematurity. Semin Perinatol 2001; 25:100–106.

150. Davi M, Sankaran K, Simons K, Simons FER, Seshia MMK, Rigatto H. Physiologic changes induced by theophylline in the treatment of apnea in preterm infants. J Pediatr 1978; 92:91–95.

151. Shannon DC, Gotay F, Stein IM, Rogers MC, Todres ID, Moylan FMB. Prevention of apnea and bradycardia in low birth weight infants. Pediatrics 1975; 55:589–594.

152. Uauy R, Shapiro DL, Smith B, Warshaw JB. Treatment of severe apnea in prematures with orally administered theophylline. Pediatrics 1975; 55:595–598.

153. Kelly DH, Shannon DC. Treatment of apnea and excessive periodic breathing in the full-term infant. Pediatrics 1981; 68:183–186.

154. Simons FER, Rigatto H, Simons KJ. Pharmacokinetics of theophylline in neonates. Semin Perinatol 1981; 5:337–345.

155. Lamm WJE, Graham MM, Albert RK. Mechanism by which the prone position improves oxygenation in acute lung injury. Am J Respir Crit Care Med 1994; 150:184–193.

156. Polgar G, Weng TR. The functional development of the respiratory system—from the period of gestation to adulthood. Am Rev Respir Dis 1979; 120:625–695.

157. Burnard ED, Grattan-Smith P, Picton-Warlow CG, Grauaug A. Pulmonary insufficiency in prematurity. Aust Paediatr J 1965; 1:12–38.

158. Pereira MR, Reis FC, Landriault LV, Cates DB, Rigatto H. Profile of alveolar gases during periodic and regular breathing in preterm infants. Biol Neonate 1995; 67:322–329.

159. Qurashi M, Khan A, Kwiatkowski K, Cates D, Rigatto H. The determinants of physical stimulation in infants with apnea of prematurity. Pediatr Res 2001; 49:379A.

160. Al-Saedi SA, Lemke RP, Haider AZ, Cates DB, Kwiatkowski K, Rigatto H. Prolonged apnea in the preterm infant is not a random event. Am J Perinatol 1997; 14:195–200.

161. Specht H, Fruhmann G. Incidence of periodic breathing in 2000 subjects without pulmonary or neurological disease. Bull Physio-Pathol Respir 1972; 8:1075–1083.

162. Pitt GN, Pembrey MS, Allen RW. Observations upon Cheyne-Stokes respiration. Med Clin Trans 1907; 90:49–85.

163. Brown HW, Plum F. The neurologic basis of Cheyne-Stokes respiration. Am J Med 1961; 30:849–860.

164. Hall MJ, Xie A, Rutherford R, Ando S-I, Floras JS, Bradley TD. Cycle length of periodic breathing in patients with and without heart failure. Am J Respir Crit Care Med 1996; 154:376–381.

165. Lange RL, Hecht HH. The mechanism of Cheyne-Stokes respiration. J Clin Invest 1962; 41:42–52.

166. Merkel G. Zur Casuistik des Cheyne-Stokes'schen Respirations-Phänomens. Dtsch Arch Klin Med 1871; viii:424–426.
167. Webb P. Periodic breathing during sleep. J Appl Physiol 1974; 37:899–903.
168. Southall DP, Richards JM, Stebbens V, Wilson AJ, Taylor V, Alexander JR. Cardiorespiratory function in 16 full-term infants with sudden infant death syndrome. Pediatrics 1986; 78:787–796.
169. Southall DP, Alexander JR, Stebbens VA, Taylor VG, Janczynski RE. Cardiorespiratory patterns in siblings of babies with sudden infant death syndrome. Arch Dis Child 1987; 62:721–726.
170. Monod N, Plouin P, Sternberg B, Peirano P, Pajot N, Flores R, Linnett S, Kastler B, Scavone C, Guidasci S. Are polygraphic and cardiopneumographic respiratory patterns useful tools for predicting the risk of sudden infant death syndrome? A 10 year study. Biol Neonate 1986; 50:147–153.
171. Kahn A, Rebuffat E, Franco P, N'Duwimana M, Blum D. Apparent life-threatening events and apnea of infancy. In: Beckerman RC, Brouillette RT, Hunt CE, eds. Respiratory Control Disorders in Infants and Children. Baltimore: Williams & Wilkins, 1992:178–189.
172. Hoppenbrouwers T, Hodgman JE, Cabal L. Obstructive apnea, associated patterns of movement, heart rate, and oxygenation in infants at low and increased risk of SIDS. Pediatr Pulmonol 1993; 15:1–12.
173. Consensus Statement. National Institutes of Health Consensus Development Conference on Infantile Apnea and Home Monitoring. Pediatrics 1987; 79:292–299.
174. Keens TG, Ward SL, Gates EP, Andree DI, Hart LD. Ventilatory pattern following diphtheria-tetanus-pertussis immunization in infants at risk for sudden infant death syndrome. Am J Dis Child 1985; 139:991–994.
175. Samuels MP. Apparent life-threatening events. Pathogenesis and management. In: Loughlin GM, Carrol J, Marcus CL, eds. Sleep and Breathing in Children. A Developmental Approach. Lung Biology in Health and Disease. New York: Marcel Dekker, 2000:423–441.
176. Hussain A, Idiong N, Lin Y-J, Kwiatkowski K, Cates D, Rigatto H. The profile and significance of periodic breathing in preterm infants. Pediatr Res 1997; 41:255A.
177. Longobardo GS, Gothe B, Goldman MD, Cherniack NS. Sleep apnea considered as a control system instability. Respir Physiol 1982; 50:311–333.
178. Waggener TB. Breathing pattern in newborn infants (PhD dissertation). Cambridge, MA: Harvard University, 1979.
179. Waggener TB, Frantz ID III, Cohlan BA, Stark AR. Mixed and obstructive apneas are related to ventilatory oscillations in premature infants. J Appl Physiol 1989; 66:2818–2826.
180. Waggener TB, Stark AR, Cohlan BA, Frantz ID III. Apnea duration is related to ventilatory oscillation characteristics in newborn infants. J Appl Physiol 1984; 57:536–544.
181. Moore SE, Walsh JK, Keenan WJ, Farrell MK, Wolske SK, Kramer M. Periodic breathing in infants with histories of prolonged apnea. Am J Dis Child 1981; 135:1029–1031.

182. Hodgman JE, Hoppenbrouwers T, Geidel S, Hadeed A, Sterman MB, Harper R, McGinty D. Respiratory behavior in near-miss sudden infant death syndrome. Pediatrics 1982; 69:785–792.

183. Oren J, Kelly DH, Shannon DC. Pneumogram recordings in infants resuscitated for apnea of infancy. Pediatrics 1989; 83:364–368.

184. Escobar GJ, Littenberg B, Petitti DB. Outcome among surviving very low birth-weight infants: a meta-analysis. Arch Dis Child 1991; 66:204–211.

185. Volpe JJ. Subplate neurons-missing link in brain injury of the premature infant? (Editorial.) Pediatrics 1996; 97:112–113.

186. Roffwarg HP, Muzio JN, Dement WC. Ontogenetic development of the human sleep-dream cycle. Science 1966; 152:604–617.

11

Apnea, Bradycardia, and Desaturation
Clinical Issues

OOMMEN P. MATHEW

Brody School of Medicine at East Carolina University
Greenville, North Carolina, U.S.A.

I. Introduction

Apnea, bradycardia, and oxygen desaturation are the most common clinical problems facing neonatologists today. These problems are seen in the critically ill infants, infants recovering from lung diseases, feeding and growing premies, and infants approaching discharge. They arise not only in spontaneously breathing infants but also in mechanically ventilated infants. Optimal clinical management of these infants depends on understanding the complex pathophysiology of these episodes. Continuous cardiorespiratory monitoring is an integral part of clinical care provided to these high-risk neonates. Cardiorespiratory monitoring in the NICU and related issues are addressed in detail in Chapter 9. The primary purpose of this chapter is to summarize the current understanding of events leading to these episodes and to offer some insights into their management. Since the pathophysiology and management of apnea of prematurity, the most common cause of these episodes, are discussed in detail in subsequent chapters, the main focus of this chapter is on other etiologies of apnea.

II. Definition and Classification

A. Apnea

Apnea is traditionally defined as absence of breathing. Unfortunately, there is no universally accepted time period that qualifies as apnea; it varies from 5 sec to

>20 sec (1–6). The American Academy of Pediatrics task force on prolonged apnea defines clinically significant apnea as apnea >20 sec or <20 sec if it is associated with bradycardia, cyanosis, or pallor (7). Apnea alarms in most NICUs are set at 15 or 20 sec.

Apnea occurs commonly in the more immature infants. Its incidence is inversely proportional to birth weight and gestational age (4,5) with essentially all infants under 1000 g experiencing at least one clinically significant apnea. Initially, the term apnea was synonymous with central apnea or absent respiratory efforts. Once other forms of apnea were recognized, the definition was expanded to include all types of apnea. The definition of apnea now is based on the absence of airflow. Three types of apneas are recognized: central, obstructive, and mixed (Figs. 1, 2). When the lack of airflow is due to the absence of respiratory efforts, it is defined as central apnea. On the other hand, respiratory efforts are present during obstructive apnea. In mixed apnea elements of both central and obstructive apnea are present during the same episode. There are significant differences in the reported incidences of various types of apnea. Largely, this discrepancy reflects differences in methodology and population studied. The general consensus now is that mixed apnea accounts for the majority of apneic spells in premature infants, followed by central apnea (4,5). Pure obstructive apnea is the least common type. Larger infants, both preterm and term, have predominantly central apnea (8).

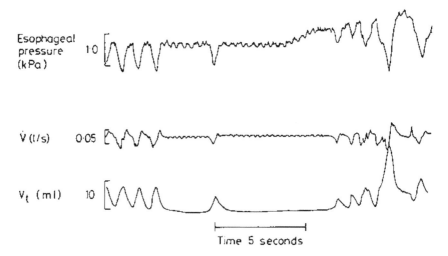

Figure 1   Central apnea. Esophageal pressure (top trace), airflow (middle), and tidal volume (bottom) are shown. Note the absence of both respiratory efforts and airflow for several seconds. Small fluctuations seen on the flow trace are due to cardiac artifacts. (From Ref. 2.)

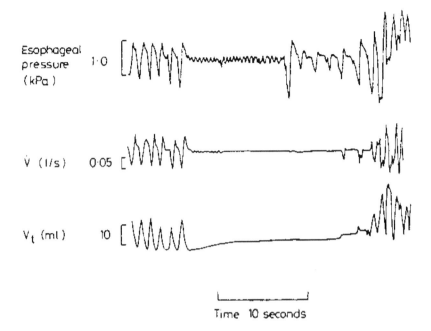

Figure 2 Mixed apnea. Traces are as in Figure 1. Airflow is absent for nearly 15 s. No respiratory efforts are seen during the initial part of this episode, whereas obstructed respiratory efforts are seen subsequently. (From Ref. 2.)

Milner and coworkers first reported the occurrence of airway closure during some central apneas on the basis of lack of cardiac artifacts in the airflow trace (2). This observation has been extended recently by Rigatto and coworkers (9). Based on the presence or absence of cardiac oscillations in the respiratory flow tracing, these investigators proposed a new definition of central, obstructive, and mixed apnea (see also Fig. 7 in the chapter on periodic breathing). It is interesting to note that some of the apneas previously defined as central would be classified as obstructive or mixed based on the new criteria. This classification is superior to the widely accepted definition in that the timing of airway occlusion can be accurately determined, providing further insight into the mechanisms involved.

Since respiration is routinely monitored in the NICU by impedance technique (and since airflow is not monitored), only central apneas and the central component of mixed apneas are clinically recognized. The limitations of thoracic impedance changes used in clinical monitoring of respiration in neonates are discussed in detail in the chapter on cardiorespiratory monitoring.

Nursing documentation of apnea is often used in daily management decisions, although it has been known for a long time that nursing documentation grossly underestimates these events. In one study, nurses documented 54% of all apneic episodes and were especially ineffective at detecting mixed and obstructive events (10). One reason is that all events witnessed by the nurses are not being documented. Another reason is that the central apnea, which triggers the alarm, may have resolved spontaneously by the time the nurse has responded. Also, she may not recognize the small, obstructed breaths; instead she records that the infant is not being apneic during the episode. Hence, nursing documentation is either lacking or misleading in a significant portion of these spells. Because of limited usefulness of nursing documentation with regard to apnea, one has to rely more on other resources in the diagnosis and management of apnea on a daily basis. The newer monitors with memory at least have the ability to document the events missed by the nurses, although it still has the inherent problem of not recognizing the obstructed breaths. Addition of nasal thermistors or respiratory inductance plethysmographs may provide further clarification of these events.

B. Bradycardia

Bradycardia is defined as a decrease in heart rate below a predetermined threshold. Generally, a heart rate < 100 beats per minute in preterm infants is defined as bradycardia (5). Several points need to be considered in determining the clinical importance of such events (see also chapter on cardiorespiratory monitoring). Suffice it to say that EKG and heart rate are typically displayed on the bedside monitor. Changes in monitored heart rate due to loose leads and movement artifacts are often easy to detect; therefore, the heart rate has been more reliable than respiration or oxygen saturation in most clinical situations.

What constitutes clinically significant bradycardia is a matter of debate. The resting heart rate is higher in preterm infants than in term infants, and heart rate increases markedly with stimulation or handling. The lowest heart rate during an episode can be calculated in a number of ways; the longest R-R interval, the longest three R-R intervals, and utilization of moving averages are used commonly in determining bradycardia. Most clinicians would agree that a heart rate < 100 bpm for 5 sec or more in an infant with resting heart rate between 140 and 160 bpm is significant. Alternatively, one could use a percentage decline from baseline (e.g., 25–33%) as a yardstick in defining significant bradycardia. This is especially true among infants with low resting heart rates. Most neonatologists would consider an instantaneous drop in heart rate to < 100 bpm for a beat or two unlikely to be meaningful or clinically significant unless one is evaluating arrhythmias. Because clinical monitoring of apnea is not reliable, bradycardia is often used as a proxy to document clinically significant episodes of apnea.

C. Oxygen Desaturation

Pulse oximetry has contributed immensely to our understanding of the pathophysiology of apnea. As a result of reduction in alveolar ventilation during the apneic period, a decrease in oxygen saturation is usually observed. Since monitoring of respiration is unreliable and the development of bradycardia, especially in the term infants, may be a late phenomenon during apnea, oxygen desaturation has become an important tool in the diagnosis of apnea in the newborn period. Pulse oximetry has been discussed in more detail in the preceding chapter. Although pulse oximetry has provided valuable insight into our understanding of the pathophysiology of apnea, it also has brought a number of difficult issues to clinical practice, the most important being false alarms. Movement artifact has been the main culprit. Ignoring the alarms or delay in responding to them has become commonplace in most NICUs, especially among infants with very labile oxygenation. Innovation in technology and algorithms are beginning to have an impact on this problem. The new Masimo monitors, for example, have decreased the false alarms significantly without sacrificing accuracy (11). Pulse oximeters are likely to continue as the mainstay in the clinical diagnosis and management of apnea in NICUs. In most centers the low saturation alarm is set between 85 and 90%. Saturation below that level for 3–5 sec can be considered desaturation. Oxygen saturation between 80% and 90% is considered mild desaturation, between 70% and 80% moderate, and <70% severe. When episodes of desaturation are prolonged and occur more frequently, they have the potential for adversely affecting the outcome of neonates.

III. Differential Diagnosis

Apnea is a symptom and not a diagnosis. Immaturity of the brainstem makes the premature infant uniquely vulnerable to apnea. As mentioned earlier, apnea of prematurity is the most common cause. Since it is a diagnosis of exclusion, other etiologies must be considered first (Table 1). Evaluation for apnea must include a review of historical facts. These include relevant maternal and neonatal history, which may give important clues as to the etiology of apnea. For example, apnea history in the immediate postpartum period alerts the physician to ask about sedatives and narcotics administered to the mother as well as any peripartum and intrapartum infections. Respiratory depression from perinatal asphyxia or intracranial hemorrhage needs to be considered in infants born after prolonged and difficult labor. Development of intracranial hemorrhage is an important etiologi-

Table 1   Causes of Apnea in the Neonatal Period

Central nervous system	Hematological
Apnea of prematurity	Severe anemia
Depression	Sepsis
Sedatives, narcotics	Bacterial
Postanesthesia	Viral
Hypoxia	Fungal
Intracranial hemorrhage	Temperature regulation
Seizures	Hypothermia
Tumors	Hyperthermia
Hyperekplexia	Airway obstruction
Hydrocephalus	Choanal atresia
Malformation	Pierre Robin sequence
Infection	Neck flexion
Meningitis	Secretions
Meningoencephalitis	Reflex
Circulatory	Passage of nasogastric tube
Patent ductus arteriosus	Vigorous suction
Heart failure	Cold stimulus to the face
Shock	Metabolic disorders
Gastrointestinal	Hypoglycemia
Nasopharyngeal reflux	Nonketotic hyperglycinemia
Gastroesophageal reflux	Urea cycle disorders
Necrotizing enterocolitis	Miscellaneous
Nipple feeding	Immunization
	Prostaglandin-E1

cal factor in the first few days of life, especially in very low-birth-weight infants. Recent administration of sedatives and narcotics to the neonate should also be investigated, whenever a sudden onset or sudden increase in frequency of apnea is noted in the neonate.

With increased survival of extremely low-birth-weight infants, nosocomial infections have become commonplace in most tertiary care units. Nosocomial infection must be foremost in one's mind while evaluating apnea in this group, because any potential delay in initiating treatment may contribute to a fatal outcome, particularly in cases of gram negative infections (12). Although bacterial infection is the primary concern, viral or fungal infections may complicate the clinical picture as well. If bacterial and fungal cultures are negative, viral infections assume greater significance, especially when sudden clustering of cases is seen (13). In winter months, infection due to respiratory syncytial virus (RSV) becomes part of the differential diagnosis. Apnea is not an uncommon presentation in the neonate with RSV. It may be the initial manifestation of RSV infection, often occurring before other respiratory signs. Apnea occurs in $\sim 20\%$ of infants hospitalized with RSV infection (14,15). Premature infants with a history of apnea are at greatest risk for developing apnea with RSV infection (16).

Although apnea is a common symptom during the onset of sepsis, the exact mechanism is still unclear. Output of the respiratory controller can be altered by changes in neural and chemical input as well as by changes in threshold or sensitivity of the controller. For example, if the sepsis is associated with infection of the airway epithelium or lung parenchyma, it is likely that the afferent input from the upper- and lower-airway mechanoreceptors would be altered. Lindgren and coworkers observed increased apnea response to laryngeal water stimulation in RSV-infected lambs (17). On the basis of this finding coupled with intact peripheral and central chemoreceptor function, these investigators suggested that sensitivity of laryngeal chemoreceptors is altered by RSV infection. In a subsequent study these investigators provided supporting histological evidence (18). Stimulation of these afferents has been well documented to have an inhibitory effect on breathing (19–22). Similarly, development of atelectasis or pneumonia is likely to alter the microenvironment of pulmonary afferents such as rapidly adapting (irritant) receptors, slowly adapting stretch receptors, and bronchial and pulmonary C-fibers. Again, alteration in the activity of these endings is known to have an immediate effect on the regulation of breathing (19–22).

The respiratory center can be affected either directly or indirectly. The role of inflammatory mediators in eliciting apnea is not entirely clear. A correlation between apnea and concentrations of interleukin 1-beta in pharyngeal secretions has been documented in RSV-infected infants (23). Infection has also been shown to alter the central respiratory response to afferent input (18,24). For example, Lindgren and coworkers (18) documented a state-dependent difference in the apnea response elicited by laryngeal stimulation in RSV-infected lambs. These investigators also noted a delay in arousal during active sleep following laryngeal chemostimulation. Apneic response to electrical stimulation of superior laryngeal nerve normally present in kittens can be elicited in adult cats following viral tracheobronchitis (24,25). This change in central response may persist even after the clinical symptoms of infection have resolved. Similarities in apnea of prematurity, upper-airway reflex apnea, and the apneas in infants with RSV infection have led Thach and coworkers to speculate that these various kinds of apnea may have related causal mechanisms (26).

Apnea is common among infants developing necrotizing enterocolitis. Since septicemia is not observed in the majority of these cases, apnea is likely to be mediated by the systemic inflammatory mediators or by the alteration of vagal afferent input. Distension of the bowel loops increases afferent input from vagal mechanoreceptors. Since abdominal distension alters pulmonary mechanics

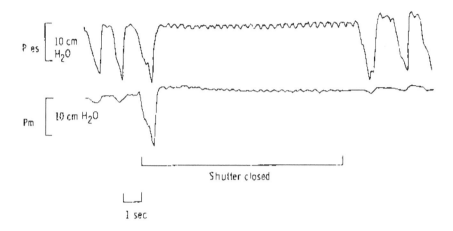

Figure 3 Apnea induced by airway occlusion. Esophageal and mouth pressures are shown. When the airway is occluded by closing a shutter attached to the face mask, the infant becomes apneic after the first obstructed effort until the shutter is released. (From Ref. 31.)

and residual lung volume, alteration of pulmonary mechanoreceptor input may contribute to the apnea as well.

Preterm infants with patent ductus arteriosus may manifest apnea. The development of pulmonary edema from left-to-right shunting is the likely mechanism. Pulmonary C-fibers are activated by pulmonary edema. Stimulation of pulmonary C-fibers is known to cause apnea and rapid shallow breathing (27–29). Hence, vagal afferents are likely to play a significant role in the initiation of apnea observed in infants with pulmonary edema.

A premature infant, whose upper airway is very small to begin with, is uniquely vulnerable to obstruction from secretions, edema, neck flexion, and mandibular hypoplasia (see also Chap. 22). The mechanism of apnea in conditions such as Pierre Robin sequence is clear. A markedly narrow pharyngeal airway predisposes infants to obstructive apnea, especially when they are supine. The greater negative pressure change seen during obstructed inspiratory effort has an inhibitory effect on breathing. It may inhibit inspiration completely, manifesting as central apnea with resultant prolongation of the apneic episode. This inhibitory reflex response has been demonstrated in animal studies by applying large negative pressures to the isolated upper airway while the animal is breathing through the tracheotomy (30). Similar reflex response has also been demonstrated in human neonates (31). Occlusion of the upper airway inducing a central apnea in a neonate is illustrated in Figure 3.

Other recognized causes of apnea include seizures, asphyxia, intracranial tumors, and metabolic disorders (32–44). The mechanism of apnea in a number of these conditions is unclear. These include some of the metabolic and electrolyte disorders. The author is unaware of any clear and convincing evidence that apnea occurs in electrolyte disorders such as hyponatremia and hypocalcemia in the absence of seizures. Seizures rarely present as apnea, or apnea can occur during or immediately following seizures (32,33). The association between anemia and apnea is discussed in Chapter 12.

An increase in the number of apneic and bradycardic episodes following immunization has been reported by several groups of investigators (45,46). For example, Sanchez et al. reported that following immunization 12% of infants experienced a recurrence of apnea and 11% had at least a 50% increase in the number of episodes (45). Apnea was attributed to the pertussis component of the vaccine. However, a recent study by the same group showed a temporal relationship between immunization and apnea in very low-birth-weight infants despite the use of acellular pertussis vaccine (47). Similarly, an increased incidence of apnea has been reported in premature infants during the postoperative period (48–50). Postanesthetic depression of the respiratory center is presumed to be responsible for this finding. Significant differences in the incidence of apnea are observed among different institutions. Methodological differences and duration of monitoring used, at least in part, account for these differences. Despite these limitations, one can conclude that postoperative apnea correlates inversely to both gestational age and postconceptional age (49). Caffeine can be used to prevent postoperative apnea and bradycardia in these growing preterm infants (51).

IV. Time of Occurrence

It is important to understand the time of occurrence of apnea and bradycardia episodes. For example, the significance of apnea, bradycardia, and desaturation spells during feeding should invoke an entirely different clinical strategy than if these episodes are occurring during sleep. The feeding-related episodes typically occur in preterm infants before 36 weeks postconceptional age. This is a reflection of brainstem immaturity in coordinating the acts of suck, swallow, and breathing, and in most cases, these spells disappear before they reach term postconceptional age (52). More mature infants may exhibit these episodes on the first day of life during bottle feeding (53,54). It is extremely rare in breast-fed infants. Infants with brochopulmonary dysplasia (BPD) and neurologically impaired infants are at increased risk for these complications (52,55,56). Respiratory control during feeding and associated disorders are discussed in detail in Chapter 16.

An increase in bradycardia and desaturation episodes may occur in the immediate postprandial period. One or more mechanisms have been implicated in these episodes. A decrease in pulmonary function has been documented immediately following feeding (56). A significant decrease in tidal volume, minute ventilation, and dynamic compliance, as well as an increase in pulmonary resistance, are observed after intermittent feedings; in comparison, the pulmonary function remains unchanged after continuous feedings (57). These findings suggest that gastric distension is an important contributing factor to the worsening pulmonary mechanics, although a contribution from a vagally mediated reflex response cannot be excluded. Another variable that needs to be considered is GE reflux (see also Chap. 21).

State of the infant is another important factor—that is, whether the infant is asleep or awake during the episodes critical to our understanding of the pathophysiology. Apnea of prematurity typically occurs during sleep; in fact, an increase in the number of spells has been documented during active sleep (58). Motor activity during apnea and bradycardia is being recognized with increasing frequency. Transient arousal or microarousal was associated with nearly a third of apneic spells in one study (59). These events are typically associated with laryngeal closure and Valsalva maneuvers. In some of these spells, the infant goes back to sleep, whereas in a minority of cases frank arousal follows. In infants with BPD and bronchomalacia, increase in positive intrathoracic pressure during expiration may lead to small-airway collapse with further worsening of hypoxia and development of bradycardia.

V. Significance of Sequence of Events

The temporal relationship among apnea, bradycardia, and oxygen desaturation provides important insight into the pathophysiology and helps us to optimize the management of infants in the NICU. However, this relationship among apnea, bradycardia, and oxygen desaturation is complex (Fig. 4). The usual cause of episodic desaturation is hypoventilation secondary to apnea. This fall in oxygen saturation triggers reflex bradycardia through carotid chemoreceptors (60,61). Apnea due to prematurity, sepsis, and CNS depression generally exhibits this sequence. Since airflow is not monitored, we may simply see oxygen desaturation followed by bradycardia. The rapidity with which desaturation develops depends on baseline oxygen saturation, pulmonary oxygen reserve, and intrapulmonary shunting. Upper-airway closure during the apnea has been suggested as an important factor in the development of bradycardia (62). In the recovery period some acceleration in heart rate may occur before a significant increase in alveolar ventilation can be documented; lung inflation has been implicated in this response (61).

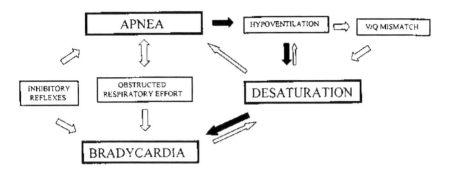

Figure 4 Apnea and its relationship with desaturation and bradycardia. The most common sequence is depicted with filled arrows. (Modified from Ref. 60.)

Another sequence is the development of bradycardia concurrently with apnea, well before the development of oxygen desaturation. This sequence of events is suggestive of inhibitory reflexes. The best example is the diving reflex, a reflex mediated through the trigeminal nerves (63). Stimulation of these nerves can reflexively induce apnea and bradycardia. Other examples of this sequence include the laryngeal and pulmonary chemoreflexes. Occurrences of apnea, bradycardia, and hypertension with laryngeal chemoreflex, and apnea, bradycardia, and hypotension with pulmonary chemoreflex have been well documented in carefully controlled animal studies (27–29,64–67). Even when apnea and bradycardia are elicited by the same stimulus, there may be a slight difference in the time of onset of each. Elicitation of pulmonary chemoreflex by intravenous administration of capsaicin, for example, showed a greater delay for cardiovascular response compared to the respiratory response (68). Lower conduction velocity of vagal efferents and/or greater number of interneurons involved in the cardiovascular response may account for this observation (68).

The inhibitory cardiorespiratory reflexes may occur spontaneously or can be elicited in the human neonate. Sudden increase in vagal or trigeminal afferent input has an inhibitory effect on both cardiovascular and respiratory output, which manifests as a sudden slowing of the heart and a decrease in breathing frequency or apnea. Passage of nasogastric tube or vigorous suctioning of the pharynx can induce both apnea and bradycardia. It has been shown that rapid passage of the nasogastric tube is more likely to be associated with apnea and bradycardia than slow passage (69). The role of laryngeal and pulmonary chemoreflexes in preterm infants is less clear. The existence of laryngeal chemoreflex has been documented; development of apnea or respiratory pause without immediate bradycardia was seen in these studies (70–72). Inhibitory reflexes can be triggered by the stimulation of laryngeal receptors during swallowing and obstructed respiratory efforts. Gastric distension and GE reflux may also elicit inhibitory reflexes.

The concept that enhanced vagal tone predisposes the infant to apnea and bradycardia is not new. Evidence supporting this concept has been emerging. An elevation in baseline parasympathetic activity was observed among infants who developed bradycardia during feeding (73). Spectral analysis of EKG signal was used to document increased vagal tone. Would prevention of the enhanced vagal tone reduce or prevent apnea in this group of patients? Intriguing results of a recently published study (74) may have shed some light on this question. Substantial reduction in the number of episodes of apnea and hypopnea, along with a reduction in the number of arousals and an increase in arterial oxyhemoglobin saturation, was achieved with atrial overdrive pacing at night in a group of adult sleep apnea patients (74). Also of interest is the observation that the vast majority of children with severe bradycardia due to breath-holding spells improved after pacing (75). These studies clearly indicate the influence of cardiac stimuli in stabilizing respiratory control.

VI. Episodic Bradycardia and Desaturation Among Intubated Infants

Not infrequently episodic desaturation and bradycardia are encountered among ventilated very low-birth-weight infants. Although there is no one pathophysiological explanation for all the desaturation episodes, there appears to be a common thread in the majority of patients. Typically these spells occur in infants with evolving BPD, often triggered by movement. In some, these desaturation episodes can be frequent and quite severe. Although no prevalence rate has been reported, desaturation episodes are not uncommon among the ventilated low-birth-weight infants during the exudative (edema) phase of BPD.

The sequence of events leading to the hypoxemia is quite complex; however, significant insight has been provided by two elegant studies (76,77). Boliver et al. studied 10 infants with episodic desaturation $\sim$ 1 month of age (76). Active expiration, evidenced by an increase in esophageal pressure, preceded both the reduction in lung volume and the decrease in tidal volume. The resulting hypoventilation was associated with a marked decrease in lung compliance and a large increase in inspiratory resistance (Fig. 5). Approximately 30 sec after the beginning of hypoventilation, the arterial oxygen saturation reaches the hypoxemic level (76). A closure of the small airways and the development of intrapulmonary shunts are likely to exacerbate the fall in oxygen saturation. Dimaguila et al. monitored tidal volume, respiratory rate, oxygen saturation, heart rate, and body movements in a similar group of infants (77). An acceleration in heart rate was observed at the onset of these episodes. Three-fourths of the

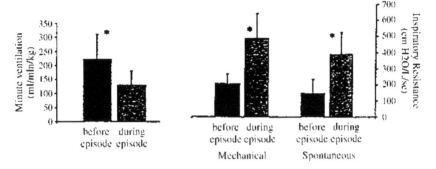

Figure 5 Minute ventilation and airway resistance before and during hypoxemic episodes in intubated infants. A marked reduction in ventilation and a marked increase in inspiratory resistance (both mechanical and spontaneous) can be seen (* $P < 0.005$). (From Ref. 76.)

desaturation spells began in association with body movements. These episodes had similarities to the apnea, bradycardia, and desaturation events observed during motor activity in nonintubated infants (59). Rarely one comes across an infant with episodic "death spells" while still being mechanically ventilated. Often these episodes are attributed to bronchospasm ("clamped down") by the nursing staff. It is likely that small-airway collapse and intrapulmonary shunting, in addition to the reduction in lung volume and ventilation, play a significant role during these severe hypoxemic spells. These spells have similarities to the observations of Southall and coworkers in more mature infants (78,79). Some of the recurrent episodes of severe hypoxemia were seen among intubated infants and were associated with continued respiratory efforts (78). Milner and Fagan suggested that active exhalation was the triggering point for the development of severe hypoxemia (80). Amato and coworkers evaluated the events associated with hypoxemia in ventilated patients with CT scan. In the supine position a decrease in lung volume elicits airways closure primarily in the posterior parts of the lower lobes. This generates local air trapping and low V/Q areas. At low FIO_2 conditions, these areas contribute to arterial hypoxemia without evident radiographic evidence. At high FIO_2 conditions, these areas promote reabsorption atelectasis with dense and visible infiltrates on CT (M. Amato, personal communication, 2002). A change in body position from supine to prone significantly decreased the frequency of the hypoxemic episodes in ventilated infants (77). An increase in the FRC, a decrease in chest wall distortion, and/or a decrease in ventilation/perfusion mismatch presumably account for this improvement (see also Chap. 10).

A small subset of ventilated low-birth-weight infants exhibit periodic desaturation on low ventilator rates. On closer observation, it becomes evident that these infants are having typical apnea of prematurity and that the decrease in desaturation is the result of marked decrease in spontaneous ventilation. Bradycardia is seldom seen in these infants. Sometime this sequence may be coupled with the movement-related spells described above. These infants respond to increasing ventilatory rate and/or the initiation of methylxanthine therapy. Successful extubation can be accomplished in most cases, once steady-state levels of methylxanthines are achieved.

Sudden onset of severe bradycardia without oxygen desaturation is seen in a small number of mechanically ventilated infants. Desaturation may develop later during the episode. Inhibitory reflexes of vagal origin are likely to be mediating these episodes. Possible sites of origin of these reflexes include the carina and the laryngeal-epilaryngeal area, both areas of dense innervation.

Infants in the exudative phase of BPD with edema and low FRC may benefit from higher PEEP and prone positioning to decrease the episodes of desaturation, whereas sleep-related apnea of prematurity with episodic decreases in spontaneous ventilation may benefit from methylxanthine therapy. These infants can be successfully extubated after initiation of methylxanthine therapy. The infants with evolving BPD, on the other hand, need to remain on the ventilator until the edema phase is resolved and the pulmonary compliance is improved, whereas the infants who manifest frequent arousal because of loud external noise and frequent hands-on interventions may benefit from minimum stimulation protocol and reduction of noise. These examples illustrate why understanding the pathophysiology of episodic events such as bradycardia and desaturation is important in their management.

VII. Apnea and Neurodevelopmental Outcome

The clinical significance of recurrent apnea on neurodevelopmental outcome remains a subject of considerable debate (61). In the absence of randomized trials specifically designed to evaluate the neurodevelopmental outcome of apneic infants, adverse outcome attributable to apnea of prematurity is difficult to quantify, especially when the clinical definition used excludes the majority of apneic spells with airway obstruction. Be that as it may, several studies have reported the developmental outcome of apneic infants with conflicting results (81–85). No adverse outcome attributable to apnea was found in some studies (81,82), whereas associations between apnea of prematurity and neurologic impairments and cerebral palsy were observed in others (83–85). Case control or cohort nature of these studies and small sample sizes render these conclusions less robust. A slightly higher rate of retrolental fibroplasia was seen in one large study (86). The facts that the above finding is the result of secondary analyses of infants enrolled in another study and that this finding could be the result of zealous treatment of apnea rather than apnea itself make this conclusion less than reassuring. Therefore, the conclusion of the 1987 National Institutes of Health Consensus Development Conference on Infantile Apnea that there is no evidence that apnea of prematurity per se causes subsequent morbidity still appears to be valid (87). The presence of persistent neonatal apnea without additional adverse perinatal events is not associated with a higher incidence of significant developmental problems (82). Long-term safety of methylxanthines, the mainstay in the treatment of apnea of prematurity, has been raised as an issue recently (88). No harmful effects of neonatal methylxanthine therapy on cognitive functioning were demonstrated at 18-month follow-up in one study (89). Davis et al. recently reported the relationship between theophylline therapy and outcome at 14 years of age in surviving preterm children (90). Theophylline therapy in the newborn period was associated with some evidence of harmful as well as helpful sensorineural effects at 14 years of age. Incidence of cerebral palsy and psychological test scores were higher in infants who received theophylline even after adjusting for potential confounding variables (90). In the final analysis, the risk of recurrent episodes of apnea or its treatment on the long-term outcome of the extremely low-birth-weight preterm infant is yet to be determined conclusively. Whether persistence of cardiorespiratory events in high-risk infants approaching discharge represents a subtle marker for neurodevelopmental delay or sleep or other disturbances of childhood is also unclear (61).

VIII. Summary

Apnea, bradycardia, and oxygen desaturation are common occurrences in NICUs. Although apnea of prematurity is by far the most common cause, the etiology of apnea in the neonatal period is quite varied. Routine monitoring of apnea by the impedance technique is not sensitive to detect obstructive apnea and therefore is not very useful by itself in evaluating or managing apnea. Detection of bradycardia is much more reliable. However, there is no consensus as to what constitutes a clinically significant bradycardia. Oxygen saturation monitoring is a sensitive measure of apnea and hypoventilation. Until recently false alarms have limited its usefulness for this purpose. The time of occurrence of these events and their sequences are important in understanding the etiology and pathophysiology of these episodes. In general, apnea of prematurity occurs during sleep, whereas feeding-related bradycardia and desaturation occur with oral feeding. Apnea of prematurity is a diagnosis of exclusion. Pathophysiology and treatment of apnea of prematurity are discussed in detail in subsequent chapters. Sudden onset of marked bradycardia (almost instantaneous) should prompt one to consider inhibitory reflexes. Oxygen desaturation seldom occurs at the onset in these cases, and recovery is usually spontaneous. Some mechanically ventilated infants develop desaturation and bradycardia, usually with forced expiration, a decrease in lung volume, and a decrease in ventilation. These episodes are generally triggered with body movement. Minimal handling, prone positioning, and increased PEEP are generally effective in minimizing these episodes.

References

1. Daily WRJ, Klaus M, Meyer HBP. Apnea in premature infants: monitoring, incidence of heart rate changes, and an effect of environmental temperature. Pediatrics 1969; 43:510–518.
2. Milner AD, Boon AW, Saunders RA, Hopkin IE. Upper airways obstruction and apnoea in preterm babies. Arch Dis Child 1980; 55:22–25.
3. Kattwinkel J, Nearman HS, Fanaroff AA, Katona PG, Klaus MH. Apnea of prematurity. Comparative therapeutic effects of cutaneous stimulation and nasal continuous positive airway pressure. J Pediatr 1975; 86:588–592.
4. Miller MJ, Carlo WA, Martin RJ. Continuous positive airway pressure selectively reduces obstructive apnea in preterm infants. J Pediatr 1985; 106:91–94.
5. Dransfield DA, Spitzer AR, Fox WW. Episodic airway obstruction in premature infants. Am J Dis Child 1983; 137:441–443.
6. Martin RJ, Miller MJ, Carlo WA. Pathogenesis of apnea in preterm infants. J Pediatr 1986; 109:733–741.
7. Task force on prolonged apnea, American Academy of Pediatrics. Pediatrics 1978; 61:651–652.
8. Lee D, Caces R, Kwiatkowski K, Cates D, Rigatto H. A developmental study on types and frequency distribution of short apneas (3 to 15 seconds) in term and preterm infants. Pediatr Res 1987; 22:344–349.
9. Lemke RP, Al-Saedi S, Alvaro R, Kwiatkowski K, Cates D, Rigatto H. Use of a magnified cardiac waveform oscillation to diagnose infant apnea: a theoretical and clinical evaluation. Am J Respir Crit Care Med 1996; 154:1537–1542.
10. Muttitt SC, Finer NN, Tierney AJ, Rossmann J. Neonatal apnea: diagnosis by nurse versus computer. Pediatrics 1988; 82:713–720.
11. Bohnhorst B, Peter CS, Poets CF. Pulse oximeters' reliability in detecting hypoxemia and bradycardia: comparison between a conventional and two new generation oximeters. Crit Care Med 2000; 28:1565–1568.
12. Stoll BJ, Gordon T, Korones SB, Shankaran S, Tyson JE, Bauer CR, Fanaroff AA, Lemons JA, Donovan EF, Oh W, Stevenson DK, Ehrenkranz RA, Papile LA, Verter J, Wright LL. Late-onset sepsis in very low birth weight neonates: a report from the National Institute of Child Health and Human Development Neonatal Research Network. J Pediatr 1996; 129:63–71.
13. Riedel F, Kroener T, Stein K, Nuesslein TG, Rieger CH. Rotavirus infection and bradycardia-apnoea-episodes in the neonate. Eur J Pediatr 1996; 155:36–40.

14. Bruhn FW, Mokrohisky ST, McIntosh K. Apnea associated with respiratory syncytial virus infection in young infants. J Pediatr 1977; 90:382–386.
15. Forster J, Schumacher RF. The clinical picture presented by premature neonates infected with the respiratory syncytial virus. Eur J Pediatr 1995; 154:901–905.
16. Church NR, Anas NG, Hall CB, Brooks JG. Respiratory syncytial virus-related apnea in infants: demographics and outcome. Am J Dis Child 1984; 138:247–250.
17. Lindgren C, Jing L, Graham B, Grogaard J, Sundell H. Respiratory syncytial virus infection reinforces reflex apnea in young lambs. Pediatr Res 1992; 31:381–385.
18. Lindgren C, Lin J, Graham BS, Gray ME, Parker RA, Sundell HW. Respiratory syncytial virus infection enhances the response to laryngeal chemostimulation and inhibits arousal from sleep in young lambs. Acta Paediatr 1996; 85:789–797.
19. Widdicombe JG. Respiratory reflexesin man and other mammalian species. Clin Sci 1961; 21:163–170.
20. Fisher JT, Sant'Ambrogio G. Airway and lung receptors and their reflex effects in the newborn. Pediatr Pulmonol 1985; 1:112–126.
21. Cross KW, Klaus M, Toley WH, Weisser K. The response of the newborn baby to inflation of the lungs. J Physiol (Lond) 1960; 151:551–565.
22. Lee JC, Stoll BJ, Downing SE. Properties of the laryngeal chemoreflex in neonatal piglets. Am J Physiol 1977; 233:R30–R36.
23. Lindgren C, Grogaard J. Reflex apnoea response and inflammatory mediators in infants with respiratory tract infection. Acta Paediatr 1996; 85:798–803.
24. Sessle BJ, Lucier GE. Functional aspect of the upper respiratory tract and larynx: a review. In: Tildon JT, Roeder LM, Steinschneider A, eds. Sudden Infant Death Syndrome. New York: Academic Press, 1983:501–529.
25. Lucier GE, Storey AT, Sessle BJ. Effects of upper respiratory tract stimuli on neonatal respiration: reflex and single neuron analyses in the kitten. Biol Neonate 1979; 35:82–89.
26. Pickens DL, Schefft GL, Storch GA, Thach BT. Characterization of prolonged apneic episodes associated with respiratory syncytial virus infection. Pediatr Pulmonol 1989; 6:195–201.
27. Coleridge JC, Coleridge HM. Afferent vagal C fibre innervation of the lungs and airways and its functional significance. Rev Physiol Biochem Pharmacol 1984; 99:1–110.
28. Roberts AM, Bhattacharya J, Schultz HD, Coleridge HM, Coleridge JC. Stimulation of pulmonary vagal afferent C-fibers by lung edema in dogs. Circ Res 1986; 58:512–522.
29. Schertel ER, Adams L, Schneider DA, Smith KS, Green JF. Rapid shallow breathing evoked by capsaicin from isolated pulmonary circulation. J Appl Physiol 1986; 61:1237–1240.
30. Mathew OP, Farber JP. Effect of upper airway negative pressure on respiratory timing. Respir Physiol 1983; 54:259–268.
31. Milner AD, Saunders RA, Hopkin IE. Apnoea induced by airflow obstruction. Arch Dis Child 1977; 52:79–82.
32. Scher MS, Painter MJ, Bergman I, Barmada MA, Brunberg J. EEG diagnoses of neonatal seizures: clinical correlations and outcome. Pediatr Neurol 1989; 5:17–24.

33. Volpe JJ. Neonatal seizure. In: Volpe JJ, ed, Neonatal Neurology. Philadelphia: W.B. Saunders, 2001:178–214.

34. Brazy JE, Kinney HC, Oakes WJ. Central nervous system structural lesions causing apnea at birth. J Pediatr 1987; 111:163–175.

35. Clarke DB, Farmer JP, Montes JL, Watters GV, Rouleau G. Newborn apnea caused by a neurofibroma at the craniocervical junction. Can J Neurol Sci 1994; 21:64–66.

36. Griffiths AD. Association of hypoglycaemia with symptoms in the newborn. Arch Dis Child 1968; 43:688–694.

37. Moore AM, Perlman M. Symptomatic hypoglycemia in otherwise healthy, breastfed term newborns. Pediatrics 1999; 103:837–839.

38. Kalhan SC, Saker F. Disorders of carbohydrate metabolism. In: Fanaroff AA, Martin RJ, eds. Neonatal Perinatal Medicine: Diseases of the Fetus and Infant, 6th ed. St. Louis; Mosby, 1997:1439–1463.

39. Summar M, Tuchman M. Proceedings of a consensus conference for the management of patients with urea cycle disorders. J Pediatr 2001; 138:S6–S10.

40. Baca CM, Milano MG, Calvo MC, Martinez VM. Apnea attacks in infants: study of 7 cases. An Esp Pediatr 1989; 30:124–126.

41. Tekinalp G, Coskun T, Oran O, Ozalp I, Figen G, Ergin H. Nonketotic hyperglycinemia in a newborn infant. Turk J Pediatr 1995; 37:57–60.

42. Nigro MA, Lim HC. Hyperekplexia and sudden neonatal death. Pediatr Neurol 1992; 8:221–225.

43. Bader D, Tirosh E, Hodgins H, Abend M, Cohen A. Effect of increased environmental temperature on breathing patterns in preterm and term infants. J Perinatol 1998; 18:5–8.

44. Perlstein PH, Edwards NK, Sutherland JM. Apnea in premature infants and incubator-air-temperature changes. N Engl J Med 1970; 282:461–466.

45. Sanchez PJ, Laptook AR, Fisher L, Sumner J, Risser RC, Perlman JM. Apnea after immunization of preterm infants. J Pediatr 1997; 130:746–751.

46. Botham SJ, Isaacs D, Henderson-Smart DJ. Incidence of apnoea and bradycardia in preterm infants following DTPw and Hib immunization: a prospective study. J Paediatr Child Health 1997; 33:418–421.

47. Goodman B, Summer J, Zeray F, Sanchez PJ. Apnea after immunization of very low birth weight infants: a second look after use of acellular pertussis vaccine (abstract). Pediatr Res 2001; 49:240A.

48. Somri M, Gaitini L, Vaida S, Collins G, Sabo E, Mogilner G. Postoperative outcome in high-risk infants undergoing herniorrhaphy: comparison between spinal and general anaesthesia. Anaesthesia 1998; 53:762–766.

49. Cote CJ, Zaslavsky A, Downes JJ, Kurth CD, Welborn LG, Warner LO, Malviya SV. Postoperative apnea in former preterm infants after inguinal herniorrhaphy. A combined analysis. Anesthesiology 1995; 82:809–822.

50. Spaeth JP, O'Hara IB, Kurth CD. Anesthesia for the micropremie. Semin Perinatol 1998; 22:390–401.

51. Henderson-Smart DJ, Steer P. Postoperative caffeine for preventing apnea in preterm infants. Cochrane Database Syst Rev 2000; (2):CD000048.

52. Mathew OP. Science of bottle feeding. J Pediatr 1991; 119:511–519.

53. Mathew OP, Clark ML, Pronske MH. Apnea, bradycardia, and cyanosis during oral feeding in term neonates. J Pediatr 1985; 106:857.

54. Bamford O, Taciak V, Gewolb IH. Coordination of sucking, swallowing and breathing in the newborn: its relationship to infant feeding and normal development. Pediatr Res 1992; 31:619–624.

55. Garg M, Kurzner SI, Bautista DB, Keens TG. Clinically unsuspected hypoxia during sleep and feeding in infants with bronchopulmonary dysplasia. Pediatrics 1988; 81:635–642.

56. Singer L, Martin RJ, Hawkins SW, Benson-Szekely LJ, Yamashita TS, Carlo WA. Oxygen desaturation complicates feeding in infants with bronchopulmonary dysplasia after discharge. Pediatrics 1992; 90:380–384.

57. Blondheim O, Abbasi S, Fox WW, Bhutani VK. Effect of enteral gavage feeding rate on pulmonary functions of very low birth weight infants. J Pediatr 1993; 122:751–755.

58. Gabriel M, Albani M, Schulte FJ. Apneic spells and sleep states in preterm infants. Pediatrics 1976; 57(1):142–147.

59. Mathew OP, Thoppil CK, Belan M. Motor activity and apnea in preterm infants. Is there a causal relationship? Am Rev Respir Dis 1991; 144:842–844.

60. Martin RJ, Fanaroff AA. Neonatal apnea, bradycardia, or desaturation: does it matter? J Pediatr 1998; 132:758–759.

61. Henderson-Smart DJ, Butcher-Puech MC, Edwards DA. Incidence and mechanism of bradycardia during apnoea in preterm infants. Arch Dis Child 1986; 61:227–232.

62. Upton CJ, Milner AD, Stokes GM. Episodic bradycardia in preterm infants. Arch Dis Child 1992; 67:831–834.

63. Jones DR. Control of the cardiovascular adjustments to diving in birds and mammals. In: Perthes G, ed. Advances in Physiological Sciences. New York: Pergamon Press, 1981; 20:307–314.

64. Johnson P, Salisbury DM, Storey AT. Apnoea induced by stimulation of sensory receptors in the larynx. In: Bosma JF, Showacre J, eds. Development of upper respiratory anatomy and function. Bethesda, MD: NIH, 1975:160–183.

65. Grogaard J, Lindstrom DP, Stahlman MT, Marchal F, Sundell H. The cardiovascular response to laryngeal water administration in young lambs. Dev Physiol 1982; 4:353–370.

66. Dawes GS, Comroe JH. Chemoreflexes from the heart and lungs. Physiol Rev 1954; 34:167–201.

67. Green JF, Schmidt ND, Schultz HD, Roberts AM, Coleridge HM, Coleridge JC. Pulmonary C-fibers evoke both apnea and tachypnea of pulmonary chemoreflex. J Appl Physiol 1984; 57:562–567.

68. Palecek F, Sant'Ambrogio G, Sant'Ambrogio FB, Mathew OP. Reflex responses to capsaicin: intravenous, aerosol, and intratracheal administration. J Appl Physiol 1989; 67:1428–1437.

69. Haxhija EQ, Rosegger H, Prechtl HF. Vagal response to feeding tube insertion in preterm infants: has the key been found? Early Hum Dev 1995; 17(41):15–25.

70. Perkett EA, Vaughan RL. Evidence for a laryngeal chemoreflex in some human preterm infants. Acta Paediatr Scand 1982; 71(6):969–972.

71. Davies AM, Koenig JS, Thach BT. Upper airway chemoreflex responses to saline and water in preterm infants. J Appl Physiol 1988; 64:1412–1420.
72. Davies AM, Koenig JS, Thach BT. Characteristics of upper airway chemoreflex prolonged apnea in human infants. Am Rev Respir Dis 1989; 139:668–673.
73. Veerappan S, Rosen H, Craelius W, Curcie D, Hiatt M, Hegyi T. Spectral analysis of heart rate variability in premature infants with feeding bradycardia. Pediatr Res 2000; 47:659–662.
74. Kelly AM, Porter CJ, McGoon MD, Espinosa RE, Osborn MJ, Hayes DL. Breath-holding spells associated with significant bradycardia: successful treatment with permanent pacemaker implantation. Pediatrics 2001; 108:698–702.
75. Garrigue S, Bordier P, Jais P, Shah DC, Hocini M, Raherisson C, De Lara MT, Haissaguerre M, Clementy J. Benefit of atrial pacing in sleep apnea syndrome. N Engl J Med 2002; 346(6):404–412.
76. Bolivar JM, Gerhardt T, Gonzalez A, Hummler H, Claure N, Everett R, Bancalari E. Mechanisms for episodes of hypoxemia in preterm infants undergoing mechanical ventilation. J Pediatr 1995; 127:767–773.
77. Dimaguila MAVT, DiFiore JM, Martin RJ, Miller MJ. Characteristics of hypoxemic episodes in very low birth weight infants on ventilatory support. J Pediatr 1996; 130:577–583.
78. Southall DP, Talbert DG, Johnson P, Morley CJ, Salmons S, Miller J, Helms PJ. Prolonged expiratory apnoea: a disorder resulting in episodes of severe arterial hypoxaemia in infants and young children. Lancet 1985; 2:571–577.
79. Southall DP, Samuels MP, Talbert DG. Recurrent cyanotic episodes with severe arterial hypoxaemia and intrapulmonary shunting: a mechanism for sudden death. Arch Dis Child 1990; 65:953–961.
80. Milner AD, Fagan DG. Prolonged expiratory apnea in children. Lancet 1985; 2:835.
81. Levitt GA, Mushin A, Bellman S, Harvey DR. Outcome of preterm infants who suffered neonatal apnoeic attacks. Early Hum Dev 1988; 16:235–243.
82. Koons AH, Mojica N, Jadeja N, Ostfeld B, Hiatt M, Hegyi T. Neurodevelopmental outcome of infants with apnea of infancy. Am J Perinatol 1993; 10:208–211.
83. Tudehope DI, Rogers YM, Burns YR, Mohay H, O'Callaghan MJ. Apnoea in very low birthweight infants: outcome at 2 years. Aust Paediatr J 1986; 22:131–134.
84. Kitchen WH, Doyle LW, Ford GW, Rickards AL, Lissenden JV, Ryan MM. Cerebral palsy in very low birthweight infants surviving to 2 years with modern perinatal intensive care. Am J Perinatol 1987; 4:29–35.
85. Taylor HG, Klein N, Schatschneider C, Hack M. Predictors of early school age outcomes in very low birth weight children. J Dev Behav Pediatr 1998; 19:235–243.
86. Purohit DM, Ellison RC, Zierler S, Miettinen OS, Nadas AS. Risk factors for retrolental fibroplasia: experience with 3,025 premature infants. Pediatrics 1985; 76:339–344.
87. National Institutes of Health Consensus Development Panel on Infantile Apnea and Home Monitoring. Consensus statement. Pediatrics 1987; 79:292–299.
88. Schmidt B. Methylxanthine therapy in premature infants: sound practice, disaster, or fruitless byway? J Pediatr 1999; 135:526–528.

89. Ment LR, Scott DT, Ehrenkranz RA, Duncan CC. Early childhood developmental follow-up of infants with GMH/IVH: effect of methylxanthine therapy. Am J Perinatol 1985; 2:223–237.
90. Davis PG, Doyle LW, Rickards AL, Kelly EA, Ford GW, Davis NM, Callanan C. Methylxanthines and sensorineural outcome at 14 years in children <1501 g birthweight. J Paediatr Child Health 2000; 36:47–50.

12

Pathophysiology of Apnea of Prematurity
Implications from Observational Studies

CHRISTIAN F. POETS

University of Tübingen
Tübingen, Germany

I. Introduction

In the past, observational studies on apnea of prematurity concentrated predominantly on an analysis of respiratory disturbances such as central and obstructive apneas (1–3). From a physiological point of view, however, it is not the apnea per se but its effect on oxygenation and/or heart rate that is relevant to the well-being of an infant. This chapter will therefore concentrate on these latter two phenomena. This is also because, at least in term infants and children, the propensity to develop intermittent episodes of oxygen desaturation decreases with age, while the frequency of spontaneous apneas remains remarkably constant (Fig. 1) (4–7). Changes in desaturation rate may therefore be a better indicator for developmental changes in respiratory control than those in apnea rate.

II. Relationship Between Apnea, Bradycardia, and Desaturation

One of the most striking findings in recordings of respiration, heart rate, and pulse oximeter saturation (SpO_2) in preterm infants is the close temporal

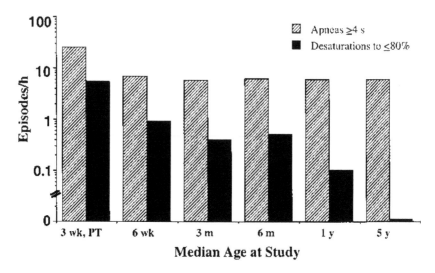

Figure 1   Data on the frequency of apnea (≥ 4 s) and desaturation ($SpO_2 \leq 80\%$) from various studies (4–7) obtained with the same methodology. Note that except for preterm infants (PT), the frequency of apneas remains remarkably constant ($\sim 6/h$), whereas that of desaturations falls from 1/h at 6 weeks to 0.1 at 1 year and to 0.0 at 5 years of age.

relationship among apnea, bradycardia, and desaturation (8). Early studies suggested that the bradycardia resulted from a chemoreceptor reflex elicited by the rapid development of hypoxemia during apnea (9,10). Subsequent investigators, however, claimed that the fall in heart rate commenced too early during the apnea to be attributed to apnea-induced hypoxemia, and suggested instead that bradycardia was caused by a reflex response to the cessation of lung inflation (11,12).

We analyzed the relationship among these three phenomena in 80 preterm infants with a mean gestational age of 32.5 weeks (SD 2.6) at birth and 36.3 weeks (2.3) at time of study. Focusing on bradycardia, which was defined as a fall in heart rate to $<2/3$ of baseline for ≥ 4 sec, we found that 86% of these (143/166) were accompanied by a fall in SaO_2 to $\leq 80\%$, and 83% by an apneic pause of 4 sec or longer (13). Analysis of the time intervals between apnea and bradycardia showed that almost all bradycardias (97%) commenced *after* the onset of apnea (median interval, 4.8 sec). In most instances (86%), bradycardia also began *after* the onset of the fall in SpO_2 (median interval, 4.2 sec). This was predominantly because the interval between the onset of apnea and that of desaturation, corrected for lung-to-toe circulation time (i.e., the time it takes for the blood to travel from the lung to the pulse oximeter sensor site) was extremely short (median 0.8 sec, Fig. 2) (13).

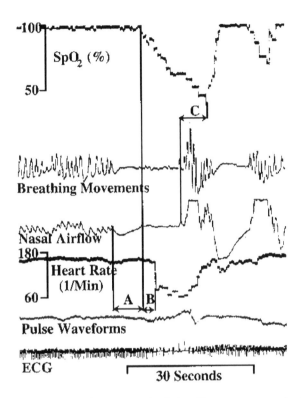

Figure 2 Example for the close temporal relationship among apnea, bradycardia, and desaturation. The delay caused by the time it takes for the blood to travel from the lung to the pulse oximeter sensor attached to the foot can be estimated from the delay between the first breath following an apnea and the onset of the recovery in SpO_2 (C). This was subtracted from the interval between the onset of apnea and that of desaturation (A) and from the interval between the onset of bradycardia and that of desaturation (B; see text).

These temporal observations support the concept that hypoxemia causes bradycardia, e.g., via stimulation of peripheral chemoreceptors (14). But why was it apparently not the hypoxemia per se, but its coincidence with an apneic pause that resulted in the development of bradycardia? The answer to this may be found in experiments by Angell-James and Daly (15). These authors performed cross-perfusion studies in dogs and showed that the fall in heart rate was far more pronounced if there was a combination of both apnea and hypoxemic excitation of arterial chemoreceptors than with either apnea or hypoxemia alone. They concluded that the appearance of bradycardia during apnea depends on there being no overriding effect from the pulmonary inflation reflex, which is known to

cause an increase in heart rate (15). One possible explanation for the comparatively high frequency of bradycardia in preterm infants, therefore, is that
bradycardia is primarily caused by hypoxemia [which is common in this age
group (16)], and that the resultant effects on heart rate are potentiated by the
concomitant cessation of lung inflation during apneic pauses. This would also
explain why, despite a similar severity of the accompanying hypoxemia, bradycardia is more common with central than with mixed or obstructive apnea (17).

III. Changes in Lung Volume During Apnea

A surprising finding in the above study (13) was the brevity of the interval
between the onset of apnea and that of desaturation. We speculate that there
would have been far less bradycardia had the hypoxemia not occurred so early
during apnea. It remains unclear, however, whether this early onset of hypoxemia
was due to preceding hypoventilation, nonapneic mechanisms, or both. Hypoventilation was suggested by Adams et al. to precede apnea (18). These authors
used inductive plethysmography to quantify tidal volume and found that 62% of
events with $SpO_2 < 80\%$ were preceded by breaths with a tidal volume of $< 50\%$
of baseline (18).

A nonapneic mechanism that could explain the early onset of hypoxemia
during apnea is a low lung volume. This is particularly relevant to young infants,
whose relaxation volume is only 10–15% of total lung capacity and thus very
close to residual volume, predisposing them to the development of airway closure
(19). To compensate for this disadvantage, both term and preterm infants actively
maintain their end-expiratory lung volume above relaxation volume (which is one
reason for their high respiratory rate) (20–22) whereas lung volume falls if
respiration ceases (23). To investigate this issue further, we measured functional
residual capacity (FRC) repeatedly in 48 "healthy" preterm infants (mean
gestational age at study 36.6 weeks, SD 2.0) during unsedated sleep using a
modified heliox/nitrogen washout technique (24). Breathing movements and
SpO_2 were recorded throughout and analyzed for apneas ($\geq 4\,\mathrm{sec}$), sighs, and
desaturations ($SpO_2 \leq 90\%$) during the last $2\,\mathrm{min}$ prior to each FRC measurement. Apneas resulted in a significant decrease in FRC: mean FRC was
$20.0\,\mathrm{mL/kg}$ (SD 6.8) following an apnea, $26.0\,\mathrm{mL/kg}$ (SD 5.8) after a sigh
($P < 0.001$), and $23.9\,\mathrm{mL/kg}$ (SD 7.7) if there had been neither a sigh or an
apnea ($P < 0.05$). The interval between the apnea and the FRC measurement had
no effect on FRC. Thus, apneas resulted in a persistent reduction in FRC, which
was restored by a sigh. These findings provide further evidence for the hypothesis
(25,26) that one of the main functions of sighs in preterm infants is to reverse falls
in lung volume caused by apneas.

What does this have to do with the interval between apnea and desaturation? The FRC serves as a buffer to stabilize oxygenation during brief periods of apnea. Lung volume is an important determinant of the speed with which desaturation develops during voluntary breath holding (27), and preapneic lung volume was found to have a strong influence on the hypoxemia that occurs during sleep apnea in adults (28). In the above study (24), we found an inverse correlation between FRC and the speed with which SpO_2 fell during desaturation; i.e., the lower the lung volume *following* an apnea, the more rapid the fall in SpO_2 *during* the apnea.

A clinical scenario in which the potential influence of lung volume on oxygenation becomes particularly evident is periodic apnea. During this respiratory pattern, SpO_2 was observed to fall twice as fast as during isolated apneas (8.4 vs. 4.3%/sec; $P < 0.005$) (8). Although other factors, e.g., a fall in mixed venous SO_2 (29), may also play a role, we hypothesize that the main reason for the more rapid fall in SpO_2 is a progressive fall in lung volume during the repeated apneas, resulting in peripheral airway closure.

Another potential consequence of the reduction in lung volume occurring during spontaneous apneas is a further inhibition of respiration via activation of the Hering-Breuer deflation reflex. In term infants this vagally mediated reflex, which acts around FRC, terminates expiration while initiating inspiration. In preterm infants, however, induction of this reflex via chest compression resulted in a shortening of inspiratory time and a tendency to have short apneas (2–5 sec) (30). A similar inhibition of breathing may result if lung volume falls spontaneously, e.g., during apnea.

These considerations provide a theoretical basis for the effectiveness of strategies that increase or stabilize lung volume in reducing the frequency and/or severity of both bradycardia and desaturation in preterm infants (31). In fact, Thibeault et al. (32) observed as long as 30 years ago that recurrent apnea may be abolished by increasing functional residual capacity via the application of negative extrathoracic pressure. The same effect can also be achieved by continuous positive airway pressure (CPAP) (33). The striking effects of CPAP on the frequency of apneic/hypoxemic episodes in preterm infants have led to suggestions that "the apnea in these infants may be related to a decreasing lung volume and increasing intrapulmonary shunt" (33).

IV. Role of Feeding and Gastroesophageal Reflux

A frequent observation in infants with apnea of prematurity (AOP), first noted almost 80 years ago (34), is that symptoms increase during and after feeding. The hypothesis that this association could be a result of "the full stomach interfering with the action of the diaphragm" was put forward in 1936 (35). Since then the effects of feeding on respiration have been studied extensively (36–46). It is now clear that some preterm infants, particularly those with bronchopulmonary dysplasia (BPD), may become severely hypoxemic during and immediately after bottle feeding (35–39), and that gavage feeding may also cause a significant reduction in blood oxygen levels (40–43). Hypoxemia *during* feeding may be caused by a reduction in minute ventilation due to an immature coordination between breathing, sucking, and swallowing (39,43,44), activation of the laryngeal chemoreceptor reflex (46), gastroesophageal reflux, diaphragmatic fatigue (47), or combinations of these mechanisms. Hypoxemia *after* feeding was suspected to be due to a reduction in lung volume and an increased work of breathing resulting from gastric distension (44). If this is true, avoidance of gastric distension via slow or continuous gavage feeding should ameliorate the problem.

To test this hypothesis, we studied the effect of bottle feeding, as compared to two methods of gavage feeding, on apnea, bradycardia, and episodic desaturation in 30 "healthy" preterm infants with a mean gestational age of 28.6 (SD 2.1) weeks at birth and 34.0 (SD 1.4) weeks at study (48). During a 9-h recording of SpO_2, ECG, breathing movements, and nasal airflow, 3×21 mL/kg of milk were administered to each infant using three different feeding techniques in random order: bottle feeding, bolus gavage feeding, and slow gavage feeding (over 1 h). Recordings were analyzed for apneas (> 4 sec, bradycardias (heart rate $< 2/3$ of baseline), and episodic desaturation ($SpO_2 \leq 80\%$). We found three times more desaturations (up to 165/h) with bottle feeding than with bolus gavage feeding ($P < 0.001$), but no further reduction with slow gavage feeding and no difference in baseline SpO_2. With all three feeding techniques there were significantly more desaturations in the hour the feeds were given than during the following 2 h. The deleterious effects of bottle feeding were most evident during the hour of feeding, but desaturation frequency remained significantly higher than with gavage feeding during the following 2 h. In contrast, there was no significant effect of feeding technique on the frequency of apnea or bradycardia (48).

Thus, bottle feeding in these premature infants conferred a significantly increased risk of episodic desaturation, which was surprisingly long-lasting. White this may be avoided by switching infants exhibiting frequent desaturation during bottle feeding to gavage feeding, we were puzzled that slow gavage feeding (over 1 h) offered no advantage over bolus gavage feeding. Gastric emptying time in preterm infants is ~30–60 min (49). We thus considered that significant gastric distension, although not specifically assessed in our study, had been avoided with slow gavage feeding. We suspected instead that gastroesophageal reflux (GER) would be the most likely explanation for the observed increase in desaturation during and immediately after feeding.

A relationship between GER and AOP has long been suspected (50,51) but was difficult to prove because most GER in this age group is nonacidic and thus undetectable by pH monitoring, the current standard for GER detection. Recently, we used the new multiple intraluminal impedance (MII) technique which allows pH-independent reflux detection via changes in impedance caused by a liquid bolus inside the esophagus to investigate whether there is a temporal relationship between GER and AOP (52). For this, 19 infants with AOP underwent recordings of MII, breathing movements, nasal airflow, ECG, and SpO_2. MII signals were analyzed, independently of cardiorespiratory (CR) signals, for reflux episodes (RE), defined as a fall in impedance in at least the two most distal channels (Fig. 3). CR signals were analyzed for CR events, i.e., apneas of ≥ 4 sec duration, desaturations to $\leq 80\%$, and falls in heart rate to $\leq 100/\text{min}$. A temporal relationship between an RE and a CR event was considered present if the two commenced within 20 sec of each other. We found high numbers of both apneas

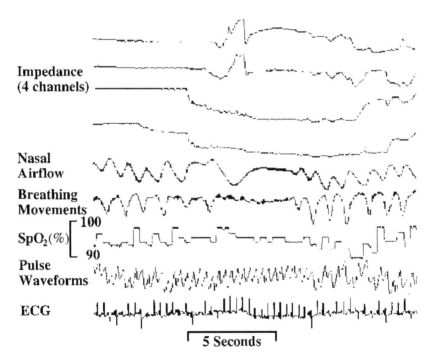

Figure 3 Example of a recording of cardiorespiratory channels and esophageal impedance. There is a fall in impedance starting at the lowest (i.e., most distal) channel, and extending orally from there. This is followed by a brief apnea in this example.

(median 67, range 10–346) and RE (25; 8–62). The frequency of apnea occurring within ± 20 s of an RE was not, however, significantly different from that found during reflux-free epochs (0.19/min (0.00–0.85) vs. 0.25/min (0.00–1.15), $P > 0.05$); the same was true for desaturations and bradycardias. Also, RE occurred similarly often within 20 sec before as after an apnea (2; 0–14 vs. 1; 0–17, $P > 0.05$). A minority of apneas (3.5%) were associated with an RE reaching the pharyngeal level; of these, significantly more (45 vs. 26; median 1; 0–10 vs. 1; 0–7, $P < 0.05$) occurred *after* rather than *before* an RE. Thus, both CR events and GER were common in these infants but, with few exceptions, did not appear to be temporally related (52).

That GER does not play a significant role in the pathogenesis of AOP was also, albeit indirectly, demonstrated in a recent study on the effects of antireflux treatment (cisapride or metoclopramide) on AOP. In this study, the documented frequency of bradycardia and hypoxemia in the last 5 days prior to treatment was similar to that in the first 5 days on treatment (53).

These studies may have practical consequences as they show that the widespread practice (54) of giving antireflux medications to infants with AOP is futile. They do not answer the question, however, why these symptoms are closely associated with feeding. A potential explanation that has so far received little study is a shift in blood flow distribution. Changes in systemic blood flow distribution after feeding were shown as long ago as 1978, when Krauss et al. measured a significant fall in peripheral blood flow 5 min after feeding in association with marked elevations in peripheral vascular resistance (55). To affect oxygenation, however, changes in pulmonary blood flow or ventilation/perfusion matching would be required. Whether such changes occur in relation to feeding remains, at best, speculative.

An alternative explanation, although initially considered unlikely, is diaphragmatic fatigue. Diaphragmatic work increases significantly after gavage feeding, whereas FRC decreases (44). Although we originally considered this explanation unlikely to account for the increase in episodic hypoxemia with slow gavage feeding (48) owing to the above data on gastric emptying (49), we cannot rule it out and have not yet found a convincing alternative to explain this observation.

V. Chest Wall Distortion, Anatomical Dead Space, and Diaphragmatic Fatigue

What is the evidence that diaphragmatic fatigue plays any role in the pathophysiology of AOP? Owing to their highly compliant chest wall, preterm infants are disadvantaged with regard to their respiratory mechanics. Chest wall distortion, clinically apparent as paradoxical breathing, is common in infants and is especially visible in preterm infants. It has been suggested that this distortion increases the volume displacement of the diaphragm during inspiration (47,56). In longitudinal studies, Heldt showed that the minute volume displacement of the diaphragm was almost twice as large as pulmonary ventilation at 29–30 weeks GA and fell to ~90% of pulmonary ventilation at 36 weeks GA. Concomitantly, diaphragmatic work was almost halved (56). The author speculated that this additional workload not only may represent a significant expenditure of calories in these infants but may also contribute to the development of diaphragmatic fatigue and apnea (56). Further contributing to this fatigue is the fact that, because of their relatively large head size, anatomical dead space is ~45% of tidal volume in newborns, compared to 25% in adults (19,22).

Circumstantial evidence that muscle fatigue may indeed be involved in neonatal apnea stems from the time course of apnea in term and preterm infants. This was already noted over 40 years ago to become more problematic toward the end of the first week of life (57), while chemoreceptor resetting, which otherwise might also explain this phenomenon, is essentially complete within ~24–48 h of birth (58). Fenner et al., studying periodic apnea, also noted that these only began after the first 2 days of life, reaching a maximum during the 2nd and 3rd weeks (59). In our own studies, we also found that preterm infants studied at ~4 weeks of age showed more desaturation than those studied during their first week of life, but at a lower postconceptional age: while the 95th centile for desaturation frequency was 8 per 12 h in the latter group, it was 61 in the former (16,60). A similar relationship between postnatal age and desaturation rate was found for term infants (Fig. 4) (4,61).

Indirect evidence for the role of muscle fatigue in AOP stems from the observation that enrichment of total parenteral nutrition (TPN) solutions with branched-chain amino acids, which improve diaphragmatic function in vitro, resulted in a decrease in the average number of episodes of apnea. These fell from 58 during standard TPN to 11 with the enriched solution infusion during matched 12-h periods ($P < 0.01$) in an open crossover study design (62). Also, frequency spectrum analysis in diaphragmatic EMG recordings in newborn infants (mean birth weight 1241 g) showed that, in 7 of 15 infants studied, EMG segments indicating diaphragmatic fatigue were followed by periods of apnea (47). A mechanism through which labored breathing may produce apnea in preterm infants is the intercostal-phrenic inhibitory reflex. This may be elicited both by rib cage distortion (63) and respiratory loading (64), and is known to inhibit respiratory effort in infants.

Thus, it is conceivable that similar to the obstructive sleep apnea syndrome in adults, where an increased work of breathing due to upper-airway obstruction may lead to an increased rate of central apneas, an increased work of breathing may also play a role in the pathophysiology of AOP.

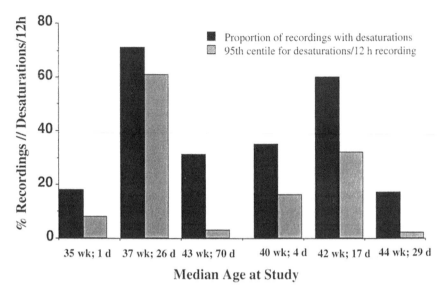

Figure 4 Data on the proportion of 12-h recordings containing prolonged episodes of desaturation (SpO$_2$ ≤ 80% for ≥ 4 s) and on the 95th centiles for desaturation rate per 12 h in various groups of term (right) and preterm (left) infants. Note that episodic desaturation in both term and preterm infants is less frequent shortly after birth than at 2–3 weeks of age and decreases again thereafter. Median age at study for each group is given both as postconceptional (left) and postnatal age (right). (From Refs. 4,8,60,61.)

VI. Upper-Airway Obstruction

Traditionally, apnea has been divided into central, obstructive, and mixed. However, analyses of artifacts on the nasal thermistor signal, produced by the transmission of cardiac impulses on the patent airway, revealed that airway obstruction may also occur during apparently central apneas (65). By amplifying these cardiac oscillations, Rigatto's group from Canada was able to assess changes in airway diameter. They analyzed these oscillations during 4456 central apneas in 41 preterm infants and found indications for airway narrowing during 585 of these, which started after only 1 sec, irrespective of the apnea duration, and with maximal narrowing usually occurring within 9 s of the onset of apnea. They speculated that their finding reflects a loss of upper-airway muscle tone during apnea (66). The same group also reported that diaphragmatic action is not needed to occlude the airway in mixed apneas, and speculated that airway closure during these apneas most likely reflects a lack of upper airway muscle tone that is not reinstated at the time the diaphragm starts to contract again.

An alternative explanation for the airway occlusion potentially occurring during apparently purely "central" apneas was given in an elegant preterm lamb study from Canada. Obtaining continuous EMG recordings of the laryngeal adductor muscle, these authors found continuous EMG activity throughout 88.4% of all apneas and 98.4% of those occurring during periodic breathing, independent of sleep state (67). EMG activity, however, was less likely to be continuous during apneas that were triggered by a sigh or a swallow. They concluded that active glottic closure, similar to that preventing outflow of lung water during the prolonged apneas that occur in utero (68), would prevent gas from flowing out freely from the lungs, thereby preserving lung volume during apnea. Although evidence for active glottic closure has also been reported during obstructive apneas in human preterm infants and in a case report on a term infant during periodic breathing (69,70), it is not yet known whether active glottic closure also generally occurs during central apneas in the human preterm infant.

Not only can apparently "central" apnea result in upper-airway obstruction, but also vice versa. Using a face mask and a pneumotachograph, including a tap that could block the mask inlet and outlet to provide an effective external obstruction, Upton et al. studied the response to airway obstruction in 23 preterm infants born at < 33 weeks gestation (71). Of 398 obstructions recorded, apnea occurred *during* the obstruction in 19%, and *upon relief* of the obstruction in 32%. This happened independently of where in the respiratory cycle the obstruction occurred. They speculated that their observation on the response to airway occlusion may be important in the prolongation of initially short respiratory pauses during which airway closure may occur (72).

Waggener et al. (73) analyzed oscillations in breath-by-breath ventilation of preterm infants, and observed that central, mixed, and obstructive apneas all occurred at the minimum phase of spontaneous ventilatory oscillations, suggesting that the three patterns had one common underlying mechanism. Hence, it appears that central, mixed, and obstructive apneas form a continuum, i.e., that obstructive components are also involved in apparently purely central apneas, and vice versa. This is probably related to the fact that the narrow upper airways of preterm infants are actively maintained open via a respiratory center input, and that it depends on which component stops being activated first (diaphragm or upper airway) whether an apnea will appear as central or obstructive. At autopsy the upper airway of young infants is closed, again suggesting that a neuromuscular mechanism is necessary to maintain airway patency during life (74). The mechanism(s) through which airway closure occurs during apnea, however, is (are) largely unclear. One factor may be flow- or pressure-sensitive airway receptors. In animal experiments, flow up and down the upper airway resulted in the maintenance of pharyngeal patency via increased genioglossus activity (73). Thus, when flow ceases, genioglossus activity falls and the airway collapses. Alternatively, cessation of respiratory drive may cause an immediate loss of lower (and probably also upper) airway tone (75), or airway closure occurs as an active reflex, as suggested from the preterm lamb data mentioned above (67). Whatever the precise mechanism for both apnea types, the strict separation into apparently purely central or purely obstructive apneas cannot be maintained in the light of these data.

VII. Hypoxic Ventilatory Depression

It has been known for almost 70 years that respiration in the fetus is diminished if oxygen supply via the placenta is reduced (76). This is in contrast to adults, who show a sustained increase in ventilation in the presence of hypoxia. While this is probably beneficial in fetal life, where respiratory movements are a waste of energy that the fetus cannot afford if oxygen supply via the placenta is reduced, this pattern is counterproductive ex utero. As shown in the classic studies by Rigatto et al. (77), the switch-over from the fetal to the adult hypoxic ventilatory response only occurs some time after birth. They also showed that the respiratory response was biphasic; i.e., an initial increase in ventilation for ∼1 min was followed by a sustained period of hypoventilation (77). This may not be true for less mature infants: in a group of infants born at 29 weeks gestation and studied at a mean age of 17 days, Alvaro et al. found a 33% reduction in minute ventilation which had already begun after 30 s and was mainly due to a fall in respiratory rate; there was no initial period of hyperventilation (78). More recently, Martin et al. showed that the neonatal hypoxic response persists at least until approximately 35 weeks postconceptional age, which correlates well with the clinical course of apnea of prematurity (79).

Below what PaO_2 level does hypoxic ventilatory depression occur? This has not been studied systematically in infants. An early study suggested, however, that breathing already becomes irregular, and apnea starts to occur, if PaO_2 falls to below 75–97 mm Hg, levels close to or even above those associated with an increased risk of retinopathy of prematurity (80). Weintraub et al. measured minute ventilation in 15 preterm infants (mean GA 29 (SD 2) weeks, age 20 (9) days) at 21, 25, 30, 35 and 40% oxygen. With the increase in FiO_2, breathing became more regular, apneas decreased, but minute ventilation did not change significantly; only breath-to-breath variability in inspiratory and expiratory times and tidal volume decreased. They concluded that oxygen facilitates the appearance of regular breathing independently of an increase in minute ventilation (81). Interestingly, their study subjects had a relatively low SpO_2 in room air (mean, 90.8%), which increased to 92.5% in 25% O_2. Even this relatively small increase in FiO_2 was associated with a decrease in apnea rate (≥ 3 sec) from 128 to 63 per hour ($P < 0.05$). Thus, although not necessarily resulting in a fall in minute ventilation, breathing irregularities and an increased propensity for short apneas may already develop at a PaO_2 < 60–90 mm Hg. Whether this response to changes in PaO_2 is mediated via the same mechanisms that elicit the hypoxic ventilatory depression, however, is not known.

An important question, well beyond the focus of this review, is which molecular mechanisms are responsible for the hypoxic ventilatory depression and how the switch-over to the adult pattern is programmed (see Chap. 5). One potential mechanism, however, should be mentioned in this context since it may have therapeutic consequences, namely the creatine-phosphocreatine (Cr-PCr) system. In the absence of oxidative phosphorylisation, provision of phosphate for generation of adenosine-triphosphate (ATP) relies predominantly on the PCr pool, before anaerobic glycolysis, with increased production of lactate and H^+, is activated (82). This is particularly relevant to tissues with a high energy metabolism such as the central nervous system. A fall in intracellular ATP is an important trigger for hypoxia-induced neuronal damage, and maintenance of ATP levels is therefore of fundamental importance for neuronal protection from hypoxic insult (83). This may also be relevant to the adaptation of ventilation during hypoxia. Investigations of the cytosolic levels of PCr during moderate hypoxia in adult rats by ^{31}P nuclear magnetic resonance spectroscopy of the brainstem showed that the occurrence of hypoxic ventilatory depression was preceded, by 30 sec, by a significant decrease in PCr levels. This reached its minimum level 30 sec after maximal respiratory depression and occurred without a significant change in ATP levels (84). In the neonatal rat brain, total creatine kinase activity increases 2–3 times over the first month of life, reflecting a doubling of PCr content during this time span (85). Thus, the neonatal brain is relatively deficient in creatine, and it is tempting to speculate that the much earlier onset of the hypoxic ventilatory depression in this age group is related to a decreased availability of PCr in the neonatal brainstem.

PCr is also important in muscle metabolism, where it serves as an energy buffer to guarantee provision of sufficient substrate for the phosphorylisation of ADP to ATP (86). Creatine levels can be increased via creatine supplementation (86). In adults, creatine supplementation was shown to result in an increased exercise performance (87) and less muscular fatigue (88,89). Wilken et al. recently showed that brainstem slices from pups of creatine-fed mice (2 g/kg/d) showed higher phosphocreatine contents and significantly less hypoxic ventilatory depression (−14 vs. −41%), than those from nonsupplemented control animals. This corresponded to nearly constant cerebral ATP levels in the former vs. a 54% decrease in the latter animals after 30 min of anoxia (90). Also, measurements of the maximal respiratory amplitudes in such pups during hypoxia showed an increase by 51%, compared to 22% in control animals (91). Thus, the newborn can be regarded as creatine deficient, and creatine supplementation may be a way to influence the characteristic hypoxic ventilatory depression seen in this age group.

VIII. Anemia

One way through which tissue hypoxia may develop is anemia. Indeed, anemia has repeatedly been implicated in the pathophysiology of AOP and also of cyanotic episodes in infants (92,93). It would thus seem logical to hypothesize that blood transfusions are an effective treatment modality in infants with AOP who are anemic. Data on the effect of blood transfusions on the frequency of these episodes, however, are conflicting. Some authors found less apnea and/or bradycardia following transfusion (94–98); others did not (99–100). None of the above studies, however, included data on the frequency of hypoxemic episodes. In an initial study on the effect of blood transfusion on episodic hypoxemia and/or bradycardia, we performed cardiorespiratory recordings in 21 spontaneously breathing preterm infants (median GA at birth 28 weeks [range 23–31], age at study 22 days [3–84]) with AOP who were mildly anemic (median hemoglobin level 109 [82–120] g/L) before and after transfusion of 20 mL/kg of packed red blood cells and found no significant changes in the frequency, severity, or duration of apnea (≥ 4 sec), bradycardia (heart rate $< 2/3$ of baseline), or desaturation ($SpO_2 \leq 80\%$) following transfusion (102).

One potential explanation for this lack of effect was that the infants studied were not sufficiently anemic, although the thresholds used to define anemia were similar to those used in studies on the effect of erythropoietin to prevent anemia of prematurity. Recently, we therefore repeated the above study (102), using thresholds to define anemia that were some 20 g/L lower than in our first study on this subject. We now recorded data in 19 preterm infants (median GA 25 weeks [range 22–30], age at study 5.5 weeks [1–13]), who had a median hemoglobin level of 78 g/L (range 63–98) (103). However, despite this more severe level of anemia, there was again no significant change in the combined frequency of bradycardia and desaturation, the primary endpoint in this study (median 6.4/h [3.0–13.5] before vs. 4.6/h [0.6–15.7] following transfusion), although there was slightly less bradycardia (0.8 [0.0–8.8] vs. 0.7/h [0.0–5.1]; $P < 0.05$). Also, in contrast to the initial study (102), there was now a significant decrease in baseline heart and respiratory rate, which decreased from 163 (140–182) and 58 (34–98), respectively, to 152 (134–172) and 55/min (36–82), $P < 0.01$, suggesting that there was at least some clinical benefit resulting from the blood transfusion. Nevertheless, blood transfusion had little effect on AOP, the condition for which it had been intended. Based on these data, we would be reluctant to recommend blood transfusion in anemic infants who exhibit frequent episodes of AOP as their only clinical symptom.

IX. Termination of Apnea

As important as the question of what causes an apnea is that of what *terminates* it. This issue, however, has received surprisingly little attention. In adults, recovery from apnea is usually associated with arousal from sleep, probably induced by activation of peripheral chemoreceptors and potentially resulting in severe sleep deprivation (104). In the preterm infant, the situation is somewhat more complex. Mathew et al. found that in 202 of 352 apneic events in 10 preterm infants, motor activity *preceded* the onset of apnea and continued during these episodes; i.e., they occurred *after* arousal rather than resulting in it (105). Similar findings have been reported by others (106,107). The majority of these awake episodes, however, did not result in bradycardia and/or hypoxemia; in fact, two-thirds of those that did, occurred during sleep (104). When looking for signs of behavioral arousal in sleep-related apneas, the same group found that such arousals were significantly more frequent during apneic than during nonapneic sleep time (0.59/h vs. 0.25/h) (108). Also, arousal was more likely to occur with longer (> 15 sec) than shorter (5–15 sec) apneas, with those that were associated with hypoxemia (SpO$_2$ < 80%) or bradycardia (HR < 100/min), and with mixed compared to central apneas. They concluded that several factors affect the occurrence of arousal during apneas in preterm infants: sleep state, severity of hypoxia/hypercapnia, airway afferent input, and sleep fragmentation/habituation resulting from previous apneic episodes (108).

One potential caveat in the above study (108), acknowledged by the authors, was the lack of EEG recordings to detect arousal. This issue was recently addressed by Wulbrand et al., who studied a group of 10 preterm infants repeatedly at 36, 40, 44 and 52 weeks postconceptional age (109). They found no changes in EEG frequency at apnea termination, but 64% of rapid eye movement (REM) and 79% of non-REM sleep apneas were terminated by a simultaneous "gasplike" activation of submental and diaphragmatic EMG. These EMG activities corresponded to a deep inspiration on the respiratory channels that was immediately preceded by a short expiration (109). Similarly, in term infants at a mean age of 9.5 weeks, McNamara et al. found EEG changes indicative of cortical arousal during only 7.9% of apneic events (110). In contrast, a more recent study examining 163 isolated apneas in 17 infants at 47 ± 4 weeks postconceptional age found increases in EEG frequency indicative of cortical arousal coinciding with termination of apnea in 61% of events (111). The reason(s) for these discrepancies between studies remain unclear, but may be related to maturity, methodology used for obtaining and interpreting the EEG, or both. The question also remains whether there is a functional difference between a cortical arousal that can be detected via surface electrodes and a subcortical arousal resulting in respiratory or behavioral but not in EEG changes. Whatever the precise arousal mechanism, the observations summarized above suggest that chemoreceptor activation plays a role in apnea termination.

X. Conclusion

Apart from the issue of hypoxic ventitatory depression, this review has focused on mechanical rather than central factors. Although there is some evidence of brainstem immaturity in infants with AOP (112), there is nothing to suggest that infants with AOP have gross deficits in respiratory control (113). As suggested by the data summarized above, it appears that the early (and frequent) occurrence of hypoxemia during apnea in preterm infants is related to their low expiratory lung volume, which falls even further during apnea, while the accompanying brady-cardia results from this combination of apnea and hypoxemia. Feeding is an important trigger for AOP. While hypoxemia *during* feeding is most likely related to an immature coordination between sucking, swallowing, and breathing, that *after* feeding may be caused by diaphragmatic fatigue; GER does not appear to play a major role. The time course of AOP, i.e., increased occurrence during the second and third rather than the first week of life, together with data from physiological studies, also suggests a role for diaphragmatic fatigue in AOP. Additional factors include upper airway obstruction and the unique response of the preterm to hypoxia. These observational data cannot provide definite answers on cause-and-effect issues. They may, however, provide a starting point for further studies into mechanisms involved in AOP and trials of new and old therapeutic interventions, such as nasal CPAP therapy or other means to stabilize the chest wall, as well as branched-chain amino acid and/or creatine supple-mentation. Thus, there is reason to hope that there will soon be better solutions to the clinical problem of AOP than there have been in the past.

References

1. Albani M, Bentele KHP, Budde C, Schulte EJ. Infant sleep apnea profile: preterm vs. term infants. Eur J Pediatr 1985; 143:261–268.
2. Daily WJR, Klaus M, Meyer HB. Apnea in premature infants: monitoring, incidence, heart rate changes, and an effect of environmental temperature. Pediatrics 1969; 43:510–518.
3. Kattwinkel J. Neonatal apnea: pathogenesis and therapy. J Pediatr 1977; 90:342–347.
4. Stebbens VA, Poets CF, Alexander JR, Arrowsmith WA, Southall DP. Oxygen saturation and breathing patterns in infancy. Full term infants in the second month of life. Arch Dis Child 1991; 66:569–573.

5. Poets CF, Stebbens VA, Alexander JR, Arrowsmith WA, Salfield SAW, Southall DP. Oxygen saturation and breathing patterns in infancy. 2. Preterm infants at discharge from special care. Arch Dis Child 1991; 66:574–578.

6. Poets CF, Stebbens VA, Southall DP. Arterial oxygen saturation and breathing movements during the first year of life. J Dev Physiol 1991; 15:341–345.

7. Poets CF, Stebbens VA, Samuels, MP, Southall DP. Oxygen saturation and breathing patterns in children. Pediatrics 1993; 92:686–690.

8. Poets CF, Southall DP. Patterns of oxygenation during periodic breathing in preterm infants. Early Hum Dev 1991; 26:1–12.

9. Girling DJ. Changes in heart rate, blood pressure, and pulse pressure during apnoeic attacks in newborn babies. Arch Dis Child 1972; 47:405–410.

10. Storrs CN. Cardiovascular effects of apnoea in preterm infants. Arch Dis Child 1977; 52:534–540.

11. Gabriel M, Albani M. Cardiac slowing and respiratory arrest in preterm infants. Eur J Pediatr 1976; 122:257–261.

12. Vyas H, Milner AD, Hopkin IE. Relationship between apnoea and bradycardia in preterm infants. Acta Paediatr Scand 1981; 70:785–790.

13. Poets CF, Stebbens VA, Samuels MP, Southall DP. The relationship between episodes of bradycardia, apnea and hypoxemia in preterm infants. Pediatr Res 1993; 34:144–147.

14. Daly M de B. Interactions between respiration and circulation. In: Fishman AP, ed. Handbook of Physiology, Section 3, Vol 2, Part 1. Bethesda, MD: American Physiological Society, 1986; 529–594.

15. Angell-James JE, Daly M de B. Cardiovascular responses in apnoeic asphyxia: role of arterial chemoreceptors and the modification of their effects by a pulmonary vagal inflation reflex. J Physiol 1969; 201:87–104.

16. Poets CF, Stebbens VA, Alexander JR, Arrowsmith WA, Salfield SAW, Southall DP. Arterial oxygen saturation in preterm infants at discharge from the hospital and 6 weeks later. J Pediatr 1992; 120:447–454.

17. Finer NN, Barrington KJ, Hayes BJ, Hugh A. Obstructive, mixed, and central apnea in the neonate: physiologic correlates. J Pediatr 1992; 121:943–950.

18. Adams JA, Zabaleta IA, Sackner MA. Hypoxemic events in spontaneously breathing premature infants: etiologic basis. Pediatr Res 1997; 42:463–471.

19. Olinsky A, Bryan MH, Bryan AC. Influence of lung inflation on respiratory control in neonates. J Appl Physiol 1974; 36:426–429.

20. Agostoni E, Mead J. Statics of the respiratory system. In: Handbook of Physiology, Respiration. Washington: American Physiology Society, 1965, Sect 3, vol 1, pp 387–409.

21. Kosch PC, Stark AR. Dynamic maintenance of end-expiratory lung volume in full-term infants. J Appl Physiol Respir Environ Exercise Physiol 1984; 57:1126–1133.

22. Numa AH, Newth CJL. Anatomic dead space in infants and children. J Appl Physiol 1996; 80:1485–1489.

23. Stark AR, Cohlan BA, Waggener TB, Frantz ID III, Kosch PC. Regulation of end-expiratory lung volume during sleep in premature infants. J Appl Physiol 1987; 62:1117–1123.

24. Poets CF, Rau GA, Neuber K, Gappa M, Seidenberg J. Determinants of lung volume in spontaneously breathing preterm infants. Am J Respir Crit Care Med 1997; 155:649–653.

25. Davis GM, Moscato J. Changes in lung mechanics following sighs in premature newborns without lung disease. Pediatr Pulmonol 1994; 17:26–30.

26. Thach BT, Taeusch HW. Sighing in newborn human infants: role of inflation-augmenting reflex. J Appl Physiol 1976; 41:502–507.

27. Henderson-Smart DJ. Vulnerability to hypoxaemia in the newborn. Sleep 1980; 3:331–342.

28. Findley LJ, Ries AL, Tisi GM, Wagner PD. Hypoxemia during apnea in normal subjects: mechanisms and impact of lung volume. J Appl Physiol Respir Environ Exercise Physiol 1983; 55:1777–1783.

29. Wilkinson MH, Berger PJ, Blanch N, Brodecky V. Effect of venous oxygenation on arterial desaturation rate during repetitive apneas in lambs. Respir Physiol 1995; 101:321–331.

30. Hannam S, Ingram DM, Milner AD. A possible role for the Hering-Breuer deflation reflex in apnea of prematurity. J Pediatr 1998; 132:35–39.

31. Speidel BD, Dunn PM. Use of nasal continuous positive airway pressure to treat severe recurrent apnoea in very preterm infants. Lancet 1976; ii:658–660.

32. Thibeault DW, Wong MM, Auld PAM. Thoracic gas volume changes in premature infants. Pediatrics 1967; 40:403–411.

33. Kattwinkel J, Nearman HS, Fanaroff AA, Katona PT, Klaus MH. Apnea of prematurity. Comparative effects of cutaneous stimulation and nasal continuous positive pressure ventilation. J Pediatr 1975; 86:588–592.

34. Bakwin H. Oxygen therapy in premature babies with anoxemia. Am J Dis Child 1923; 25:157–162.

35. Phillips S. Cyanosis in infancy. J Ark Med Soc 1936; 33:99–102.

36. Garg M, Kurzner SI, Bautista DB, Keens TG. Clinically unsuspected hypoxia during sleep and feeding in infants with bronchopulmonary dysplasia. Pediatrics 1988; 81:635–642.

37. Singer L, Martin RJ, Hawkins SW, Benson-Szekely LJ, Yamashita TS, Carlo WA. Oxygen desaturation complicates feeding in infants with bronchopulmonary dysplasia after discharge. Pediatrics 1992; 90:380–384.

38. Guilleminault C, Coons S. Apnea and bradycardia during feeding in infants weighing > 2000 gm. J Pediatr 1984; 104:932–935.

39. Rosen CL, Glaze DG, Frost JD. Hypoxemia associated with feeding in the preterm infant and full-term neonate. Am J Dis Child 1984; 138:623–628.

40. Shivpuri CR, Martin RJ, Carlo WA, Fanaroff AA. Decreased ventilation in preterm infants during oral feeding. J Pediatr 1983; 103:285–289.

41. Wilkinson A, Yu VYH. Immediate effects of feeding on blood-gases and some cardiorespiratory functions in ill newborn infants. Lancet 1974; i:1083–1085.

42. Patel BD, Dinwiddie R, Kumar SP, Fox WW. The effects of feeding on arterial blood gases and lung mechanics in newborn infants recovering from respiratory disease. J Pediatr 1977; 90:435–438.

43. Blondheim O, Abbasi S, Fox WW, Bhutani VK. Effect of enteral gavage feeding rate on pulmonary functions of very low birth weight infants. J Pediatr 1993; 122:751–755.

44. Heldt GP. The effect of gavage feeding on the mechanics of the lung, chest wall, and diaphragm of preterm infants. Pediatr Res 1988; 24:55–58.

45. Mathew OP. Respiratory control during nipple feeding in preterm infants. Pediatr Pulmonol 1988; 5:220–224.

46. Davies AM, Koenig JS, Thach BT. Characteristics of upper airway chemoreflex prolonged apnea in human infants. Am Rev Respir Dis 1989; 139:668–673.

47. Lopes JM, Muller NL, Bryan MH, Bryan AC. Synergistic behavior of inspiratory muscles after diaphragmatic fatigue in the newborn. J Appl Physiol 1981; 51:547–551.

48. Poets CF, Langner M, Bohnhorst B. Effects of nipple feeding and 2 different methods of gavage feeding on oxygenation in preterm infants. Acta Paediatr 1997; 86:419–423.

49. Ewer AK, Durbin GM, Morgan MEI, Booth IW. Gastric emptying in preterm infants. Arch Dis Child 1994; 71:F24–F27.

50. Herbst JJ, Minton SD, Book LS. Gastroesophageal reflux causing respiratory distress and apnea in newborn infants. J Pediatr 1979; 95:763–768.

51. Menon AP, Schefft GL, Thach BT. Apnea associated with regurgitation in infants. J Pediatr 1985; 106:625–629.

52. Peter CS, Sprodowski N, Bohnhorst B. Gastroesophageal reflux and apnea of prematurity: No temporal relationship. Pediatrics 2002; 109:8–11.

53. Kimball AL, Carlton DP. Gastroesophageal reflux medications in the treatment of apnea in premature infants. J Pediatr 2001; 138:355–360.

54. Ward RM, Lemons JA, Molteni RA. Cisapride: a survey of the frequency of use and adverse events in premature newborns. Pediatrics 1999; 103:469–472.

55. Krauss AN, Brown J, Waldman S, Gottlieb G, Auld PA. Pulmonary function following feeding in low-birth-weight infants. Am J Dis Child 1978; 132:139–142.

56. Heldt GP. Development of stability of the respiratory system in preterm infants. J Appl Physiol 1988; 65:441–444.

57. Miller HC, Behrle FC, Smull NW. Severe apnea and irregular respiratory rhythms among premature infants. Pediatrics 1959; 23:676–685.

58. Calder NA, Williams BA, Kumar P, Hanson MA. The respiratory response of healthy term infants to breath-by-breath alternations in inspired oxygen at two postnatal ages. Pediatr Res 1994; 35:321–324.

59. Fenner A, Schalk U, Hoenicke H, Wendenburg A, Roehling T. Periodic breathing in premature and neonatal babies: incidence, breathing pattern, respiratory gas tensions, response to changes in the composition of ambient air. Pediatr Res 1973; 7:174–183.

60. Richard D, Poets CF, Neale S, Stebbens VA, Alexander JR, Southall DP. Arterial oxygen saturation in preterm neonates without respiratory failure. J Pediatr 1993; 123:963–968.

61. Poets CF, Stebbens VA, Lang JA, O'Brien L, Boon A, Southall DP. Arterial oxygen saturation in healthy term neonates. Eur J Pediatr 1996; 155:219–223.

62. Blazer S, Reinersman GT, Askanazi J, Furst P, Katz DP, Fleischman AR. Branched-chain amino acids and respiratory pattern and function in the neonate. J Perinatol 1994; 14:290–295.

63. Knill R, Bryan AC. An intercostal-phrenic inhibitory reflex in human newborn infants. J Appl Physiol 1976; 40:352–356.

64. Knill R, Andrews W, Bryan AC, Bryan MH. Respiratory load compensation in infants. J Appl Physiol 1976; 40:357–361.

65. Milner AD, Boon AW, Saunders RA, Hopkin IE. Upper airway obstruction and apnoea in preterm babies. Arch Dis Child 1980; 55:22–25.

66. Lemke RP, Idiong N, Al-Saedi S, Kwiatkowski K, Cates DB, Rigatto H. Evidence of a critical period of airway instability during central apneas in preterm infants. Am J Respir Crit Care Med 1998; 157:470–474.

67. Renolleau S, Letourneau P, Niyonsenga, Praud J-P. Thryoarytenoid muscle electrical activity during spontaneous apneas in preterm lambs. Am J Respir Crit Care Med 1999; 159:1296–1404.

68. Klanicka I, Diaz V, Dorion D, Praud JP. Coordination between glottic adductor muscle and diaphragm EMG activity in the fetal lamb in utero. J Appl Physiol 1998; 84:1560–1565.

69. Ruggins NR, Milner AD. Site of upper airway obstruction in preterm infants with problematical apnoea. Arch Dis Child 1991; 66:787–792.

70. Ruggins NR, Milner AD. Site of upper airway obstruction in infants following an acute life-threatening event. Pediatrics 1993; 91:595–601.

71. Upton CJ, Milner AD, Stokes GM. Response to external obstruction in preterm infants with apnea. Pediatr Pulmonol 1992; 14:233–238.

72. Abu-Osba YK, Mathew OP, Thach BT. An animal model for airway sensory deprivation producing obstructive apnea with postmortem findings of sudden infant death syndrome. Pediatrics 1981; 68:796–801.

73. Waggener TB, Frantz ID, Cohlan BA, Stark AR. Mixed and obstructive apneas are related to ventilatory oscillations in premature infants. J Appl Physiol 1989; 66:2818–2826.

74. Mathew OP. Maintenance of upper airway patency. J Pediatr 1985; 106:863–869.

75. Mitchell RA, Herbert DA, Baker DG. Inspiratory rhythm in airway smooth muscle tone. J Appl Physiol 1985; 58:911–920.

76. Eastman NJ. Fetal blood studies. Am J Obstet Gynecol 1936; 31:563–572.

77. Rigatto H, Brady JP, De la Torre Verduzco R. Chemoreceptor reflexes in preterm infants. I. The effect of gestational and postnatal age on the ventilatory response to inhalation of 100% and 15% oxygen. Pediatrics 1975; 55:604–613.

78. Alvaro R, Alvarez J, Kwiatkowski K, Cates D, Rigatto H. Small preterm infants (< 1500 g) have only a sustained decrease in ventilation in response to hypoxia. Pediatr Res 1992; 32:403–406.

79. Martin RJ, DiFiore JM, Davis RL, Miller MJ, Coles SK, Dick TE. Persistence of the biphasic ventilatory response to hypoxia in preterm infants. J Pediatr 1998; 132:960–964.

80. Lagercrantz H, Ahlström H, Jonson B, Lindroth M, Svenningsen N. A critical oxygen level below which irregular breathing occurs in preterm infants. In: Von

Euler C, Lagercrantz H, eds. Central Nervous Control Mechanisms in Breathing. Oxford: Pergamon Press, 1978:161–164.

81. Weintraub Z, Alvaro R, Kwiatkowski K, Cates D, Rigatto H. Effects of inhaled oxygen (up to 40%) on periodic breathing and apnea in preterm infants. J Appl Physiol 1992; 72:116–120.

82. Bessman SP, Carpenter CL. The creatine-creatinephosphate energy shuttle. Annu Rev Biochem 1985; 54:831–862.

83. Wilken B, Ramirez JM, Probst I, Richter DW, Hanefeld F. Creatine protects the central respiratory network of mammals under anoxic conditions. Pediatr Res 1998; 43:8–14.

84. Pierard C, Champagnat J, Denavit-Saubie MA, Gillet B, Beloeil JC, Guezennec CY, Barrere B, Peres M. Brain stem energy metabolism response to acute hypoxia in anaesthetized rats: a ^{31}P NMR study. NeuroReport 1995; 7:281–285.

85. Lolley R, Balfour W, Samson F. The high energy phosphates in developing brain. J Neurochem 1961; 7:289–297.

86. Balsom PD, Söderlund K, Ekblom B. Creatine in humans with special reference to creatine supplementation. Sports Med 1994; 18:268–280.

87. Greenhaff PL, Casey A, Short AH, et al. Influence of oral creatine supplementation on muscle tone during repeated bouts of maximal voluntary exercise in man. Clin Sci 1993; 84:565–571.

88. Sahlin K, Tonkonogi M, Söderlund K. Energy supply and muscle fatigue in humans. Acta Physiol Scand 1998; 162:261–266.

89. Green AL, Hultman E, Macdonald IA, Sewell DA, Greenhaff PL. Carbohydrate ingestion augments skeletal muscle creatine accumulation during creatine supplementation in humans. Am J Physiol 1996; 271:E821–E826.

90. Wilken B, Ramirez JM, Probst I, Richter DW, Hanefeld F. Anoxic ATP depletion in neonatal brainstem is prevented by creatine supplementation. Arch Dis Child Fetal Neonatal Ed 2000; 82:F224–F227.

91. Wilken B, Ramirez JM, Richter DW, Hanefeld F. Supplemental creatine enhances hypoxic augmentation in vivo by preventing ATP depletion (abstract). Eur J Pediatr 1998; 157:178.

92. Pohl CA, Epstein M, Kaplon D, Gibson E. Role of a screening hematocrit for pathologic apnea and bradycardia in healthy preterm infants. Pediatr Pulmonol 1998; 26:445.

93. Poets CF, Samuels MP, Wardrop CAJ, Picton-Jones E, Southall DP. Reduced haemoglobin levels in infants presenting with apparent life-threatening events—a retrospective investigation. Acta Paediatr 1992; 81:319–321.

94. Bifano EM, Smith F, Borer J. Relationship between determinants of oxygen delivery and respiratory abnormalities in preterm infants with anemia. J Pediatr 1992; 120:292–296.

95. DeMaio JG, Harris MC, Deuber C, Spitzer AR. Effect of blood transfusion on apnea frequency in growing premature infants. J Pediatr 1989; 114:1039–1041.

96. Joshi A, Gerhardt T, Shandloff P, Bancalari E. Blood transfusion effect on the respiratory pattern of preterm infants. Pediatrics 1987; 80:79–84.

97. Sasidharan P, Heimler R. Transfusion induced changes in the breathing patterns of healthy preterm anemic infants. Pediatr Pulmonol 1992; 12:170–173.
98. Stute H, Greiner B, Linderkamp O. Effect of blood transfusion on cardiorespiratory abnormalities in preterm infants. Arch Dis Child 1995; 72:F194–F196.
99. Blank JP, Sheagren TG, Vajaria J, Mangurten HH, Benawra RS, Puppala BL. The role of RBC transfusion in the premature infant. Am J Dis Child 1984; 138:831–833.
100. Keyes WG, Donohue PK, Spivak JL, Jones MD, Oski FA. Assessing the need for transfusion of premature infants and role of hematocrit, clinical signs, and erythropoietin level. Pediatrics 1989; 84:412–417.
101. Meyer J, Sive A, Jacobs P. Empiric red cell transfusion in asymptomatic preterm infants. Acta Paediatr 1993; 82:30–34.
102. Poets CF, Pauls U, Bohnhorst B. Effect of blood transfusion on apnea, bradycardia and hypoxemia in preterm infants. Eur J Pediatr 1997; 156:311–316.
103. Westkamp E, Adrian S, Soditt V, Bohnhorst B, Poets CF. Bluttransfusionen bei Frühgeborenenapnoen und ausgeprägter Anämie. Z Geburtsh Neonatol 2001; 205:S39.
104. Sullivan CE, Issa FG. Obstructive sleep apnea. Clin Chest Med 1985; 6:633–650.
105. Mathew OP, Thoppil CK, Belan M. Motor activity and apnea in preterm infants. Am Rev Respir Dis 1991; 144:842–844.
106. Abu-Osba YK, Broulliette RT, Wilson SL, Thach BT. Breathing pattern and transcutaneous oxygen tension during motor activity in preterm infants. Am Rev Respir Dis 1982; 125:382–387.
107. Weintraub Z, Alvaro R, Mills S, Cates D, Rigatto H. Short apneas and their relationship to body movements and sighs in preterm infants. Biol Neonate 1994; 66:188–194.
108. Thoppil CK, Belan MA, Cowen CP, Mathew OP. Behavioral arousal in newborn infants and its association with termination of apnea. J Appl Physiol 1991; 70:1479–1484.
109. Wulbrand H, Von Zezschwitz G, Bentele KHP. Submental and diaphragmatic muscle activity during and at resolution of mixed and obstructive apneas and cardiorespiratory arousal in preterm infants. Pediatr Res 1995; 38:298–305.
110. McNamara F, Issa FQ, Sullivan CE. Arousal pattern following central and obstructive breathing abnormalities in infants and children. J Appl Physiol 1996; 81:2651–2657.
111. Vecchierini MF, Curzi-Dascalova L, Trang-Pham H, Bloch J, Gaultier C. Patterns of EEG frequency, movement, heart rate, and oxygenation after isolated short apneas in infants. Pediatr Res 2001; 49:220–226.
112. Henderson-Smart DJ, Pettigrew AG, Campbell DJ. Clinical apnea and brain-stem neural function in preterm infants. N Engl J Med 1983; 308:353–357.
113. Upton CJ, Milner AD, Stokes GM. Response to tube breathing in preterm infants with apnea. Pediatr Pulmonol 1992; 12:23–28.

13

Pharmacotherapy of Apnea of Prematurity

ALISON GRAHAM and NEIL N. FINER

University of California, San Diego
San Diego, California, U.S.A.

I. Introduction

Idiopathic apnea of prematurity is a condition that affects a large percentage of premature infants. It is especially common in the very low and extremely low birth weight infants. In infants <1000 g up to 90% will be affected by apnea of prematurity (1,2), and one study found significant apnea in all infants of <34 weeks gestational age (3). This is due mainly to the immature development of both the brain and the respiratory system. Idiopathic apnea is not solely due to a central event, but rather up to 50% of events have an obstructive component (4). Apnea by definition is the cessation of breathing for up to 10 sec or greater, which may be associated with bradycardia and/or oxygen desaturation (5). While mechanical ventilation and continuous positive airway pressure (CPAP) are used to treat apnea of prematurity, pharmacotherapy is the commonest treatment utilized. Methylxanthines (caffeine and theophylline) have been the mainstay of therapy. Doxapram, not commonly used in the United States, has also been shown to be an effective therapy and may be useful for the treatment of apnea resistant to methylxathinines.

II. Theophylline

A. Mechanisms of Action

The exact mechanism by which theophylline acts to reduce apnea of prematurity is unknown. Theophylline is known to increase ventilation and increase the sensitivity to carbon dioxide, which is thought to occur through lowering the threshold of central chemoreceptors (6–8), and is mediated at the level of the brainstem and may involve the action of the neurochemical dopamine (9). Theophylline also exerts significant behavioral effects, which are thought to occur as a result of antagonism of endogenous adenosine and central nervous system excitation. The respiratory stimulant effects of xanthines are linked to phosphodiesterase inhibition and to the antagonism of adenosine (10,11). In addition, it has been demonstrated that theophylline can enhance respiratory muscle activity and decrease muscle fatigue through a mechanism involving excitation-contraction coupling mechanisms (12–16), although some studies in animals and neonates have failed to confirm such an effect (17–20).

B. Evidence of Efficacy

The initial studies demonstrating the efficacy of theophylline were done in the 1970s, were not blinded placebo-controlled trials, and used infants as their own controls (21–25). The first placebo-controlled trial appeared ~7 years after the first reported use of this agent for neonatal apnea and noted that 66% of the 15 patients treated with theophylline had a decrease in apnea, as defined by nursing observations, for a period of up to 48 h (26). The following year Jones et al. compared theophylline to CPAP, using a continuous recording technique and found a greater reduction in short (<10 sec) apnea frequency and bradycardia with theophylline. In addition, 5/18 theophylline-treated infants compared with 12/14 CPAP infants required mechanical ventilation (27). In 1985, Sims et al. performed the first placebo-controlled trial, which included 43 preterm infants. While theophylline did reduce respiratory failure and apneic episodes in the preterm infant, the study identified a subgroup of infants who were unresponsive to theophylline (28).

The only double-blind, randomized, controlled study was done by Peliowski and Finer (29) in 1990. The study included the continuous monitoring of the heart rate, impedance respiratory rate, oxygen saturation and/or transcutaneous oxygen pressure, and end-tidal CO_2. In the past the efficacy of theophylline had been based on bedside heart rate and impedance monitoring and nursing observations (29). This methodology has been shown to miss a large number of significant apneas (30). In addition to being placebo controlled, Peliowski's study also evaluated the use of doxapram and provided a crossover if either of the study drugs was not effective. The results revealed that doxapram and theophylline were effective both individually and together in reducing the incidence of apneas on a short-term basis.

C. Pharmacokinetics

The pharmacokinetics of theophylline have been described in a number of studies, which led to widely discrepant recommendations for dosing of this agent. The standardization of theophylline dosing was difficult owing to the immaturity of the cytochrome P450 system in preterm infants as well as the extended half-life. The FDA attempted to standardize the dose of theophylline and provided a dosing guideline (31). However, Gillman and Gal (32) challenged this guideline. Their study revealed that following this guideline resulted in subtherapeutic levels of theophylline in 80% of the study population. Similarly Murphy et al. (33) commented that in their experience the volume of distribution was greater than that noted by the FDA. Their infants also received larger loading and maintenance doses, while remaining in the therapeutic range. Other studies have attempted to individualize the dose of theophylline through the use of several equations (34,35). Bhatt-Mehta et al. (34,35) first compared two equations using postnatal and gestational age to determine maintenance dosage of theophylline. Infants were placed into two categories: infants <30 days and infants >30 days of life. They found that using these two equations did not provide reliable standard maintenance dosing. However, they used this knowledge to create two new equations, which they prospectively evaluated in 54 infants at 27–34 weeks gestation. Bhatt-Mehta et al. determined that by using equations that included gestational age, weight, and postnatal age they were successful in reaching their target concentration in 74% of the infants. The failure to reach their target concentration was thought to be due to interindividual variation (35).

D. Metabolism

Theophylline is metabolized by the hepatic cytochrome P450 enzyme system. It is methylated in the neonate to form caffeine (36,37). Bory et al. (37) evaluated the transformation of theophylline to caffeine in the premature infant. They found that the caffeine level increased from day 1 to day 7. In addition, they determined that while both drugs decreased after discontinuation of theophylline, caffeine remained present in the blood 9 days following discontinuation. The metabolism of this agent increases during the first 6 months of age and the half-life appears to decrease with increasing postnatal age (38,39). Theophylline levels should be monitored very closely as the drug has a very narrow therapeutic window and toxicity can rapidly occur. The therapeutic level ranges from 6 to 12 mg/L, although some infants may require levels up to 20 mg/L (40).

E. Side Effects and Toxicity

The most common side effects of theophylline are tachycardia (41), feeding intolerance, jitteriness, and exacerbation of gastroesophageal reflux (42). Because of the narrow therapeutic window and iatrogenic misadventures, cases of theophylline toxicity have been reported with plasma theophylline levels >13 mg/L (43,44). Infants can present with jitteriness, seizures, feeding intolerance, electrolyte imbalance, vomiting, and abdominal distension (45). While the mainstay of therapy for theophylline overdose includes discontinuation of the drug and intravenous hydration, both activated charcoal and exchange transfusion have been used in the management of severe theophylline overdose (46–48). There have been no controlled trials to evaluate the effectiveness or the safety of these procedures in preterm infants. While the use of activated charcoal and exchange transfusions appears to be safe in the case reports, they should be considered only after all other methods of treatment have been exhausted in a severely affected and symptomatic neonate.

F. Routes of Administration

In addition to oral and intravenous dosing, theophylline can also be administered rectally. While early experiences suggested that it was difficult to achieve uniformity of dose using suppositories (49), one group has produced and administered a rectal gel, which appears to provide consistent blood levels (50). In addition, Evans et al. (51) have demonstrated that aminophylline may be administered percutaneously to preterm infants with satisfactory blood levels being achieved for up to 20 days.

III. Caffeine

Caffeine citrate, a methylxanthine like theophylline, has been used in infants for the treatment of apnea for over 20 years. In the past theophylline use was favored, even though its therapeutic index was much smaller and the risk of toxicity was greater, owing to the lack of a standard formula for caffeine. If caffeine was to be used it had to be created by each individual hospital pharmacy. This changed in 1999 with the development of a standard oral and injectable preparation of caffeine citrate. Caffeine is now regarded as a first-line therapy for the treatment of apnea of prematurity.

A. Mechanism of Action

Caffeine's mechanism of action for the reduction of apnea of prematurity is generally unknown (52,53). It antagonizes adenosine receptors, inhibits phosphodiesterase, and mobilizes intracellular calcium (54). It also affects many different organ systems in the body, including the brain, the lungs, the kidneys, and the heart.

Caffeine is known to stimulate the central respiratory system in the brain, resulting in increased pulmonary blood flow, increased respiratory rate, and minute volume. Similar to theophylline, caffeine improves diaphragmatic muscle contractility and lessens fatigue. Caffeine, however, does not require extracellular calcium for this action, unlike theophylline (55). Some studies have suggested that caffeine may be more potent than theophylline in improving contractility and reducing diaphragmatic fatigue (56).

The effect on the cardiovascular system is well documented in adults. Robertson et al. described an increase in blood pressure, serum renin, norepinephrine, and epinephrine (57). In neonates a study by Walther et al. measured left ventricular outflow, stroke volume, and heart rate by Doppler echo and mean arterial blood pressure by oscillometry. Although they noted no changes in heart rate, both left ventricular outflow and stroke volume were increased during day 1 through day 7 of the study. Mean blood pressure increased on day 3 of the study and returned to normal by day 7 of the study. This inotropic and pressor effect was noted in infants at 25 to 33 weeks gestation and is thought to be due to the increase in cyclic adenosine monophosphate via inhibition of phosphodiesterase and the release of calcium and the antagonism of adenosine receptor (58). Rothberg et al. also found no change in heart rate in neonates receiving caffeine (59).

Renal effects include increased urine flow rate, creatine clearance, and water output-to-input ratio (60). Clinical studies which evaluated urine output did not report large diuresis associated with caffeine administration.

B. Evidence of Efficacy

Aranda et al. reported a significant decrease in the number of apneas after loading the infants with 20 mg/kg of caffeine citrate and providing premature infants with a maintenance dose between 5 and 10 mg/kg 1–3 times per day depending on their clinical response (61). Murat et al. compared 18 premature infants of ∼30 weeks gestation. They randomized infants to caffeine or no therapy (control group) and found the apnea index to be lower for the caffeine-treated infants on days 1 and 5 of therapy (62). Anwar et al. used 23 infants as their own controls. Pneumograms were performed before caffeine and then 10 days later (63). The recent study by Erenberg et al. is the only double-blind, placebo-controlled, multicenter trial to evaluate the efficacy and the safety of caffeine citrate (64). Eighty-five infants between 28 and 32 weeks gestation were enrolled at 24 hours of life after they had at least six apneic events. They were loaded on 10 mg/kg of caffeine base IV and then received 10 days of maintenance caffeine at 2.5 mg/kg/day. Those that failed were provided with open-label rescue. The study did show a 70% reduction in the number of apneas in the study group. However, the placebo group did show a remarkable reduction of 40% from baseline in the number of apneas, demonstrating that infants benefit from enrollment in clinical trials (65).

C. Side Effects and Toxicity

Caffeine has a wide therapeutic index, relatively few side effects, and few reported cases of overdose. The studies done with a loading dose of 20 mg/kg caffeine citrate and maintenance of 5 mg/kg/dose reveals few if any side effects. One study by Lee et al. used intravenous caffeine at 30 mg/kg after a loading dose of 60 mg/kg and found it to be well tolerated. Infants were noted to tolerate serum levels >70 mg/L (66).

The side effects that have been reported include jitteriness, irritability, and restlessness. Romagnoli et al. reported hyperglycemia, vomiting, regurgitation, and tachycardia when compared to an age-matched control. Significant tachycardia was observed in infants who received 5 mg/kg/day of caffeine (67). Bauer et al. recently reported an increase in oxygen consumption and a reduction in weight gain as compared to infant controls that did not receive caffeine (68).

Toxicities have been reported in the literature, but are generally due to massive overdoses. Perrin et al. reported an acute poisoning after 10 times the prescribed dose of caffeine which resulted in tremors, hypertonia, opisthotonos posture, and crying (69). The serum caffeine level was 160 mg/L. Likewise, Van den Anker reported an overdose with a serum level of 346 mg/L, which resulted in tachypnea, tachycardia, vomiting, and seizures (70).

D. Pharmacokinetics

The pharmacokinetics of caffeine in the neonate were initially reported in the late 1970s and found that postnatal age, birth weight, and gestational age had no influence on clearance or half-life of caffeine (71,72). However, Thomson et al. evaluated 60 neonates and found that clearance was influenced by both body weight and postnatal age, but no factors influenced the volume of distribution (73). Using current guidelines, >70% of the neonates would fall into the target range of 25–100 mnol/L (73). Lee et al. described an association between clearance and volume of distribution and body weight and postnatal age (66). Le Guennec et al. found that infants <30 weeks gestation had a longer half-life than those >33 weeks. They concluded that it is better to use the postconceptual age than the postnatal age to indicate maturation, and that this change in half-life is due to hepatic maturation (74). The half-life of caffeine has been noted to be much longer than in adults and has been described to be anywhere from 75 to 144 h while the clearance has been reported to be 8.5–8.9 mL/kg/h (75,76). This prolongation in both clearance and half-life in premature infants is thought to be related to the immature liver and decreased activity of the hepatic cytochrome P450 mono-oxygenase system.

The standard dosage has been 20 mg/kg load of caffeine citrate intravenously followed by 5 mg/kg/day given as a single dose (52,54). The therapeutic range is between 8 and 20 mg/L. Lee et al. stated that this recommendation is too conservative and would result in maintenance levels that are <15 mg/L (66). As noted above, higher loading and maintenance doses have been noted in the literature and appear to be well tolerated and more effective in reducing the incidence of apnea of prematurity. Some have recommended that levels be checked once or twice per week, but the majority of users do not evaluate or rely on such levels.

E. Comparison of Theophylline and Caffeine

A number of studies have evaluated the comparative effects of theophylline and caffeine. Scanlon et al. placed infants in three study groups (41). Group 1 was loaded with caffeine at 12.5 mg/kg and given an oral maintenance of 3 mg/kg. Group 2 was loaded with caffeine at 25 mg/kg and given an oral maintenance of 6 mg/kg. Group 3 was placed on theophylline, loaded with 7.5 mg/kg, and given a maintenance dose of 3 mg/kg. The infants were then evaluated for 48 h for apneas. Although all three groups of infants showed a reduction in the number of apneas by 24 h, only the higher-dose caffeine and the theophylline groups showed a 50% reduction in apneas at 24 h and significant improvement at 8 h of life (41). Fuglsang et al. designed a double-blind and randomized trial to compare caffeine and theophylline. They found the two drugs to be equally effective in reducing apnea and bradycardia (77). Likewise, Bairam et al. (78) and Brouard et al. (79) compared the two methylxanthines and had similar findings. Yet, unlike previous studies, Bairam et al. found that caffeine had an earlier effect on the respiratory system. The infants on caffeine increased their mean respiratory rate from 43 bpm before the administration of the drug to 52 bpm on day 1 ($P < 0.05$), while those infants receiving theophylline did not have a significant increase (78). Most investigators have concluded that they would rather administer caffeine owing to the ease of administration and the marked reduction in potential serious side effects.

Two studies evaluated caffeine for apnea that was unresponsive to theophylline. Davis et al. placed infants who had breakthrough apnea despite an adequate theophylline level on caffeine. They found a reduction in the number of apneic events by 88% ($P < 0.01$). Similarly, Harrison et al. noted that 14 of 16 infants who failed theophylline therapy, responded to caffeine (81).

IV. Doxapram

Doxapram is an analeptic agent which has been used effectively in central hypoventilatory syndrome (82,83), in acute respiratory failure in adults (84,85), and as a respiratory stimulant postanesthesia (86–88).

A. Mechanism of Action

Doxapram acts on the central nervous system as a nonspecific stimulant. Doxapram is thought to act mainly through stimulation of the carotid chemoreceptors in small doses, with larger doses having a direct effect on stimulation of the medullary respiratory neurons (89,90). This agent increases ventilation and the sensitivity to carbon dioxide in normal adults (91) and in neonates with apnea of prematurity (92).

B. Evidence of Efficacy

Initial use of this agent in the newborn was to stimulate breathing after birth (93). The first report of its use in neonatal apnea was that of Burnard et al. (94). The majority of subsequent studies documented the effectiveness of doxapram in treating infants who had failed to respond to methylxanthines (92,95–98). Bairam et al. used a continuous infusion of doxapram in eight premature infants. They found a significant decrease in the number of apneas on days 1 and 2 ($P < 0.001$) and an increase in the apneic events following cessation of the drug. They also suggest a dose response, i.e., 1 mg/kg/h being more effective than 0.25 mg/kg/h. However, this study was limited both in the small study group and in the noncontrolled nature of the trial (99). Poets et al. found that doxapram resulted in a significant decrease in the apnea frequency (22 [range 11–27] vs. 14 [7–23]/h, $P < 0.01$), bradycardia (3 [0–7] vs. 1 [0–3]/h, $P < 0.01$) and hypoxaemia (8 [0–18] vs. 2 [0–17]/h, $P < 0.01$) after 1 day of treatment an improvement that was sustained throughout the 6-day study period (100). Side effects included an increase in the proportion of time spent awake (5 [0–24] vs. 12% [3–28], $P < 0.01$) and in gastric residuals (0% of feeding volume [0–5] vs. 4% [0–19], $P < 0.05$). They had to switch to intravenous doxapram in three of their nine infants because of gastrointestinal side effects.

Peliowski et al. provided the only blinded, randomized, placebo-controlled trial of doxapram. They compared 31 infants with significant apnea and randomized them to doxapram, placebo, or theophylline. The doxapram dose was 2.5 mg/kg/h. These authors found essentially no significant difference between the responses to theophylline and doxapram. In the second part of the study 10 infants who had apneas despite theophylline were then treated with doxapram. Eight of the 10 infants showed a beneficial response (29). Several other studies have also evaluated the use of doxapram to promote earlier extubation from the ventilator in the premature infant (101–103). However, these trials failed to show significant benefits, although doxapram did reduce apnea.

C. Pharmacokinetics

Both Beaudry and Jamali et al. initially described the pharmacokinetics of doxapram (104,105). The half-life was 6.6–8.17 h. Plasma clearance was 0.2–0.56 L/kg/h. After these evaluations and calculations the recommended dose for doxapram was a loading dose of 3 mg/kg by Beaudry et al. (104) and 5.5 mg/kg by Jamali et al. (105), followed by a maintenance dose of 1 mg/kg/h. The previous studies have used anywhere from 0.25 to 2.5 mg/kg/h of doxapram. Although Bairam et al. found that doxapram was effective at the low dose of 0.25 mg/kg/h, there does appear to be a dose response. Barrington et al. reported that 47% of the neonates had a significant response to doxapram at 0.5 mg/kg/h, with the percent responding increasing up to 89% at 2.5 mg/kg/h (106). Hayakawa et al. found that six of their 12 patients responded to doxapram doses of 0.5–0.8 mg/kg/h, while three responded to the higher dose of 1–1.5 mg/kg/h (107). While it appears that higher doses of doxapram are more effective in reducing the incidence of apnea of prematurity, it also appears that these higher doses (>1.5 mg/kg/h) are associated with increased side effects (107).

Doxapram may be administered orally in the neonate, but because of poor absorption it must be given in large doses up to 24 mg/kg every 6 h using the intravenous preparation (108). Oral doxapram has been shown to be effective in controlling apnea resistant to methylxanthines, and Poets noted that they had to revert to intravenous treatment in one-third of their infants (100).

D. Side Effects of Doxapram

The side effects of doxapram include a significant increase in blood pressure (106), abdominal distension, irritability, jitteriness, vomiting, and increased gastric residuals and feeding intolerance (100,107). De Villiers et al. expressed concern that doxapram could be linked to prolonged QT syndrome in a published case report using the intravenous preparation (109). A major concern with respect to the use of doxapram in the United States is that it is prepared with benzyl alcohol. A dosage of 2–2.5 mg/kg/h would deliver ~20–30 mg/kg/day of benzyl alcohol as a preservative, significantly less than that reported to be associated with the gasping syndrome, but nevertheless a significant concern with respect to its administration. Brion et al. used the form of doxapram with benzyl alcohol and found no increase in morbidity or mortality in these infants (95). If one uses the lower doses of doxapram that have been found to be efficacious, the amount of benzyl alcohol delivered would be even less, and certainly compatible with that found in other agents commonly used for the newborn, including phenobarbital.

V. Gastroesophageal Reflux and Apnea

While idiopathic apnea of prematurity is largely thought to be due to an immature brain and respiratory system, there is strong belief that reflux may cause apnea. Few studies support this widely held belief. While significant and severe reflux may trigger obstructive apnea (110,111), there is no good evidence that supports the view that apnea and reflux are temporally or causally related (112) and that the use of antireflux medications including cisapride and metoclopramide decrease apneas in neonates (113).

Cisapride, a gastrointestinal prokinetic agent, was commonly used in the neonatal nursery to decrease episodes of reflux. While it has been found to be effective in reducing symptoms of gastroesophageal reflux, it does not appear to reduce apnea associated with reflux (114). Its side effect of prolongation of the QTc interval became widely reported in the late 1990s (115–118), and the drug is no longer marketed in the United States.

Metoclopramide, a dopamine antagonist, is not well studied in the neonate. There is mixed evidence as to its effectiveness in the reduction of gastroesophageal reflux (119,120). However, there are no randomized trials to evaluate its role in the reduction of apnea in preterm neonates. Cases of metoclopramide-induced methemoglobinemia and increased serum aldosterone have been reported (121,122).

VI. Conclusion

Idiopathic apnea of prematurity will remain a common problem as neonatologists care for increasing numbers of surviving very low birth weight and extremely low birth weight infants. While methylxanthines remain the mainstay of pharmacologic therapy, there is a shift to the use of caffeine over theophylline due to its wider safety index and ease of use. Doxapram, while not a preferred agent in the United States, may be useful for a number of infants and should be considered as a second-line agent. CPAP and noninvasive methods of ventilatory support including nasal synchronous intermittent mechanical ventilation may be useful in infants whose apneas are resistant to pharmacologic treatments, and particularly helpful in those infants that have problematic apneas with a large obstructive component (123). These therapies are more fully discussed elsewhere in this volume. Perhaps the most significant question regarding apnea of prematurity is whether treatment of this disorder improves the longer-term outcomes of the most immature infants. While there are a number of reports of series of infants who were treated with single or multiple agents (124,125), there are no studies to date that have compared outcomes in infants treated with any agent compared to a similar group of infants with similar occurrences of apnea without such treatment. It is unlikely that such studies will ever be performed. Current studies under way will hopefully shed more light on this important issue.

References

1. Alden ER, Mandelkorn T, Woodrum DE, Wennberg RP, Parks CR, Hudson,WA. Morbidity and mortality of infants weighing less than 1,000 grams in an intensive care nursery. Pediatrics 1972; 50:40–49.
2. Daily WJR, Klaus M, Meyer HBP. Apnea in premature infants: monitoring, incidence, heart rate changes, and an effect of environmental temperature. Pediatrics 1967; 43:510–518.
3. Barrington K, Finer N. The natural history of the appearance of apnea of prematurity. Pediatr Res 1991; 29(4 Pt 1):372–375.
4. Finer NN, Barrington KJ, Hayes BJ, Hugh A. Obstructive, mixed and central apnea in the neonate: Physiologic correlates. J Pediatr 1992; 121:943–950.
5. Aranda JV, Turmen T. Methylxanthines in apnea of prematurity. Clin Perinatol 1979: 6(1):87–108.
6. Gerhardt T, McCarthy J, Bancalari E. Aminophylline therapy for idiopathic apnea in premature infants: effects on lung function. Pediatrics 1978; 62:801–804.
7. Gerhardt T, McCarthy J, Bancalari E. Effect of aminophylline on respiratory center activity and metabolic rate in premature infants with idiopathic apnea. Pediatrics 1979; 63:537–542.
8. Davi MJ, Sankaran K, Simons KJ, Simons FER, Seshia MM, Rigatto H. Physiologic changes induced by theophylline in the treatment of apnea of preterm infants. J Pediatr 1978; 92:91–95.
9. Eldridge FL, Millhorn DE, Waldrop TG, Kiley JP. Mechanism of respiratory effects of methylxanthines. Respir Physiol 1983; 53(2):239–261.
10. Howell LL. Comparative effects of caffeine and selective phosphodiesterase inhibitors on respiration and behavior in rhesus monkeys. J Pharmacol Exp Ther 1993; 266:894–903.
11. Eldridge FL, Millhorn DE, Kiley JP. Antagonism by theophylline of respiratory inhibition induced by adenosine. J Appl Physiol 1985; 59:1428–1433.
12. Aubier M, De Troyer A, Sampson M, Macklem PT, Roussos C. Aminophylline improves diaphragmatic contractility. N Engl J Med 1981; 305(5):249–252.
13. Gauthier AP, Yan S, Sliwinski P, Macklem PT. Effects of fatigue, fiber length, and aminophylline on human diaphragm contractility. Am J Respir Crit Care Med 1995; 152(1):204–210.
14. Vinogradova IA, Shevchenko AI. The pharmacological correction of respiratory musculature fatigue. Eksp Klin Farmakol 1997; 60(4):35–37.
15. Prostran M, Todorovic Z, Varagic VM. Some new evidence on antifatigue action of aminophylline on the isolated hemidiaphragm of the rat. Gen Pharmacol 1993; 24(1):225–232.
16. Heyman E, Ohlsson A, Heyman Z, Fong K. The effect of aminophylline on the excursions of the diaphragm in preterm neonates. A randomized double-blind controlled study. Acta Paediatr Scand 1991; 80(3):308–315.
17. Levy RD, Nava S, Gibbons L, Bellemare F. Aminophylline and human diaphragm strength in vivo. J Appl Physiol 1990; 68(6):2591–2596.

18. Mayock DE, Standaert TA, Watchko JF, Woodrum DE. Effect of aminophylline on diaphragmatic contractility in the piglet. Pediatr Res 1990; 28(3):196–198.

19. Janssens S, Derom E, Reid MB, Tjandramaga TB, Decramer M. Effects of theophylline on canine diaphragmatic contractility and fatigue. Am Rev Respir Dis 1991; 144(6):1250–1255.

20. Polaner DM, Kimball WR, Fratacci MD, Wain JC, Torres A, Kacmarek RM, Zapol WM. Effects of aminophylline on regional diaphragmatic shortening after thoracotomy in the awake lamb. Anesthesiology 1992; 77(1):93–100.

21. Kuzemko JA, Paala J. Apnoeic attacks in the newborn treated with aminophylline. Arch Dis Child 1973; 48:404–406.

22. Shannon DC, Gotay F, Stein IM. Prevention of apnea and bradycardia in low-birthweight infants. Pediatrics 1975; 55:589–594.

23. Uauy R, Shapiro DL, Smith B, Warshaw JP. Treatment of severe apnea in prematures with orally administered theophylline. Pediatrics 1975; 55:595–598.

24. Bednarek FJ, Roloff DW. Treatment of apnea of prematurity with aminophylline. Pediatrics 1976; 58:335–339.

25. Peabody JL, Neese AL, Lucey JF. Decreased hypoxic, hyperoxic and bradycardic episodes as responses of neonates to theophylline. Pediatr Res 1977; 11:419.

26. Gupta JM, Mercer HP, Koo WWK. Theophylline in treatment of apnoea of prematurity. Aust Paediatr J 1981; 17:290–291.

27. Jones RAK. Apnoea of immaturity: a controlled trial of theophylline and face mask continuous positive airways pressure. Arch Dis Child 1982; 57:761–765.

28. Sims ME, Yau G, Rambhatla S. Limitations of theophylline in the treatment of apnea of prematurity. Am J Dis Child 1985; 139:567–570.

29. Peliowski A, Finer NN. A blinded, randomized placebo-controlled trial to compare theophylline and doxapram for the treatment of apnea of prematurity. J Pediatr 1990; 116:648–653.

30. Muttitt SC, Finer NN, Tierney AJ, Rossmann J. Neonatal apnea: diagnosis by nurse versus computer. Pediatrics 1988; 82(5):713–720.

31. U.S. Departement of Health and Human Services. Use of theophylline in infants. FDA Drug Bull 1985; 15:16–17.

32. Gilman JT, Gal P. Inadequacy of FDA dosing guidelines for theophylline use in neonates. Drug Int Clin Pharm 1986; 20:481–484.

33. Murphy JE, Erkan NV, Fakhreddine F. New FDA guidelines for theophylline dosing in infants. Clin Pharm 1986; 5:16.

34. Bhatt-Mehta V, Johnson CE, Donn SM. Accuracy and reliability of dosing equations to individualize theophylline treatment of apnea of prematurity. Pharmacotherapy 1995; 15(2):246–250.

35. Bhatt-Mehta V, Donn SM, Schork MA. Prospective evaluation of two dosing equations for theophylline in premature infants. Pharmacotherapy 1996; 16(5):769–776.

36. Bonati M, Latini R, Marra G. Theophylline metabolism during the first month of life and development. Pediatr Res 1981; 15:304.

37. Bory C, Baltassat P, Porthault M. Metabolism of theophylline to caffeine in premature newborn infants. J Pediatr 1979; 94:988–993.

38. Dothey CI, Tserng KY, Kaw S, King KC. Maturational changes of theophylline pharmacokinetics in preterm infants. Clin Pharmacol Ther 1989; 45:461–468.
39. Martin ES III. The population pharmacokinetics of theophylline during the early postnatal period. J Pharmacokinet Biopharm 1991; 19:59S–77S.
40. Bhatia J. Current options in the management of apnea of prematurity. Clin Pediatr 2000; 39:327–336.
41. Scanlon JEM, Chin KC, Morgan MEI, Durbin GM, Hale KA, Brown SS. Caffeine or theophylline for neonatal apnoea? Arch Dis Child 1992; 67:425–428.
42. Vandenplas Y, De Wolf D, Sacre L. Influence of xanthines on gastroesophageal reflux in infants at risk for sudden death syndrome. Pediatrics 1986; 77:807–810.
43. Robertson WO. Index of suspicion case 1. Pediatr Rev 1992; 13(3):113–114.
44. Strauss AA, Modanlou HD, Komatsu G. Theophylline toxicity in a preterm infant: selected clinical aspects. 1985; 5:209–212.
45. Simons FE, Friesen FR, Simons KJ. Theophylline toxicity in term infants. Am J Dis Child 1980; 134:39–41.
46. Shannon M, Amitai Y, Lovejoy FH. Multiple dose activated charcoal for theophylline poisoning in young infants. Pediatrics 1987; 80:368–370.
47. Ginoza GW, Strauss AA, Iskra MK. Potential treatment of theophylline toxicity by high surface area activated charcoal. J Pediatr 1987; 111:140–142.
48. Osborn HH, Henry G, Wax P. Theophylline toxicity in a premature neonate-elimination kinetics of exchange transfusion. Clin Toxicol 1993; 31(4):639–644.
49. Waxler SH, Schack JA. Administration of aminophylline (theophylline ethylenediamine). JAMA 1950; 143:736–740.
50. Cooney S, Dillon S, Bennett G, Trehane C. Rectal aminophylline gel in treatment of apnoea in premature newborn babies. Lancet 1991; 337:1351.
51. Evans NJ, Rutter N, Hadgraft J, Parr G. Percutaneous administration of theophylline in the preterm infant. J Pediatr 1985; 307–311.
52. Kriter KE, Blanchard J. Management of apnea in infants. Clin Pharm 1989; 8:577–587.
53. Assael BM, Bonati M, Latini R. Clinical use of methylxanthines in the treatment of apnea in the premature neonate. In: Soyka LF, Redmond GP, eds. Drug Metabolism in the Immature Human. New York: Raven Press, 1981:249–263.
54. Aranda JV, Cook CE, Gorman W. Pharmacokinetic profile of caffeine in the premature newborn infant with apnea. J Pediatr 1979; 94:663–668.
55. Aubier M, Murciano D, Viires N, Lecocguic Y, Pariente R. Diaphragmatic contractility enhanced by aminophylline: role of extracellular calcium. J Appl Physiol 1983; 54(2):460–464.
56. Golgeli A, Ozesmi C, Ozesmi M. The effects of theophylline and caffeine on the isolated rat diaphragm. Acta Physiol Pharmacol Ther Latinoam 1995; 45(2):105–113.
57. Robertson D, Frolich JC, Carr RK. Effects of caffeine on plasma renin activity, catecholamines and blood pressure. N Engl J Med 1978; 298:181–186.
58. Walther FJ, Erickson R, Sims ME. Cardiovascular effects of caffeine therapy in preterm infants. Am J Dis Child 1990; 144:1164–1166.

59. Rothberg AD, Marks KH, Ward RM. The metabolic effects of caffeine in the newborn infant. Pediatr Pharm 1981; 1:181–186.

60. Gillot I, Gouyon JB, Guignard JP. Renal effects of caffeine in preterm infants. Biol Neonate 1990; 58:133–136.

61. Aranda JV, Gorman W, Bergsteinsson H. Efficacy of caffeine in treatment of apnea in the low-birth-weight infant. J Pediatr 1977; 90:467–472.

62. Murat I, Moriette G, Blin MC. The efficacy of caffeine in the treatment of recurrent idiopathic apnea in premature infants. J Pediatr 1981; 99:984–989.

63. Anwar M, Mondestin H, Mojica N. Effect of caffeine on pneumogram and apnoea of infancy. Arch Dis Child 1986; 61:891–895.

64. Erenberg A, Leff RD, Haack DG. Caffeine citrate for the treatment of apnea of prematurity: a double-blinded, placebo-controlled study. Pharmacotherapy 2000; 20:644–652.

65. Schmidt B, Gillie P, Caco C. Do sick newborn infants benefit from participation in a randomized clinical trial? J Pediatr 1999; 134:151–155.

66. Lee TC, Charles B, Steer P. Population pharmacokinetics of intravenous caffeine in neonates with apnea of prematurity. Clin Pharm Ther 1997; 61:628–640.

67. Romagnoli C, De Carolis MP, Muzii U. Effectiveness and side effects of two different doses of caffeine in preventing apnea in premature infants. Ther Drug Monit 1992; 14:14–19.

68. Bauer J, Maier K, Linderkamp O. Effect of caffeine on oxygen consumption and metabolic rate in very low birth weight infants with idiopathic apnea. Pediatrics 2001; 107:660–663.

69. Perrin C, Debruyne D, Lacotte J. Treatment of caffeine intoxication by exchange transfusion in a newborn. Acta Paediatr Scand 1987; 76:679–681.

70. Van den Anker JN, Jongejan HTM, Sauer PJJ. Severe caffeine intoxication in preterm neonates. Eur J Pediatr 1992; 151:466–468.

71. Aranda JV, Cook CE, Gorman W. Pharmacokinetic profile of caffeine in the premature newborn infant with apnea. J Pediatr 1979; 94:663–668.

72. Gorodisher R, Karplus M. Pharmacokinetic aspects of caffeine in premature infants with apnoea. Eur J Clin Pharm 1982; 22:47–52.

73. Thomson AH, Kerr S, Wright S. Population pharmacokinetics of caffeine in neonates and young infants. Ther Drug Monit 1996; 18:245–253.

74. Le Guennec J-C, Billon B, Pare C. Maturational changes of caffeine concentrations and disposition in infancy during maintenance therapy for apnea of prematurity: influence of gestational age, hepatic disease, and breast-feeding. Pediatrics 1985; 76:834–840.

75. Aranda JV, MacLeod SM, Renton KW. Hepatic microsomal drug oxidation and electron transport in newborn infants. J Pediatr 1974; 85:534.

76. Neims AH, Warner M, Loughnan PM. Developmental aspects of cytochrome P450 mono-oxygenase system. Annu Rev Pharmacol 1976; 16:427.

77. Fuglsang G, Nielsen K, Nielsen LK. The effect of caffeine compared with theophylline in the treatment of idiopathic apnea in premature infants. Acta Paediatr Scand 1989; 78:786–788.

78. Bairam A, Boutroy MJ, Badonnel Y, Vert P. Theophylline versus caffeine: comparative effects in treatment of idiopathic apnea in the preterm infant. J Pediatr 1987; 110:636–639.
79. Brouard C, Moriette G, Murat I. Comparative efficacy of theophylline and caffeine in the treatment of idiopathic apnea in premature infants. Am J Dis Child 1985; 139:698–700.
80. Davis JM, Spitzer AR, Stefano JL. Use of caffeine in infants unresponsive to theophylline in apnea of prematurity. Pediatr Pulmonol 1987; 3:90–93.
81. Harrison H. Apnea of prematurity: theophylline vs caffeine. Alaska Med 1992; 34:173–176.
82. Lugliani R, Whipp BJ, Wasserman K. Doxapram hydrochloride: a respiratory stimulant for patients with primary alveolar hypoventilation. Chest 1979; 76:414–419.
83. Hunt CE, Inwood RJ, Shannon DC. Respiratory and nonrespiratory effects of doxapram in congential central hypoventilation syndrome. Am Rev Respir Dis 1979; 119:263–269.
84. Moser KM, Luchsinger PC, Adamson JS. Respiratory stimulation with intravenous doxapram in respiratory failure. N Engl J Med 1973; 288:427–431.
85. Edwards G, Lond MB. A double-blind trial of five respiratory stimulants in patients with acute ventilatory failure. Lancet 1967; ii:226–229.
86. Robertson GS, MacGregor, Jones CJ. Evaluation of doxapram for arousal from general anaesthesia in outpatients. Br J Anaesth 1977; 49:133–140.
87. Noe FE, Borrillo N, Greifenstein FE. Use of a new analeptic, doxapram hydro-chloride, during general anesthesia and recovery. Anesth Analg 1965; 44:206–213.
88. Council on Drugs. A new analeptic agent. JAMA 1966; 196:147–148.
89. Mitchell RA, Herbert DA. Potencies of doxapram and hypoxia in stimulating carotid-body chemoreceptors and ventilation in anesthetized cats. Anesthesiology 1975; 42:559–566.
90. Burki NK. Ventilatory effects of doxapram in conscious human subjects. Chest 1984; 85(5):600–604.
91. Calverley PMA, Robson RH, Wraith PK. The ventilatory effects of doxapram in normal man. Clin Sci 1983; 65:65–69.
92. Barrington KJ, Finer NN, Peters KL, Barton J. Physiologic effects of doxapram in idiopathic apnea of prematurity. J Pediatr 1986; 108(1):124–129.
93. Gupta PK, Moore J. The use of doxapram in the newborn. J Obstet Gynaecol Br Commun 1973; 80:1002–1006.
94. Burnard ED, Moore RG, Nichol H. A trial of doxapram in the current apnea of prematurity. In: Stern L, Oh W, Friis-Hansen B, eds. Intensive Care in the Newborn. II. New York: Masson, 1976:143–148.
95. Brion LP, Vega-Rich C, Reinersman G. Low-dose doxapram for apnea unresponsive to aminophylline in very low birthweight infants. J Perinatol 1991; 11:359–364.
96. Alpan G, Eyal F, Sagi E. Doxapram in the treatment of idiopathic apnea of prematurity unresponsive to aminophylline. J Pediatr 1984; 104:634–637.
97. Barrington KJ, Finer NN, Peters KL. Physiologic effects of doxapram and aminophylline. Arch Dis Child 1984; 59:281–283.

98. Sagi E, Eyal F, Alpan G. Idiopathic apnoea of prematurity treated with doxapram and aminophylline. Arch Dis Child 1984; 59:281–283.
99. Bairam A, Faulon M, Monin P. Doxapram for the initial treatment of idiopathic apnea of prematurity. Biol Neonate 1992; 61:209–213.
100. Poets CF, Darraj S, Bohnhorst B. Effect of doxapram on episodes of apnoea, bradycardia and hypoxaemia in preterm infants. Biol Neonate 1999; 76:207–213.
101. Huon C, Rey E, Mussat P. Low dose doxapram for treatment of apnea following early weaning in very low birthweight infants: a randomized, double-blinded controlled study. Acta Paediatr 1998; 87:1180–1184.
102. Barrington KJ, Muttitt SC. Randomized, controlled, blinded trial of doxapram for extubation of the very low birthweight infant. Acta Paediatr 1998; 87:191–194.
103. Eyal F, Alpan G, Sagi E. Aminophylline versus doxapram in idiopathic apnea of prematurity: a double-blinded controlled study. Pediatrics 1985; 75:709–713.
104. Beaudry MA, Bradley JM, Gramlich LM. Pharmacokinetics of doxapram in idiopathic apnea of prematurity. Dev Pharm Ther 1988; 11:65–72.
105. Jamali F, Barrington KJ, Finer NN. Doxapram dosage regimen in apnea of prematurity based on pharmacokinetic data. Dev Pharm Ther 1988; 11:253–257.
106. Barrington KJ, Finer NN, Torok-Both G. Dose-response relationship of doxapram in the therapy for refractory idiopathic apnea of prematurity. Pediatrics 1987; 80:22–27.
107. Hayakawa F, Hakamada S, Kuno K. Doxapram in the treatment of idiopathic apnea of prematurity: desirable dosage and serum concentrations. J Pediatr 1986; 109:138–140.
108. Bairam A, Akramoff-Gershan L, Beharry K. Gastrointestinal absorption of doxapram in neonates. Am J Perinatol 1991; 8:110–113.
109. De Villiers GS, Walele A, Van der Merwe P-L. Second-degree atrioventricular heart block after doxapram administration. J Pediatr 1998; 133:149–150.
110. Newell SJ, Booth IW, Morgan MEI. Gastro-oesophageal reflux in preterm infants. Arch Dis Child 1989; 64:780–786.
111. Marino AJ, Assing E, Carbone MT. The incidence of gastroesophageal reflux in preterm infants. J Perinatol 1995; 15:369–371.
112. Menon AP, Schefft GL, Thach BT. Apnea associated with regurgitation in infants. J Pediatr 1985; 106:625–629.
113. Kimball AL, Carlton DP. Gastroesophageal reflux medications in the treatment of apnea in premature infants. J Pediatr 2001; 138(3):355–360.
114. Ariagno RL, Kikket MA, Mirmiran M. Cisapride decreases gastroesophageal reflux in preterm infants. Pediatrics 2001; 107:58–71.
115. Dubin A, Kikkert M, Mirmiram M, Ariagno R. Cisapride Associated with QTc prolongation in very low birth weight preterm infants. Pediatrics 2001; 107:1313
116. Hill SL, Evangelista JK, Pissi AM. Proarrhythmia associated with cisapride in children. Pediatrics 1998; 101:1053–1056.
117. Lewin MB, Bryant RM, Fenrich AL. Cisapride-induced long QT interval. J Pediatr 1996; 128:279–281.
118. Bernardini S, Semama DS, Huet F. Effects of cisapride on QTc interval in neonates. Arch Dis Child Fetal Neonatal Ed 1997; 77:F241–F243.

119. Tolia V, Calhoun J, Kuhns L, Kauffman RE. Randomized, prospective double-blind trial of metoclopramide and placebo for gastroesophageal reflux in infants. Pediatr Pharm Ther 1989; 115:141–145.

120. Noerr B. Metoclopramide. Neonat Net 1993; 12:77–78.

121. Kearns GL, Fiser DH. Metoclopramide-induced methemoglobinemia. Pediatrics 1988; 82:364–366.

122. Fanning S, Ishisaka DY, Merritt TA. Possible metoclopramide-induced increase in serum aldosterone in a premature infant. Am J Health Syst Pharm 1995; 52:316–319.

123. Barrington KJ, Bull D, Finer NN. Randomized trial of nasal synchronized intermittent mandatory ventilation compared with continuous positive airway pressure after extubation of very low birth weight infants. Pediatrics 2001; 107(4):638–641.

124. Cheung PY, Barrington KJ, Finer NN, Robertson CM. Early childhood neurodevelopment in very low birthweight infants with predischarge apnea. Pediatr Pulmonol 1999; 27:14–20.

125. Mathew OP. Neurodevelopmental outcome of apneic infants treated with doxapram. Pediatr Res 2001; 49:379A.

14

Nonpharmacological Management of Idiopathic Apnea of the Premature Infant

EDWARD E. LAWSON

Johns Hopkins University School of Medicine
Baltimore, Maryland, U.S.A.

I. Introduction

This chapter is a review of nonpharmacological means to manage infants having obstructive, central and mixed apnea related to prematurity. While many of these management strategies may be effective for apnea of other etiologies, the chapter will not directly discuss management of those other causes.

Breathing activity in newborns, children, and adults results from neuronal signals that originate in the brainstem and transmit excitatory signals causing contraction of various respiratory muscles. These neuronal signals originate from a network of brainstem neurons that oscillate between three states of activity—inspiration, postinspiration, and expiration (1–3). The outputs from these neurons innervate (often via intermediary neurons) muscles of the upper airway, chest, diaphragm, and abdomen. Periodic contraction of these muscles controls inhalation and exhalation of air. Inspiration is the phase where the upper airway and larynx dilate by contraction of upper-airway dilator muscles, and then lungs expand by contraction of the diaphragm and inspiratory intercostal muscles. In postinspiration, the larynx is closed or partially closed controlling air flow across the vocal cords. Postinspiration actively restricts expiratory pulmonary airflow. During the expiratory phase, passive relaxation or active contraction of intercostal, abdominal, and airway muscles results in outward flow of air from the lungs.

The major principle behind most nonpharmacological methods of apnea management is that apnea is often secondary to lack of sufficient neuronal activity in the brainstem centers for the respiratory network to oscillate between the three stages of respiration. Some evidence suggests that when failure of oscillation occurs, postinspiratory activity (4) due either to lack of neuronal inputs or to direct stimulation of the postinspiratory neurons prevents oscillation through the other phases. In any case whether postinspiratory activity is the root cause of central apnea is unimportant in understanding the mechanisms of pharmacological and nonpharmacological apnea therapies. The concept that effective therapies often work by generating excitatory neuronal activity in the brainstem centers such that these centers oscillate between the various respiratory stages is sufficient mechanistic understanding for the clinician. In effect, any nonspecific neuronal activity impinging upon the brainstem respiratory centers acts to give "momentum" to the oscillation between the various respiratory states. In turn, lack of nonspecific and specific (e.g., chemosensory) input to the brainstem allows dissolution of the oscillating momentum, resulting in respiratory apnea. Further, reduced neuronal output to the upper airway muscles to maintain sufficient tone is one physiologic mechanism resulting in obstructive or mixed obstructive/central apnea. Another important concept regarding obstructive apnea is that the obstruction occurs in the pharynx (or perhaps the larynx) secondary to structural characteristics of the small airway in premature infants in addition to loss of neuronal drive to the airway-dilating muscles of the upper airway.

Lack of neurologic activity in the brainstem respiratory control centers derives from reduced excitatory influences that counterbalance inhibitory influences. Neurons in the brainstem of newborn infants, in particular premature infants, are characterized by higher density of inhibitory receptors and transmitters than excitatory receptors and transmitters. Additionally, fewer neurons are present, so maintaining synchronous oscillatory neuronal activity appears more difficult than in older subjects. Other mechanisms associated with apnea in newborns are: various sleep stages that result in reduced excitatory and increased inhibitory inputs to the brainstem, lack of nonspecific neuronal inputs from peripheral sensory inputs, strong inhibitory inputs from vagal and laryngeal receptors, and various causes of hypoxemia. Finally, obstructive apnea in newborns is particularly common secondary to structural issues unique to the premature infant. The size of the upper airway allows easy closure of the pharynx if sleep, anesthetics, sedatives, etc., inhibit the airway muscles (5). Also, neck flexion easily results in airway closure secondary to the small diameter of the airway and the high compliance of these structures (6).

II. Positioning

A. Prone vs. Supine

One of the apparent inconsistencies in management of premature infants is the frequent use of prone positioning in the neonatal intensive care unit and the recommendation to parents that infants are placed on their backs for sleep at home. This apparent conflict arises from older research that demonstrated improved pulmonary function in preterm infants when placed on their stomach (7–9), as well as the historical teaching of the American Academy of Pediatrics that infants should be placed prone in order to prevent aspiration during sleep. The research regarding pulmonary function improvement when prone was limited to premature infants recovering from respiratory distress syndrome and breathing without aid of mechanical devices (e.g., continuous positive airway pressure or mechanical ventilation). Nevertheless, the recommendation was generalized and many premature infants are regularly placed prone on their stomachs in incubators and bassinets while in hospitals. More recent information indicates that the incidence of apnea among preterm infants is not affected by supine or prone position (10). Another recent report indicates that term healthy infants have improved lung volume and decreased upper-airway resistance when placed supine rather than prone (11).

Other work has demonstrated that infants sleeping at home are at increased risk for sudden infant death syndrome (SIDS) when placed to sleep in the prone position (12–14). This has led to the recommendation for supine positioning of infants when they are sleeping. The mechanism of death is uncertain, but likely relates to rebreathing of exhaled air leading to hypercapnia and carbon dioxide narcosis. Data supporting this hypothesis derive from epidemiological, anecdotal, human, and animal studies (15–19). Another possibility is that covering the face results in obstructive apnea, especially in a head-down position in infants too young to allow head lifting if they arouse in response to the acute airway obstruction (18). Another hypothesis is that swallowing is inhibited in the prone position and therefore laryngeal receptors are more likely to be stimulated resulting in apnea (20).

Removing soft bedding, pillows, sheepskins, and crib "bumpers" prevents accidental entrapment and face-covering situations (15–17). Again, common practices in the NICU are often at odds with recommendations to parents. Physicians and nurses should be aware of the different circumstances leading to use of soft bedding materials and sheepskins in the NICU that are inconsistent with home care needs.

B. Head/Neck Flexion

Neck flexion has been shown to result in airway closure, particularly in premature infants, but also in term infants (6). It has been long recommended that to prevent obstructive apnea and cardiac arrest during procedures such as lumbar puncture the holder should place the caudal hand on the shoulders in order to flex the back, but to avoid flexing the neck. In premature infants another cause of neck flexion is the common practice of placing the infant on an inclined surface to reduce gastroesophageal reflux. An active infant may creep down the incline and then its head may further droop resulting in airway occlusion and apnea (21). Treatment of this form of apnea is based on a high index of suspicion given the clinical situation.

C. Gastroesophageal Reflux (GER)

Whether gastroesophageal reflux results in apnea is controversial. Most current literature indicates a lack of direct correlation of reflux episodes with apnea events (22–24) as well as lack of improvement in apnea events following onset of effective therapy (25). However, using a newer technique of intraluminal impedance, Wenzl et al. (26) demonstrated a positive correlation of GER with apnea in premature infants, but this is not in agreement with similar studies by Peter et al. (24).

Despite the general lack of correlation of GER and apnea, many clinicians invoke various therapies to reduce or minimize GER in premature infants in order to reduce apnea events. Thickening feeds by adding cereal to formula and placing the infant on an inclined surface (reverse Trendelenberg) are the two most common nonpharmacological therapies. As mentioned above, the inclined plane may result in obstructive apnea if the head flexes due to gravitational forces. A surgical procedure to create a one-way valve from the lower esophagus into the stomach (Nissen procedure) is the extreme therapy to prevent GER. However, this procedure should not be performed to manage apnea without careful evaluation that clearly establishes the correlation of GER with apnea in the individual patient. This evaluation would at minimum include simultaneous polysomnography with esophageal pH monitoring and the newer multiple intraluminal impedance technique (24,26). Since stomach pH in infants is frequently > 4, regurgitated material in the esophagus may not register as reflux when using simple pH monitoring.

GER is likely to be very overmanaged with the current medications and nonpharmacological management techniques. Indeed, it is reasonable to suggest that in absence of clear evidence of aspiration events or esophagitis, the usual GER may be a mild if not benign problem in otherwise normal preterm infants. In this case one should not provide antireflux medical management unless the reflux is actually interfering with nutritional intake and growth.

III. Nonpharmacological Mechanisms to Stimulate the Central Nervous System

Respiratory drive originates in neuronal clusters of the brainstem that spontaneously oscillate between the various states of respiration. Specific neuronal inputs such as inhibitory and excitatory reflexes (e.g., vagal stretch receptors from the lungs) and chemosensory information derived from oxygen sensors in the carotid body and carbon dioxide sensors in the brainstem provide important modulation of this respiratory oscillator. Another source of important neuronal activity that also excites the respiratory neurons is nonspecific neural activity deriving from myriad sensors throughout the body, as well as excitatory and inhibitory inputs from the higher brain. Neuronal activity from body sensors may derive from any of the peripheral tactile, stretch and thermal sensors in skin, muscle, and joints. Inhibition or accentuation by influences of the higher brain due to wakefulness, sleep, speech, eating, muscle commands, etc., from mid- or higher-brain centers also interacts at the brainstem level, affecting the drive to these oscillating neuronal pools. The following sections review common practices for preventing apnea and for interrupting apnea once initiated using stimulation techniques.

A. Cutaneous/Muscle/Joint Stimulation

Initiation of respiratory activity in the delivery room is classically associated with onset of massive cutaneous and thermal stimuli. The cutaneous stimuli derive from poking, prodding, and rubbing by mother and associated caretakers shortly after delivery. Observations of the effects of these stimuli have resulted in clinical practices such as mild shaking, rubbing, and patting of feet and hands to stimulate an infant once apnea has persisted for a designated period. In modern times the act of drying infants in the delivery room provides a great amount of cutaneous stimulation, often resulting in initiation of respiratory activity.

An old-time classic means for preventing apnea of the premature infant was to attach a string or tape to the leg of a premature infant and then to periodically pull the leg, resulting in prevention of apnea for a short period. This technique presumably stimulated joint receptors as well as cutaneous sensors, resulting in a burst of stimulatory activity in the brainstem (27). Mild apnea was stopped and the effect lasted for a brief time following each pull of the tape. This technique was apparently widely accepted in the 1970s, but has been supplanted by use of methylxanthine therapy. Other problems with the technique were a perception that the technique could interfere with normal sleep patterns as the stimulation also resulted in arousal of sleeping infants.

B. Kinesthetic Stimulation—Oscillating Waterbeds/Airbeds

Following the understanding that cutaneous and joint stimuli resulted in prevention of apnea for brief periods, many neonatologists began searching for an automated technique that would provide continuous central nervous system stimulation to prevent or reduce apnea events. The logical technique to try was stimulation of vestibular receptors (kinesthetic stimulation), the logic being that these receptors are quiet when the infant is not moving and that any movement of the infant would result in a nonspecific excitatory stimulus to the brainstem.

Indeed, the technique was shown to work utilizing an electric oscillating bed (28–33). The sleep surface of the infant was tilted from front to back or from side to side in order to stimulate the vestibular system. Modifications of this system included use of waterbeds and a bladder underneath the mattress that was periodically inflated by a spare mechanical ventilator, and most recently airbeds (34). Each system had advocates, and each was shown to reduce the incidence of apnea over periods of several hours. Unfortunately, with protracted use of these devices, apnea gradually recurred, indicating loss of effectiveness of these devices. Except for a recent report of use of gentle rocking to prevent obstructive apnea (35), these devices have fallen out of routine clinical practice (36).

Ignoring the physiological mechanism of central nervous system accommodation was the critical error in attempts to utilize these devices. Accommodation is the neural mechanism by which a repetitive stimulus to the brain is ultimately inhibited so that the previous stimulatory effect becomes negated. Neural accommodation is essentially a learning mechanism and it develops over hours. While the new stimulus remains unique, many of the peripheral stimulatory techniques initially worked but then ultimately lost their therapeutic effects. Unfortunately, the initial enthusiastic reports of efficacy measured incidence of apnea only for the first few hours after initiation of the repetitive stimulation. In contrast, other peripheral stimulatory techniques continue to be effective because they are irregularly applied or are unique in each application. Recognizing that accommodation resulted in loss of efficacy of the oscillating bed, several groups investigated use of a randomly oscillating bed. These devices had similar effects to the regularly oscillating bed, though perhaps a slightly longer period of time was required for accommodation to occur (33). They too are no longer widely utilized.

C. Facial Air Jets

Air jets, directed at the face or nares, result in arousal from sleep. At least one group postulated in a preliminary fashion that an air jet stimulus following onset of protracted apnea may be an effective remedy by inducing arousal (personal communication). Though the technique can be automated in response to apneas and may be set to respond to only protracted apneas, this technique has not been developed widely as a tool for prevention of apnea in premature infants. Reasons for this may be twofold. First, if the stimulus is repetitively applied, then it may lose the stimulatory effect with repetitive exposure. Second, the face also is richly innervated with receptors that stimulate an inhibitory respiratory effect known as the "dive response." This reflex results in profound apnea, bradycardia, and redistribution of blood flow from peripheral organs to central organs. The possibility of initiating such a reflex when attempting to reverse central or obstructive apnea of the premature infant is clearly not desired, especially when other, similar techniques, such as cutaneous stimulation, are known to be effective.

D. Audible Alarms

Numerous people have questioned the efficacy of audible alarms for reinitiating respiratory efforts; most recently a report of home monitoring questioned whether alarms resulted in premature termination of protracted apnea events (37). In the clinical environment of the modern NICU, electronic cardiorespiratory and oxygen saturation monitoring devices often initiate a rather loud alarm in response to apnea, bradycardia, or protracted arterial hemoglobin desaturation in order to alert caretaking personnel that an apnea event is occurring. Whether the auditory alarm may independently effect recovery from the apnea event is an area of some interest. In the clinical NICU, most infants are managed within a closed incubator that reduces transmission of sound into the infant's environment. Consequently, one would predict that without an audible alarm within the incubator, audible alarms would generally be ineffective in the NICU.

In contrast, many susceptible infants are in open bassinets or cribs, and the auditory alarm may indeed bring about recovery without other intervention. The strongest evidence to date for this hypothesis comes from the recently completed CHIME trial of recorded home monitors, wherein reinitiating of respiration was observed to frequently follow onset of the alarm without other intervention (37). This finding, however, may not be relevant to the premature infant with idiopathic apnea as the alarms were louder than tolerable in an NICU, the infants were generally of older postconceptual age than the usual premature infant in an NICU, and the apnea events were not occurring with sufficient frequency to be of concern regarding the possibility of accommodation.

E. Neuronal Entrainment Techniques—"Breathing Bear"

Various stimuli have been used to entrain respiratory efforts or to stabilize respiratory function. Two reports of devices indicate that there may be some improvement in apnea when audible or vestibular devices are used at a pace similar to that of normal respiratory frequency. One device, the "breathing" teddy bear (38), emits a sound that "is a source of optional rhythmic stimulation that reflects the breathing rate of the individual infant it is with." This device was shown to entrain premature infants' breathing efforts, resulting in more regular respiratory rhythm. Another device uses gentle rocking with an audible sound to mimic in utero sounds, and claims improved outcomes as well as reduced incidence of apnea (39). Those advocating cobedding of infants and mothers have described similar effects, but this has not been proven in studies (40).

IV. Thermal Environment

A. Neutral Thermal Environment

The thermoneutral environment is defined as the external temperature at which a warm-blooded animal maintains normal body temperature using the minimal amount of metabolism to generate heat. In an environment either warmer or cooler, greater metabolism is necessary to maintain normal body temperature. One principle of nursing infants, particularly ill premature infants, is to maintain a thermoneutral environment to minimize metabolism necessary to maintain body temperature. Under these circumstances, growth and injury repair may theoretically proceed despite limited external metabolic supply. Under normal NICU circumstances the thermoneutral environment is maintained through use of an incubator or radiant warming device. The incubator ambient temperature may be regulated using a predetermined target depending on gestational age and body mass. Alternatively, skin temperature may be used as a proxy for core temperature and then the ambient temperature in the incubator, or the heating source of a radiant warmer may be servocontrolled.

B. Relationship of Body Core Temperature to Respiratory Control

Wide Swings in Ambient/Core Temperature

Clinical experience indicates that respiratory pattern abnormalities, including apnea, occur when infants have abnormally low body temperature or when they are somewhat overheated (41). Apnea seems particularly prevalent when an infant is increasing core temperature above the normal 37°C. Mechanisms for this effect are entirely speculative, but may include inhibition from midbrain thermal regulatory centers excited by changes in core temperature. Alternatively, high core temperatures may initiate panting activity that results in hyperventilation, causing hypocapnea and apnea. Infants under radiant warmers may be particularly prone to varying core temperature (42), particularly if they are in an area susceptible to drafts that would accentuate changes in skin temperature independent of core temperature. Of course many standard nursing practices are used to prevent this possibility, including: reflective and insulating patches over the thermode, placement of the thermode over the liver (a high-heat-source solid organ), placement of the infant in prone position with the thermode between the infant and the radiant heat source, prevention of drafts, and development of incubators having dual radiant and ambient temperature regulation possibilities (Giraffe, Ohmeda Medical).

Skin Core Temperature Gradient

When an infant has a stable core temperature and is in a thermoneutral ambient environment, an old technique for decreasing the density of apnea events is to lower the ambient temperature by $\sim 0.5°C$. Evidence for this comes from work of Daily et al., who demonstrated that preterm infants in an incubator with a skin temperature set-point at $36°C$ had less apnea than when the set-point was $36.8°C$ (41). Similarly, at least two groups have shown that higher ambient temperatures (between $20–24°C$ and $30°C$) result in higher incidence of apnea despite little change in rectal/core temperature (43,44). The theory is that increased ambient temperature, within the thermoneutral range, decreases the skin core temperature gradient, resulting in loss of nonspecific thermal related neuronal signals to the brainstem. The positive effect of lowering ambient temperature presumably depends on skin thermal receptors being relatively activated by this change in temperature gradient hence resulting in increased nonspecific neural information impinging upon the brainstem and the respiratory centers.

The SIDS literature is replete with many articles that indicate hyperthermia as a mechanism causing apnea and associated with sudden unexpected death of older infants (44,45). These data may be relevant to the care of premature infants with apnea as well. Overwrapping and face covering (18) are associated with changes in body temperature and apnea. Mild increases in environmental temperature of preterm infants at term as well as term infants results in increased incidence of apnea during sleep (43). Attention to amounts of wrapping and to environmental temperature allowing adequate self-regulation of temperature is likely to result in simple means to reduce the incidence of apnea.

V. Oxygen

A. Oxygen Effects on Apnea

As is discussed in Chapter 12, the respiratory response to hypoxia in infants (particularly premature infants) less than a few weeks of age is different from that of older children and adults. The respiratory response is "biphasic" with an initial phase of increased respiratory activity followed shortly by a phase of declining breathing secondary to loss of drive to the diaphragm (46–48). This loss of drive may actually be a central inhibition of the brainstem respiratory centers by higher central nervous system structures (49). In any case, the lack of sustained respiratory response may lead even to apnea in some infants with significant hypoxia of sufficient duration. One tenet of managing apnea in premature infants is then to avoid situations that may lead to hypoxemia that would initiate the sequence of respiratory inhibition. Infants with pulmonary failure secondary to respiratory distress syndrome and pneumonia may present with apnea due to their relative hypoxemia. To avoid hypoxemia, use of supplemental oxygen is frequently done by nasal cannula or by enriching the inhaled air by use of a hood or oxygen directly flowing into an incubator.

On the other hand, otherwise well premature infants may develop a respiratory pattern identified as periodic breathing (50–53). Periodic breathing is characterized by repetitive periods of relatively high ventilation interspersed with periods of no respiratory activity; occasionally the respiratory pauses will last long enough to trigger the electronic monitoring system or even convert to a true mixed or central apnea. In these situations, the one attractive explanation for the cause is a peripheral oxygen-sensing system that has a higher output than is appropriate (54). In this case the carotid body senses hypoxemia, the infant hyperventilates, carbon dioxide drops, and peripheral oxygen increases, thus reducing the chemical drive to breathe at both peripheral and central sensing systems. This is followed by the respiratory pause during which carbon dioxide rises and blood oxygen falls, leading the central respiratory system to over-ventilate again. These seemingly wide shifts in respiratory drive are thought to be secondary to a carotid body that is too responsive to mild reductions in blood oxygen. Weintraub et al. (54) have demonstrated that simply increasing the inhaled oxygen to 0.40 FiO_2 may stop the periodic or irregular breathing patterns. This may be accomplished by use of either hood oxygen or nasal prongs. Alternatively, the mechanism for the effect of increased ambient oxygen is actual relief of central nervous system hypoxia in the face of inadequate carotid body response to peripheral hypoxemia (55,56).

Management of apnea with oxygen is not without risk. One obvious issue is whether increased ambient oxygen may predispose small premature infants to retinopathy of the premature. This issue is not clear, though the levels of oxygen recommended to reduce apnea and periodic breathing should not achieve blood levels associated with ROP. Continuous percutaneous arterial hemoglobin satura-tion (SpO_2) monitoring is recommended to ensure that the infants do not have persistent hyperoxemia. A second concern is that external oxygen may actually accentuate the periodic pattern leading to prolonged apnea, an effect recently reported by Berger et al. (57).

B. Carbon Dioxide Effects on Apnea

Newborn infants increase respiratory activity in response to increased ambient carbon dioxide (58,59), but the increase is not as great as for older infants and children (corrected for size). Hence, carbon dioxide levels in blood do affect respiratory drive. In the awake state, normal spontaneous ventilation maintains blood carbon dioxide levels below the threshold to drive ventilation. However, in non-REM sleep, the infant becomes completely dependent on the chemical stimulus to breathe exerted by carbon dioxide and oxygen blood levels. Infants may exhibit apnea secondary to low blood carbon dioxide levels, but usually only in circumstances such as controlled mechanical ventilation. When apnea is noted but not desired in the ventilated infant, a reduction in minute ventilation will usually result in onset of spontaneous breaths.

Only one report of examining carbon dioxide administration to ameliorate apnea in newborns is available (60). Otherwise, administration of carbon dioxide has not been used in the clinical environment to affect breathing patterns on a routine basis. Concerns regarding the effects of respiratory acidosis and the effects of high levels of carbon dioxide on cerebral blood flow (61,62) limit its use.

In contrast, hypercapnia due to rebreathing or face-covered circumstances that may occur when the face is buried in soft bedding in the prone position or the face is covered by bed sheets or blankets, is one of the major theories explaining the mechanism for SIDS (19,63). In these circumstances carbon dioxide in animal models has been shown to increase to levels associated with carbon dioxide narcosis that may result in death (16).

C. Erythrocyte Transfusion

Anemia has long been associated with an increase in incidence of periodic breathing and apnea in premature infants. Those who invoke anemia as a cause of apnea tend to suggest that tissue hypoxia secondary to lack of red blood cells results in central nervous system "depression" as the mechanism (56). They then suggest that transfusion of small amounts of packed red blood cells that reverses anemia would also ameliorate apnea. As one would suspect, this thesis resulted in a rather extensive literature with both proponents of transfusion (56,64,65) and those who have not found transfusion (66–68) to be an effective means to manage apnea.

Proponents of transfusion to ameliorate apnea in otherwise well premature infants suggest that the hematocrit should be < 25% to be effective. The clinician considering transfusion to treat apnea should evaluate the following issues:

1. Is the apnea new in origin or has it been longstanding?
2. Has the apnea incidence increased as anemia worsened?
3. Is the child receiving oxygen or other ventilatory support?
4. Has heart rate increased?
5. Are other respiratory rhythm changes, such as periodic breathing, more prominent?

Association of these signs with apnea would support a trial of transfusion. The clinician may also consider whether management with erythropoietin would be preferable to a transfusion. Erythropoietin has been shown to be an effective means to maintain hematocrit higher than the nadir that would ordinarily occur (64). However, erythropoietin is not suitable for acute management of anemia.

Now that blood banks can supply packed red blood cells from a single donor for a period as long as a month, the clinician may have a lower threshold for transfusion if exposure to another donor is not being considered.

D.   Patent Ductus Arteriosus (PDA) Closure

Patent ductus arteriosus with apnea secondary to intractable congestive heart failure has been cited as an indication for surgical ligation. The mechanism is likely to be relative central nervous system hypoxia causing inhibition of respiratory drive. PDA as a cause of apnea is mentioned mostly in older literature (69) as apnea seems no longer to be a major indicator for closure of the ductus. Reasons for this may be that newer modalities for diagnosis of a PDA, such as bedside echocardiography, and wide acceptance of early indomethacin usage, now result in only the very rare case of clinically significant progressive heart failure. PDA should remain in the differential diagnosis of apnea, but certainly surgical closure to manage apnea will remain an unusual indication.

VI.   Mechanical Airway Support

A.   Nasal Cannulas

Nasal cannulas are frequently used to administer oxygen in increased concentration without relegating the infant to a closed environment. The mechanism by which this common clinical practice prevents apnea is not entirely clear. It is clear that use of either 100% oxygen at low flow rates (0.25 L/min or lower) or varying concentrations of oxygen at higher flow rates often result in stabilization of irregular respiratory patterns and often dramatically reduce the incidence of apnea in an individual infant (54). However, on occasion we note infants in whom we are unable to remove the nasal cannulas even when only 21% oxygen is being administered. This seeming paradox has not been explained satisfactorily in the literature. Three possible mechanisms may be posited. First, the nasal cannula may act like an air jet and provide a stimulus that activates the central respiratory control system. This is unlikely, as one would certainly expect accommodation to eventually reduce the effectiveness of the signal. Second, the 1–2.5 liter per minute flow through the cannula results in a functional nasal continuous positive airway pressure that may result in increased blood oxygen levels or may prevent obstructive events (70). A third hypothesis (J. Pomerance, personal communication) is that the flow of air into the upper airway effectively reduces airway dead space such that the infant's ventilation results in slightly higher blood oxygen level sufficient to prevent apnea secondary to hypoxemia. Such an effect could be sleep/wake state dependent.

B. Oral and Nasal Airways

Apnea secondary to anatomic obstruction may occasionally be treated by fashioning a nasal or oral airway allowing passage of air around or through an anatomic obstruction. A nasal endotracheal tube is often adequate for this process on a temporary basis. Various infant-size oral devices are commercially marketed for this purpose. However, experience indicates that these devices are adequate for temporary use, but are often inadequate for long-term usage. All these devices are inadequate for management of apnea of premature infants whether obstructive or central in origin. Permanent anatomic obstruction that may not be surgically approached for a period of time is best bypassed by use of a tracheostomy. These are difficult to manage in newborns.

C. Continuous Positive Airway Pressure (CPAP)

When apnea is resistant to the mild stimulation techniques and is demonstrated to be obstructive or mixed obstructive/central, then delivery of continuous positive airway pressure is often highly effective in preventing further episodes (27,71–73). Obstructive apneas may be detected by careful physical examination—particularly pulmonary auscultation to demonstrate obstructed breaths. Alternatively, multichannel recording of airflow at the nose or use of inductance plethysmography may also demonstrate more rigorously the diagnosis of obstructive apnea components. Finally, one can simply apply nasal CPAP and demonstrate efficacy, thus establishing that obstructive apnea was the problem.

Providing positive airway pressure preventing closure of the pharynx may appropriately treat persistent apnea with an obstructive component (73–77). In this circumstance the positive airway pressure results in reduced upper-airway resistance (78) and expansion of the larynx. These positive forces counteract passive tendencies to close the pharynx, as well as negative pressures generated by inspiration that augment closure (71,79). Effective pressure may be generated using many different techniques. The most common of these is use of a short pronged nasal cannula that generates pressure through many different techniques. Continuous flow to the nasal prongs with a resistance generator (e.g., a ventilator or simply a bottle of water) develops adequate pressure, but the airflow should be two to three times greater than the maximal inspiratory airflow. This elevated flow rate is necessary to prevent rebreathing of the baby's exhaled breath. The original description of a continuous positive airway generator is by Gregory et al. (80) and was originally described for treatment of respiratory distress syndrome. A device that generates variable flow continuous airway pressure using a Venturi effect has also been patented and may be more effective than conventional nasal CPAP (72).

Other airway techniques to generate CPAP include use of an endotracheal tube positioned just above the epiglottis in the pharynx (76), long silastic thin prongs that extend from the nares to the nasopharynx, and face masks (81). While face masks may provide adequate pressure to adequately treat obstructive apnea, they have been associated with posterior fossa hemorrhage secondary to skull deformation of the tight bands needed to provide sufficient force to seal the mask to the face. The endotracheal tube technique requires increased surveillance, as airway secretions tend to accumulate and require suctioning. The long prong technique has its advocates, as the devices tend to stay in place well and may reduce nasal trauma due to their softness and the reduced pressure needed to apply them to the nose.

CPAP should not be attempted with an intubated patient for protracted periods. An intubated patient is unable to generate the airway closure necessary to produce sighs that result in maintenance of functional residual capacity. In the case of protracted intubation without intermittent positive pressure ventilation, functional residual capacity inevitably declines over time resulting in inadequate ventilation.

D. Intermittent Positive Pressure Ventilation

When CPAP fails (and in the case of central apnea when methylxanthines, and possibly doxapram, fail) then the affected infant having many significant apnea episodes requires mechanical ventilation. Intermittent positive pressure breaths delivered through a nasal cannula may be effective initial therapy. The earliest reports of nasal intermittent positive pressure ventilation (NIPPV) indicated no advantage over nasal CPAP alone (82), but more recent reports demonstrate NIPPV to be effective therapy in treating respiratory distress syndrome, and presumably would also be effective in treatment of resistant clinical apnea (72,83). Effective techniques to synchronize and deliver positive pressure during an infant's inspiratory effort have led to the development of synchronized nasal intermittent positive pressure ventilation using the normal nasal CPAP device (84,85). The acronym that I prefer for this technique is "SNIPPV" (we need another snappy acronym!). This technique has been shown to very effectively prevent extubation failure (e.g., apnea) in infants.

The final nonpharmacological technique for management of apnea of prematurity is intubation and mechanical ventilation. In infants with intractable apneas despite optimizing nonpharmacological and pharmacological management, this technique may be utilized. Most infants in this circumstance have relatively normal pulmonary compliance; hence low pressures and low ventilatory rates may be utilized simply to provide minimal "backup" ventilation for the infant having many episodes of desaturation. Synchronized intermittent mandatory ventilation or assist control ventilatory styles may be less traumatic to the lungs than conventional intermittent mandatory ventilation. Mechanical ventilation seems most commonly needed in extremely low birth weight infants whose pulmonary function is otherwise normal yet whose chest wall compliance is quite low, resulting in inability to maintain functional residual capacity causing hypoxemia. Clinically, this may be recognized a "fatigue" or "retractions" by medical staff. SNIPPV may be a preferred alternative as we gain experience with these newer techniques.

VII. Concluding Remarks

Regular respiratory rhythm depends on a set of brainstem neurons constantly oscillating between phases of activity that regulate inspiration, postinspiration, and expiration. Both pharmacological and nonpharmacological methods to prevent apnea in premature infants are based on stimulating these neurons to maintain their rhythm. In many circumstances the techniques utilized are designed to activate these respiratory neurons, but some techniques are also designed to prevent inhibition of the neuronal network.

Many infants also have episodic airway obstruction due to anatomic and neurologic differences in the upper airway. In the latter case, in addition to increasing neural activity, nonpharmacological methods are designed to prevent airway closure. Astute clinicians utilize both nonpharmacological and pharmacological approaches in various combinations to reduce the incidence of apnea in infants.

References

1. Richter DW, Ballantyne D, Remmers JE. How is the respiratory rhythm generated? A model. News Physiol Sci 1986; 1:109–112.
2. Richter DW, Ballanyi K, Schwarzacher S. Mechanisms of respiratory rhythm generation. Curr Opin Neurobiol 1992; 2:788–793.
3. Ramirez JM, Telgkamp P, Elsen FP, Quellmalz UJ, Richter DW. Respiratory rhythm generation in mammals: synaptic and membrane properties. Respir Physiol 1997; 110(2–3):71–85.
4. Czyzyk-Krzeska MF, Lawson EE. Synaptic events in ventral respiratory neurones during apnoea induced by laryngeal nerve stimulation in neonatal pig. J Physiol (Lond) 1991; 436:131–147.
5. Hwang J, St. John WM, Bartlett D Jr. Respiratory-related hypoglossal nerve activity: influence of anesthetics. J Appl Physiol 1983; 55:785–792.
6. Stark AR, Thach BT. Mechanisms of airway obstruction leading to apnea in newborn infants. J Pediatr 1976; 89:982–985.
7. Martin RJ, Herrell N, Rubin D, Fanaroff A. Effect of supine and prone positions on arterial oxygen tension in the preterm infant. Pediatrics 1979; 63(4):528–531.
8. Mizuno K, Aizawa M. Effects of body position on blood gases and lung mechanics of infants with chronic lung disease during tube feeding. Pediatr Int 1999; 41(6):609–614.

9. Wolfson MR, Greenspan JS, Deoras KS, Allen JL, Shaffer TH. Effect of position on the mechanical interaction between the rib cage and abdomen in preterm infants. J Appl Physiol 1992; 72(3):1032–1038.

10. Keene DJ, Wimmer JE Jr, Mathew OP. Does supine positioning increase apnea, bradycardia, and desaturation in preterm infants? J Perinatol 2000; 20(1):17–20.

11. Shen XM, Zhoa W, Huang DS, Lin FG, Wu SM. Effect of positioning on pulmonary function of newborns: comparison of supine and prone position. Pediatr Pulmonol 1996; 21(3):167–170.

12. Mitchell EA, Tuohy PG, Brunt JM, et al. Risk factors for sudden infant death syndrome following the prevention campaign in New Zealand: a prospective study. Pediatrics 1997; 100(5):835–840.

13. Cote A, Gerez T, Brouillette RT, Laplante S. Circumstances leading to a change to prone sleeping in sudden infant death syndrome victims. Pediatrics 2000; 106(6):E86.

14. Oyen N, Markestad T, Skaerven R, et al. Combined effects of sleeping position and prenatal risk factors in sudden infant death syndrome: the Nordic Epidemiological SIDS Study. Pediatrics 1997; 100(4):613–621.

15. Kemp JS, Unger B, Wilkins D, et al. Unsafe sleep practices and an analysis of bedsharing among infants dying suddenly and unexpectedly: results of a four-year, population-based, death-scene investigation study of sudden infant death syndrome and related deaths. Pediatrics 2000; 106(3):E41.

16. Kemp JS, Thach BT. A sleep position–dependent mechanism for infant death on sheepskins. Am J Dis Child 1993; 147:642–646.

17. Kemp JS, Thach BT. Sudden death in infants sleeping on polystyrene-filled cushions. N Engl J Med 1991; 324:1858–1864.

18. Skadberg BT, Markestad T. Consequences of getting the head covered during sleep in infancy. Pediatrics 1997; 100(2):E6.

19. Kemp JS, Kowalski RM, Burch PM, Graham MA, Thach BT. Unintentional suffocation by rebreathing: a death scene and physiologic investigation of a possible cause of sudden infant death. J Pediatr 1993; 122:874–880.

20. Jeffery HE, Megevand A, Page H. Why the prone position is a risk factor for sudden infant death syndrome. Pediatrics 1999; 104(2 Pt 1):263–269.

21. Thach BT, Stark AR. Spontaneous neck flexion and airway obstruction during apneic spells in preterm infants. J Pediatr 1979; 94:275–281.

22. Arad-Cohen N, Cohen A, Tirosh E. The relationship between gastroesophageal reflux and apnea in infants. J Pediatr 2000; 137(3):321–326.

23. Kahn A, Rebuffat E, Sottiaux M, Dufour D, Cadranel S, Reiterer F. Lack of temporal relation between acid reflux in the proximal oesophagus and cardio-respiratory events in sleeping infants. Eur J Pediatr 1992; 151:208–212.

24. Peter CS, Sprodowski N, Bohnhorst B, Silny J, Poets CF. Gastroesophageal reflux and apnea of prematurity: no temporal relationship. Pediatrics 2002; 109(1):8–11.

25. Kimball AL, Carlton DP. Gastroesophageal reflux medications in the treatment of apnea in premature infants. J Pediatr 2001; 138(3):355–360.

26. Wenzl TG, Schenke S, Peschgens T, Silny J, Heimann G, Skopnik H. Association of apnea and nonacid gastroesophageal reflux in infants: investigations with the intraluminal impedance technique. Pediatr Pulmonol 2001; 31(2):144–149.

27. Kattwinkel J, Nearman HS, Fanaroff AA, Katona PG, Klaus MH. Apnea of prematurity. Comparative therapeutic effects of cutaneous stimulation and nasal continuous positive airway pressure. J Pediatr 1975; 86(4):588–592.

28. Korner AF, Guilleminault C, Van den Hoed HJ, Baldwin RB. Reduction of sleep apnea and bradycardia in preterm infants on oscillating water beds: a controlled polygraphic study. Pediatrics 1978; 61(4):528–533.

29. Tuck SJ, Monin P, Duvivier C, May T, Vert P. Effect of a rocking bed on apnoea of prematurity. Arch Dis Child 1982; 57(6):475–477.

30. Jirapaet K. The effect of vertical pulsating stimulation on apnea of prematurity. J Med Assoc Thai 1993; 76(6):319–326.

31. Jones RA. A controlled trial of a regularly cycled oscillating waterbed and a non-oscillating waterbed in the prevention of apnoea in the preterm infant. Arch Dis Child 1981; 56(11):889–891.

32. Osborn DA, Henderson-Smart DJ. Kinesthetic stimulation for treating apnea in preterm infants. Cochrane Database Syst Rev 2000; (2):CD000499.

33. Henderson-Smart DJ, Osborn DA. Kinesthetic stimulation for preventing apnea in preterm infants. Cochrane Database Syst Rev 2000; (2):CD000373.

34. Svenningsen NW, Wittstrom C, Hellstrom-Westas L. OSCILLO-oscillating air mattress in neonatal care of very preterm babies. Technol Health Care 1995; 3(1):43–46.

35. Groswasser J, Sottiaux M, Rebuffat E, et al. Reduction in obstructive breathing events during body rocking: a controlled polygraphic study in preterm and full-term infants. Pediatrics 1995; 96(1 Pt 1):64–68.

36. Saigal S, Watts J, Campbell D. Randomized clinical trial of an oscillating air mattress in preterm infants: effect on apnea, growth, and development. J Pediatr 1986; 109(5):857–864.

37. Ramanathan R, Corwin MJ, Hunt CE, et al. Cardiorespiratory events recorded on home monitors: comparison of healthy infants with those at increased risk for SIDS. JAMA 2001; 285(17):2199–2207.

38. Ingersoll EW, Thoman EB. The breathing bear: effects on respiration in premature infants. Physiol Behav 1994; 56(5):855–859.

39. Gatts JD, Wallace DH, Glasscock GF, McKee E, Cohen RS. A modified newborn intensive care unit environment may shorten hospital stay. J Perinatol 1994; 14(5):422–427.

40. Richard CA, Mosko SS, McKenna JJ. Apnea and periodic breathing in bed-sharing and solitary sleeping infants. J Appl Physiol 1998; 84(4):1374–1380.

41. Daily WJ, Klaus M, Meyer HB. Apnea in premature infants: monitoring, incidence, heart rate changes, and an effect of environmental temperature. Pediatrics 1969; 43(4):510–518.

42. LeBlanc MH. Thermoregulation: incubators, radiant warmers, artificial skins, and body hoods. Clin Perinatol 1991; 18(3):403–422.

43. Bader D, Tirosh E, Hodgins H, Abend M, Cohen A. Effect of increased environmental temperature on breathing patterns in preterm and term infants. J Perinatol 1998; 18(1):5–8.

44. Franco P, Szliwowski H, Dramaix M, Kahn A. Influence of ambient temperature on sleep characteristics and autonomic nervous control in healthy infants. Sleep 2000; 23(3):401–407.

45. Guntheroth WG, Spiers PS. Thermal stress in sudden infant death: is there an ambiguity with the rebreathing hypothesis? Pediatrics 2001; 107(4):693–698.

46. Rigatto H, Brady JP, De la Torre Verduzco R. Chemoreceptor reflexes in preterm infants. I. The effect of gestational and postnatal age on the ventilatory response to inhalation of 100% and 15% oxygen. Pediatrics 1975; 55:604–613.

47. Rigatto H, Brady JP. Periodic breathing and apnea in preterm infants. II. Hypoxia as a primary event. Pediatrics 1972; 50:219–228.

48. Martin RJ, DiFiore JM, Jana L, et al. Persistence of the biphasic ventilatory response to hypoxia in preterm infants. J Pediatr 1998; 132(6):960–964.

49. Lawson EE, Long WA. Central origin of biphasic breathing pattern during hypoxia in newborns. J Appl Physiol 1983; 55:483–488.

50. Finer NN, Barrington KJ, Hayes B. Prolonged periodic breathing: significance in sleep studies. Pediatrics 1992; 89:450–453.

51. Barrington KJ, Finer NN. Periodic breathing and apnea in preterm infants. Pediatr Res 1990; 27:118–121.

52. Glotzbach SF, Baldwin RB, Lederer NE, Tansey PA, Ariagno RL. Periodic breathing in preterm infants: incidence and characteristics. Pediatrics 1989; 84:785–792.

53. Hodgman JE, Gonzales F, Hoppenbrouwers T, Cabal LA. Apnea, transient episodes of bradycardia, and periodic breathing in preterm infants. Am J Dis Child 1990; 144:54–57.

54. Weintraub Z, Alvaro R, Kwiatkowski K, Cates D, Rigatto H. Effects of inhaled oxygen (up to 40%) on periodic breathing and apnea in preterm infants. J Appl Physiol 1992; 72:116–120.

55. Donnelly DF, Haddad GG. Prolonged apnea and impaired survival in piglets after sinus and aortic nerve section. J Appl Physiol 1990; 68(3):1048–1052.

56. Joshi A, Gerhardt T, Shandloff P, Bancalari E. Blood transfusion effect on the respiratory pattern of preterm infants. Pediatrics 1987; 80(1):79–84.

57. Berger PJ, Skuza EM, Brodecky V, Cranage SM, Adamson TM, Wilkinson MH. Unusual respiratory response to oxygen in an infant with repetitive cyanotic episodes. Am J Respir Crit Care Med 2000; 161(6):2107–2111.

58. Frantz ID III, Adler SM, Thach BT, Taeusch HW Jr. Maturational effects on respiratory responses to carbon dioxide in premature infants. J Appl Physiol 1976; 41:41–45.

59. Rigatto H, Brady JP. Chemoreceptor reflexes in preterm infants. II. The effect of gestational and postnatal age on ventilatory response to inhaled carbon dioxide. Pediatrics 1975; 55:614–620.

60. Al Aif S, Alvaro R, Manfreda J, Kwiatkowski K, Cates D, Rigatto H. Inhalation of low (0.5%–1.5%) CO_2 as a potential treatment for apnea of prematurity. Semin Perinatol 2001; 25(2):100–106.

61. Menke J, Michel E, Rabe H, et al. Simultaneous influence of blood pressure, P_{CO_2}, and P_{O_2} on cerebral blood flow velocity in preterm infants of less than 33 weeks' gestation. Pediatr Res 1993; 34:173–177.

62. Beulen P, Rotteveel J, De Haan A, Liem D, Mullaart R. Ultrasonographic assessment of congestion of the choroid plexus in relation to carbon dioxide pressure. Eur J Ultrasound 2000; 11(1):25–29.

63. Harper RM, Kinney HC, Fleming PJ, Thach BT. Sleep influences on homeostatic functions: implications for sudden infant death syndrome. Respir Physiol 2000; 119(2–3):123–132.

64. Ross MP, Christensen RD, Rothstein G, et al. A randomized trial to develop criteria for administering erythrocyte transfusions to anemic preterm infants 1 to 3 months of age. J Perinatol 1989; 9(3):246–253.

65. Sasidharan P, Heimler R. Transfusion-induced changes in the breathing pattern of healthy preterm anemic infants. Pediatr Pulmonol 1992; 12(3):170–173.

66. Bifano EM, Smith F, Borer J. Relationship between determinants of oxygen delivery and respiratory abnormalities in preterm infants with anemia. J Pediatr 1992; 120:292–296.

67. Keyes WG, Donohue PK, Spivak JL, Jones MD Jr, Oski FA. Assessing the need for transfusion of premature infants and role of hematocrit, clinical signs, and erythropoietin level. Pediatrics 1989; 84(3):412–417.

68. Poets CF, Pauls U, Bohnhorst B. Effect of blood transfusion on apnoea, bradycardia and hypoxaemia in preterm infants. Eur J Pediatr 1997; 156(4):311–316.

69. Coran AG, Cabal L, Siassi B, Rosenkrantz JG. Surgical closure of patent ductus arteriosus in the premature infant with respiratory distress. J Pediatr Surg 1975; 10(3):399–404.

70. Sreenan C, Lemke RP, Hudson-Mason A, Osiovich H. High-flow nasal cannulae in the management of apnea of prematurity: a comparison with conventional nasal continuous positive airway pressure. Pediatrics 2001; 107(5):1081–1083.

71. Miller MJ, Martin RJ. Apnea of prematurity. Clin Perinatol 1992; 19:789–808.

72. Courtney SE, Pyon KH, Saslow JG, Arnold GK, Pandit PB, Habib RH. Lung recruitment and breathing pattern during variable versus continuous flow nasal continuous positive airway pressure in premature infants: an evaluation of three devices. Pediatrics 2001; 107(2):304–308.

73. Sullivan CE, McNamara F, Waters KA, et al. Nasal CPAP—state of the art. Nasal CPAP: use in the management of infantile apnea. Sleep 1993; 16(suppl):S108–S113.

74. Annibale DJ, Hulsey TC, Engstrom PC, Wallin LA, Ohning BL. Randomized, controlled trial of nasopharyngeal continuous positive airway pressure in the extubation of very low birth weight infants. J Pediatr 1994; 124:455–460.

75. Gaon P, Lee S, Hannan S, Ingram D, Milner AD. Assessment of effect of nasal continuous positive pressure on laryngeal opening using fibre optic laryngoscopy. Arch Dis Child Fetal Neonatal Ed 1999; 80(3):F230–F232.

76. Kurz H. Influence of nasopharyngeal CPAP on breathing pattern and incidence of apnoeas in preterm infants. Biol Neonate 1999; 76(3):129–133.

77. McNamara F, Sullivan CE. Effects of nasal CPAP therapy on respiratory and spontaneous arousals in infants with OSA. J Appl Physiol 1999; 87(3):889–896.

78. Miller MJ, DiFiore JM, Strohl KP, Martin RJ. Effects of nasal CPAP on supraglottic and total pulmonary resistance in preterm infants. J Appl Physiol 1990; 68(1):141–146.

79. Martin RJ, Miller MJ, Carlo WA. Pathogenesis of apnea in preterm infants. J Pediatr 1986; 109:733–741.

80. Gregory GA, Kitterman JA, Phibbs RH, Tooley WH, Hamilton WK. Treatment of the idiopathic respiratory-distress syndrome with continuous positive airway pressure. N Engl J Med 1971; 24:1333–1340.

81. Henderson-Smart DJ, Subramanian P, Davis PG. Continuous positive airway pressure versus theophylline for apnea in preterm infants. Cochrane Database Syst Rev 2000; (2):CD001072.

82. Ryan CA, Finer NN, Peters KL. Nasal intermittent positive-pressure ventilation offers no advantages over nasal continuous positive airway pressure in apnea of prematurity. Am J Dis Child 1989; 143(10):1196–1198.

83. Lemyre B, Davis PG, De Paoli AG. Nasal intermittent positive pressure ventilation (NIPPV) versus nasal continuous positive airway pressure (NCPAP) for apnea of prematurity. Cochrane Database Syst Rev 2000; (3):CD002272.

84. Khalaf MN, Brodsky N, Hurley J, Bhandari V. A prospective randomized, controlled trial comparing synchronized nasal intermittent positive pressure ventilation versus nasal continuous positive airway pressure as modes of extubation. Pediatrics 2001; 108(1):13–17.

85. Barrington KJ, Bull D, Finer NN. Randomized trial of nasal synchronized intermittent mandatory ventilation compared with continuous positive airway pressure after extubation of very low birth weight infants. Pediatrics 2001; 107(4):638–641.

15

Maturation of Respiratory Control

ERIC C. EICHENWALD and ANN R. STARK

Harvard Medical School and Brigham and Women's Hospital
Boston, Massachusetts, U.S.A.

I. Introduction

The control of breathing, like many other physiologic functions, differs greatly in the newborn infant from the older child and adult, and imposes important challenges. The most profound challenge occurs at birth, with the switch from irregular, episodic, nonrespiratory fetal breathing movements to the sustained respiratory rhythm essential to extrauterine life. Although the structural, anatomic, and cellular mechanisms for ventilatory homeostasis are in place at birth, the newborn must compensate for neurophysiologic immaturity and the mechanical disadvantages of the immature chest wall.

The infant born prematurely has even greater challenges than the term infant. The preterm infant is vulnerable to frequent apneas that are often associated with hypoxemia and bradycardia. This disorder, known as apnea of prematurity, results from immaturity in central respiratory drive, respiratory reflexes, and chemoreceptor and mechanoreceptor function. Research into the mechanisms underlying apnea of prematurity has enhanced our understanding of the maturation of respiratory control.

The study of the control of breathing soon after birth and its maturation in infancy has inherent difficulties. Most studies of breathing in newborns are performed during sleep, typically in the supine position. A face mask or nasal prongs with a device to measure airflow or airway pressure, a procedure that would not be tolerated by an awake infant, can be applied to a sleeping newborn. Thus, understanding the effects of both behavioral state and body position on breathing is important to the interpretation of studies of breathing and its control. In addition, in contrast to measurements in newborns, most studies in adults are typically performed during wakefulness. This limits the comparisons that can be made between newborns and adults. As a result, much of our understanding of the maturation of respiratory control in humans comes from comparisons of premature to term newborns or to older infants.

This chapter will review the effects of sleep state on respiratory muscle activity in the newborn, and maturation and development of neuromuscular and reflex responses of the respiratory pump muscles and the upper airway. Special consideration will be given to the disorder of apnea of prematurity as a model for maturation of respiratory control. The issues of ventilatory patterns, periodic breathing, and the effect of maturation on chemical control of breathing will be discussed elsewhere (see Chapters 4 and 10).

II. Sleep and Breathing

A. Definitions of Sleep State

Respiratory control is profoundly influenced by sleep state. Understanding the effects of sleep state on breathing is especially important in newborn infants, who spend most of the time sleeping. The development of sleep states is addressed in detail elsewhere in this book (see Chapter 6) and will be considered briefly here.

In the adult, stable and well-defined states of wakefulness, non–rapid eye movement (NREM) sleep, and rapid eye movement (REM) sleep are readily identified using neurophysiological measurements (1). Recordings are made of encephalographic activity (electroencephalogram, EEG), eye movements (electrooculogram, EOG), and postural muscle electromyogram (EMG). Based on these recordings, distinct states of neurophysiological organization can be recognized as NREM and REM sleep. NREM sleep is characterized by a synchronized high-voltage low-frequency EEG pattern, low levels of tonic postural muscle tone, and little or no eye movement on EOG. REM sleep is characterized by desynchronized low-voltage high-frequency EEG patterns similar to the awake state, lack of postural muscle tone, and rapid conjugate eye movements.

Neurophysiological criteria can be used to determine sleep state in the infant born at term (40 weeks' gestation). Cyclic organization of NREM and REM sleep, as defined by EEG, EOG, and EMG criteria, is present after 36–37 weeks' gestational age (2,3). However, full maturation of NREM sleep into true slow-wave sleep that is similar to the adult does not occur until several weeks after birth. Before 36 weeks' gestation, NREM sleep is poorly organized, with a discontinuous EEG pattern.

In contrast to NREM sleep, REM sleep can be identified earlier in gestation. Continuous, organized REM sleep EEG patterns are first recognized in the human as early as 32 weeks' gestation, and become fully mature at 34–35 weeks (3). Other neurophysiologic measurements, such as the EOG and postural muscle EMG, are not useful to discriminate state until after 32–33 weeks' gestation (4).

Because of the difficulties in using neurophysiological criteria during early human development, behavioral criteria have been widely used to determine sleep state (5). Two distinct states, active and quiet sleep, have been characterized using observations of body and eye movements and respiratory patterns. These states correspond to REM and NREM sleep, respectively. Respiratory patterns are especially useful, because variability of respiratory cycle time has been shown to be almost as accurate as neurophysiological criteria in the determination of sleep state in the term infant (6). Using behavioral criteria, *active* and *quiet* sleep can be differentiated as early as 30 weeks' gestation (3). With behaviorally defined states, premature infants spend 50–80% of the time in active sleep; term infants spend slightly less time in that state. A significant proportion of sleep time in newborns, especially those born preterm, may be indeterminate, that is, neither active nor quiet.

B. Sleep State Effects on Respiratory Muscle Activity in the Newborn

Intercostal Muscles and Diaphragm

The function of the entire motor system is dramatically altered by sleep, especially REM sleep. During REM, or active, sleep, tonic postural muscle activity ceases (7). In contrast, in NREM, or quiet, sleep, tonic postural muscle activity persists. These effects have significant consequences to respiratory muscle activity and control of breathing. Loss of tonic intercostal muscle activity and depression of phasic activity during REM sleep results in a further increase in compliance in the newborn's already highly compliant chest wall (Fig. 1). During REM sleep, as the diaphragm shortens with inspiration, the rib cage moves inward and abdominal displacement increases, leading to the characteristic "paradoxical" breathing during this state (Fig. 1). This is especially pronounced in the preterm infant, whose chest wall is more compliant than that of the term infant. Indeed, increased activity of the intercostal muscles may not be sufficient to offset the increased flexibility of the rib cage in the preterm infant. As a result, preterm infants may continue to demonstrate paradoxical chest movement during neurophysiologically determined NREM sleep (8).

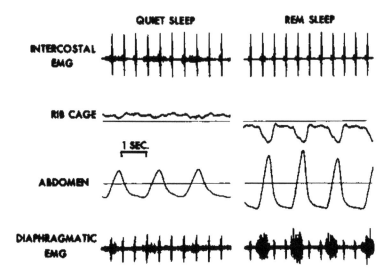

Figure 1 Diaphragm and intercostal muscle EMGs and rib cage and abdominal motion measured with magnetometers in a preterm infant in quiet and REM sleep. Note the paradoxical rib cage and abdominal movement and increased abdominal excursion during REM sleep. In REM sleep, phasic intercostal EMG activity markedly decreases, and diaphragm EMG activity increased compared to quiet sleep. (From Ref. 14.)

With maturation, rib cage distortion decreases, resulting in improved mechanical stability of the respiratory system (9). In NREM sleep, tonic and phasic activity of the intercostal muscles helps to stabilize and "stiffen" the chest wall (12) (Fig. 1). As noted above, the amount of time spent in REM sleep also decreases with maturation. As a result, the rib cage contribution to tidal volume increases with development (10,11).

Diaphragm contraction is not subject to the generalized inhibition of skeletal muscle activity that occurs during REM sleep. In contrast to other respiratory muscles, phasic diaphragmatic EMG activity may increase during active sleep (13). This may represent a compensatory response to the loss of the intercostal muscle contribution to ventilation (14). In newborns, however, a significant proportion of diaphragmatic work may be expended on distortion of the chest wall. This inefficiency may be more problematic with decreasing maturity. In preterm infants, diaphragmatic volume displacement during paradoxical breathing can be up to twice the volume change of the lung, leading to inefficient diaphragmatic work (15). Some have hypothesized that this inefficiency in diaphragmatic activity may lead to muscle fatigue, which may contribute to apneic spells (16).

Although the phasic activity of the diaphragm is similar across sleep states, differences exist in both its tonic and postinspiratory activity. These changes can affect the infant's ability to maintain end-expiratory lung volume above the mechanically determined level (17). The basal level of diaphragm tone is lower in REM than in NREM sleep (18,19). In addition, postinspiratory inspiratory activity (PIIA) is considerably more variable in REM sleep than NREM. The reduction in PIIA is evident in both preterm (20) and term infants (17).

The mechanism of this variability in PIIA is uncertain. It may be a centrally mediated state-related phenomenon or secondary to changes in peripheral afferent input. The latter is supported by studies in preterm infants during REM sleep. During this state, neural inspiratory time and PIIA are shortened with increased chest wall distortion (21). However, if the rib cage is stabilized with continuous positive airway pressure, both inspiratory time and PIIA increase. These results suggest that changes in diaphragmatic activity that occur with sleep may be mediated indirectly by changes in mechanical feedback, such as differences in chest distortion or lung volume.

Upper-Airway Muscles

The upper airway, specifically the larynx, pharynx, and nose, contributes significantly to total pulmonary resistance to airflow (22). Similar to other respiratory muscles, the muscles of the upper airway are subject to state-related modulation of their activity.

It is likely that total upper-airway resistance is increased in REM compared to NREM sleep (23), but the contribution of changes in laryngeal aperture versus other upper-airway structures to this increase is unclear. Respiratory activity of the posterior cricoarytenoid (PCA) muscle, the sole abductor of the vocal cords, mimics that of the diaphragm during different states of sleep. In studies in preterm infants in which PCA EMG activity was measured with an esophageal surface electrode, tonic and phasic activity increased during NREM sleep (19), which should result in decreased inspiratory resistance.

Expiratory resisistance may also be influenced by increased activity of the thyroarytenoid muscle, the principal adductor of the larynx. In newborn animals, phasic activity of the thyroarytenoid is increased during NREM sleep; this results in glottic narrowing and slowing of expiratory airflow (24). Demonstration of active laryngeal adduction in human infants is difficult because the thyroarytenoid is not accessible to surface EMG measurements. In newborn infants, however, expiratory flow patterns suggest that active laryngeal narrowing may contribute to establishment of lung volume immediately after birth (25). Active adduction of the larynx also occurs during expiratory "grunting" observed in newborn infants with lung disease.

The muscles of the pharynx are also affected by sleep state. Loss of phasic and tonic activity of the pharyngeal dilators may make upper airway collapse more likely during REM sleep (26). The pharynx is the most common site of upper-airway obstruction during spontaneous mixed or obstructive apnea in preterm infants (27). In one study in preterm infants, increased negative pressure generated during inspiratory efforts against an added elastic load resulted in a higher frequency of upper-airway obstruction during active compared to quiet sleep (28).

The stability of the upper airway increases with development. Although airway obstruction appears more likely during REM sleep when considered on mechanical factors alone, experimental data suggest that reflexes that promote upper-airway patency continue to operate during sleep in more mature infants. For example, term infants, in contrast to those born prematurely, are able to maintain airway patency during active sleep despite increased negative pressures generated during occluded efforts (29,30).

III. Maturation of Neuromuscular Reflex Responses

A. Control of Lung Volume

One of the most striking features of the respiratory system in the newborn is the highly compliant chest wall (31). Inward recoil of the lung is only slightly less than that of the adult. However, this opposes the minimal outward recoil of the chest wall. As a result, the passively determined functional residual capacity (FRC) in the newborn is $\sim 10\%$ of total lung capacity, and below its closing capacity (32). However, measurements in newborn infants show that end-expiratory volume is substantially higher than the passively determined FRC during quiet sleep (33). Newborns maintain an elevated end-expiratory lung volume by actively interrupting expiration and initiating inspiration before passive deflation is complete. This interruption is accomplished by shortening expiratory time, retarding expiratory airflow by PIIA activity of the diaphragm, and/or laryngeal narrowing (Fig. 2) (17,20,34). End-expiratory lung volume is lower during active sleep, owing in part to loss of these active mechanisms (33). Decreased intercostal muscle tone that helps to stiffen the chest wall also plays a role. Lower end-expiratory lung volume during REM sleep leads to lower and less stable oxygen tensions in newborn infants (35) and a more rapid decline in oxygen saturation than is seen in adults during the brief periods of apnea and hypoventilation that are characteristic of this sleep state (36).

Mechanical stability of the respiratory system is a bigger challenge in preterm infants, owing in part to their more compliant chest wall. Although many of the breathing strategies used by term infants to defend lung volume are operative (17,34,37), the vulnerability of preterm infants is increased by the longer time spent in active sleep, greater irregularity of respiratory rhythm, and

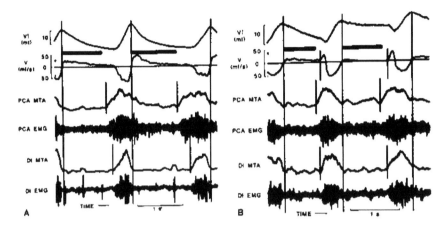

Figure 2 Example of expiratory braking in a full term infant in quiet sleep. In panel (A) expiration is passive, in contrast to panel (B), where there is marked slowing of expiratory airflow. Note that expiratory EMG activity of the posterior cricoarytenoid (PCA), quantified by the moving time average (MTA), is high in panel (A), and low in panel (B), indicative of glottic narrowing slowing expiratory airflow. (V = airflow; V↑ = tidal volume; DI = diaphragm). (From Ref. 34.)

frequent apneas. Reduced lung volume and the lower, more variable oxygen levels during active sleep may lead to rapid development of hypoxemia even during brief respiratory pauses (Fig. 3) (36). Mechanical support of the chest wall achieved by placing preterm infants prone rather than supine improves the rib

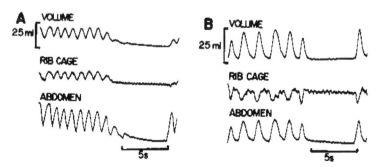

Figure 3 Recordings of volume, rib cage, and abdominal motion during breathing and unobstructive apnea in a preterm infant. (A) Quiet sleep; (B) active sleep. End-expiratory lung volume during apnea falls from that during breathing in quiet sleep and remains unchanged in active sleep. (From Ref. 20.)

cage contribution to tidal volume and the ventilatory response to inhaled carbon dioxide (38). However, this intervention does not appear to be associated with a decrease in the frequency of apnea (39).

With maturation, chest wall compliance decreases and the mechanical advantage of the chest wall muscles improves, enhancing the mechanical stability of the respiratory system (9). Motor activity, such as sitting and crawling, increases abdominal and intercostal muscle strength, and progressive mineralization of the rib cage stiffens the chest wall. The transition from a dynamically maintained end-expiratory lung volume to one determined passively occurs by ~1 year of age (Figs. 4, 5) (40). A substantial increase in expiratory time also occurs in this time frame (41), and allows older infants to breathe from their relaxed FRC.

B. Upper Airway

The tendency of the preterm infant to develop obstructive apnea demonstrates the central role of upper-airway muscle activity in ensuring regular breathing. Reflex protection of the upper airway occurs through several mechanisms, including inhibition of pump muscle activity. Negative suction pressure applied to the upper airway during inspiration, as might occur during airway obstruction, inhibits respiratory pump muscle activity and shortens inspiratory time in normal newborns (42,43). In tracheotomized infants, whose upper airways are isolated

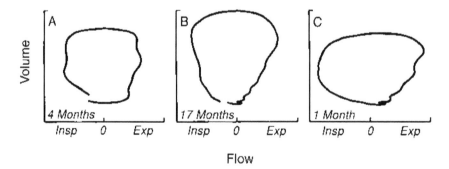

Figure 4 Examples of flow-volume loops of tidal breaths obtained by respiratory inductance plethysmography at three different ages demonstrating transition from a dynamically maintained to a relaxed end-expiratory lung volume. (A) Tidal breath in a 4-month-old infant in which airflow is interrupted above the relaxation volume; (B) tidal breath in a 17-month-old child with the expiratory limb continuing uninterrupted to zero flow; (C) tidal breath in a 1-month-old infant in which the flow pattern (interrupted or relaxed) could not be determined. (From Ref. 40.)

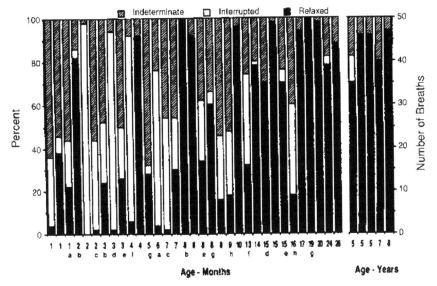

Figure 5 Distribution of relaxed (expiratory flow uninterrupted to zero flow), interrupted (expiratory flow interrupted before reaching relaxation volume), and indeterminate breaths shown as number of breaths (right) or percent of breaths (left). The percent of breaths with dynamic maintenance of end-expiratory volume above relaxation volume decreased with maturation. (From Ref. 40.)

from their lower airways, negative pressure spontaneously generated during inspiratory efforts against an upper airway occlusion also depressed ventilation (43).

These upper-airway inhibitory reflexes may be important in the recovery from obstructive apnea. During apnea, inspiration in the face of upper-airway obstruction increases negative pressure below the site of obstruction. Reflex inhibition of diaphragmatic contraction due to increasing negative pressure in the airway lumen would result in a decrease in luminal pressure, helping the airway to reopen. It is likely that similar reflexes are active in preterm infants, although their tendency to have frequent obstructive apnea suggests that this protective effect may increase with maturation.

Immaturity may also disturb the relationship of the timing of onset of upper-airway and pump muscle activity, predisposing the immature infant to airway obstruction. In the normal sequence of inspiration, activation of the upper-airway muscles occurs before the diaphragm. This promotes a decrease in upper-airway resistance prior to the onset of inspiratory airflow. Activation of the upper-airway muscles first also stabilizes the pharynx from the negative pressure generated by pump muscle activity and protects against upper-airway collapse.

In a study comparing timing of PCA activation (measured by esophageal surface EMG electrode) to that of the diaphragm (also measured by surface EMG electrodes), preterm infants were found to have frequent "uncoupled" breaths in which diaphragm EMG activity preceded PCA activity (44). Although this uncoupling of PCA and diaphragm activity was also observed in term newborns, it occurred significantly less frequently than in the preterm infants.

Development also affects other upper-airway muscle reflex responses that promote airway patency. Upper-airway muscle activity increases more than pump muscle activity during experimental airway occlusions in both preterm and term newborns (45,46), as well as in older infants (29). However, differences were observed between preterm infants who had frequent apnea spells from those who did not. Upper-airway closure occurred more commonly with nasal occlusion in preterm infants with apnea than in those without (30,47). In addition, preterm infants with apnea were less likely to recruit genioglossus muscle activity during airway occlusion compared to those without apnea (48). Finally, in preterm infants chemoreceptor stimulation appears to accentuate diaphragmatic activity to a greater extent than upper-airway muscles (49). This might predispose preterm infants to upper-airway obstruction during the enhanced diaphragm activity associated with increased ventilatory drive. Differential response of the respiratory muscles to hypercapnia may explain the observation in preterm infants of several obstructed inspiratory efforts that may follow a central apnea.

C. Laryngeal Reflexes

Upper-airway protective mechanisms involving the pharynx and larynx include coughing, sneezing, swallowing, and laryngeal or pharyngeal closure. The laryngeal chemoreflex appears to be active in the newborn and may be clinically important. This reflex can be elicited by dripping a small amount of fluid (water or saline) into the hypopharynx of a newborn infant. The response includes central apnea, swallowing, and obstructed breaths (Fig. 6) (50–52). Cough, the most prominent adult response to similar stimulation of the larynx, is rarely elicited. Preterm infants demonstrate a stronger protective response than term infants, with a higher frequency of obstructive and central apnea, as well as more prolonged apneas with associated bradycardia (Fig. 6) (51). Hypoxia appears to reinforce this reflex response (53). The response to stimulation of the laryngeal chemoreflex in preterm infants is similar to observations during spontaneously occurring apneas, suggesting that this reflex may contribute to the etiology of some apneic spells. Swallows, which are prominent in both induced and spontaneous apneas in preterm infants, are more common during apneas than in periods of quiet breathing during sleep (54), and do not occur during periodic breathing (55). This reflex response to apnea may be important in reestablishing pharyngeal airway patency by reducing adhesion forces in the collapsed tissues.

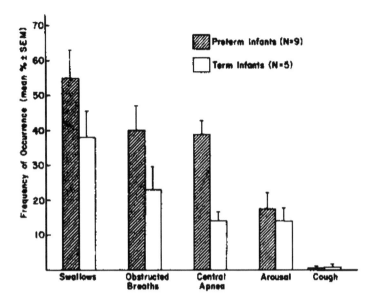

Figure 6 Frequency of swallows, obstructed breaths, central apnea, arousal, and cough to saline bolus pharyngeal stimuli in preterm and term infants. (From Ref. 51.)

IV. Maturation of Respiratory Control: Resolution of Apnea of Prematurity

The major clinical correlate of immaturity of respiratory control is the disorder known as apnea of prematurity. Studies of its pathophysiology and resolution have added to our understanding of the development of respiratory control. This condition is one of the most frequent diagnoses in newborn intensive care units, and delay in its resolution may prolong the hospital stay (56,57). The pathogenesis of apnea of prematurity is multifactorial, as detailed in Chapter 12. Thus, the resolution of recurrent apneic spells involves the maturation of multiple interactive aspects that influence respiratory control, and remains poorly understood. It is not surprising, therefore, that the time required for apnea of prematurity to resolve varies greatly in infants born at different gestational ages. It is clear, however, that maturation of respiratory control occurs in parallel with other measures of physiologic maturity, including feeding behavior (56,57). Cessation of apnea of prematurity may be a reflection of overall brainstem maturation (58), although it is likely that changes in respiratory muscle function and reflex activity also play a role.

In infants born at 35–36 weeks' gestational age, apnea of prematurity is not usually a clinical problem. In infants delivered at a gestational age > 28 weeks, apnea typically resolves by 35–36 weeks' postmenstrual age (59,60). This suggests that the maturational processes leading to development of respiratory control in the preterm infant continue as they would have in the fetus. However, infants born at extremely early gestational ages (24–28 weeks) have a longer time course to resolution of their apnea than infants born after 28 weeks (56,60). Apnea in these younger infants frequently persists beyond 40 weeks' postmenstrual age (Fig. 7), indicating that respiratory control of infants who are very immature at birth may develop more slowly. Similar results were found in a smaller study of preterm infants discharged with a home cardiorespiratory monitor (61). In that study, the mean postmenstrual age of resolution of apnea was ∼41 weeks, although no correlation between the degree of prematurity and the postmenstrual age at last apnea was observed. In infants born at 24–28 weeks' gestation, bronchopulmonary dysplasia was associated with later resolution of apnea (56). This suggests that lung disease may influence the maturation of peripheral and central respiratory control in ways that are poorly understood. Consistent with this hypothesis is the observation that maturation of chemo-receptor function is delayed in preterm infants with a prolonged requirement for

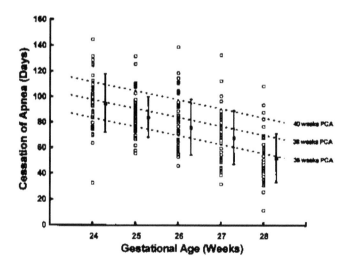

Figure 7 Individual (□) and mean (■) (±SD) values for last postnatal day with a documented apnea and/or bradycardia event of any type for cohort of infants delivered at 24–28 weeks. Dotted lines indicate when infants in each gestational age group reach 36, 38, and 40 weeks' postmenstrual age. Apnea of prematurity frequently persisted beyond term gestation for all gestational ages. (From Ref. 56.)

oxygen supplementation compared to infants with no supplemental oxygen need after birth (62).

The time course of resolution of apnea of prematurity appears to have a consistent natural history. Severe apnea events that require intervention (tactile stimulation or positive pressure ventilation with oxygen) are the first to disappear, followed by episodes that resolve spontaneously without intervention. Transient spontaneously resolving episodes of bradycardia without associated observed apnea are the last to disappear (Fig. 8) (56). These results are confounded, however, by variability in monitoring practices and the inability of standard cardiorespiratory monitors to detect obstructive apnea (63).

Continuous cardiorespiratory recordings prior to hospital discharge demonstrate that preterm infants continue to have significant abnormalities of breathing patterns, apneic events, and bradycardias, although their clinically apparent apnea was thought to have resolved (64–67). Similarly, preterm infants who are monitored at home have persistent abnormalities of ventilatory control documented on home monitor memory recordings (68,69). In the largest longitudinal study of cardiorespiratory events to date in infants monitored at home (69), asymptomatic preterm infants were shown to be at higher risk for significant breathing abnormalities than healthy term infants until ~43 weeks' postmen-

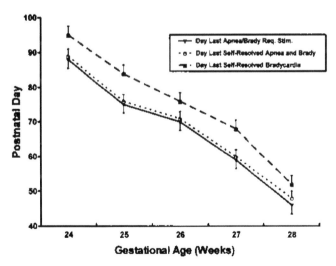

Figure 8 Mean (± SE) for the last postnatal day with a documented apnea/bradycardia event requiring tactile stimulation or other intervention (▼), self-resolved apnea and bradycardia event (○), and self-resolved bradycardia without documented apnea (■) for the same subject cohort as Figure 7. Note the similar progress of resolution of apnea for the different gestational ages. (From Ref. 56).

strual age. In this study, 20% of asymptomatic preterm infants experienced one or more episodes of severe apnea of at least 30 sec duration or heart rate < 60 bpm for at least 10 sec duration during the 6 months of home monitoring. The clinical significance of these events remains uncertain. However, these findings indicate that respiratory control, even when thought to be mature by conventional measures, may remain unstable in infants born prematurely, even when they reach a postmenstrual age of 40 weeks or older.

V. Conclusions

Newborn infants are presented with several challenges to their control of breathing. Their highly compliant chest wall puts them at a mechanical disadvantage that is worsened by the inhibitory effects of sleep on respiratory muscle activity. Respiratory reflexes, such as upper-airway responses to negative pressure, which are adaptive in the adult, may depress ventilation in the newborn. In no other species do newborns display prolonged respiratory pauses that resolve with maturation.

Understanding the maturation of respiratory control in the newborn has been enhanced by research into the pathophysiology of apnea of prematurity. Growth and development bring greater stability of respiratory control, but the preterm infant remains vulnerable to disturbances of breathing well beyond term postmenstrual age, suggesting that premature birth may slow the course of maturation that occurs during fetal development. Further research on how maturation affects the developing respiratory system will enhance our understanding of its disorders in early infancy.

References

1. Rechtschaffen A, Kales A. Manual of Standardized Terminology. Techniques and Scoring System for Sleep Stages in Human Subjects. Washington, National Institutes of Health 1968, No. 204.
2. Dreyfus-Brisac C. Ontogenesis of sleep in human prematures after 32 weeks of conceptional age. Dev Psychobiol 1970; 3:91–121.
3. Dreyfus-Brisac C. Neurophysiological studies in human premature and full-term newborns. Biol Psychiatry 1975; 10:485–496.
4. Parmalee AH Jr, Stern E. Development of states in infants. In: Clement CD, Purpura DP, Mayer FE, eds. Sleep and the Maturing Nervous System. New York: Academic Press, 1972.
5. Prechtl HFR. The behavioral states of the newborn infant (a review). Brain Res 1974; 76:185–212.
6. Haddad GG, Jeng HJ, Lai TL, Mellins RB. Determination of sleep state in infants using respiratory variability. Pediatr Res 1987; 21:556–562.

7. Jouvet M. Neurophysiology of the states of sleep. Physiol Rev 1967; 47:117–177.

8. Davi M, Sankaran K, MacCullum M, Cates D, Rigatto H. Effect of sleep state on chest distortion and on the ventilatory response to CO_2 in neonates. Pediatr Res 1979; 13:982–986.

9. Heldt GP. Development of stability of the respiratory system in preterm infants. J Appl Physiol 1988; 65:441–444.

10. Honma Y, Wilkes D, Bryan MH, Bryan AC. Rib cage and abdominal contributions to ventilatory response to CO_2 in infants. J Appl Physiol 1984; 56:1211–1216.

11. Hershenson MB, Colin AA, Wohl MEB, Stark AR. Changes in the contribution of the rib cage to tidal breathing during infancy. Am Rev Respir Dis 1990; 141:922–925.

12. Thach BT, Abroms IF, Frantz ID III, Sotrel A, Bruce EN, Goldman MD. Intercostal muscle reflexes and sleep breathing patterns in the human infant. J Appl Physiol 1980; 48:139–146.

13. Muller N, Gulston G, Cade D, Whitton J, Froese AB, Bryan MH, Bryan AC. Diaphragmatic muscle fatigue in the newborn. J Appl Physiol 1979; 46:688–695.

14. Bryan AC, Bowes G, Maloney JE. Control of breathing in the fetus and newborn. In: Handbook of Physiology, Section 3. The Respiratory System, Vol II. Control of Breathing, Part 2. Washington: American Physiological Society, 1986.

15. Heldt DP, McIlroy MB. Distortion of the chest wall and work of diaphragm in preterm infants. J Appl Physiol 1987; 62:164–169.

16. Lopes JM, Muller NL, Bryan MH, Bryan AC. Importance of inspiratory muscle tone in maintenance of FRC in the newborn. J Appl Physiol 1981; 51:830–834.

17. Kosch PC, Stark AR. Dynamic maintenance of end-expiratory lung volume in full-term infants. J Appl Physiol 1984; 57:1126–1133.

18. Prechtl HFR, Van Eykem LA, O'Brien MJ. Respiratory muscle EMG in newborns: a non-intrusive method. Early Hum Dev 1977; 1:265–283.

19. Eichenwald EC, Stark AR. Respiratory motor output: effect of state and maturation in early life. In: Haddad GG, Farber JP, eds. Developmental Neurobiology of Breathing. Lung Biology in Health and Disease, New York: Marcel Dekker, 1991:551–587.

20. Stark AR, Cohlan BA, Waggener TB, Frantz ID III, Kosch PC. Regulation of end-expiratory lung volume during sleep in premature infants. J Appl Physiol 1987; 62:1117–1123.

21. Hagan R, Bryan AC, Bryan MH, Gulston G. Neonatal chest wall afferents and regulation of respiration. J Appl Physiol 1977; 42:362–367.

22. Van Lunteren E, Strohl KP. The muscles of the upper airways. Clin Chest Med 1986; 7:171–188.

23. Lopes JM, Tabachnik E, Muller NL, Levison H, Bryan AC. Total airway resistance and respiratory muscle activity during sleep. J App. Physiol 1983; 54:773–777.

24. England SJ, Kent G, Stogryn HAF. Laryngeal muscle and diaphragmatic activities in conscious dog pups. Respir Physiol 1985; 60:95–108.

25. Mortola JP, Fisher JT, Smith JB, Fox GS, Weeks S, Willis D. Onset of respiration in infants delivered by cesarean section. J Appl Physiol, 1982; 52:716–724.

26. Hudgel DW, Hendricks C. Palate and hypopharynx—sites of inspiratory narrowing of the upper airway during sleep. Am Rev Respir Dis 1988; 138:1542–1547.
27. Mathew OP, Roberts JL, Thach BT. Pharyngeal airway obstruction in preterm infants during mixed and obstructive apnea. J Pediatr 1982; 100:964–968.
28. Knill R, Andrews W, Bryan AC, Bryan MH. Respiratory load compensation in infants. J Appl Physiol 1976; 40:357–361.
29. Roberts JL, Reed WR, Mathew OP, Menon AP, Thach BT. Assessment of pharyngeal airway stability in normal and micrognathic infants. J Appl Physiol 1985; 58:290–299.
30. Cohen G, Henderson-Smart DJ. Upper airway stability and apnea during nasal occlusion in newborn infants. J Appl Physiol 1986; 60:1511–1517.
31. Gerhardt T, Bancalari E. Chestwall compliance in full-term and premature infants. Acta Pediatr Scand 1980; 69:359–364.
32. Agostoni E. Volume-pressure relationships of the thorax and lung in the newborn. J Appl Physiol 1959; 14:909–913.
33. Henderson-Smart, DJ, Read DJC. Reduced lung volume during behavioral active sleep in the newborn. J Appl Physiol 1979; 46:1081–1085.
34. Kosch PC, Hutchinson AA, Wozniac JA, Carlo WA, Stark AR. Posterior crico-arytenoid and diaphragm activities during tidal breathing in neonates. J Appl Physiol 1988; 64:1968–1978.
35. Martin RJ, Okken A, Rubin D. Arterial oxygen tension during active and quiet sleep in the normal neonate. J Pediatr 1979; 94:271–274.
36. Henderson-Smart DJ. Vulnerability to hypoxaemia during sleep in the newborn. Sleep 1980; 1:195–208.
37. Eichenwald EC, Ungarelli RA, Stark AR. Hypercapnia increases expiratory braking in preterm infants. J Appl Physiol 1993; 75(6):2665–2670.
38. Martin RJ, DiFiore, JM, Korenke CB, Randal H, Miller MJ, Brooks LJ. Vulnerability of respiratory control in healthy preterm infants placed supine. J Pediatr 1995; 127:609–614.
39. Keene DJ, Wimmer JE Jr, Mathew OP. Does supine positioning increase apnea, bradycardia, and desaturation in preterm infants? J Perinatol 2000; 20(1):17–20.
40. Colin AA, Wohl MEB, Mead J, Ratjen FA, Glass G, Stark AR. Transition from dynamically maintained to relaxed end-expiratory volume in human infants. J Appl Physiol 1989; 67:2107–2111.
41. Ratjen FA, Colin AA, Stark AR, Mead J, Wohl MEB. Changes of time constants during infancy and childhood. J Appl Physiol 1989; 67:2112–2115.
42. Thach BT, Menon AP, Schefft GL. Effects of negative upper airway pressure on pattern of breathing in sleeping infants. J Appl Physiol 1989; 66(4):1599–1605.
43. Thach BT, Schefft GL, Pickens DL, Menon AP. Influence of upper airway negative pressure reflex on response to airway occlusion in sleeping infants. J Appl Physiol 1989; 67(2):749–755.
44. Eichenwald EC, Howell RG III, Kosch PC, Ungarelli RA, Lindsey J, Stark AR. Developmental changes in sequential activation of laryngeal abductor muscle and diaphragm in infants. J Appl Physiol 1992; 73(4):1425–1431.

45. Carlo WA, Miller MJ, Martin, RJ. Differential response of respiratory muscles to airway occlusion in infants. J Appl Physiol 1985; 59:847–852.
46. Gauda EB, Miller MJ, Carlo WA, DiFiore JM, Martin RJ. Genioglossus and diaphragm activity during obstructive apnea and airway occlusion in infants. Pediatr Res 1989; 26(6):583–587.
47. Cohen G, Henderson-Smart DJ. Upper airway muscle activity during nasal occlusion in newborn babies. J Appl Physiol 1989; 66:1328–1335.
48. Gauda EB, Miller MJ, Carlo WA, Difiore JM, Johnsen DC, Martin RJ. Genioglossus response to airway occlusion in apneic versus nonapneic infants. Pediatr Res 1987; 22:683–687.
49. Carlo WA, Martin RJ, DiFiore JM. Differences in CO_2 threshold of respiratory muscles in preterm infants. J Appl Physiol 1988; 65(6):2434–2439.
50. Davies AM, Koenig JS, Thach BT. Characteristics of upper airway chemoreflex prolonged apnea in human infants. Am Rev Res Dis 1989; 139:668–673.
51. Pickens DL, Schefft GL, Thach BT. Pharyngeal fluid clearance and aspiration preventive mechanisms in sleeping infants. J Appl Physiol 1989; 66(3):1164–1171.
52. Davies AM, Koenig JS, Thach BT. Upper airway chemoreflex responses to saline and water in preterm infants. J Appl Physiol 1988; 64:1412–1420.
53. Wennergren G, Hertzberg T, Milerad J, Bjure J, Lagercrantz H. Hypoxia reinforces laryngeal reflex bradycardia in infants. Acta Pediatr Scand 1989; 78:11–17.
54. Menon AP, Schefft GL, Thach BT. Frequency and significance of swallowing during prolonged apnea in infants. Am Rev Respir Dis 1984; 130(6):969–973.
55. Miller MJ, DiFore JM. A comparison of swallowing during apnea and periodic breathing in premature infants. Pediatr Res 1995; 37(6):796–799.
56. Eichenwald EC, Aina A, Stark AR. Apnea frequently persists beyond term gestation in infants delivered at 24 to 28 weeks. Pediatrics 1997 100:354–359.
57. Eichenwald EC, Blackwell M, Lloyd JS, Tran T, Wilker RE, Richardson D. Inter-neonatal intensive care unit variation in discharge timing: influence of apnea and feeding management. Pediatrics 2001; 108:928–933.
58. Henderson-Smart DJ, Pettigrew AG, Campbell DJ. Clinical apnea and brain stem neural function in preterm infants. N Engl J Med 1983; 308:353–357.
59. Henderson-Smart DJ. The effect of gestational age on the incidence and duration of recurrent apnoea in newborn babies. Aust Pediatr J 1981; 17:273–276.
60. Darnall RA, Kattwinkel J, Nattie C, Robinson M. Margin of safety for discharge after apnea in preterm infants. Pediatrics 1997; 100(5):795–801.
61. Tauman R, Sivan Y. Duration of home monitoring for infants discharged with apnea of prematurity. Biol Neonatel 2000; 78(3):168–173.
62. Katz-Salamon M, Lagercrantz H. Hypoxic ventilatory defence in very preterm infants: attenuation after long term oxygen treatment. Arch Dis Child Fetal Neonatal Ed 1994; 70:F90.
63. Warburton D, Stark AR, Taeusch HW. Apnea monitor failure in infants with upper airway obstruction. Pediatrics 1977; 60:742–744.
64. Poets CF, Stebbens VA, Richard D, Southall DP. Prolonged episodes of hypoxemia in preterm infants undetectable by cardiorespiratory monitors. Pediatrics 1995; 95(6):860–863.

65. Barrington KJ, Finer N, Li D. Predischarge respiratory recordings in very low birth weight newborn infants. J Pediatr 1996; 129(6):934–940.
66. Razi NM, Humphreys J, Pandit PB, Stahl GE. Pediatr Pulmonol 1999; 27:113–116.
67. Subhani M, Katz S, DeCristofaro, JD. Prediction of postdischarge complications by predischarge event recordings in infants with apnea of prematurity. J Perinatol 2000; 20(2):92–95.
68. Cote A, Hum C, Brouillette R, Themens M. Frequency and timing of recurrent events in infants using home cardiorespiratory monitors. J Pediatr 1998; 312:783–789.
69. Ramanathan R, Corwin MJ, Hunt CE, Lister G, Tinsaley LR, Baird T, Silvestri JM, Crowell DH, Hufford D, Martin RJ, Neuman MR, Weese-Mayer DE, Cupples LA, Peucker M, Willinger M, Keens TG, Cardiorespiratory events recorded on home monitors: comparison of healthy infants with those at increased risk for SIDS. JAMA 2001; 285(17):2199–2207.

16

Respiratory Control During Oral Feeding

OOMMEN P. MATHEW

Brody School of Medicine at East Carolina University
Greenville, North Carolina, U.S.A.

I. Introduction

Oral feeding in the neonate is usually accomplished in one of two ways: breast or bottle feeding. Achieving full oral feeding is an important milestone prior to discharge. Feeding-related bradycardia and desaturation are common among premature infants and infants with chronic lung disease. Before discussing the pathophysiology of feeding-related bradycardia and desaturation, an understanding of the following concepts is vital.

1. The upper airway constitutes a common conduit to both respiratory and digestive tracts.
2. Feeding and breathing present conflicting priorities.
3. Oral feeding in the neonatal period consists of sucking and swallowing into which the act of breathing is integrated.
4. Contraction of a number of upper-airway muscles occurs during this complex motor act.
5. Unless the airway can be protected during oral feeding, aspiration ensues.

For optimal performance of this complex motor act, sequential and coordinated activation of the upper-airway muscles is a must. Regulation of the activity of these muscles during development is discussed in detail in Chapter 5. In order to better understand the interplay of sucking and swallowing on breathing, the motor acts of sucking and swallowing and their development are reviewed first. Changes in the breathing pattern observed during oral feeding and the factors implicated in the etiology of this ventilatory depression are discussed next. The primary focus of this chapter is on feeding-related changes in the control of respiration.

II. Sucking

Sucking has been documented in fetal life by week 15 of gestation (1) and rarely, neonates are born with sucking blisters. Gryboski described an immature suck-swallow pattern in newborn infants between 32 and 34 weeks' gestation and a mature sucking pattern, which consists of multiple swallows during a sucking burst, in these infants by 6–12 postnatal weeks (2). Among infants born at 34–36 weeks, a mature pattern was observed by 2 weeks of age (2). Hack et al. (3), on the other hand, reported mouthing movements in infants at 28 weeks, a clear burst-pause pattern by 32 weeks, and a stable rhythm by 34 weeks.

Two types of sucking have been recognized: nutritive and nonnutritive. Nonnutritive sucking has been observed from the time of birth in both healthy and sick neonates. The newborn infant is capable of sucking and breathing simultaneously. This can be accomplished by functionally isolating the oral cavity from the pharynx. Physiological studies reveal that negative pressure changes are produced within the oral cavity during sucking (4–10). Suction pressure is generated by the rhythmic contractions of jaw muscles. These studies on sucking have also documented the presence of positive pressure changes in the oral cavity. These negative and positive pressure changes have been termed suction and expression components, respectively. During nutritive sucking, milk is expressed from the breast or bottle into the oral cavity. The relative importance of negative and positive pressures has been the focus of several investigators. Based on cineradiographic studies, Ardran and coworkers suggested that infants express milk by squeezing (11,12) and attributed greater importance on positive pressures. Pressure measurements by Colley and Creamer (13), on the other hand, indicated that suction pressure created by the pistonlike movements of the tongue and jaw is the critical factor in milk expression. Recent ultrasonographic studies, which permit visualization in both horizontal and transverse planes (14–17), indicate that suction component is the critical factor in milk expression, even in breastfeeding (14).

A number of factors determine how much milk is expressed per suck; these include the integrity of the labial, facial and palatal muscles to create a seal around the nipple, as well as the magnitude of contraction of the pressure-generating muscles. Decreased milk flow observed with the paralysis of facial muscles, inability of infants with cleft palate to generate negative sucking pressure, and reduced pressure changes seen among infants born to mothers receiving sedation during labor (4,18) support this line of reasoning. The volume of milk expressed per suck depends, in addition, on the characteristics of the container system. Rigid glass vs. collapsible containers, presence or absence of vent holes, as well as the shape, consistency, and size of feedhole all have an effect on milk flow (19). Nipples for premature infants in general have a softer consistency and a larger feedhole than nipples for term infants (20). Wide variability in milk flow is observed within and among the different nipple types; this is primarily attributable to the variability in the size of the feedhole (21). Variability in milk flow within a given nipple type can be significantly reduced by decreasing the variability in the size of the feedhole (22), for example, by utilizing technological innovations during the manufacturing process.

One should balance the work of sucking against the potential detrimental effect of greater milk flow. One could easily choke the infant by exceeding his/her autoregulatory capacity or increase the work of sucking by markedly restricting flow. Reduced variability in the size of feedhole is essential to ensure uniform milk flow in any given nipple type. A flow rate of 0.15–0.20 mL per suck would be adequate for most newborn infants, corresponding to the suck volume observed at the beginning of a feed in breastfed babies (23). Nipple units with lower or higher flow may have a role in feeding infants who generate markedly higher or lower sucking pressure than average so that milk flow/suck can be maintained within the range of autoregulation.

Infants usually suck vigorously and continuously at the beginning of the feed. This initial period, continuous sucking phase, often lasts >30 sec and is typically followed by a period in which the sucking bursts alternate with periods of rest or pause, termed intermittent sucking phase. In breastfed infants a linear relationship between milk flow and sucking frequency has been demonstrated (24). Sucking pressures vary markedly (4). In term infants, sucking pressure during bottle-feeding decreases when flow rate increases (13). A decrease in sucking pressure and an increase in time between sucking clusters are seen towards the end of the feeding. These findings suggest that term infants exhibit an autoregulatory mechanism during feeding. The premise for a larger feedhole for preterm infants is that higher milk flow compensates for the lower sucking pressures. However, when nipples for term and preterm infants are compared, no significant difference in sucking pressures or frequency is seen in preterm infants (10), suggesting that preterm infants are unable to autoregulate milk flow. An alternative explanation for this finding is that the variability in milk flow within the two types of nipples tested is too great. In fact, studies with laser-cut nipples with less variable feedhole sizes show a significant difference in sucking pressures between high and low flow nipple units among preterm infants (22).

This finding supports the notion that preterm infants have at least a limited ability to autoregulate milk flow. Drooling during oral feeding is more common at high flow in both preterm and term infants, but it is more prominent in preterm infants (25). The fact that drooling was more common in preterm infants likely reflects the decreased ability of these infants to adequately regulate milk flow. Nevertheless, according to these investigators, the ability to drool while continuing to feed may be a mark of feeding competence, rather than incompetence (25).

In recent years, several groups of investigators have studied the developmental pattern of nutritive sucking. Gewolb and coworkers (26) showed that the percentage of sucks organized into run increased with increasing postmenstrual age (PMA). Similarly stability of suck rhythm expressed as a coefficient of variation of suck-suck interval showed a significant relationship to increasing postmenstrual age. However, these changes showed no relationship to postnatal age, suggesting an intrinsic maturational pattern rather than a learned behavior (26). Lau et al. (27) showed that the premature sucking pattern consisted primarily of the expression component. With age, infants shifted to more frequent use of the term sucking pattern with the rhythmic alternation of suction/expression. These investigators also observed a positive correlation between different stages of sucking and postmenstrual age (28). Bu'Lock (16) also showed that adequate neuromuscular coordination during oral feeding is more a function of gestational maturity than of postnatal sucking experience. In a longitudinal study of term infants, Gewolb et al. showed that suck rate, percentage of suck aggregated into runs, and length of suck runs increased over the first 4 weeks (29). Further increase in sucking rate with increasing postnatal age was reported by McGowan (30) in older term infants. However, stability of sucking rhythm is established by 40 weeks, and no significant change occurs between infants at term and at 1 month of age (29).

Ability to alter sucking rate has been demonstrated by several groups of investigators. Schrank et al. observed that preterm infants responded similarly to term infants with respect to increased suck and swallow activity in response to increases in milk flow (25). A decrease in the rate of both sucking and swallowing frequency was noted during oral feeding in acute hypercapnia, suggesting that increased ventilatory drive may directly inhibit nutritive feeding behavior of premature infants (31). However, no difference in sucking frequency was seen between BPD and non-BPD infants, although suck rhythm was less stable in BPD infants (32). This difference in sucking rates between the two studies may be attributable to chronic hypercapnia of the BPD group.

III. Swallowing

Sequential activation of various upper-airway muscles is critical for suck-swallow coordination. Three distinct phases of swallowing have been recognized:

oral, pharyngeal, and esophageal. Detailed discussion of these phases is beyond the scope of this chapter, and readers are referred to excellent reviews on this topic (33–35). Nutritive sucking constitutes the oral phase of swallowing in neonates. In the pharyngeal stage, the bolus is propelled through the pharynx into the esophagus. The esophageal phase is a continuation of the pharyngeal motion and begins as the bolus enters the esophagus. The pharyngeal and esophageal phases are under involuntary control. Slowly adapting mechanoreceptors located in the mucosa of the pharynx and larynx responding to water and light touch initiate swallowing (36).

Neurophysiological influences of swallowing on central control of breathing have been studied in both adult and neonatal animals. In general, breathing is transiently inhibited during swallowing (37). Respiratory activity of some neurons in the reticular activating system is abolished during swallow. These neurons may exhibit a burst of impulses with swallowing and often remain silent for 1.0–2.0 sec; respiratory discharges then resume. Other neurons may cease firing during repetitive swallowing. A similar pattern has been seen in phrenic motoneurons as well (38).

The mechanical act of swallowing has been studied extensively by cineradiography, ultrasonography, and electromyography. Findings of earlier cineradiographic studies have been confirmed recently by ultrasonography (15). Horizontal transbuccal, as well as transverse and longitudinal submental projections show a depression in the posteromedial aspect of the tongue along the median raphe. Expressed milk is conveyed posteriorly toward the pharynx, while the lateral portion of the tongue encloses the nipple and the bolus. A number of events occur during swallowing. These include closure of velopharynx, closure of the glottis, and relaxation of the cricoesophageal sphincter. Velopharyngeal closure prevents pharyngonasal reflux, glottic closure prevents aspiration into the trachea, and relaxation of the cricoesophageal sphincter allows propulsion of the bolus into the esophagus. In addition, the pharynx moves anteriorly and cranially, while the larynx is pulled forward and upward. The muscles contracting at the onset of swallow are the superior pharyngeal constrictor, genioglossus, styloglossus, stylohyoid, geniohyoid, and mylohyoid. The sequence of activation of these muscles during swallowing has also been investigated extensively by electromyography (39,40).

A. Dysphagia

A number of clinical conditions are associated with dysphagia in neonates; some are congenital, others are acquired. Symptoms of dysphagia include difficulty in sucking and swallowing, vomiting, nasal regurgitation, cough, stridor, and hoarseness. Congenital structural abnormalities of the nasal airway, face, palate, pharynx, larynx, and neck may frequently result in dysphagia. For example, palatal and laryngeal clefts, pharyngeal and laryngeal cysts, choanal atresia, macroglossia, and esophageal atresia often cause dysphagia. Some neuromuscular diseases such as muscular dystrophy and myasthenia gravis as well as prematurity can also be included here. Acquired causes include cerebral palsy and acquired causes of mental retardation and developmental delay.

The evaluation of the swallowing mechanism may yield important diagnostic information about airway dysfunction. Video fluoroscopy of swallowing, also known as the modified barium swallow, is ideal for the evaluation of the swallowing mechanism. The oral cavity, the pharynx, and the larynx are evaluated using small amounts of liquids of various viscosities. Preterm neonates exhibit immature feeding skills and discoordinated swallowing and respiratory functions. Preterm babies usually develop sufficient airway protective mechanisms to allow feeding without aspiration by 36 weeks. In preterm infants with bradycardia and oxygen desaturation during oral feeding, video fluoroscopy is rarely needed before 36 weeks. If the infant aspirates with thin liquids, semithick and thickened liquids can be tried. Additionally, feeding positions can be changed, and oral support maneuvers can be attempted to alter the swallowing dysfunction during the fluoroscopic examination. The single most important aspect of this examination is the determination of the immediate effects of feeding intervention performed during the procedure, as it may allow parents and caretakers to modify feeding habits. Nasal regurgitation, also termed pharyngonasal reflux, may occur in premature infants (41). It appears to be rare, but its prevalence has not been documented.

Swallow rhythm is established by 32 weeks PMA; it stabilizes well before the stabilization of suck rhythm. The stability of swallow rhythm does not change from 32 weeks PMA to term (26,29). Timms et al. (31) reported a decrease in swallow frequency in preterm infants during acute hypercapnia. This is likely to be a secondary effect of decreased sucking frequency. However, no decrease in swallow frequency was seen in a group of BPD infants (32). A difference in the response between acute and chronic hypercapnia may account for this observed discrepancy. Nevertheless, swallow rhythm, expressed as the percentage of swallows aggregated into runs and average length of swallow runs, was decreased in BPD infants when compared to non-BPD infants of similar postmenstrual age (32). This may be indicative of dysmaturity rather than immaturity. It is not clear whether this observation has any value in predicting adverse neurological outcome.

IV. Breathing

Coordination of breathing and feeding poses fundamental challenges, since these two vital functions utilize a common pathway. As mentioned earlier, swallowing and breathing are mutually exclusive, and swallowing has an inhibitory influence on the respiratory center. Breathing, however, can continue during the sucking phase. This can be accomplished by maintaining a nasopharyngeal airway and by compartmentalizing the sucking to the oral cavity.

As mentioned earlier, sucking can be categorized as nutritive or nonnutritive. Even nonnutritive sucking has an effect on breathing. Expiratory duration during the sucking burst is shorter, resulting in an increase in breathing frequency (9). An increase in transcutaneous oxygen tension has been reported during nonnutritive sucking (42). However, this finding cannot be attributed to an increase in minute ventilation, since breathing frequency, tidal volume, and minute ventilation for the entire nonnutritive period remain unchanged (9). Hence, this increase in transcutaneous oxygen tension can only be explained as a result of a decrease in ventilation-perfusion mismatch.

Unlike sucking, swallowing interrupts breathing. Until the cineradiographic studies by Ardran and Kemp (11) showed that airway closure occurs during swallowing, infants were believed to be capable of breathing during swallowing. This followed the suggestion by Negus (43) that many herbivorous animals are able to pass food through the pharynx without interrupting breathing. The fact that the epiglottis is rather long in neonates and can even overlap the soft palate added credence to this notion. Recent studies unequivocally show that airflow is interrupted during swallowing in humans (4,44–46). Accurate measurement of ventilation during feeding is not easy, and significant methodological and analytic differences exist between studies (4). Nevertheless, it is clear from these studies that the minute ventilation decreases markedly during nipple feeding. Ventilation decreases dramatically during the initial continuous sucking phase (7,47). A reduction in both frequency and tidal volume is seen. Partial recovery occurs in premature infants during the intermittent sucking period (Figs. 1 and 2), and this recovery is greater in the more mature infants (47). Mathew et al. observed a

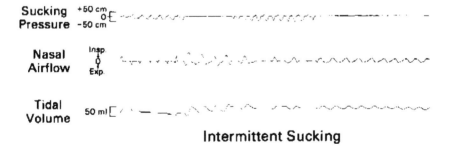

Intermittent Sucking

Figure 1 Breathing pattern of a term infant during intermittent sucking phase. Ventilation is markedly reduced during the sucking period. Note that most of the ventilation occurs during the pause in sucking. (From Ref. 7.)

complete recovery of ventilation in term infants during the intermittent sucking period (7). However, a marked difference in ventilation can be seen even within the intermittent sucking period; minute ventilation, breathing frequency, and tidal volume are significantly lower during the sucking burst compared to the pause period (Fig. 1). In fact, the overall recovery in term and preterm infants depends on the duration of these pauses and the infants' ability to increase ventilation during these periods (7,47). Interestingly, Mizuno et al. (48) documented that feeding in the prone position may reduce some of the disadvantages of oral feeding on ventilation. Better oxygenation and larger tidal volume, when compared to the traditional supine positioning, were observed in the prone position (48).

Newborn infants have limited ability to regulate milk flow during feeding. What are its implications on breathing pattern and ventilation? Several of the studies documenting a reduction in ventilation were conducted with a reservoir

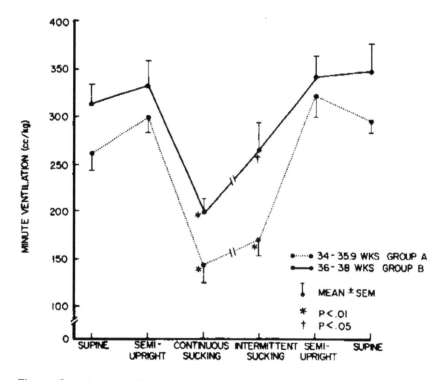

Figure 2 Minute ventilation during feeding in two groups of premature infants. Ventilation during the continuous sucking phase is significantly lower than control in both groups. Note that greater reduction in ventilation occurs in the more immature group of infants. (From Ref. 47.)

nipple system (7,47). In this system, milk is delivered from the container through a tube into the oral cavity, essentially bypassing the nipple. Although it is true that milk flow depends on sucking pressure, the flow rate in this system is at least twice the flow through the nipple (10). Hence, it is difficult to determine from these studies how much of the decrease in ventilation is flow dependent. A significant insight into this issue can be obtained by evaluating breastfed infants. It is a well-known fact that milk flow is low during the first few days of breastfeeding. Breathing pattern was only minimally altered during the first few days of breastfeeding, whereas marked alteration in breathing pattern was observed during formula feeding (5). However, this difference became minimal when expressed breast milk was fed from a bottle. This finding indicates that the difference in ventilation between formula feeding and breastfeeding is not primarily due to differences in composition but rather to a difference in flow rate. It is also in agreement with the results of the study using low and high flow laser-cut nipples (49). A greater reduction in ventilation occurred with high-flow nipples (49).

In a more recent study, physiological stability of infants during cup feeding was compared to breast and bottle feeding (50). No significant differences were observed between bottle and cup feeding with respect to feeding time, amount ingested, heart rate, respiratory rate, or oxygen saturation. However, physiological stability was greater during breast feeding than in the other two regimens (50). Breast feeding time was significantly longer, which suggests that the flow rate was low during breast feeding and consequently, the effect on ventilation smaller.

As mentioned above, a marked decrease in ventilation occurs during nipple feeding in both preterm and term infants. Several factors have been implicated in the etiology of this ventilatory depression. These include laryngeal chemoreflex, repeated swallowing, prolonged airway obstruction, and behavioral overriding. Ventilatory response to inhaled CO_2 is reduced during feeding (51). Durand et al. attributed this reduction in ventilatory response to behavioral overriding (51). Since the cortical influences are similar in nutritive and nonnutritive sucking, and since no alteration in minute ventilation is seen during nonnutritive sucking, Mathew et al. (9) concluded that the reduction in ventilation during feeding is not due to behavioral overriding.

Johnson and coworkers showed that the breathing pattern of human neonates is altered during nipple feeding and suggested that laryngeal chemo-receptors are likely to be responsible for this phenomenon (52). Studies in neonatal animals have shown that instillation of distilled water into the larynx of newborn animal elicits apnea. Superior laryngeal nerve afferents mediate this reflex response (53,54). Elegant studies by Boggs and Bartlett subsequently showed that lack of small anions such as chloride is responsible for the laryngeal chemoreflex (54). Davies et al. (55) and Perkett and Vaughn (56) provided further support for the existence of the laryngeal chemoreflex in human neonates by showing that instillation of distilled water into the pharynx alters breathing pattern compared to saline. Nevertheless, the marked difference in breathing pattern between human milk and artificial formula reported by Johnson and his colleagues has not been replicated by others (5,57). Guilleminault and Coons (57), as well as Mathew and Bhatia (5), were unable to show a marked difference in breathing pattern between human milk and formula feeding. It should be pointed out that chloride ions are low in both human milk and formula. Furthermore, chloride ions are even lower in human milk than in cow milk and formula (4). Therefore, the laryngeal chemoreflex does not appear to be the primary factor in the reduction of ventilation during feeding. In some infants it may play a contributory role.

Vocal cord closure during swallowing interrupts nasal airflow. The duration of this flow interruption of individual swallow varies from 0.35 to 0.70 sec (45). Often, there is a 1 : 1 correlation between sucking and swallowing during the continuous sucking period. Since neonates are capable of swallowing up to 30 times per minute (19), the time for ventilation is substantially reduced during nipple feeding. An inverse relationship between the frequency of swallowing and ventilation (Fig. 3) has been documented (45). In a subsequent study, the same

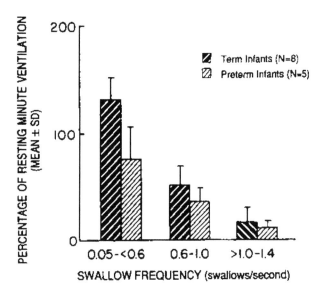

Figure 3   Relationship between swallow frequency and minute ventilation. For term and preterm infants minute ventilation decreases as swallow frequency increases. (From Ref. 45.)

group of investigators (58) showed that increased formula consumption is associated with reduced ventilation, a predictable consequence of increased swallowing fre-quency. Additionally, when consumption rate is high, the infant increases swallowing volume. Similarly, at low consumption rate, swallowing frequency is reduced, resulting in an increase in the suck-to-swallow ratio. These findings indicate that infants can autoregulate milk flow (through alteration of sucking pressure) as well as volume per swallow. This ventilation sparing strategy can be considered as a protective response.

The airway normally reopens in a cephalocaudal sequence at the end of the swallow and ventilation resumes. However, sometimes the airway fails to reopen. Such episodes can result in prolonged airway closure, not an uncommon finding during feeding (45). Two types of obstructed breaths have been observed during feeding: a small-amplitude swallow breath occurring before the swallow, and normal or increased amplitude respiratory efforts occurring at any time (45). A teleological explanation of the swallow breath is to remove air from the pharynx and prevent air swallowing. In this regard these swallow breaths appear to be inefficient in preventing aerophagia, since almost all infants need burping following feeding. Factors implicated in prolonged airway closure are mucosal adhesive forces, continued activation of pharyngeal constrictors, and insufficient activation of airway dilators.

Feeding efficiency and respiratory integration have been evaluated in older infants with bronchiolitis (59). These infants spent less time sucking than healthy controls. Mean volume per suck was lower during their illness. Unlike newborn infants in whom swallowing frequency is maintained at the expense of eupnea, feeding is subordinate to breathing in these infants. This finding is similar to the observation reported by Timms et al. that sucking and swallowing frequency decrease when respiratory drive increases (31).

Changes in pulmonary function following feeding have been the focus of several studies (60–64). The results of these studies have been conflicting; differences in birth weight, postnatal age, and lung disease status may account for some of these discrepancies. For example, differences in baseline pulmonary function among the study infants can be attributed to the fact that some of these infants were normal whereas others were recovering from acute lung disease or were suffering from chronic lung disease. Overall, these studies tend to suggest that the impact of feeding on pulmonary mechanics is likely to be greater in infants with poorly compliant lungs, compliant chest wall, and collapsible airways. Blondheim et al. (65) studied a group of low birth weight infants recovering from respiratory distress syndrome and showed that tidal volume decreased by 38%, minute ventilation by 44%, and dynamic compliance by 28% immediately following gavage (over 15–20 min) feeding. No such change in pulmonary function was seen following continuous nasogastric feeding. Abdominal loading is the likely basis of for the deterioration in pulmonary function (61).

Although functional residual capacity was not measured in the above study (65), a decrease in lung volume after feeding has been documented in neonates recovering from lung disease (64). These changes in pulmonary mechanics may result in apnea, cyanosis, and/or oxygen desaturation (66,67). Therefore, a continuous feeding appears to be advantageous for infants with chronic lung disease as well as for infants recovering from acute respiratory distress.

V. Disorders of Breathing During Feeding

Apnea, bradycardia, and oxygen desaturation during feeding have become common clinical problems in neonatal intensive care units. It can be attributed in part to an overzealous feeding regimen in a group of vulnerable infants. As discussed earlier, ventilation decreases significantly during nipple feeding in all neonates. This reduction in ventilation that occurs during feeding decreases PO_2 and increases PCO_2 (6,47). However, this change in ventilation with feeding is likely to have a greater impact in preterm infants and in sick term infants (4). Greater breathing difficulties during initiation of oral feeding are often seen among infants following prolonged intubation and tracheostomy. Laryngeal penetration of formula in these infants with transient laryngeal dysfunction probably accounts for this observation. Development of apnea and bradycardia during nipple feeding (Fig. 4) is a common occurrence in preterm infants (6,57,68). Similarly, a higher incidence of oxygen desaturation is seen during oral feeding in infants with chronic lung disease (69). Preterm infants breathed more during sucking bursts in breast-feeding sessions than in bottle-feeding sessions, and had fewer episodes of oxygen desaturation during breast feeding (70).

Mature infants without any underlying pulmonary disease usually tolerate oral feeding without developing any apnea or bradycardia. Occurrence of apnea and bradycardia is rare, especially beyond the first few days of life. Even during the first 48 h, apnea and bradycardia in term neonates are usually limited to the first feeding (71) or when the milk flow is very high (8). However, the normal term infant has little coordination between swallowing and breathing rhythms before 48 h and maintains rhythmic swallowing at the expense of eupnea (72). Mild transient oxygen desaturation without bradycardia is not uncommon among term infants during the first 48 h (72).

Understanding the mechanisms leading to the development of these symptoms is important in providing optimal clinical care. Because of the monitoring technique used, apnea is difficult to detect in the usual clinical setting, unless it is central. Prolonged airway occlusions often go undetected. Decrease in ventilation, either due to apnea or hypopnea, results in a decrease in oxygen saturation. How quickly it becomes clinically significant depends on two factors: baseline oxygenation prior to feeding, and pulmonary oxygen reserve. If

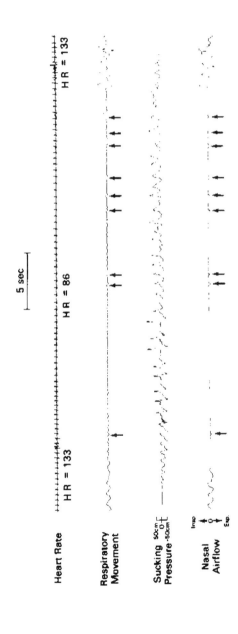

Figure 4 Apnea and bradycardia during feeding. Inspiratory airflow is absent during the sucking phase. Small obstructed respiratory efforts are indicated by arrows. Brief expiratory airflow can be seen during these obstructed respiratory efforts. (From Ref. 4.)

baseline oxygenation is borderline, hypoxemia may develop quickly, because it is on the linear portion of the oxygen dissociation curve. Similarly, infants with parenchymal lung disease may develop desaturation rapidly as a result of limited pulmonary oxygen reserve.

Timing of bradycardia during feeding is also important in understanding the pathophysiology. Oxygen desaturation and bradycardia usually develop during the initial continuous sucking phase in term infants (8). It may occur at any time in preterm infants; often they may have recurrent episodes during the same feeding (6). In term infants oxygen desaturation occurs first, followed by cyanosis. Bradycardia often occurs last, at much lower oxygen saturation levels than in preterm infants. It is not clear whether the bradycardia is a direct effect of hypoxia on SA node or mediated through the peripheral chemoreceptors. If bradycardia occurs early, especially when it occurs with normal oxygen saturation, it is unlikely to be due to a decrease in ventilation. A reflex bradycardia is more likely. Vagal afferents are presumed to mediate this response. An elevated level of baseline parasympathetic activity has been noted in the group of premature infants suffering from bradycardia during feeding (73). Stimulation of vagal afferents can induce both apnea and bradycardia in neonatal animals and in human neonates (74). In these cases, oxygen desaturation follows the onset of bradycardia and is likely to be delayed by several seconds. Even when the apnea and bradycardia responses are elicited by the same stimuli, respiratory and cardiovascular responses may not occur simultaneously. In animal studies, the respiratory responses preceded the cardiac response by approximately 0.5 sec (75). In addition to the occurrence of apnea, bradycardia, and desaturation during nipple feeding, these episodes may be observed shortly after feeding. A number of mechanisms have been implicated. A decrease in pulmonary function has been noted immediately following feeding (76). Abdominal loading is likely to decrease lung volume. Increase in feeding-related bradycardia observed within 24 h of their screening examination for retinopathy of prematurity may have a similar basis as well. Decreased gastric motility due to the effects of mydriatic agents is associated with decreased gastric emptying, resulting in increased gastric residuals, episodes of emesis, and abdominal distension (77). In addition, the gastric distension increases vagal afferent feedback. Rarely GE reflux may also induce some of these events.

Feeding-related bradycardia and desaturation can be managed in a number of ways. If these spells are severe and occur with every feed, nipple feeding should be postponed. This is particularly true in premature infants. Preterm infants who are normally oxygenated in room air but have significant desaturation during bottle feeding can be managed effectively by gavage feeding. Slow gavage feeding, however, offers no advantage over bolus gavage feeding with respect to oxygen desaturation (78). In less severe cases nipple feeding should be limited to once or twice a shift, until these infants are more mature. Continuous sucking, owing to the dramatic reduction in ventilation, has more detrimental effects on infants' breathing than intermittent sucking (4,79). Interruption of feeding by removing the nipple from the mouth for a few seconds, essentially converting this long continuous sucking into more stable intermittent sucking, is often sufficient. Whether the preterm infants' limited ability to regulate milk flow contributes to the development of these events is not known. The extent of the ventilatory depression can be attenuated by the use of low-flow nipple units (49). Although certain type of nipple units have high flow, it is impossible to predict the flow in an individual nipple with certainty. Mechanically drilled feedholes have the highest variability.

Feeding-related respiratory control may have some relevance in SIDS. In 1976 Steinschneider and Rabbuzzi reported two infants with feeding-related bradycardia subsequently dying of SIDS (80). Increased incidence of apnea/ airway obstruction during feeding was seen in the neonatal period among SIDS victims in a subsequent prospective study by the same group of investigators (81). However, this finding was not sufficiently discriminating to identify SIDS victims prospectively. Nevertheless, it must be pointed out, no one has tested the hypothesis that persistence of feeding-related apnea increases the risk for SIDS.

VI. Maturation

Respiratory control matures as myelination advances. Changes in the ventilatory responses to hypoxia and hypercapnia as well as changes in the auditory evoked response can be utilized in evaluating the maturation of the respiratory control system. Issues related to the maturation of respiratory control are discussed in greater length in Chapter 15. Henderson-Smart showed that conduction time decreases as myelination in the auditory pathways increases (82). This coincided with maturation of the brainstem respiratory center as reflected by the resolution of apnea (82). The inhibitory effect of afferent feedback from the upper airway on respiration is greater in the neonate (83). That more immature infants experience greater respiratory depression with the same feeding regimen (47) is consistent with this line of reasoning. Similarly, apnea duration associated with swallowing decreased as infants matured along with the number and length of episodes of multiple-swallow apnea (84). Maturation of respiratory control during feeding, in general, appears to be related to postmenstrual age rather than postnatal age or feeding experience (26,84). It is not complete at term gestation. Prolonged episodes of apnea associated with swallowing remained significantly more frequent in preterm infants reaching term postconceptual age compared to term infants (84), suggesting that myelination may be somewhat delayed in infants born markedly prematurely. A delay in the maturation of vagal function in preterm infants has been reported by Suess et al. (85). They studied two groups of premature infants at 33 weeks PMA. The less prematurely born infants exhibited expected decreases in respiratory sinus arrhythmia during feeding and returned to prefeed levels (85). The more prematurely born infants, on the other hand, did not return to prefeed levels during the study period. It is intriguing to note that earlier maturation has been seen in breast-fed infants (86).

VII. Summary

Nipple feeding is a complex motor act consisting of sucking and swallowing into which the act of breathing is integrated. Sequential and coordinated contractions of a number of upper-airway muscles are essential for optimal performance of nipple feeding. Ventilation decreases markedly during oral feeding. Greater reduction in ventilation occurs during the initial continuous sucking phase when compared to the intermittent sucking phase. Both tidal volume and breathing frequency decrease during oral feeding. The decrease in ventilation is greater in the more immature infants. Several factors have been implicated in the etiology of this ventilatory depression. These include repeated swallowing, laryngeal chemoreflex, prolonged airway obstruction, and behavioral overriding. Reduction in ventilation results in a decrease in oxygen saturation. How quickly it becomes clinically significant depends on baseline oxygenation prior to feeding and pulmonary oxygen reserve. Feeding-related bradycardia and desaturation are common in premature infants. Infants with chronic lung disease are also at higher risk for feeding-related bradycardia and desaturation. Frequency of sucking and swallowing decreases when respiratory drive increases acutely. Feeding related abnormalities of respiration typically resolve near term PMA, reflecting the maturation of the brainstem.

References

1. Ianniruberto A, Tejani E. Ultrasound study of fetal movements. Semin Perinatol 1981; 5:175–181.
2. Gryboski JD. Suck and swallow in the premature infant. Pediatrics 1969; 43:96–102.
3. Hack M, Estabrook MM, Roberston SS. Development of sucking rhythm in preterm infants. Early Hum Dev 1985; 11:133–140.
4. Mathew OP. Regulation of breathing pattern during feeding: role of suck, swallow and nutrients. In: Mathew OP, Sant'Ambrogio G, eds. Respiratory Function of the Upper Airway. New York: Marcel Dekker, 1988:535–560.
5. Mathew OP, Bhatia J. Sucking and breathing patterns during breast- and bottle-feeding in term neonates. Effects of nutrient delivery and composition. Am J Dis Child 1989; 143:588–592.
6. Mathew OP. Respiratory control during nipple feeding in preterm infants. Pediatr Pulmonol 1988; 5:220–224.

7. Mathew OP, Clark ML, Pronske ML, Luna-Solarzano HG, Peterson MD. Breathing pattern and ventilation during oral feeding in term newborn infants. J Pediatr 1985; 106:810–813.
8. Mathew OP, Clark ML, Pronske MH. Apnea, bradycardia, and cyanosis during oral feeding in term neonates. J Pediatr 1985:106:857.
9. Mathew OP, Clark ML, Pronske MH. Breathing pattern of neonates during non-nutritive sucking. Pediatr Pulmonol 1985; 1:204–206.
10. Mathew OP, Belan MA, Thoppil CK. Sucking pattern of neonates during bottle feeding: comparison of different nipple units. Am J Perinatol 1992; 9:265–269.
11. Ardran GM, Kemp FH, Lind J. A cineradiographic study of bottle feeding. Br J Radiol 1958; 31:11–22.
12. Ardran GM, Kemp FH, Lind J. A cineradiographic study of breast feeding. Br J Radiol 1958; 31:156–162.
13. Colley JRT, Creamer B. Sucking and swallowing in infants. Br Med J 1958; 2:422–423.
14. Smith WL, Erenberg A, Nowak A. Imaging evaluation of the human nipple during breast-feeding. Am J Dis Child 1988; 142:76–78.
15. Bosma JF, Hepburn LG, Josell SD, Baker K. Ultrasound demonstration of tongue movements during suckle feeding. Dev Med Child Neurol 1990; 32:223–229.
16. Bu'Lock F, Woolridge MW, Baum JD. Development of co-ordination of sucking, swallowing, and breathing: ultrasound study of term and preterm infants. Dev Med Child Neurol 1990; 32:669–678.
17. Smith WL, Erenberg A, Nowak A, Franken EA. Physiology of sucking in the normal term infant using real-time US. Radiology 1985; 156:379–381.
18. Kron, RE, Stein M, Goddard KE. Newborn sucking behavior affected by obstetric sedation. Pediatrics 1966; 37:1012–1016.
19. Mathew OP. Science of bottle feeding. J Pediatr 1991; 119:511–519.
20. Mathew OP. Nipple units for newborn infants: a functional comparison. Pediatrics 1988; 81:688–691.
21. Mathew OP. Determinants of milk flow through nipple units. Am J Dis Child 1990; 144:222–224.
22. Mathew OP. Milk flow variability is reduced among laser-cut nipple units. Pediatr Res 1991; 29:226A.
23. Woolridge MW, How TV, Drewett RF, Rolfe P, Baum JD. The continuous measurement of milk intake at a feed in breast-fed babies. Early Hum Dev 1982; 6:365–373.
24. Bowen-Jones A, Thompson C, Drewett RF. Milk flow and sucking rates during breast feeding. Dev Med Child Neurol 1982; 24:626–633.
25. Schrank W, Al-Sayed LE, Beahm PH, Thach BT. Feeding responses to free-flow formula in term and preterm infants. J Pediatr 1998; 132(3):426–430.
26. Gewolb IH, Vice FL, Scheiter-Kenney EL, Taciak VL, Bosma JF. Developmental patterns of rhythmic suck and swallow in preterm infants. Dev Med Child Neurol 2001; 43:22–37.
27. Lau C, Sheena HR, Shulman RJ, Schanler RJ. Oral feeding in low birth weight infants. J Pediatr 1997; 130:561–569.

28. Lau C, Alagugurusamy R, Schanler RJ, Smith EO, Shulman RJ. Characterization of the developmental stages of sucking in preterm infants during bottle feeding. Acta Paediatr 2000; 89(7):846–852.

29. Qureshi MA, Vice FL, Taciak VL, Bosma JF, Gewolb IH. Changes in rhythmic suckle feeding in term infants in the first month of life. Dev Med Child Neurol 2002; 44:34–39.

30. McGowan JS, Marsh RR, Fowler SM, Levy SE, Stallings VA. Developmental patterns of normal nutritive sucking in infants. Dev Med Child Neurol 1991; 33:891–897.

31. Timms BJ, DiFiore JM, Martin RJ, Miller MJ. Increased respiratory drive as an inhibitor of oral feeding of preterm infants. J Pediatr 1993; 123:127–131.

32. Gewolb IH, Bosma JF, Taciak VL, Vice FL. Abnormal developmental patterns of suck and swallow rhythms during feeding in preterm infants with bronchopulmonary dysplasia. Dev Med Child Neurol 2001; 43:454–459.

33. Bosma JF. Deglutition: pharyngeal stage. Physiol Rev 1957; 37:275–300.

34. Doty RW. Neural organization of deglutition. In: Handbook of Physiology, Section 6, Vol 4. Washington: Alimentary Canal American Physiological Society, 1968:1861–1902.

35. Miller AJ. Deglutition. Physiol Dev 1982; 62:129–184.

36. Storey AT. Laryngeal initiation of swallowing. Exp Neurol 1968; 20:359–365.

37. Clark GA. Deglutition apnoea. J Physiol (Lond) 1920; 54:59.

38. Sumi T. Coordination of neural organization of respiration deglutition: its change with post-natal maturation. In: Bosma JF, Showacre J, eds. Development of Upper Respiratory Anatomy and Function. Bethesda, MD: U.S. Dept. of Health, Education, and Welfare publication (NIH) 75–941, 1975:145–159.

39. Cunningham DP, Basmajian JV. Electromyography of genioglossus and geniohyoid muscles during deglutition. Anat Rec 1969; 165:401–410.

40. Doty RW, Bosma JF. An electromyographic analysis of reflex deglutition. J Neurophysiol 1956; 19:44–60.

41. Ostreich AE, Dunbar JS. Pharyngonasal reflex: spectrum and significance in early childhood. AJR 1984; 141:923–925.

42. Paladetto R, Roberson SS, Hack H, Shivpuri CR, Martin RJ. Transcutaneous oxygen tension during non-nutritive sucking in preterm infants. Pediatrics 1984; 74:539–542.

43. Negus V. The mechanism of swallowing. J Laryngol Otol 1943; 58:46–59.

44. Nishino T, Yonezawa T, Honda Y. Effects of swallowing on the pattern of continuous respiration in human adults. Am Rev Respir Dis 1985; 132:1219–1222.

45. Koenig JS, Davies AM, Thach BT. Coordination of breathing, sucking and swallowing during bottle feedings in human infants. J Appl Physiol 1990; 69:1623–1629.

46. Wilson SL, Thach BT, Brouillette RT, Abu-Osba YK. Coordination of breathing and swallowing in human infants. J Appl Physiol Respir Environ Exercise Physiol 1981; 50:851–858.

47. Shivpuri CR, Martin RJ, Carlo WA, Fanarof AA. Decreased ventilation in preterm infants during oral feeding. J Pediatr 1983; 103:285–289.

48. Mizuno K, Inoue M, Takeuchi T. The effects of body positioning on sucking behaviour in sick neonates. Eur J Pediatr 2000; 159:827–831.
49. Mathew OP. Breathing patterns of preterm infants during bottle feeding: role of milk flow. J Pediatr 1991; 119:960–965.
50. Howard CR, de Blieck EA, ten Hoopen CB, Howard FM, Lanphear BP, Lawrence RA. Physiologic stability of newborns during cup- and bottle-feeding. Pediatrics 1999; 104:1204–1207.
51. Durand M, MacCallum M, Cates DB, Rigatto H, Chernick V. Effect of feeding on the chemical control of breathing in the newborn infant. Pediatr Res 1981; 15:1509–1512.
52. Johnson P, Salisbury DM. Sucking and breathing during artificial feeding in the human neonate. In: Bosma JF, Showacre J, eds. Development of Upper Respiratory Anatomy and Function. Bethesda, MD: U.S. Dept. of Health, Education, and Welfare publication (NIH) 75–941, 1975:206–211.
53. Johnson P, Salisbury DM, Storey AT. Apnea induced by stimulation of sensory receptors in the larynx. In: Development of Upper Respiratory Anatomy and Function. Bethesda, MD: U.S. Dept. of Health, Education, and Welfare publication (NIH) 75–941, 1975:160–178.
54. Boggs DF, Bartlett D Jr. Chemical specificity of a laryngeal apneic reflex in puppies. J Appl Physiol 1983; 53:455–463.
55. Davies AM, Koenig JS, Thach BT. Upper airway chemoreflex responses to saline and water in preterm infants. J Appl Physiol 1988; 64:1412–1420.
56. Perkett EA, Vaughan RL. Evidence for a laryngeal chemoreflex in some human preterm infants. Acta Paediatr Scand 1982; 71:969–972.
57. Guilleminault C, Coons S. Apnea and bradycardia during feeding in infants weighing > 2000 gm. J Pediatr 1984; 104:932–935.
58. Al-Sayed LE, Schrank WI, Thach BT. Ventilatory sparing strategies and swallowing pattern during bottle feeding in human infants. J Appl Physiol 1994; 77:78–83.
59. Pinnington LL, Smith CM, Ellis RE, Morton RE. Feeding efficiency and respiratory integration in infants with acute viral bronchiolitis. J Pediatr 2000; 137:523–526.
60. Feather EA, Russell G. Respiratory mechanics in infants of low birthweight. Arch Dis Child 1971; 46(247):398.
61. Heldt GP. The effect of gavage feeding on the mechanics of the lung, chest wall, and diaphragm of preterm infants. Pediatr Res 1988; 24:55–58.
62. Russell G, Feather EA. Effects of feeding on respiratory mechanics of healthy newborn infants. Arch Dis Child 1970; 45:325–327.
63. Krauss AN, Brown J, Waldman S, Gottlieb G, Auld PA. Pulmonary function following feeding in low-birth-weight infants. Am J Dis Child 1978; 132:139–142.
64. Pitcher-Wilmott R, Shutack JG, Fox WW. Decreased lung volume after nasgogastric feeding of neonates recovering from respiratory disease. J Pediatr 1979; 95:119–121.
65. Blondheim O, Abbasi S, Fox WW, Bhutani VK. Effect of enteral gavage feeding rate on pulmonary functions of very low birth weight infants. J Pediatr 1993; 122:751–755.
66. Patel BD, Dinwiddie R, Kumar SP, Fox WW. The effects of feeding on arterial blood gases and lung mechanics in newborn infants recovering from respiratory disease. J Pediatr 1977; 90:435–438.

67. Wilkinson A, Yu VY. Immediate effects of feeding on blood-gases and some cardiorespiratory functions in ill newborn infants. Lancet 1974; 1(7866):1083–1085.
68. Rosen CR, Glaze DG, Frost SD Jr. Hypoxemia associated with feeding in the preterm and fullterm neonate. Am J Dis Child 1984; 138:623–628.
69. Garg M, Kurzner SI, Bautista DB, Keens TG. Clinically unsuspected hypoxia during sleep and feeding in infants with bronchopulmonary dysplasia. Pediatrics 1988; 81:635–642.
70. Dowling DA. Physiological responses of preterm infants to breast-feeding and bottle-feeding with the orthodontic nipple. Nurs Res 1999; 48:78–85.
71. Burnard ED. Apnea and cyanosis during feeding in the neonate. Proceedings of Eighth Singapore-Malaysia Congress of Medicine 1973; 8:220–222.
72. Bamford O, Taciak V, Gewolb IH. Coordination of sucking, swallowing and breathing in the newborn: its relationship to infant feeding and normal development. Pediatr Res 1992; 31:619–624.
73. Veerappan S, Rosen H, Craelius W, Curcie D, Hiatt M, Hegyi T. Spectral analysis of heart rate variability in premature infants with feeding bradycardia. Pediatr Res 2000; 47:659–662.
74. Haxhija EQ, Rosegger H, Prechtl HF. Vagal response to feeding tube insertion in preterm infants: has the key been found? Early Hum Dev 1995; 41:15–25.
75. Palacek F, Sant'Ambrogio G, Sant'Ambrogio FB, Mathew OP. Reflex responses to capsaicin: intravenous, aerosol, and intratracheal administration. J Appl Physiol 1989; 67:1428–1437.
76. Singer L, Martin RJ, Hawkins SW, Benson-Szekely LJ, Yamashita TS, Carlo WA. Oxygen desaturation complicates feeding in infants with bronchopulmonary dysplasia after discharge. Pediatrics 1992; 90:380–384.
77. Bonthala S, Sparks JW, Musgrove KH, Berseth CL. Mydriatics slow gastric emptying in preterm infants. J Pediatr 2000; 137:327–330.
78. Poets CF, Langner MU, Bohnhorst B. Effects of bottle feeding and two different methods of gavage feeding on oxygenation and breathing patterns in preterm infants. Acta Paediatr 1997; 86:419–423.
79. Shiao SY. Comparison of continuous versus intermittent sucking in very-low-birth-weight infants. J Obstet Gynecol Neonatal Nurs 1997; 26:313–319.
80. Steinschneider A, Rabuzzi DD. Apnea and airway obstruction during feeding and sleep. Laryngoscope 1976; 86:1359–1366.
81. Steinschneider A, Weinstein SL, Diamond E. Sudden infant death syndrome and apnea/obstruction during neonatal sleep and feeding. Pediatrics 1982; 70:858–863.
82. Henderson-Smart DJ, Pettigrew AG, Campbell DJ. Clinical apnea and brain-stem neural function in preterm infants. N Engl J Med 1983; 308:353–357.
83. Mathew OP, Sant'Ambrogio FB. Laryngeal reflexes. In: Mathew OP, Sant'Ambrogio G, eds. Respiratory Function of the Upper Airway. New York: Marcel Dekker, 1988: 259–302.
84. Hanlon MB, Tripp JH, Ellis RE, Flack FC, Selley WG, Shoesmith HJ. Deglutition apnoea as indicator of maturation of suckle feeding in bottle-fed preterm infants. Dev Med Child Neurol 1997; 39:534–542.

85. Suess PE, Alpan G, Dulkerian SJ, Doussard-Roosevelt J, Gewolb IH. Respiratory sinus arrhythmia during feeding: a measure of vagal regulation of metabolism, ingestion, and digestion in preterm infants. Dev Med Child Neurol 2000; 42:169–173.

86. Amin SB, Merle KS, Orlando MS, Dalzell LE, Guillet R. Brainstem maturation in premature infants as a function of enteral feeding type. Pediatrics 2000; 106:318–322.

17

Idiopathic Congenital Central Hypoventilation Syndrome

DEBRA E. WEESE-MAYER and JEAN M. SILVESTRI

Rush Children's Hospital
Chicago, Illinois, U.S.A.

I. Introduction

Idiopathic congenital central hypoventilation syndrome (CCHS) is a rare entity with abundant case reports, but likely fewer than 200 living children worldwide. Children with CCHS typically present in the newborn period with symptoms including duskiness or cyanosis upon falling asleep, and decreasing oxyhemoglobin saturation with increasing carbon dioxide levels, yet no increase in breathing frequency or awakening. While some infants appear to have diminutive chest wall movement, others will appear apneic both awake and asleep.

II. Differential Diagnosis

If a diagnosis of CCHS is considered, studies must be performed to rule out primary neuromuscular, lung, or cardiac disease, or an identifiable brainstem lesion. Because CCHS may mimic other diseases, the possibility of a discrete congenital myopathy, myasthenia gravis, altered airway or intrathoracic anatomy, diaphragm dysfunction, congenital cardiac disease, a structural hindbrain or brainstem abnormality, or Mobius syndrome should be considered. Specific metabolic diseases such as Leigh disease, pyruvate dehydrogenase deficiency, and discrete carnitine deficiency should also be considered in the differential diagnosis. Confounding variables including asphyxia, infection, trauma, tumor, and infarction should be distinguished from the unique diagnosis of CCHS.

III. Initial Evaluation

The initial evaluation should include a detailed neurologic assessment that may require a muscle biopsy, chest x-ray, fluoroscopy of the diaphragm, broncho-scopy, electrocardiogram, Holter recording, echocardiogram, and an MRI of the brain/brainstem. Serum and urinary carnitine levels to rule out an inborn error in fatty acid metabolism should be obtained from a laboratory with known expertise in their assessment. The infant with carnitine deficiency may require a muscle biopsy for diagnostic confirmation. A detailed ophthalmologic evaluation should be performed to assess pupillary reactivity and optic disk anatomy. A rectal biopsy should be considered in the event of abdominal distension and delayed defecation to assess for Hirschsprung disease.

IV. Control of Breathing Deficit

CCHS is characterized by generally adequate ventilation while the child is awake, but alveolar hypoventilation with monotonous respiratory rates, shallow breathing (diminished tidal volume), and progressive hypercapnia and hypoxemia during sleep (1–18). However, more severely affected children hypoventilate both awake and asleep, with improved ventilation in rapid eye movement (REM) sleep compared with non-REM (NREM) (3). During sleep, ventilatory sensitivity to hypercarbia is negligible or absent, and ventilatory sensitivity to hypoxemia is variable or absent (2–16). These children lack an arousal response to the endogenous challenges of isolated hypercarbia, hypoxemia, and to the combined stimulus of hypercarbia and hypoxemia (2). Awake ventilatory responsiveness to hypercarbia and hypoxemia is generally absent (2,3,19), as is the perception of asphyxia (i.e., behavioral awareness of hypercarbia and hypoxemia), even when awake minute ventilation is adequate.

Each infant should be studied in detail in a pediatric respiratory physiology laboratory to evaluate spontaneous breathing during sleep (NREM and REM) and wakefulness. The recording montage should include at a minimum tidal volume (pneumotachograph), movement of the chest and abdomen (respiratory induc-tance plethysmography), hemoglobin saturation with pulse waveform, end tidal carbon dioxide, and electrocardiogram. Careful observation should be made of the infant's tidal volume and respiratory frequency response to the endogenous challenges of hypercarbia and hypoxemia both awake and asleep. Such endogenous challenges during spontaneous breathing awake and asleep may preclude the need for exogenous challenge testing. The distinction of need for artificial ventilatory support asleep only, or awake and asleep, should be made after *several* detailed evaluations in a controlled laboratory setting.

V. Associated Conditions

Conditions associated with CCHS include Hirschsprung disease (1,2,7,8,16, 17,20–25), ganglioneuroma (26), neuroblastoma (16), ganglioneuroblastoma (2,8,9), lack of heart rate variability (2,8,27–29), and eye abnormalities (2,30) including diminished pupillary light response. Feeding difficulty with esophageal dysmotility in infancy, breath-holding spells, poor temperature regulation with the basal body temperature typically <98°F, and sporadic profuse sweating episodes with cool extremities have been described anecdotally (1). Children with CCHS lack a perception of dyspnea but maintain conscious control of breathing (31) (i.e., ability to "take a big breath" when asked). During exercise these children may be at risk for hypercarbia and hypoxemia, though the degree of exercise and the severity of the CCHS likely impact on the response for each child (32–34). Perception of anxiety is also decreased among children with CCHS (35).

VI. Autonomic Nervous System Dysfunction in CCHS

Abnormalities of the autonomic regulation of cardiovascular and/or respiratory function have long been postulated in children with CCHS (1,7,8,12). Supportive cardiac measure data include the above-cited decreased heart rate beat-to-beat variability, increased ratios of low-frequency band to high-frequency band spectral power and transient asystoles, and an attenuated heart rate response to exercise. Supportive respiratory measures include the above-cited alveolar hypoventilation, lack of normal ventilatory and arousal responses to hypercarbia and hypoxemia, and limited breath-to-breath variability.

Children with CCHS often have additional symptoms compatible with altered physiologic regulation of the autonomic nervous system (ANS), and in one report, "autonomic crises" with and without elevated urinary catecholamines have been described (36). A recent report of manifestations of potential ANS dysfunction among 56 children with CCHS [through meticulous review of their medical records and a scripted questionnaire (37)] indicated remarkably prevalent symptoms of ANS dysfunction (ANSD). Incidences among the more prevalent symptoms (experienced by >15% of CCHS probands) are indicated below. It should be noted that among age-, race-, and gender-matched control subjects the median percent of children with any of the symptoms listed below was 0, with a range of 2–4% affected for only seven of the symptoms listed below.

Symptom of ANS dysfunction	Percent of affected CCHS probands
Alveolar hypoventilation	100
Altered temperature regulation	68
Altered sweating	66
Decreased heart rate variability	55
Nonreactive/sluggish pupils	55
Altered perception of pain	50
Constipation without Hirschsprung disease	43
Altered lacrimation	41
Extreme breath-holding spells	39
Dysrhythmia	39
Dysphagia	38
Anisocoria	27
Altered perception of anxiety	27
Vasovagal syncope with normal SaO_2 and CO_2	23
Miosis	21
Gastroesophageal reflux	21
Hirschsprung disease	21
Facial pallor	18
Headache with normal SaO_2 and CO_2	16
Diarrhea without Hirschsprung disease	16

Many children with CCHS also have anatomic findings compatible with altered development of neural crest–derived structures, including the above-cited Hirschsprung disease and tumors of neural crest origin. Finally, neuropathologic findings that support the notion of deficient ANS function/structure include neuronal loss of the reticular nuclei and nearby cranial nerve nuclei (nucleus ambiguus, hypoglossal, dorsal motor nuclei of the vagus) in one child (11). These physiologic, anatomic, and neuropathologic observations reflect a reduced capability for a homeostatic, compensatory response among children with CCHS.

VII. Familial Occurrence of CCHS

Data on familial occurrence include reports describing one case each of mono-zygotic (MZ) female twins (10), sisters (8), male–female half-sibs (20), and male–female sibs (2) with CCHS. The MZ female twins are the only cases reported of familial recurrence of CCHS without Hirschsprung disease in at least one sib.

The association of Hirschsprung disease [a common malformation characterized by the absence of parasympathetic intrinsic ganglion cells of the hindgut and regarded as a neurocristopathy (38)] with CCHS has provided an important avenue for studying genetic mutations that might account for the complex phenotype of CCHS. Mutations in several genetic loci have been identified in Hirschsprung disease, including receptor tyrosine kinase (RET) (39,40), endothelin signaling pathway genes (41–44), and glial-derived neurotrophic factor (GDNF), a ligand of the RET proto-oncogene (45–47). Two discrete mutations in RET have also been reported in two unrelated CCHS patients (48,49) and the unaffected father of one. A mutation in endothelin-3 was reported in a third patient (50), and a mutation in GDNF was reported in another patient and his unaffected mother (48). A mutation in brain-derived neurotrophic factor (BDNF) was reported in a patient with CCHS and in his non-CCHS father with symptoms of ANS dysfunction (50b).

A segregation analysis of 50 families with a CCHS index case provided further data consistent with familiality of CCHS, although multifactorial and major locus models could not be distinguished statistically, probably owing to a lack of statistical power (51). In that segregation analysis, two ANSD symptoms were investigated (constipation and Hirschsprung disease); heterogeneity tests found no significant differences in the genetic analysis results between those families whose index case had Hirschsprung disease or chronic constipation and those who did not (51). The variable expression of a respiratory control defect in RET-/-homozygous mice when exposed to increased carbon dioxide (52) supports the consideration of a genetic origin of CCHS and diseases of the ANS and neural crest.

A recent report of a child with CCHS born to a woman who had neuroblastoma as an infant (53) provides evidence for a transmitted component in the relationship between CCHS and the ANS. Likewise, two and potentially three infants born to four young women with idiopathic CCHS illustrate transmission of altered respiratory control by CCHS into the next generation. Further, one of the three infants has confirmed CCHS (53b).

VIII. Familial Occurrence of ANSD

Results from a recent study utilizing a scripted questionnaire administered to families of 56 CCHS cases and 56 age-, race-, and gender-matched controls support the hypothesis that findings consistent with ANSD are more likely to be found in relatives of CCHS cases than in controls or relatives of controls (37). Furthermore, relatives of the CCHS cases tended to manifest a milder form of ANSD, with fewer systems and/or fewer symptoms than the cases (37). To our knowledge, this represents the first study of ANSD in families of children with CCHS.

A subsequent study designed to test the hypothesis that CCHS is the most severe manifestation of general autonomic nervous system dysfunction (ANSD) applied a case control family study design to determine if the familiality of ANSD was consistent with a genetic pattern among 52 probands with CCHS as well as 52 age-, race-, and gender-matched controls (54). ANSD phenotypic features were characterized in the cases, controls, and their family members. We performed major locus segregation analysis of ANSD utilizing regressive models. CCHS probands were assumed to be affected; controls and relatives were designated as affected if they had two or more relevant symptoms. The hypothesis of "no transmission and no familial effects" was rejected in both case and control families. Case families were consistent with transmission of a major effect; control families were not (the difference in the pattern of results was significant; $P < 0.0001$). In the total dataset, the best-fitting model was codominant Mendelian inheritance of a major gene for ANSD. The case control family studies support the hypothesis that CCHS is the most severe manifestation of a general ANS dysfunction, with a family pattern consistent with Mendelian transmission.

Further clarification of the complex phenotype for primary generalized ANS dysfunction as a unique entity and as expressed in kindreds with CCHS index cases is timely as many of the children with CCHS are reaching reproductive age. Although there are some indirect leads for specific candidate genetic loci for ANSD, results thus far with those candidates have not been uniform in CCHS subjects, and need to be further investigated. After the relationship between ANSD and CCHS is more clearly delineated, the identified differences can be applied to better understand the physiology of the ANS dysfunction.

IX. Ventilatory Support Options

As soon as a diagnosis of CCHS is confirmed, a tracheostomy should be performed by a pediatric otolaryngologist. A transition to a home mechanical ventilator should be made to allow ample time for parental training prior to discharge. Arrangement for discharge to home with the primary mechanical ventilator and a backup ventilator should be completed, and requests for adequate home nursing care made. Typically 24-h/day care with highly trained registered nurses is required to optimize patient management in the home. Discharge with a pulse oximeter and an end-tidal carbon dioxide monitor is an essential part of the home management of a child with CCHS. These monitors often provide objective evidence for early deterioration of ventilation or "outgrowing" of ventilator settings, in both cases preventing clinical deterioration, risk for prolonged hospitalization, and risk of cor pulmonale. Because these patients do not demonstrate dyspnea in response to chronic hypoventilation or acute pulmonary infection, objective measures of physiologic compromise are necessary to assure early clinical intervention.

Several ventilatory support options are available for the infant and child with CCHS. Typically the infant who requires ventilatory support 24 h/day will have a tracheostomy and use a home mechanical ventilator in the pressure-plateau mode. As the infant becomes ambulatory, the possibility of diaphragm pacing by phrenic nerve stimulation (55,56) should be considered to allow for increased mobility and improved quality of life. The paced older infants and toddlers may use a Passy-Muir one-way speaking valve while awake, allowing for vocalization and use of the upper airway on exhalation, but only after thorough assessment in a pediatric respiratory physiology laboratory. The paced child may also be assessed for capping of the tracheostomy tube during pacing while awake, allowing for inspiration and exhalation via the upper airway. Again, the capped tracheostomy during pacing should be carefully assessed in a pediatric respiratory physiology laboratory before introducing it into clinical management. Nonetheless, these 24-h/day-supported patients will still require a tracheostomy for the nighttime mechanical ventilation. Though not yet accomplished, the older child with an entirely normal airway may be able to rely on pacing awake and Bi-Pap mask ventilation asleep eliminating the need for a tracheostomy. In the event of severe pneumonia requiring more aggressive ventilatory management, such a child would require interim endotracheal intubation to allow for adequate ventilation.

Those children who consistently require ventilatory support during sleep only (as opposed to sleep and wakefulness) and who are able to cooperate can be considered as candidates for noninvasive ventilation with either Bi-Pap or a negative pressure ventilator. If successful, a tracheal decanulation can be considered, but with the recognition that in the event of an overwhelming pneumonia the child may require interim endotracheal intubation, and may require ventilatory assistance awake and asleep during an intercurrent illness.

Regardless of the method of ventilatory support, the goal is to optimize oxygenation and ventilation for each child. Typically the recommendation is for hemoglobin saturation values ≥95%. The end-tidal carbon dioxide range may be broad with limits of 30–45 mm Hg, allowing for variation with sleep position. The rationale for achieving relative hyperventilation in the respiratory physiology laboratory is to ensure that when the child is later exposed to potentially suboptimal conditions at home or school, end carbon dioxide values will never be worse than in the normal range of 35–45 mm Hg. The goal for chronic care is thus to minimize exposure to hypoventilation, not to achieve hyperventilation. The value of long-term hyperventilation with low end-tidal carbon dioxide values during sleep (25–35 mm Hg) versus "normal" values (35–45 mm Hg) has not been studied prospectively.

For each of the above-described modalities, the goal is to match the patient with the optimal technology for her/his lifestyle needs. Although diaphragm pacing is not typically recommended in the young child who requires only nighttime support (the benefits do not outweigh the risks), in the older child this might be an appropriate consideration.

X. Long-Term Comprehensive Management

Meticulous follow-up and coordination of care by the family in conjunction with the local pulmonologist and the physicians in a center with recognized expertise in CCHS are vital to the successful outcome of each child. Ideally, infants and young children should be evaluated every 1–2 months by their local pulmonologist and pediatrician, and every 6 months by a center with recognized expertise in CCHS. The local evaluations should include assessment of growth, speech, and mental and motor development. The evaluations every 6 months should include an in-hospital evaluation with detailed recording during sleep and wakefulness in a pediatric respiratory physiology laboratory to monitor the adequacy of ventilation. Since many infants appear to "acquire" awake hypoventilation at 2–3 years of age when the natural decrease in respiratory frequency occurs, toddlers in this age group must be closely monitored to assure adequate ventilatory support. With advancing age, physiologic assessment of oxygenation and ventilation during exercise and recovery from exercise should be performed on a routine basis. After ~ 3 years of age the child can be seen for the detailed center evaluation on an annual basis. An echocardiogram should be performed every 6 months to evaluate for right ventricular hypertrophy and pulmonary hypertension, occurring as the result of unrecognized hypoxemia. A Holter recording should be considered annually to assess for transient asystole, and especially in the event of dizziness or syncope. A bronchoscopy should be performed every 12–18 months to assess for suprastomal granulation tissue and/or adenotonsillar hypertrophy that may interfere with successful use of the Passy-Muir one-way speaking valve or mask nocturnal ventilation. Detailed developmental and ophthalmologic assessments should be performed every 12 months to verify that the child is on track and/or to provide guidance for intervention. Pulmonary function testing should be performed as needed to identify and follow the status of reactive airway disease.

XI. Long-Term Outcome

Published data show prolonged survival of children with CCHS as well as overall good quality of life (2,4,57,58). Long-term follow-up and neurodevelopmental outcome reveal a broad range of results, with a great deal of variability. Sadly, many children demonstrate findings that may be related to sequelae of intermittent hypoxemia. Thus it is difficult to determine whether neurodevelopmental outcome is related to a diffuse central nervous system process specific to CCHS or is secondary to intermittent hypoxemia. These studies of neurodevelopmental follow-up serve to emphasize the importance of early diagnosis, ongoing vigilant care in the day-to-day management of these special children with CCHS, and management in collaboration with a center with broad experience with CCHS. It should be noted that with meticulous management, several of the children with CCHS have demonstrated excellent neurodevelopmental outcome.

XII. Key to the Successful Management of the Child with CCHS

Management of CCHS requires a cooperative and diligent effort on the part of the parents and other family members, home health care personnel, and referring physicians. With an increasing awareness of the disease entity, patients will be recognized and referred earlier than in the past. With earlier diagnosis and referral to centers with known expertise in the management and research of CCHS, vigilant management of ventilation, and rigorous efforts to support an age-appropriate and progressively independent lifestyle, the outcome for these children is encouraging.

Because these patients are not like other children on home ventilators, they must be managed with extreme vigilance owing to their lack of responsiveness to hypoxemia and hypercarbia. Likewise, these patients are not like normal children with adequate responses to exercise and infection. Special consideration with regard to normal childhood activities and infections must be considered in their management. Guided by maximally conservative management, these children should be participating in noncontact sports with a moderate level of activity and frequent rest periods; they should not be swimming, even in those cases where the tracheostomy has been removed. Recalling that they do not perceive the challenges of hypoxemia and hypercarbia even with adequate awake ventilation, these children with CCHS will likely swim farther and longer than their friends without sensing their physiologic compromise (hypoxemia, hypercarbia, and acidosis). Infection is another key area where children with CCHS will differ from the non-CCHS ventilator-dependent child. Children with CCHS do not typically increase their respiratory rate or have dyspnea in response to pneumonia. The absence of these symptoms does not preclude severe respiratory compromise. Likewise, they rarely develop a fever in spite of an infection. These limitations emphasize the importance of three key factors:

1. The objective measures of hemoglobin saturation and end tidal carbon dioxide by noninvasive monitoring in the home

2. Highly skilled and consistent caretakers in the home
3. The need for ongoing care by a center with known expertise in CCHS allowing for close supervision of each child.

Early intervention is clearly in the best interest of the child, the family, and the health care provider with the goals of optimal neurodevelopmental outcome balanced with a satisfactory quality of life.

XIII. Limitations to Optimal Care for the Child with CCHS

The diagnosis of CCHS is often delayed because the practitioners may never have seen a case. Further, ongoing care may be inappropriately commensurate with a chronically ventilated child without attention to the unique needs of the child with CCHS. Finally, limitations of financial resources imposed by health care providers often prevent these children from receiving optimal evaluation and long-term care in pediatric referral centers that have expertise in CCHS from both the diagnostic and treatment perspectives, and have the interest and expertise to provide and/or coordinate the long term follow-up. The introduction of a written statement from the ATS has increased the knowledge base of the practitioner, minimized delays in diagnosis, standardized the initial evaluation and subsequent management, and will hopefully optimize the outcome of these special children by tailoring their care to their individual needs.

References

1. Weese-Mayer DE, Shannon DC, Keens TG, Silvestri JM. American Thoracic Society statement on the diagnosis and management of idiopathic congenital central hypoventilation syndrome. Am J Respir Crit Care Med 1999; 160:368–373.
2. Weese-Mayer DE, Silvestri JM, Menzies LJ, Morrow-Kenny AS, Hunt CE, Hauptman SA. Congenital central hypoventilation syndrome: diagnosis, management, and long-term outcome in thirty-two children. J Pediatr 1992; 120:381–387.
3. Fleming PJ, Cade D, Bryan MH, Bryan AC. Congenital central hypoventilation and sleep state. Pediatrics 1980; 66(3):425–428.
4. Oren J, Kelly DH, Shannon DC. Long-term follow-up of children with congenital central hypoventilation syndrome. Pediatrics 1987; 80(3):375–380.
5. Coleman M, Boros SJ, Huseby TL, Brennom WS. Congenital central hypoventilation syndrome. Arch Dis Child 1980; 55:901–903.
6. Deonna T, Arczynska W, Torrado A. Congenital failure of automatic ventilation (Ondine's curse). J Pediatr 1974; 84(5):710–714.
7. Guilleminault C, McQuitty J, Ariagno RL, Challamel MJ, Korobkin R, McClead RE Jr. Congenital central alveolar hypoventilation syndrome in six infants. Pediatrics 1982; 70(5):684–694.

8. Haddad GG, Mazza NM, Defendini R, Blanc WA, Driscoll JM, Epstein MAF, Epstein RA, Mellins RB. Congenital failure of automatic control of ventilation, gastrointestinal motility and heart rate. Medicine 1978; 57(6):517–526.

9. Hunt CE, Matalon SV, Thompson TR, Demuth S, Loew JM, Liu HM, Mastri A, Burke B. Central hypoventilation syndrome. Experience with bilateral phrenic nerve pacing in 3 neonates. Am Rev Respir Dis 1978; 118:23–28.

10. Khalifa MM, Flavin MA, Wherrett BA. Congenital central hypoventilation syndrome in monozygotic twins. J Pediatr 1988; 113(5):853–855.

11. Liu HM, Loew JM, Hunt CE. Congenital central hypoventilation syndrome: a pathological study of the neuromuscular system. Neurology 1978; 28:1013–1019.

12. Mellins RB, Balfour HH Jr, Turino GM, Winters RW. Failure of automatic control of ventilation (Ondine's curse). Medicine 1970; 49(6):487–504.

13. Ruth V, Pesonen E, Raivio KO. Congenital central hypoventilation syndrome treated with diaphragm pacing. Acta Paediatr Scand 1983; 72:295–297.

14. Shannon DC, Marsland DW, Gould JB, Callahan B, Todres ID, Dennis J. Central hypoventilation during quiet sleep in two infants. Pediatrics 1976; 57(3):342–346.

15. Wells HH, Kattwinkel J, Morrow JD. Control of ventilation in Ondine's curse. J Pediatr 1980; 96(5):865–867.

16. Bower RJ, Adkins JC. Ondine's curse and neurocristopathy. Clin Pediatr 1980; 19(10):665–668.

17. Minutillo C, Pemberton PJ, Goldblatt J. Hirschsprung's disease and Ondine's curse: further evidence for a distinct syndrome. Clin Genet 1989; 36:200–203.

18. Nattie EE, Bartlett D Jr, Rozycki AA. Central alveolar hypoventilation in a child: an evaluation using a whole body plethysmograph. Am Rev Respir Dis 1975; 112:259–266.

19. Paton JY, Swaminathan S, Sargent CW, Keens TG. Hypoxic and hypercapnic ventilatory responses in awake children with congenital central hypoventilation syndrome. Am Rev Respir Dis 1989; 140:368–372.

20. Hamilton J, Bodurtha JN. Congenital central hypoventilation syndrome and Hirschsprung's disease in half sibs. J Med Genet 1989; 26:272–274.

21. O'Dell K, Staren SE, Bassuk A. Total colonic aganglionosis (Zuelzer-Wilson syndrome) and congenital failure of automatic control of ventilation (Ondine's curse). J Pediatr Surg 1987; 22:1019–1020.

22. Stern M, Erttmann R, Hellwege HH, Kuhn N. Total aganglionosis of the colon and Ondine's curse (letter to editor). Lancet 1980; April:877–878.

23. Weese-Mayer DE, Brouillette RT, Naidich TP, McClone DG, Hunt CE. Magnetic resonance imaging and computerized tomography in central hypoventilation. Am Rev Respir Dis 1988; 137:393–398.

24. Mukhopadhyay, S, Wilkinson PW. Cerebral arteriovenous malformation, Ondine's curse and Hirschsprung's disease. Dev Med Child Neurol 1990; 32:1087–1089.

25. Verloes A, Elmer C, Lacombe D, Heinrichs C, Rebuffat E, Demarquez JL, Moncla A, Adam E. Ondine–Hirschsprung syndrome (Haddad syndrome). Further delineation in two cases and review of the literature. Eur J Pediatr 1993; 152:75–77.

26. Swaminathan S, Gilsanz V, Atkinson J, Keens TG. Congenital central hypoventilation syndrome associated with multiple ganglioneuromas. Chest 1989; 96:423–424.

27. Woo MS, Woo MA, Gozal D, Jansen MT, Keens, TG, Harper RM. Heart rate variability in congenital central hypoventilation syndrome. Pediatr Res 1992; 31:291–296.
28. Ogawa T, Kojo M, Fukushima N, Sonoda H, Goto K, Ishawa S, Ishiguro M. Cardio-respiratory control in an infant with Ondine's curse: a multivariate autoregressive modeling approach. J Autonom Nerv Syst 1993; 42:41–52.
29. Silvestri JM, Hanna BD, Volgman AS, Jones JP, Barnes SD, Weese-Mayer DE. Cardiac rhythm disturbances among children with idiopathic congenital central hypoventilation syndrome. Pediatr Pulmonol 2000; 29:351–358.
30. Goldberg DS, Ludwig IH. Congenital central hypoventilation syndrome: ocular findings in 37 children. J Pediatr Ophthalmol Strabismus 1996; 33:176–181.
31. Shea SA, Andres LP, Paydarfar D, Banzett RB, Shannon DC. Effect of mental activity on breathing in congenital central hypoventilation syndrome. Respir Physiol 1993; 94:251–263.
32. Shea SA, Andres LP, Shannon DC, Banzett RB. Ventilatory responses to exercise in humans lacking ventilatory chemosensitivity. J Physiol 1993; 468:623–640.
33. Paton JY, Swaminathan S, Sargent CW, Hawksworth A, Keens TG. Ventilatory response to exercise in children with congenital central hypoventilation syndrome. Am Rev Respir Dis 1993; 147:1185–1191.
34. Silvestri JM, Weese-Mayer DE, Flanagan EA. Congenital central hypoventilation syndrome: cardiorespiratory responses to moderate exercise, simulating daily activity. Pediatr Pulmonol 1995; 20(2):89–93.
35. Pine DS, Weese-Mayer DE, Silvestri JM, Davies M, Whitaker AH, Klein DF. Anxiety and congenital central hypoventilation syndrome. Am J Psychiatry 1994; 151:864–870.
36. Commare MC, François B, Estournet B, Barois A. Ondine's curse: a discussion of five cases. Neuropediatrics 1993; 24:313–318.
37. Weese-Mayer DE, Silvestri JM, Huffman AD, Smok-Pearsall SM, Kowal MH, Maher BS, Cooper ME, Marazita ML. Case-control family study of ANS dysfunction in idiopathic congenital central hypoventilation syndrome. Am J Med Genet 2001; 100:237–245.
38. Bolande RP. The neurocristopathies a unifying concept of disease arising in neural crest maldevelopment. Hum Pathol 1974; 5:409–429.
39. Angrist M, Bolk S, Thiel B, Puffenberger EG, Hofstra R, Buys H, Cass D, Chakravarti A. Mutation analysis of the RET receptor tyrosine kinase in Hirsch-sprung disease. Hum Mol Genet 1995; 4:821–830.
40. Attié T, Pelet A, Edery P, Eng C, Mulligan LM, Amiel J, Boutrand L, Beldjord C, Nihoul-Fékété C, Munnich A, Ponder BAJ, Lyonnet S. Diversity of RET proto-oncogene mutations in familial and sporadic Hirschsprung disease. Hum Mol Genet 1995; 4:1381–1386.
41. Puffenberger EG, Hosoda K, Washington SS, Nakao K, de Wit D, Yanagisawa N, Chakravarti A. A missense mutation of the endothelin-B receptor gene in multigenic Hirschsprung's disease. Cell 1994; 79:1257–1266.
42. Attié T, Till M, Pelet A, Amiel J, Edery P, Boutrand L, Munnich A, Lyonnet S. Mutation of the endothelin-receptor B gene in the Waardenburg-Hirschsprung disease. Hum Mol Genet 1995; 4:2407–2409.

43. Edéry P, Attié T, Amiel J, Pelet A, Eng C, Hofstra RMW, Bidaud C, Lyonnet S. Mutation of the endothelin-3 gene in the Waardenburg- Hirschsprung disease. Nat Genet 1996; 12:442–444.

44. Amiel J, Attié T, Jan D, Pelet A, Edery P, Bidaud C, Lacombe D, Tam P, Simeoni J, Flori E, Nihoul-Fékété C, Munnich A, Lyonnet S. Heterozygous endothelin receptor B (EDNRB) mutations in isolated Hirschsprung disease. Hum Mol Genet 1996; 5:355–357.

45. Durbec P, Marcos-Gutierrez CV, Kilkenny C, Grigoriou M, Wartiowaara K, Suvanto P, Smith D, Ponder B, Costantini F, Saarma M, Sariola H, Pachnis V. GDNF signaling through the Ret receptor tyrosine kinase. Nature 1996; 381:789–793.

46. Salomon R, Attié T, Pelet A, Bidaud C, Amiel J, Sarnacki S, Goulet C, Ricour C, Nihoul-Fékété C, Munnich A, Lyonnet S. Germline mutations of the RET ligand GDNF are not sufficient to cause Hirschsprung disease. Nat Genet 1996; 14:345–347.

47. Angrist M, Bolk S, Halushka M, Lapchak PA, Chakravarti A. Germline mutations in glial cell line–derived neurotrophic factor (GDNF) and RET in a Hirschsprung disease patient. Nat Genet 1996; 14:341–344.

48. Amiel J, Salomon R, Attié T, Pelet A, Trang H, Mokhtari M, Gaultier C, Munnich A, Lyonnet S. Mutations of the RET-GDNF signaling pathway in Ondine's curse. Am J Hum Genet 1998 62:715–717.

49. Sakai T, Wakizaka A, Matsuda H, Nirasawa Y, Itoh Y. Point mutation in exon 12 of the receptor tyrosine kinase proto-oncogene RET in Ondine–Hirschsprung syndrome. Pediatrics 1998; 101:924–926.

50. Bolk S, Angrist M, Xie J, Yanagisawa M, Silvestri JM Weese-Mayer DE, Chakravarti A. Endothelin-3 frameshift mutation in congenital central hypoventilation syndrome. Nat Genet 1996; 3:395–396.

50b. Weese-Mayer DE, Bolk S, Silvestri JM, Chakravarti A: Idiopathic congenital central hypoventilation syndrome: evaluation of brain-derived neurotrophic factor genomic DNA sequence. Am J Med Genet 107:306–310, 2002.

51. Weese-Mayer DE, Silvestri JM, Marazita ML, Hoo JJ. Congenital central hypoventilation syndrome: inheritance and relation to sudden infant death syndrome. Am J Med Genet 1993; 47:360–367.

52. Burton MD, Kawashima A, Brayer JA, Kazemi H, Shannon DC, Schuchardt A, Costantini F, Pachnis V, Kinane TB. RET proto-oncogene is important for the development of respiratory CO_2 sensitivity. J Autonom Nerv Syst 1997; 63:137–143.

53. Devriendt K, Fryns J, Naulaers G, Devlieger H, Alliet P. Neuroblastoma in a mother and congenital central hypoventilation in her daughter: variable expression of the same genetic disorder? Am J Med Genet 2000; 90:430–431.

53b. Silvestri JM, Chen ML, Weese-Mayer DE, McQuitty JM, Carveth HJ, Nielson DW, Borowitz D, Cerny F: Idiopathic congenital central hypoventilation syndrome: the next generation. Am J Med Genet 112:46–50, 2002.

54. Marazita MM, Maher BS, Cooper ME, Silvestri JM, Huffman AD, Smok-Pearsall SM, Kowal MH, Weese-Mayer DE. Genetic segregation analysis of autonomic

nervous system dysfunction in families of probands with congenital central hypoventilation syndrome. Am J Med Genet 2001; 100:229–236.

55. Weese-Mayer DE, Hunt CE, Brouillette RT, Silvestri JM. Diaphragm pacing in infants and children. J Pediatr 1992; 120(1):1–8.

56. Weese-Mayer DE, Silvestri JM, Kenny AS, Ilbawi MN, Hauptman SA, Lipton JW, Talonen PP, Garrido Garcia H, Watt JW, Exner G, Baer GA, Elefteriades JA, Peruzzi WT, Alex CG, Harlid R, Vincken W, Davis GM, Decramer M, Kuenzle C, Sæterhaug A, Schöber JG. Diaphragm pacing with a quadripolar phrenic nerve electrode: an international study. PACE 1996; 19:1311–1319.

57. Silvestri JM, Weese-Mayer DE, Nelson MN. Neuropsychologic abnormalities in children with congenital central hypoventilation syndrome. J Pediatr 1992; 120:388–393.

58. Marcus CL, Jansen MT, Poulsen MK, Keens SE, Nield TA, Lipsker LE, Keens TG. Medical and psychosocial outcome of children with congenital central hypoventilation syndrome. J Pediatr 1991; 19:888–895.

18

Regulation of Breathing in Neuromuscular Diseases

OOMMEN P. MATHEW

Brody School of Medicine at East Carolina University
Greenville, North Carolina, U.S.A.

I. Introduction

Respiratory muscle function can be affected in many ways by neuromuscular diseases, which in turn may manifest as abnormalities in mechanical output and/or in their control. These diseases can be classified as those originating in the central nervous system, at the level of the lower motor neuron, the peripheral (cranial) nerves, the neuromuscular junction, or the muscles. Hypoventilation and apnea are the most commonly manifested respiratory abnormalities; they occur primarily during sleep. Occurrences of obstructive apnea are, at least in part, due to upper airway muscles weakness, which is further aggravated by the physiological inhibition of these muscles during rapid eye movement (REM) sleep. Respiratory control abnormalities may result in central apnea. Failure to propagate the respiratory signals from the brainstem or to convert them into mechanical output due to impairment of the neural pathway or muscle function may also manifest as breathing abnormalities.

Sleep influences breathing profoundly (1,2). Inhibitory influences dominate in the neonate, especially in premature infants because of neuroanatomic constraints. Neonates spend more time in REM sleep than older children (2). The preterm infant has some distinct mechanical disadvantages to breathing, and these disadvantages are exaggerated during sleep (especially in REM sleep). Lung immaturity, poor lung compliance, residual lung disease, compliant chest wall, and decreased intercostal muscle activity contribute to this unique vulnerability. The thoracic contribution to the tidal volume is less in the newborn because the ribs are nearly horizontal and, therefore, intercostal muscles are less effective in expanding the rib cage. Furthermore, lack of rib cage mineralization reduces outward recoil and increases compliance, often resulting in paradoxical breathing during wakefulness, especially in preterm infants. Neonates are primarily abdominal breathers. Their functional residual capacity is near the closing volume. Postinspiratory activity of the diaphragm, believed to be an important mechanism for maintaining lung volume, decreases in REM sleep (3). Activities of intercostal and upper-airway muscles are also inhibited markedly (especially during REM sleep), increasing ribcage deformation; the decrease in lung volume approximates 30% (3). Changes in breathing pattern during sleep are discussed in detail in Chapter 10.

Generalized hypotonia, weakness, and feeding difficulties are common symptoms of neuromuscular diseases in neonates and infants. Signs and symptoms of respiratory distress due to neuromuscular diseases are nonspecific. These infants often exhibit tachypnea, intercostal retractions, and paradoxical breathing. A bell-shaped thorax is usually seen with the prenatal onset of the disease. The degree of respiratory abnormalities can be assessed by oxygen saturation monitoring during wakefulness and sleep, serial blood gases, pulmonary function tests, and polysomnography. Patients with diaphragmatic weakness have decreased maximal inspiratory pressures. Abdominal muscle weakness reduces maximal expiratory pressures. Vital capacity reduction also suggests respiratory muscle weakness. However, these measurements are often impractical in the neonate. In the vast majority of neuromuscular diseases, respiratory abnormalities do not manifest during the neonatal period. A detailed discussion of these disorders is beyond the scope of this chapter; readers are referred to excellent recent reviews (1,2). Focus of this chapter is on neuromuscular diseases beginning in the neonatal period; comparisons to diseases in children and adults are made when appropriate.

Progression of respiratory abnormalities in adults with neuromuscular diseases is well documented (2). Initial abnormalities, noted exclusively during REM sleep, may remain relatively stable for several years depending on the progression of the underlying disease and its complications and may progress later to involve non-REM (NREM) sleep. Respiratory abnormalities during wakefulness, such as hypercarbia, decreased mean oxygen saturation, and constitutional symptoms (fatigue, morning headache), may follow. Finally, respiratory failure ensues during wakefulness. Progression of respiratory abnormalities is less well defined in infants and children with neuromuscular diseases. The type and extent of disease clearly plays a role in this population as well.

Diaphragmatic involvement generally indicates earlier onset and greater severity (4). Neonatal respiratory failure due to neuromuscular diseases is associated with markedly increased mortality (5).

II. Central Nervous System

Neurological causes of respiratory failure and apnea in the neonate are listed in Chapters 8 and 11. Apnea of prematurity and congenital central hypoventilation syndrome are the focus of several preceding chapters. Central hypoventilation syndrome (CHS) in Arnold-Chiari malformation (ACM), a neurological disease often exhibiting neonatal respiratory abnormalities, will be highlighted in this section.

Central hypoventilation syndromes may be congenital or acquired. The differential diagnosis and workup of these disorders are discussed in Chapter 17. Idiopathic CHS and CHS associated with ACM account for the majority of congenital disorders. ACM is commonly seen in infants with myelomeningocele and hydrocephalus. The importance of folic acid supplementation before and during early pregnancy in reducing the incidence of neural tube defects is clear (6–8). The low incidence of neural tube defects in the folic acid supplemented groups probably reflects the genetically determined rate of occurrence. Both the American Academy of Pediatrics and the U.S. Public Health Service recommend that "all women capable of becoming pregnant consume 0.4 mg of folic acid daily to prevent neural tube defects" (9).

Acquired causes of hypoventilation syndromes, including encephalitis, brain tumors, rupture of vascular malformations, and cerebrovascular accidents, are rare during infancy (10). Brainstem damage can result in respiratory control abnormalities; however, the pattern depends on the site of injury and extent of the lesion (11). If the damage is associated with injury to the motor tracts, weakness of the respiratory muscles may be seen.

ACM is a congenital malformation of the hindbrain. The major features are inferior displacement of the medulla and the fourth ventricle, elongation and thinning of the lower pons and upper medulla, inferior displacement of the lower cerebellum through the foramen magnum, and a variety of bony defects of the foramen magnum, occiput, and cervical vertebra (12). Other anomalies of the CNS in these patients include hypoplasia of the falx and tentorium, low placement of the tentorium, abnormalities of the septum pellucidum, thickened interthalamic connections, and widened foramen magnum. Another common feature is impaired neuronal migration; cortical dysplasia was seen in 90% of patients in one neuropathological study, with polymicrogyria being present in nearly half (13).

Several brainstem malformations, such as defective myelination, hypoplasia of cranial nerve nuclei, and hypoplasia or aplasia of olives and basal pontine nuclei, have been documented in ACM patients (13). Congenital malformation or compression of the brainstem may cause brainstem dysfunction. Infants with ACM may exhibit clinically significant hypoventilation, obstructive apnea, stridor, and breath-holding spells (14–16). Abnormal vocal cord motion from laryngeal paralysis (17) and/or reduced pharyngeal muscle response (18) predispose these infants to obstructive apnea. Infants with stridor and obstructive apnea generally respond to reduced intracranial pressure (16,19) but the role of additional decompressive therapy is less clear (16,19–21). Some patients respond to posterior fossa decompression (20). In a group of 17 symptomatic infants with functioning ventricular shunts, upper cervical laminectomy resulted in resolution of symptoms in 15 infants (22). In a group of myelomeningocele patients, Waters et al. (23) reported five or more respiratory events per hour of sleep in nearly 20% (17/83). Nearly 40% of the patients evaluated had posterior fossa decompression prior to the study. Infants with severe symptoms are less likely to respond (16,19), suggesting an underlying malformation or irreversible damage.

Abnormal ventilatory patterns during sleep occur in infants with ACM. Central apnea, hypoventilation, and hypoxia during sleep are the typical abnormalities (20). Even the vast majority of infants without clinically apparent apnea or hypoventilation had abnormal two-channel pneumograms (24). There was no relationship between abnormalities during sleep and the neural tube defect level (24). Waters et al. (23) investigated the prevalence of sleep-disordered breathing in myelomeningocele patients. Some degree of abnormality was seen in nearly two-thirds of the patients; 20% exhibited moderate or severe abnormalities. The sleep-related respiratory abnormalities were worse during REM sleep. Sleep-disordered breathing was higher in children with brainstem malformations, scoliosis, restrictive lung disease, and spina bifida lesions at the level of the thorax or higher (23). Also, life-threatening apneic spells may occur during the transition to REM sleep in infants (25).

Ventilatory responses to hypoxia and hypercapnia have been investigated in patients with ACM (26–28). During wakefulness and sleep, ventilatory responses to hypercapnia are significantly lower in children with ACM (26). Abnormal ventilatory responses to CO_2 were observed in 60% of newborns with myelomeningocele (27) and 61% of children with spina bifida (29). A correlation between abnormal CO_2 response and brainstem dysfunction was also noted (29). In contrast, hypoxic ventilatory response was not significantly different between myelomeningocele patients with ACM and the control group (26,28). Some patients with ACM, however, had markedly low ventilatory response to hypoxia (26,28). Gozal and coworkers suggested that central chemosensitivity and central integration of chemoreceptor output are altered in ACM (28). These abnormal ventilatory responses persist into adolescence and adulthood (26). Scoliosis, low lung volume, and limited rib cage excursion can result in ventilation/perfusion mismatches, which may be further aggravated during sleep (30).

Arousal from sleep is an important defense mechanism. In the absence of intact arousal responses to hypoxia and hypercapnia, infants with hypoventilation and apnea are at an increased risk for both morbidity and mortality. Aspiration resulting from dysfunctional swallowing complicates the pulmonary problems. In children with ACM, impaired arousal responses to hypoxia and hypercarbia (31) may also result in aspiration. In one large study, ventilatory dysfunction was documented in nearly 6% infants and children with ACM (32). Two-thirds of these patients died; apnea, stridor, and/or aspiration were the primary cause of death in the majority. These findings indicate that hypoventilation and sleep-disordered breathing contribute significantly to both morbidity and mortality. A severe form of the breath-holding spell has been reported in this population. These spells occur during wakefulness, resulting in hypoxia, hypercarbia, and even sudden death (16,20). Tracheostomy does not improve these spells (16,20).

Respiratory control abnormalities in patients with myelomeningocele and ACM may be caused by abnormalities of brainstem nuclei and/or their mechanical compression. No intervention can improve the function of abnormally developed nuclei. However, relief of mechanical obstruction should be undertaken promptly, since marked improvement in symptoms has been noted in some patients following surgery (16,19,21,22). If the symptoms persist after controlling the intracranial pressure, posterior fossa decompression should be considered to prevent further damage to the brainstem. These infants need to be watched closely for hypoventilation. Chronic ventilatory assistance is often required to improve the quality of life. Continuous positive airway pressure (CPAP) and mechanical ventilation during sleep may be useful adjuncts in their management.

III. Anterior Horn Cells

Anterior horn cell diseases account for 20–25% of arthrogryposis multiplex congenita and can be divided into dysgenetic, destructive, and degenerative types (12). The dysgenetic type results from a decrease in the number or migration of neurons. The destructive type usually results from an intrauterine ischemic event. Several autosomal-recessive syndromes cause the degenerative type. During the neonatal period, spinal muscular atrophy predominates among the anterior horn cell diseases.

A. Spinal Muscular Atrophy

Spinal muscular atrophy (SMA) is an autosomal-recessive disorder involving the anterior horn cells. It is divided into three types based on the time of onset (12,33). Type 1 SMA, also known as Werdnig Hoffman disease, is the most severe. The gene defect involves the q13 region of chromosome 5 (34). DNA testing is available. Clinical signs are present at birth in nearly a third of cases and in the first 2 months in another third (35). Decreased fetal movements are reported in neonates with signs at birth or early in the neonatal period. Prenatal onset with ventilatory compromise at birth and death by 3 months is noted in a subset of these patients, and some investigators suggest type 0 designation for this group (36).

Clinical features of type I SMA include severe hypotonia, severe generalized weakness, weak cry, difficulty in sucking and swallowing, and areflexia (33). The anterior horn cells are diffusely affected in severe cases. Cranial nerves involved are VII, IX, X, XI, and XII. Diaphragmatic function is relatively preserved, whereas intercostal muscles are weak. The chest wall is often collapsed. These infants exhibit intercostal and subcostal retractions and develop partial airway obstruction during sleep. Aspiration is a frequent complication, especially among infants with cranial nerve involvement. Tube feedings are instituted to provide adequate nutrition, and tracheostomy may be needed for positive pressure breathing.

Type 1 SMA infants have progressive respiratory failure, with most dying before 2 years (12). In type 2 SMA, the onset may be delayed up to 18 months. These infants do not develop the ability to stand, and death occurs after 2 years. In type 3 SMA, symptoms begin after 18 months. These infants can stand and walk; death typically occurs in adulthood. Distinction between types 1 and 2 can be difficult, especially when marked muscle weakness develops before 6 months. Given the significant difference in clinical course and prognosis between the two types, the decision to initiate ventilatory assistance is a difficult one. Primary respiratory insufficiency, secondary to diaphragmatic involvement, is reported in a variant of infantile SMA (37).

Sleep studies performed early in the disease in infants with type 1 SMA reveal tachypnea, hypocapnia, and decreased baseline oxygen saturation (38). Children with type 2 disease may manifest hypoventilation and oxygen desaturation during sleep (39); these signs are generally not recognized initially. Respiratory failure is usually precipitated by infection (39). In at least one report on type 2 SMA, mild to moderate hypercarbia and low oxygen saturation during sleep were documented in all children (40). One child had obstructive apnea as well (40)

B. Spinal Cord Injury

Injury to the spinal cord is rare in neonates. Such injury is often associated with difficult labor and delivery. The onset of respiratory symptoms is immediate, and the severity depends on the level of the lesion; preservation of diaphragmatic function is seen in injuries below C5. There are no published polysomnographic studies in neonates with spinal cord injuries. Infants who do not die during the neonatal period usually require long-term ventilation (41).

IV. Nerves, Neuromuscular Junction, and Muscles

Muscle weakness in these disorders is due to nerve injury, neuromuscular junction abnormalities, or intrinsic disorders of muscles themselves. Diaphragmatic paralysis, transient myasthenia gravis, and myotonic dystrophy are the prototype of these disorders in the neonatal period. These infants often exhibit respiratory problems during the neonatal period.

A. Diaphragmatic Paralysis

Diaphragmatic paralysis in the neonate is almost always associated with brachial plexus injury. Phrenic nerve involvement occurs in 5–10% of cases of brachial plexus injury (12,42). Intercostal muscles are intact in these cases. The onset of symptoms is immediately after birth. These infants hypoventilate in spite of their tachypnea. With ventilatory assistance, they tend to stabilize or improve over the next several days. The clinical course is biphasic in some infants. Further deterioration in respiratory status occurs after several days or weeks owing to the development of atelectasis or infection (12). Most infants recover over the next several months (43,44). Mortality is ~10%. The vast majority of infants improve over time with expectant management, but some infants need surgical plication of the diaphragm. Expectant management is generally advocated for at least 2 months before performing surgical plication (45). The improvement of symptoms over time is related primarily to recovery of diaphragmatic function. Increased thoracic contribution to breathing from maturation of the intercostal muscles and increased stiffness of the ribcage may also help. In the rare infant with bilateral diaphragmatic involvement, respiratory failure is invariably present from birth. Nearly 50% of these infants die (43–45).

B. Neonatal Transient Myasthenia Gravis

Approximately 10% of infants born to myasthenic mothers are affected (46). In autoimmune myasthenia gravis, there is a decrease in available acetylcholine receptors at the postsynaptic membrane due to circulating antibody. The affected infants show increased levels of antiacetylcholine receptor antibody (47), which may be antifetal or antiadult. A high ratio of antifetal/antiadult antibody levels in the mother is generally predictive of neonatal transmission (48). However, host factors also play a role in the pathogenesis (12).

Most affected neonates develop clinical symptoms within the first few hours of birth, and invariably within the first 72 hours (49). Generalized muscle weakness and hypotonia are present. Feeding disturbances typically include sucking and swallowing difficulties (49). Ptosis and occulomotor problems are infrequent. On the other hand, respiratory difficulties are very common (49) and are due to respiratory muscle weakness as well as the infant's inability to handle secretions. Nearly a third of affected patients need ventilatory assistance. Polyhydraminos, pulmonary hypoplasia, and neonatal death are common in the most severely affected patients (46). The diagnosis is confirmed by demonstrating the myasthenic phenomenon on electrophysiological testing. The vast majority of infants with neonatal onset require anticholineesterase therapy for 7–10 days (46). Exchange transfusion (50,51) and high-dose intravenous immunoglobulin (52,53) have been used as adjunct therapy with variable results. The mean duration of illness is 18 days.

C. Congenital Myasthenic Syndromes

These syndromes are caused by presynaptic, synaptic, or postsynaptic abnormalities. The observed abnormalities include defects in acetylcholine synthesis, packaging, decrease in synaptic vesicles, and deficiency of acetylcholine or its receptors. Familial infantile myasthenia is a rare autosomal-recessive disorder with onset during the neonatal period (54,55). The defect involves synthesis or packaging of acetylcholine into the vesicles (55,56).

The affected infants are typically hypotonic, exhibit facial weakness, have significant feeding problems, and often require resuscitation at birth (54,55). Episodes of apnea are not uncommon. These infants generally require anticholinesterase medication. In spite of significant neonatal problems, spontaneous remission occurs in subsequent months. The disease may worsen in infancy with infection. Anticholinesterase therapy is recommended for a year to avoid apnea and sudden death (12). In general, the disease improves over time.

D. Hypermagnesemia

Hypermagnesemia in neonates is related to maternal treatment of preeclampsia with magnesium sulfate. High serum levels of magnesium can affect the function of several organ systems. Neonatal serum levels correlate well with maternal serum levels (57). High serum magnesium levels cause muscle weakness, hypotonia, and hyporeflexia (58). High levels may also depress the central nervous system. Term infants with hypermagnesemia (cord Mg level $4.15 \pm 0.74\,mg/dL$) showed no respiratory embarrassment, suggesting intact diaphragmatic function (57). However, these infants had poorer sucking and cry responses than the control infants. Their oral intake was also significantly lower. These findings suggest weakness of some skeletal muscles. Hypermagnesemia also depresses smooth muscle function, resulting in abdominal distension. Pathogenesis is impairment of presynapatic mobilization of acetylcholine (12).

Management is supportive. Hypocalcemia, if present, should be treated aggressively.

E. Congenital Myotonic Dystrophy

Congenital myotonic dystrophy is by far the most common myopathic disorder seen in the neonatal period. This is an autosomal-dominant disorder. Significant insight into this disease has been provided by molecular genetic studies (12,33,59–61). The defect is located on chromosome 19q13 involving the myotonin–protein–kinase encoding gene (61). Abnormal triplet sequence in the gene increases in length in successive generations. The gene defect alters the function of several organs since it is not tissue specific (60).

Polyhydraminos is common during pregnancy and is a sign of severe involvement of the fetus (62,63). Pregnancy may result in abortion or premature birth (33,62,64). The clinical symptoms often manifest during the first few hours and days. Severe respiratory involvement at birth may result in birth asphyxia, in which case the myopathic origin of the asphyxia is often overlooked initially. The congenital form of myotonic dystrophy has distinctive differences from that seen in adults; it is characterized by severe hypotonia rather than myotonia. Besides the generalized hypotonia and respiratory distress, these infants also exhibit feeding problems, facial diplegia, areflexia, muscle atrophy, and arthogryposis (33,62,63). The respiratory difficulties are due to respiratory muscles weakness and difficulty handling secretions due to impaired swallowing. Hypotonia and facial weakness are the most common clinical manifestations in less severe cases.

Overall mortality is ~10–15%; however, it is nearly 50% in severely affected infants (12). Infants requiring ventilation for >30 days have a poor prognosis (65). Muscle strength improves in surviving infants. There is no correlation between the severity of illness during the neonatal period and the severity of illness during later life. Surviving infants almost invariably show mental retardation (33,63). Cardiac involvement is common in adult patients with myotonic dystrophy (see below). However, onset of cardiomyopathy during the neonatal period has been reported (66). Poorly developed diaphragm and pharyngeal muscles are noted at autopsy (65).

The adult (classic) form of myotonic dystrophy is caused by the same genetic defect as the neonatal form but has fewer triplet repeats. This type of myotonic dystrophy presents with muscle weakness, myotonia, and muscle wasting. These patients may also exhibit excessive sleepiness, cardiac dysrhythmias, and psychiatric problems as well as endocrine and gastrointestinal dysfunctions. The most frequent arrhythmias are atrial and ventricular extrasystoles, atrial flutter and fibrillation, and ventricular tachycardia. The mechanisms underlying ventricular arrhythmias are conduction disturbances, prolongation of the QT interval, and impaired autonomic function. Cognitive function is often normal

(67). Some of these patients are prone to develop malignant hyperthermia, which may result in postoperative respiratory failure and even sudden death (68,69).

Unlike in the neonatal form, more data on respiratory function abnormalities are available in patients with the classic form of myotonic dystrophy. Pulmonary function tests in these patients show a decrease in maximal voluntary ventilation, decrease in vital capacity, and elevated awake CO_2 levels (70–72). Decreased maximal voluntary ventilation suggests inspiratory muscle weakness. Higher transdiaphragmatic pressures that were observed during normal breathing are attributed to expiratory muscle myotonia (73). However, in other studies, myotonia of the respiratory muscles was observed only at higher ventilation levels (74). Decreased vital capacity and decreased inspiratory and expiratory pressures indicate a restrictive abnormality (72).

Alveolar hypoventilation and sleep-disordered breathing are documented in this population (70). The available evidence suggests that hypoventilation in myotonic dystrophy is probably caused by diaphragmatic weakness. However, an impairment of conduction in the respiratory motor pathways occurs in some patients (75). Sleep apnea is a common finding in these patients. A potential mechanism for sleep apnea (76) involves muscle weakness during the neonatal period, which limits the growth of the mandible and face, resulting in a small airway. An increased apnea index and oxygen desaturation are seen during sleep in young adults with myotonic dystrophy (70). Sleep-disordered breathing evidenced by increased apnea/hypopnea index was also reported by Veale and coworkers. Irregular breathing pattern, present during wakefulness, is not observed during slow wave sleep, suggesting there is no underlying central control abnormality in the medulla (72). An intact central drive and a normal afferent limb are suggested by other studies as well (77). Central apneas occur in all sleep stages (78). Obstructive apnea is less frequent. Hypoxic and hypercapneic responses are abnormal (2).

F. Congenital Muscular Dystrophy

Congenital muscular dystrophy is a group of disorders with common clinical and myopathological features (12,79,80). Typically they are divided into two types: those with only myopathy, and those with myopathy and CNS involvement. Among the former, often termed classic, or merosin-positive muscular dystrophy, the common symptoms are hypotonia; weakness involving the face, trunk, and proximal limbs; and contractures (12,81). Respiratory difficulty and dysphagia are less frequent (81). Involvement of diaphragm and intercostal muscles occurs later in infancy and childhood (82). Although the severity of hypotonia and weakness is greater in the subgroup of myopathic infants with CNS involvement, ventilatory problems are not common during the neonatal period.

Histologically the myopathies include central core disease and nemaline, myotubular, mitochondrial, metabolic, and other specific congenital myopathies. Myopathies with neonatal respiratory abnormalities will be highlighted here. In central core disease, respiratory difficulties are unlikely during the neonatal period. In the more common form of nemaline myopathy, weakness and hypotonia are not prominent features (83–85). However, in the less common form, marked hypotonia, weakness, and severe respiratory problems are the norm (12,84,86). These infants may need resuscitation at birth. Weakness of the respiratory muscles predisposes these infants to respiratory failure requiring ventilatory assistance. Some infants die during the neonatal period or early in infancy (5,87,88). The most common defect involves nebulin on chromosome 2, whereas the clinically severe disease has a defect of alpha-actin on chromosome 1 (89–91). Two forms of myotubular myopathy have been described. Again, the common form is the milder one; the less common form is the more severe, with marked hypotonia and respiratory failure (89,92–94). Polyhydraminos, decreased fetal movements, and birth asphyxia are commonly observed (95). The gene defect has been linked to Xq28 (96,97), which encodes myotubularin.

In older children, pulmonary function tests reveal a reduced vital capacity consistent with restrictive lung diseases (98–100). These patients developed apnea and marked oxygen desaturation during sleep. Improvement in symptoms was noted following positive pressure ventilation.

Mitochondrial myopathies result from primary abnormalities of mitochondrial structure and function (12). Biochemically, mitochondrial myopathies can be divided into defects of substrate utilization, oxidation-phosphorylation coupling, and defects of the respiratory chain. Respiratory chain disturbances typically manifest during the neonatal period. Cytochrome-c oxidase deficiency accounts for the majority of neonatal disorders and is inherited as an autosomal-recessive disorder. Common neonatal signs are hypotonia, lethargy, feeding and respiratory difficulties, failure to thrive, psychomotor delay, seizures, and vomiting. Lactic acidosis is a distinct feature of cytochrome-c oxidase deficiency. Laboratory studies show increased levels of lactate, an increased lactate/pyruvate ratio, hypoglycemia, and elevated ketone bodies. Respiratory failure is often seen during the neonatal period, with death occurring in the first year of life (101,102). A benign form of the diseases has also been reported (103,104).

V. Summary

The vast majority of neuromuscular diseases become clinically apparent beyond the neonatal period. However, diseases that manifest during this period, regardless of etiology, have some common characteristics. These include generalized hypotonia, muscle weakness, and feeding difficulties. The most severely affected infants often require resuscitation at birth and may even exhibit contractures. Mortality in this group of infants is significant. The surviving infants are particularly vulnerable to develop hypoxia and hypercapnia during sleep, and polysomnography is useful in assessing the severity of the disease. Pulmonary functions tests have very limited value. Supportive care is the only available treatment option.

References

1. Loughlin GM, Carroll JL, Marcus CL, eds. Sleep and Breathing in Children, Vol 147. New York: Marcel Dekker, 2000.
2. Saunders NA, Sullivan CE, eds. Sleep and Breathing, 2nd ed, Vol 71. New York: Marcel Dekker, 1994.
3. Henderson-Smart DJ, Read DJ. Reduced lung volume during behavioral active sleep in the newborn. J Appl Physiol 1979; 46(6):1081–1085.
4. Sivan Y, Galvis A. Early diaphragmatic paralysis. In infants with genetic disorders. Clin Pediatr (Phila) 1990; 29(3):169–171.
5. Martinez BA, Lake BD. Childhood nemaline myopathy: a review of clinical presentation in relation to prognosis. Dev Med Child Neurol 1987; 29(6):815–820.
6. Laurence KM, James N, Miller MH, Tennant GB, Campbell H. Double-blind randomised controlled trial of folate treatment before conception to prevent recurrence of neural-tube defects. Br Med J (Clin Res Ed) 1981; 282(6275):1509–1511.
7. Smithells RW, Sheppard S, Schorah CJ, Seller MJ, Nevin NC, Harris R, Read AP, Fielding DW. Possible prevention of neural-tube defects by periconceptional vitamin supplementation. Lancet 1980; 1(8164):339–340.
8. MRC Vitamin Study Research Group. Prevention of neural tube defects: results of the Medical Research Council Vitamin Study. Lancet 1991; 338(8760):131–137.
9. American Academy of Pediatrics. Committee on Genetics. Folic acid for the prevention of neural tube defects. Pediatrics 1999; 104(2 Pt 1):325–327.
10. Beckerman RC, Hunt CE. In: Beckerman RCD, Brouillette RT, Hunt CE, eds. Respiratory Control Disorders in Infants and Children. Baltimore: Williams and Wilkins, 1992:251–270.
11. Keens TG, Ward SLD. Syndromes affecting respiratory control during sleep. In: Loughlin GM, Carroll JL, Marcus CL, eds. Sleep and Breathing in Children, Vol 147. New York: Marcel Dekker, 2000:525–553.
12. Volpe JJ. Neurology of the Newborn. 4th ed. Philadelphia: W.B. Saunders, 2001.
13. Gilbert JN, Jones KL, Rorke LB, Chernoff GF, James HE. Central nervous system anomalies associated with meningomyelocele, hydrocephalus, and the Arnold-Chiari malformation: reappraisal of theories regarding the pathogenesis of posterior neural tube closure defects. Neurosurgery 1986; 18(5):559–564.
14. Fitzsimmons JS. Laryngeal stridor and respiratory obstruction associated with meningomyelocele. Arch Dis Child 1965; 40(214):687–688.

15. Hesz N. Vocal-cord paralysis and brainstem dysfunction in children with spina bifida. Dev Med Child Neurol 1985; 27(4):528–531.
16. Cochrane DD, Adderley R, White CP, Norman M, Steinbok P. Apnea in patients with myelomeningocele. Pediatr Neurosurg 1990–91; 16(4–5):232–239.
17. Ruff ME, Oakes WJ, Fisher SR, Spock A. Sleep apnea and vocal cord paralysis secondary to type I Chiari malformation. Pediatrics 1987; 80(2):231–234.
18. Doherty MJ, Spence DP, Young C, Calverley PM. Obstructive sleep apnoea with Arnold-Chiari malformation. Thorax 1995; 50(6):690–691.
19. Charney EB, Rorke LB, Sutton LN, Schut L. Management of Chiari II complications in infants with myelomeningocele. J Pediatr 1987; 111(3):364–371.
20. Oren J, Kelly DH, Todres ID, Shannon DC. Respiratory complications in patients with myelodysplasia and Arnold-Chiari malformation. Am J Dis Child 1986; 140(3):221–224.
21. Kirk VG, Morielli A, Gozal D, Marcus CL, Waters KA, D'Andrea LA, Rosen CL, Deray MJ, Brouillette RT. Treatment of sleep-disordered breathing in children with myelomeningocele. Pediatr Pulmonol 2000; 30(6):445–452.
22. Vandertop WP, Asai A, Hoffman HJ, Drake JM, Humphreys RP, Rutka JT, Becker LE. Surgical decompression for symptomatic Chiari II malformation in neonates with myelomeningocele. J Neurosurg 1992; 77(4):541–544.
23. Waters KA, Forbes P, Morielli A, Hum C, O'Gorman AM, Vernet O, Davis GM, Tewfik TL, Ducharme FM, Brouillette RT. Sleep-disordered breathing in children with myelomeningocele. J Pediatr 1998; 132(4):672–681.
24. Ward SL, Jacobs RA, Gates EP, Hart LD, Keens TG. Abnormal ventilatory patterns during sleep in infants with myelomeningocele. J Pediatr 1986; 109(4):631–634.
25. Wealthall SR, Whittaker GE, Greenwood N. The relationship of apnoea and stridor in spina bifida to other unexplained infant deaths. Dev Med Child Neurol 1974; 16(6 suppl 32):107–116.
26. Swaminathan S, Paton JY, Ward SL, Jacobs RA, Sargent CW, Keens TG. Abnormal control of ventilation in adolescents with myelodysplasia. J Pediatr 1989; 115(6):898–903.
27. Petersen MC, Wolraich M, Sherbondy A, Wagener J. Abnormalities in control of ventilation in newborn infants with myelomeningocele. J Pediatr 1995; 126(6):1011–1015.
28. Gozal D, Arens R, Omlin KJ, Jacobs RA, Keens TG. Peripheral chemoreceptor function in children with myelomeningocele and Arnold-Chiari malformation type 2. Chest 1995; 108(2):425–431.
29. Worley G, Oakes WJ, Spock A. CO_2 response test in children with spina bifida. Am Acad Cereb Palsy Dev Med 1985; 40A.
30. Carstens C, Paul K, Niethard FU, Pfeil J. Effect of scoliosis surgery on pulmonary function in patients with myelomeningocele. J Pediatr Orthop 1991; 11(4):459–464.
31. Ward SL, Nickerson BG, Van der Hal A, Rodriguez AM, Jacobs RA, Keens TG. Absent hypoxic and hypercapneic arousal responses in children with myelomeningocele and apnea. Pediatrics 1986; 78(1):44–50.
32. Hays RM, Jordan RA, McLaughlin JF, Nickel RE, Fisher LD. Central ventilatory dysfunction in myelodysplasia: an independent determinant of survival. Dev Med Child Neurol 1989; 31(3):366–370.

33. Dubowitz V. Muscle Disorders in Childhood. Philadelphia; W.B. Saunders, 1995.
34. Morrison KE. Advances in SMA research: review of gene deletions. Neuromuscul Disord 1996; 6:397–408.
35. Thomas NH, Dubowitz V. The natural history of type I (severe) spinal muscular atrophy. Neuromuscul Disord 1994; 4(5–6):497–502.
36. Dubowitz V. Very severe spinal muscular atrophy (SMA type 0): an expanding clinical phenotype. Eur J Paediatr Neurol 1999; 3(2):49–51.
37. Novelli G, Capon F, Tamisari L, Grandi E, Angelini C, Guerrini P, Dallapiccola B. Neonatal spinal muscular atrophy with diaphragmatic paralysis is unlinked to 5q11.2-q13. J Med Genet 1995; 32(3):216–219.
38. Given DC. Sleep and breathing in children with neuromuscular disease In: Loughlin GM, Carroll JL, Marcus CL, eds. Sleep and Breathing in Children, Vol 147. New York: Marcel Dekker, 2000:691–735.
39. Bach JR, Wang TG. Noninvasive long-term ventilatory support for individuals with spinal muscular atrophy and functional bulbar musculature. Arch Phys Med Rehabil 1995; 76(3):213–217.
40. Canani SF, Given D, Weibke J, Eigan H. Does nasal positive pressure ventilation improvepulmonary function in patients with non-progressive neuromuscular disease? Am J Respir Crit Care Med 1997; 155:A709.
41. MacKinnon JA, Perlman M, Kirpalani H, Rehan V, Sauve R, Kovacs L. Spinal cord injury at birth: diagnostic and prognostic data in twenty-two patients. J Pediatr 1993; 122(3):431–437.
42. Eng GD. Brachial plexus palsy in newborn infants. Pediatrics 1971; 48(1):18–28.
43. Greene W, L'Heureux P, Hunt CE. Paralysis of the diaphragm. Am J Dis Child 1975; 129(12):1402–1405.
44. Zifko U, Hartmann M, Girsch W, Zoder G, Rokitansky A, Grisold W, Lischka A. Diaphragmatic paresis in newborns due to phrenic nerve injury. Neuropediatrics 1995; 6(5):281–284.
45. Aldrich TK, Herman JH, Rochester DF. Bilateral diaphragmatic paralysis in the newborn infant. J Pediatr 1980; 97(6):988-991.
46. Papazian O. Transient neonatal myasthenia gravis. J Child Neurol 1992; 7(2):135–141.
47. Keesey J, Lindstrom J, Cokely H. Anti-acetylcholine receptor antibody in neonatal myasthenia gravis. N Engl J Med 1977; 296(1):55.
48. Gardnerova M, Eymard B, Morel E, Faltin M, Zajac J, Sadovsky O, Tripon P, Domergue M, Vernet–Der Garabedian B, Bach JF. The fetal/adult acetylcholine receptor antibody ratio in mothers with myasthenia gravis as a marker for transfer of the disease to the newborn. Neurology 1997; 48(1):50–54.
49. Namba T, Brown SB, Grob D. Neonatal myasthenia gravis: report of two cases and review of the literature. Pediatrics 1970; 45(3):488–504.
50. Pasternak JF, Hageman J, Adams MA, Philip AG, Gardner TH. Exchange transfusion in neonatal myasthenia. J Pediatr 1981; 99(4):644–646.
51. Donat JF, Donat JR, Lennon VA. Exchange transfusion in neonatal myasthenia gravis. Neurology 1981; 31(7):911–912.

52. Tagher RJ, Baumann R, Desai N. Failure of intravenously administered immuno-globulin in the treatment of neonatal myasthenia gravis. J Pediatr 1999; 134(2):233–235.

53. Bassan H, Spirer Z. Intravenous immunoglobulin in neonatal myasthenia gravis. J Pediatr 1999; 135(6):790.

54. Engel AG. Congenital myasthenic syndromes. J Child Neurol 1988; 3(4):233–246.

55. Misulis KE, Fenichel GM. Genetic forms of myasthenia gravis. Pediatr Neurol 1989; 5:205–210.

56. Mora M, Lambert EH, Engel AG. Synaptic vesicle abnormality in familial infantile myasthenia. Neurology 1987; 37(2):206–214.

57. Rasch DK, Huber PA, Richardson CJ, L'Hommedieu CS, Nelson TE, Reddi R. Neurobehavioral effects of neonatal hypermagnesemia. J Pediatr 1982; 100(2):272–276.

58. Lipsitz PJ. The clinical and biochemical effects of excess magnesium in the newborn. Pediatrics 1971; 47(3):501–509.

59. Shelbourne P, Davies J, Buxton J, et al. Direct diagnosis of myotonic dystrophy with a disease-specific DNA marker. N Engl J Med 1993; 328(7):471–475.

60. Ptacek LJ, Johnson KJ, Griggs RC. Genetics and physiology of the myotonic muscle disorders. N Engl J Med 1993; 328(7):482–489.

61. Tsilfidis C, MacKenzie AE, Mettler G, Barcelo J, Korneluk RG. Correlation between CTG trinucleotide repeat length and frequency of severe congenital myotonic dystrophy. Nat Genet 1992; 1(3):192–195.

62. Pearse RG, Howeler CJ. Neonatal form of dystrophia myotonica. Five cases in preterm babies and a review of earlier reports. Arch Dis Child 1979; 54(5):331–338.

63. Hageman AT, Gabreels FJ, Liem KD, Renkawek K, Boon JM. Congenital myotonic dystrophy; a report on thirteen cases and a review of the literature. J Neurol Sci 1993; 115(1):95–101.

64. Rudnik-Schoneborn S, Nicholson GA, Morgan G, Rohrig D, Zerres K. Different patterns of obstetric complications in myotonic dystrophy in relation to the disease status of the fetus. Am J Med Genet 1998; 80(4):314–321.

65. Rutherford MA, Heckmatt JZ, Dubowitz V. Congenital myotonic dystrophy: respiratory function at birth determines survival. Arch Dis Child 1989; 64(2):191–195.

66. Igarashi H, Momoi MY, Yamagata T, Shiraishi H, Eguchi I. Hypertrophic cardiomyopathy in congenital myotonic dystrophy. Pediatr Neurol 1998; 18(4):366–369.

67. Tuikka RA, Laaksonen RK, Somer HV. Cognitive function in myotonic dystrophy: a follow-up study. Eur Neurol 1993; 33(6):436–441.

68. Reardon W, Newcombe R, Fenton I, Sibert J, Harper PS. The natural history of congenital myotonic dystrophy: mortality and long term clinical aspects. Arch Dis Child 1993; 68(2):177–181.

69. Alberts MJ, Roses AD. Myotonic muscular dystrophy. Neurol Clin 1989; 7(1):1–8.

70. Guilleminault C, Cummiskey J, Motta J, Lynne-Davies P. Respiratory and hemo-dynamic study during wakefulness and sleep in myotonic dystrophy. Sleep 1978; 1(1):19–31.

71. Kilburn KH, Eagan JT, Seiker HO, Heyman A. Cardiopulmonary insufficiency in myotonic and progressive muscular dystrophy. N Engl J Med 1959; 261:1089–1096.

72. Veale D, Cooper BG, Gilmartin JJ, Walls TJ, Griffith CJ, Gibson GJ. Breathing pattern awake and asleep in patients with myotonic dystrophy. Eur Respir J 1995; 8(5):815–818.

73. Begin R, Bureau MA, Lupien L, Bernier JP, Lemieux B. Pathogenesis of respiratory insufficiency in myotonic dystrophy: the mechanical factors. Am Rev Respir Dis 1982; 125(3):312– 318.

74. Rimmer KP, Golar SD, Lee MA, Whitelaw WA. Myotonia of the respiratory muscles in myotonic dystrophy. Am Rev Respir Dis 1993; 148(4 Pt 1):1018– 1022.

75. Zifko UA, Hahn AF, Remtulla H, George CF, Wihlidal W, Bolton CF. Central and peripheral respiratory electrophysiological studies in myotonic dystrophy. Brain 1996; 119(Pt 6):1911–1922.

76. Culebras A. Sleep and neuromuscular disorders. Neurol Clin 1996; 14(4):791–805.

77. Clague JE, Carter J, Coakley J, Edwards RH, Calverley PM. Respiratory effort perception at rest and during carbon dioxide rebreathing in patients with dystrophia myotonica. Thorax 1994; 49(3):240–244.

78. Cirignotta F, Mondini S, Zucconi M, Barrot-Cortes E, Sturani C, Schiavina M, Coccagna G, Lugaresi E. Sleep-related breathing impairment in myotonic dystrophy. J Neurol 1987; 235(2):80–85.

79. Voit T. Congenital muscular dystrophies: 1997 update. Brain Dev 1998; 20(2):65–74.

80. Parano E, Pavone L, Fiumara A, Falsaperla R, Trifiletti RR, Dobyns WB. Congenital muscular dystrophies: clinical review and proposed classification. Pediatr Neurol 1995; 13(2):97–103.

81. Kobayashi O, Hayashi Y, Arahata K, Ozawa E, Nonaka I. Congenital muscular dystrophy: clinical and pathologic study of 50 patients with the classical (Occidental) merosin-positive form. Neurology 1996; 46(3):815–818.

82. McMenamin JB, Becker LE, Murphy EG. Congenital muscular dystrophy: a clinicopathologic report of 24 cases. J Pediatr 1982; 100(5):692–697.

83. Wallgren-Pettersson C, Pelin K, Hilpela P, Donner K, Porfirio B, Graziano C, Swoboda KJ, Fardeau M, Urtizberea JA, Muntoni F, Sewry C, Dubowitz V, Iannaccone S, Minetti C, Pedemonte M, Seri M, Cusano R, Lammens M, Castagna-Sloane A, Beggs AH, Laing NG, De la Chapelle A. Clinical and genetic heterogeneity in autosomal recessive nemaline myopathy. Neuromuscul Disord 1999; 9(8):564–572.

84. Wallgren-Pettersson C. Congenital myopathies. Eur J Paediatr Neurol 2001; 5(2):87–88.

85. North KN, Laing NG, Wallgren-Pettersson C. Nemaline myopathy: current concepts. The ENMC International Consortium and Nemaline Myopathy. J Med Genet 1997; 34(9):705–713.

86. Sasaki M, Takeda M, Kobayashi K, Nonaka I. Respiratory failure in nemaline myopathy. Pediatr Neurol 1997; 16(4):344–346.

87. Shahar E, Tervo RC, Murphy EG. Heterogeneity of nemaline myopathy. A follow-up study of 13 cases. Pediatr Neurosci 1988; 14(5):236–240.

88. Schmalbruch H, Kamieniecka Z, Arroe M. Early fatal nemaline myopathy: case report and review. Dev Med Child Neurol 1987; 29(6):800–804.

89. Wallgren-Pettersson C. Genetics of the nemaline myopathies and the myotubular myopathies. Neuromuscul Disord 1998; 8(6):401–404.

90. Sewry CA, Brown SC, Pelin K, Jungbluth H, Wallgren-Pettersson C, Labeit S, Manzur A, Muntoni F. Abnormalities in the expression of nebulin in chromosome-2 linked nemaline myopathy. Neuromuscul Disord 2001; 11(2):146–153.

91. Ilkovski B, Cooper ST, Nowak K, Ryan MM, Yang N, Schnell C, Durling HJ, Roddick LG, Wilkinson I, Kornberg AJ, Collins KJ, Wallace G, Gunning P, Hardeman EC, Laing NG, North KN. Nemaline myopathy caused by mutations in the muscle alpha-skeletal-actin gene. Am J Hum Genet 2001; 68(6):1333–1343.

92. Hung FC, Huang SC, Jong YJ. Neonatal myotubular myopathy with respiratory distress: report of a case. J Formos Med Assoc 1991; 90(9):844–847.

93. Buj-Bello A, Biancalana V, Moutou C, Laporte J, Mandel JL. Identification of novel mutations in the MTM1 gene causing severe and mild forms of X-linked myotubular myopathy. Hum Mutat 1999; 14(4):320–325.

94. Bucher HU, Boltshauser E, Briner J, Gnehm HE, Janzer RC. Severe neonatal centronuclear (myotubular) myopathy: an X-linked recessive disorder. Helv Paediatr Acta 1986; 41(4):291–300.

95. Barth PG, Van Wijngaarden GK, Bethlem J. X-linked myotubular myopathy with fatal neonatal asphyxia. Neurology 1975; 25(6):531–536.

96. Laporte J, Biancalana V, Tanner SM, Kress W, Schneider V, Wallgren-Pettersson C, Herger F, Buj-Bello A, Blondeau F, Liechti-Gallati S, Mandel JL. MTM1 mutations in X-linked myotubular myopathy. Hum Mutat 2000; 15(5):393–409.

97. Janssen EA, Hensels GW, Van Oost BA, Hamel BC, Kemp S, Baas F, Weber JW, Barth PG, Bolhuis PA. The gene for X-linked myotubular myopathy is located in an 8 Mb region at the border of Xq27.3 and Xq28. Neuromuscul Disord 1994; 4(5–6):455–461.

98. Riley DJ, Santiago TV, Daniele RP, Schall B, Edelman NH. Blunted respiratory drive in congenital myopathy. Am J Med 1977; 63(3):459–466.

99. Heckmatt JZ, Loh L, Dubowitz V. Nocturnal hypoventilation in children with nonprogressive neuromuscular disease. Pediatrics 1989; 83(2):250–255.

100. Maayan C, Springer C, Armon Y, Bar-Yishay E, Shapira Y, Godfrey S. Nemaline myopathy as a cause of sleep hypoventilation. Pediatrics 1986; 77(3):390–395.

101. DiMauro S, Mendell JR, Sahenk Z, Bachman D, Scarpa A, Scofield RM, Reiner C. Fatal infantile mitochondrial myopathy and renal dysfunction due to cytochrome-c-oxidase deficiency. Neurology 1980; 30(8):795–804.

102. Tritschler HJ, Bonilla E, Lombes A, Andreetta F, Servidei S, Schneyder B, Miranda AF, Schon EA, Kadenbach B, DiMauro S. Differential diagnosis of fatal and benign cytochrome c oxidase–deficient myopathies of infancy: an immunohistochemical approach. Neurology 1991; 41(2 Pt 1):300–305.

103. DiMauro S, Nicholson JF, Hays AP, Eastwood AB, Papadimitriou A, Koenigsberger R, DeVivo DC. Benign infantile mitochondrial myopathy due to reversible cytochrome c oxidase deficiency. Ann Neurol 1983; 14(2):226–234.

104. Zeviani M, Peterson P, Servidei S, Bonilla E, DiMauro S. Benign reversible muscle cytochrome c oxidase deficiency: a second case. Neurology. 1987; 37(1):64–67.

19

Regulation of Breathing in Acute Ventilatory Failure

ANNE GREENOUGH

Guy's, King's and St Thomas' School of Medicine and King's College Hospital
London, England

I. Introduction

During mechanical respiratory support for acute ventilatory failure, neonates may be apneic. The majority of infants, however, do exhibit respiratory activity. Distinct patterns of spontaneous respiration with positive pressure inflations can be seen (1), and generally are the result of provocation of respiratory reflexes. In this chapter, the patterns of respiratory activity, the physiological mechanisms underlying them, and the factors influencing which pattern occurs will be described. Methods of detecting respiratory activity during mechanical ventilation and their role in the management of infants with acute ventilatory failure will be discussed, and the impact of respiratory activity on the outcome of ventilated infants will be considered.

II. Respiratory Activity During Mechanical Ventilation

A. Apnea

During the acute stages of respiratory distress, apnea is uncommon except in heavily sedated and/or very immature infants. It is more likely to occur when fast rates are used, particularly when infants are supported by high-frequency oscillation (2). After the perinatal period, spontaneous respiratory activity is less common in infants who are fully supported by mechanical ventilation (3). Possible explanations include that respiratory reflexes are less likely to be provoked in older infants or in infants with compliant lungs.

B. Patterns of Respiratory Activity

Four distinct patterns have been described:
  1.   Prolongation of the spontaneous expiratory period during positive pressure inflation (Fig. 1); this is due to stimulation of the Hering Breuer inflation reflex.
  2.   Active expiration against positive pressure inflation (Fig. 2); this is also due to stimulation of the Hering Breuer inflation reflex.
  3.   Larger inspiratory effort provoked by positive pressure inflation (Fig. 3); this is due to provocation of an augmented inspiration, likened to Head's paradoxical reflex (4).

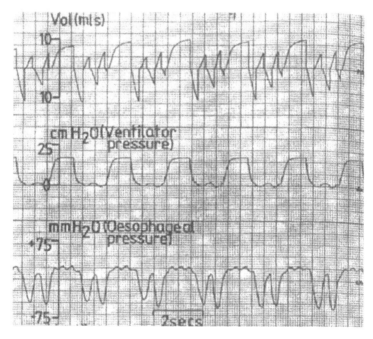

Figure 1   Hering Breuer inflation reflex. Between positive pressure inflations, the infant breathes well (note narrow negative deflections in esophageal pressure trace). Each positive pressure inflation, however, causes a brief period of apnea (flat esophageal trace during positive pressure inflation). (From Ref. 1.)

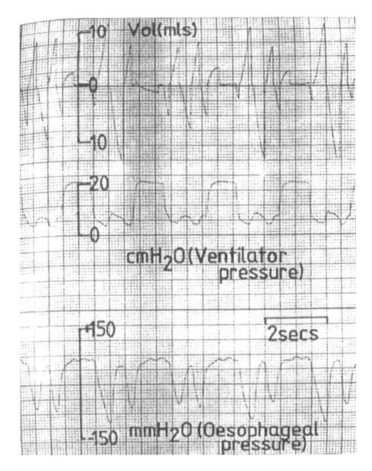

Figure 2 Active expiratory effort against positive pressure inflation. Between positive pressure inflations, the infant breathes well (narrow negative deflections in esophageal pressure tracing and large inspiratory and expiratory volume changes). Each ventilator inflation, however, is associated with a small amount of air entry into the infant's chest (upward deflection), and after this the infant is able to inhibit further air entry into the chest (resetting of integrator at zero airflow to zero during positive pressure inflation, despite maintenance of the peak pressure). During one positive pressure inflation, an active expiratory effort by the infant causes air to leave lungs (downward deflection in volume tracing) despite positive pressure inflation continuing. (From Ref. 1.)

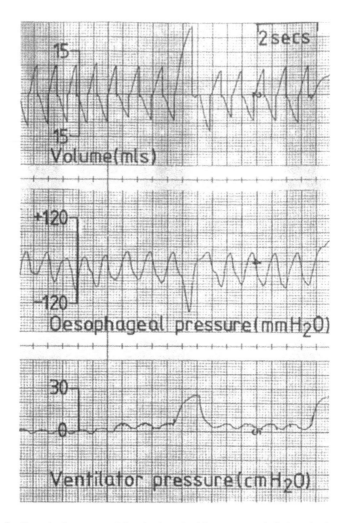

Figure 3 Provoked augmented inspiration. Positive pressure inflation (in the center of the tracing) provokes a large negative deflection in the esophageal tracing at least twice that caused by spontaneous inspiration. (From Ref. 1.)

4. Coincidence of inspiration with positive pressure inflation (Fig. 4); this interaction is described as synchrony. Infants may breathe synchronously with each or a proportion of positive pressure inflations, that is, with every second or third inflation when fast ($\geq$60 breaths/min) ventilator rates are used.

When examined during a short period of time (1), infants' respiratory patterns were persistent, provided the blood gases remained in the therapeutic

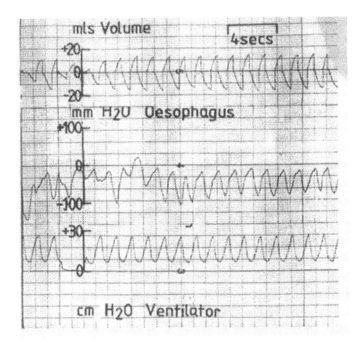

Figure 4 Synchrony. The recording shows that the baby makes a spontaneous inspiration (negative deflection in esophageal pressure tracing) synchronously with each positive pressure inflation. (From Ref. 1.)

range, the infants were not disturbed by nursing procedures, and the ventilator settings not altered (1). Usually only one respiratory pattern was seen but, on 28 of the 120 study occasions on which infants were assessed, provoked augmented inspirations occurred with one other respiratory pattern (1). Uncommonly, infants exhibit chaotic respiratory activity, which has no relationship to positive pressure inflation; this can occur when infants are hypoxic and/or hypercarbic.

III. Respiratory Reflexes

A. Hering Breuer Reflexes

Hering and Breuer (5) reported that distension of the lungs in anesthetized animals decreased the frequency of inspiration (the Hering Breuer inflation reflex), and if the inflation was prolonged, an active expiratory effort was provoked. The reflex is mediated by pulmonary slowly adapting stretch receptors, whose afferents run in the vagus nerve to the nucleus solitarius. The reflex is volume dependent; larger volume changes in early rather than late inspiration are required to halt inspiration and inhibition increases with increasing tidal volumes (6), as evidenced by the duration of the expiratory apnea being proportional to the inflating volume (7). The reflex is an important respiratory control mechanism in premature infants with immature higher centers, whereas in older children and adults it may not operate in the tidal volume range. The reflex was first demonstrated in human neonates by Cross and colleagues in 1960 (4). Bag and mask inflation of the infants' lungs provoked the reflex. Similarly, positive pressure inflations of mechanical ventilation can provoke the reflex (8). Lung inflation resulting from the application of negative pressure around the chest, as occurs during continuous negative pressure ventilation, also provokes the Hering Breuer inflation reflex, as evidenced by an increase in expiratory time (9,10).

Hering and Breuer also demonstrated that deflation of the lungs caused stronger and more frequent inspirations, the Hering and Breuer deflation reflex (5). The reflex, as evidenced by an increased respiratory rate and inspiratory force, has been reported following acute lung deflation in adult patients with pneumothoraces and in situ chest drains (11). Whether this reflex occurs in ventilated infants has not been formally tested, but it can be provoked in healthy infants by rapid lung volume reduction using an inflatable jacket (12). It has been suggested that the reflex may be of physiological importance only during exercise or coughing (13), but others (12) hypothesized that it might have a role in infancy in protecting functional residual capacity.

B. Provoked Augmented Inspirations

Head (14) described a lengthened and stronger contraction of the diaphragm on rapid inflation of the lung when vagal conduction was partially blocked (Head's paradoxical reflex). It is likely that this reflex is mediated via vagally innervated, rapidly adapting irritant receptors, which are spread throughout the epithelial cells of the trachea and bronchi, but most are in the large airways. Stimulation of these irritant receptors can augment inspiratory activity and cause coughing or rapid shallow breathing. Irritant receptor stimulation may also initiate the augmented breaths or sighs that occur periodically during normal breathing and maintain lung expansion. Cross et al. (4), using a bag and mask to inflate the lungs, were able to provoke augmented inspirations, which they likened to Head's paradoxical reflex. Positive pressure inflations during mechanical ventilation also provoke augmented inspirations (15). In the first few days after birth, augmented inspirations aid establishment of a functional residual capacity. The increase in lung volume is presumed to be due to opening of alveolar units (16). Provoked augmented inspirations improve lung compliance (17,18).

IV. Factors Influencing Respiratory Activity

A. Gestational Age

In ventilated infants, the Hering Breuer reflex can be identified by an increase in the spontaneous expiratory time (apnea) provoked by the volume change of positive pressure inflations (8). It is not possible, using such a technique, to determine whether the strength of the reflex is influenced by gestational age, as the length of apnea cannot be used to quantify the reflex (19). The reflex, however, was present in ventilated infants as immature as 25 weeks' gestation, and the frequency of elicitation of the reflex did not correlate with gestational age (8). Using an end-inspiratory occlusion technique, the strength of the Hering Breuer reflex was found to decrease with increasing gestational age in 26 preterm ventilated infants with and without respiratory distress syndrome (RDS) (20). This is consistent with data from nonventilated infants (21,22). Olinsky et al. (22) demonstrated that the reflex was present in infants of gestational age of 29 weeks and stronger in premature than term infants. The extrauterine environment was associated with a significant delay in the disappearance of the reflex with increasing maturity (21). In those studies (21,22), an end-expiratory airway occlusion technique was used to provoke the reflex. When the airway is occluded at end expiration, respiratory efforts produce no volume change, so there can be no stretch receptor stimulation. If inspiration is usually terminated by stretch receptor stimulation, that is, the Hering Breuer reflex is present, then end-expiratory occlusion will be associated with a prolonged inspiratory time. Others, however, have used the end-expiratory technique and arrived at different conclusions regarding the influence of gestational age on the Hering Breuer reflex. Bodegard (23) found the reflex to be infrequent in infants of 32 weeks' gestational age, to increase to a maximum strength at a postmenstrual age of 36–38 weeks and then the strength of the reflex to decline. No significant relationship of the occurrence of provoked augmented inspirations to gestational age was noted in ventilated infants (8).

B. Postnatal Age

The influence of postnatal age on the Hering Breuer reflex may differ between ventilated and nonventilated infants and with respect to maturity at birth. Whereas in ventilated, preterm infants the reflex persisted throughout the first 11 days after birth (8), in term infants requiring no form of respiratory support studied serially at 10, 60, and 90 min and a few days of age, prolongation of the inspiratory time during end-expiratory occlusions was less as the infant's age increased (24). The Hering Breuer reflex does persist during tidal breathing beyond the neonatal period, with apparently no statistically significant change in its strength during the first 2 months after birth in healthy infants during natural sleep (25). In addition, the reflex can be provoked in nonventilated (26) and ventilated children (27) and anesthetized adults (28,29). The significant volume-related inhibition of inspiratory muscle activity during mechanical ventilation (30) is not dependent on afferent information from the rib cage, as it is seen in both normal and quadriplegic patients (31). The reflex, however, may become less easy to provoke with increasing age. In ventilated children, an inverse relationship of the reflex with postnatal age was demonstrated (27). In conscious adults, the reflex was only provoked outside the tidal range (6). Using CO_2-induced increased ventilation, no change in inspiratory duration in conscious adult humans was demonstrated until the tidal volumes were twice the resting values (6). Widdicombe (32) also found that the Hering Breuer reflex was weak or absent in awake adult subjects.

The active expiratory component of the Hering Breuer inflation reflex is less prominent in older ventilated, prematurely born infants. Assessment of the respiratory interactions of 27 preterm ventilated infants during the first 14 days after birth demonstrated that the active expiration was only seen in the first few days (3). In the second week, ~50% of the infants were apnoeic and, despite studying the infants at a series of rates (30, 60, and 120 bpm), active expiration was rarely provoked (3). The change in the occurrence of the reflex, however, may be explained by a change in respiratory compliance (33) rather than an effect of advancing postnatal age per se. When studied in the second week, the infants had recovered from RDS and thus would be predicted to have less stiff lungs than when examined in the perinatal period. Those data (3) highlight that, after the first week after birth, it is usually unnecessary to manipulate ventilator rate to avoid active expiration, and may explain why there is a low pneumothorax rate in ventilated infants after the perinatal period.

In ventilated preterm infants, provoked augmented inspirations were seen only in the first 5 postnatal days regardless of gestational age (8). Similar results have been reported in nonventilated infants born at term (4). Augmented inspirations occurred most frequently soon after birth (4) and were commoner during the first day of life than on subsequent days (16). The activity of the reflex was noted to decrease during the first 5 days after birth (4).

C. Respiratory Function

In ventilated, prematurely born infants, the active expiratory component of the Hering Breuer reflex is commoner in infants with noncompliant lungs (33). The strength of the Hering Breuer inflation reflex was also noted to decline at a slower rate with increasing gestational age in ventilated infants who had a low respiratory compliance or RDS (20). Those data are consistent with the findings that, in adult animals, decreased lung compliance caused an increased discharge from the stretch receptors of the lungs (34), and that in nonventilated infants with stiff lungs, neither increasing postnatal age nor maturity affected the strength of the Hering Breuer inflation reflex (35). It seems likely, then, that the level of lung compliance is the most important determinant of the strength of the reflex. In support of that hypothesis is the finding that in spontaneously breathing infants, the correlation of the strength of the inspiratory inhibitory reflex to pulmonary compliance was stronger than the correlation between reflex strength and gestational age (36). In addition, serial examination of two healthy newborns and four with respiratory problems revealed a decrease in the strength of the reflex as the compliance increased (36).

Provoked augmented inspiration is also commoner in infants with noncompliant lungs. In one series (15), provoked augmented inspirations were only seen in infants with a lung compliance of $<2 \, \text{mL/cmH}_2\text{O}$. In addition, the frequency of elicitation of the reflex was inversely proportional to the lung compliance (Fig. 5), as was the ventilator pressure provoking the reflex. An inverse relationship between the sensitivity of Head's paradoxical reflex and lung compliance has also been demonstrated in cats (37).

D. Blood Gases

No chemoreceptor influence on the occurrence of the Hering Breuer reflex has been demonstrated in ventilated infants (8,20). In one of the studies (20), an end-

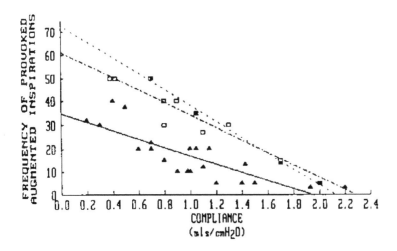

Figure 5 The frequency of elicitation of provoked augmented inspirations related to dynamic compliance. ▲, Babies on no medication except antibiotics; □, babies recovering from paralysis with pancuronium; ■, babies receiving treatment with theophylline. Each subpopulation is associated by its regression line. A higher incidence of augmented inspirations was seen in infants receiving theophylline or recovering from paralysis with pancuronium. (From Ref. 15.)

inspiratory occlusion technique was used, but in the other (8) the results may have been biased by failure to maintain ventilator inflation until the breakpoint of the reflex was reached. In both studies, the majority of infants had blood gases within the normal range, which may have further influenced the results. In nonventilated infants, there is disagreement regarding the effect of blood gases on the strength of the reflex. The inspiratory time during an occlusion has been demonstrated to correlate significantly with carbon dioxide tensions in healthy newborns (36), but this has not been a consistent finding (19,38) and it has not been seen in cats (19).

No relationship of the occurrence of provoked augmented inspirations to blood gases was noted in preterm, ventilated infants (15). That is not inconsistent with the finding that in mature cats the frequency of augmented breaths increased with increasing levels of hypercapnia and hypoxia, as hypoxia was a very potent stimulus (39), and only a minority of the preterm infants studied were hypoxic (arterial oxygen tension <40 mm Hg) (15). In addition, the infants studied were born very prematurely, and complex pathways of chemoreceptor influence modifying mechanical reflexes (40) may not be present in such infants during the first days after birth.

E. Medication

Administration of theophylline in prematurely born infants has been associated with an increase in the strength of the Hering Breuer reflex (41), as has caffeine administration in anesthetised newborn rabbits aged 2–7 days (42). Those data perhaps indicate an alteration in the phasic vagal afferent impulses from pulmonary stretch receptors. In a subsequent study (43), however, there was a significant reduction in the strength of the Hering Breuer reflex when preterm infants were given caffeine. Overall, a significant inverse relationship was found between the infants' compliance of the respiratory system and the strength of the Hering Breuer reflex. Thus, the decrease in the strength of the reflex is likely to be explained by the improvement in compliance the caffeine-treated infants experienced, rather than an effect of caffeine administration per se. Methylxanthine administration enhanced the frequency of provoked augmented inspirations in preterm ventilated infants (Fig. 5) (15,44). Theophylline increases diaphragmatic contractility and so may improve the efferent part of the reflex. The increase in reflex strength resulting from methylxanthine administration may be one of the mechanisms by which this therapy facilitates early extubation (45).

Infants thought to be actively expiring have been paralyzed to prevent the development of air leaks (46). Nowadays, the preferred option is to sedate infants or to administer analgesics with the hope that this will suppress respiratory activity. When formally tested, however, sedation was shown to have no effect on the strength on the Hering Breuer reflex, but only infants born at term were studied (47). Infants recovering from neuromuscular blockade with pancuronium in the first day after birth have been shown to have a high frequency of provoked augmented inspirations (15). Pancuronium has effects on autonomic ganglia, although minimal (48), and can cause tachycardia by partial vagal blockade (49). Possibly, this causes a differential effect on vagal conduction during recovery, such as is seen during cooling (14), and other reflex loops are selectively blocked to enhance the elicitation of the reflex.

Maternal administration of corticosteroids has been associated with a reduction in RDS and neonatal mortality. In addition, infants exposed to corticosteroids antenatally and exogenous surfactant postnatally have more compliant lungs; as a consequence, respiratory reflexes are less likely to be provoked (see above). The respiratory activity of ventilated infants routinely exposed to antenatal corticosteroids and postnatal "surfactant," however, has not been systematically examined.

F. Mode of Ventilation

Continuous Positive Airway Pressure (CPAP)/Positive End-Expiratory Pressure (PEEP)

Elevation of the PEEP or CPAP level can result in prolongation of expiratory time and slowing of the respiratory rate (50,51). Application of 0, 3, and 6 cmH$_2$O of CPAP resulted in a progressive increase in FRC and expiratory time, with a fall in respiratory rate in term infants (52). Elevation of end-expiratory lung volume by administration of continuous negative pressure also results in an increase in the duration of expiration and a reduction in respiratory rate (10). The mechanism of slowing of the respiratory rate is that elevation of lung volume stimulates the Hering Breuer reflex.

Conventional Ventilation

During conventional ventilation, ventilator rate has an important influence on which respiratory pattern occurs. Active expiration is more common in infants ventilated with slow rates (53). At slow rates, long-duration positive pressure inflations are frequently employed; such inflations are particularly likely to stimulate active expiration (33). The mean spontaneous inspiratory time of prematurely born infants studied in the perinatal period is ~0.3 s (54). Thus, a long positive pressure inflation results in inflation extending into expiration; this has been termed asynchrony, and leads to active expiration and airleak. Active expiration also occurs when the commencement of a square wave positive pressure inflation is in a spontaneous respiratory window (±0.2 sec) around the end of inspiration (55). Positive pressure inflations are only "square wave" at relatively low frequencies (56); this may be another explanation for the association of active expiration and slow-rate conventional ventilation. Increasing ventilator rate and by necessity reducing inflation time, however, does not universally suppress the active component of the Hering Breuer inflation reflex (53).

Augmented inspirations only occur when slow ventilator rates are used. In one series (15), augmented inspirations were only provoked if the ventilator rate was 15 bpm or less. In anesthetised cats (39) and rabbits (57), the inspiration-augmenting reflex has also been shown to have a relatively long refractory period. This refractoriness relates to the accompanying increase in end-expiratory volume following a provoked augmented inspiration. In contrast, synchrony is more common at fast rates, that is, 60 bpm or greater (58). Examination of 24 prematurely born infants at a series of ventilator rates (30, 60, and 120 bpm) (58) revealed that 17 became synchronous at a rate of 120 bpm and a smaller number (four) at 60 bpm. Two infants were only synchronous if ventilated at their own spontaneous respiratory rate, and one infant was asynchronous throughout the study. The 17 infants synchronous at 120 bpm were less mature and had a faster spontaneous respiratory rate than those synchronous at 60 bpm. Those data are consistent with the findings that the spontaneous respiratory rate of preterm infants in the first days after birth was inversely proportional to their gestational age (58) (Fig. 6) and that smaller animals have been shown to breathe faster than larger ones, possibly due to a stronger Hering Breuer reflex (34). To entrain infants' respiratory activity to positive pressure inflations and hence induce synchrony, the ventilator rate must be faster than, but similar to, the infants' respiratory frequency. Thus, rates of 120 bpm did not induce synchrony in more mature infants (58).

High-Frequency Oscillation (HFO)

At the very fast frequencies employed during HFO, animals are apneic (59); this is the consequence of lowered carbon dioxide tensions and is reversed by vagotomy (59). In anesthetised cats, rhythmic phrenic discharge inhibited by HFO reappears following neuromuscular blockade (60). Those data suggest that the apnea during HFO results from inspiratory inhibition mediated by chest wall and vagal afferents. A possible source for the vagal inhibition is stimulation of slowly adapting stretch receptors. In neonates, spontaneous respiratory rate was shown to significantly decrease on transfer from conventional ventilation to HFO, but only a minority of the infants became apneic (2). It has been suggested that spontaneous respiratory activity during HFO usually occurs in response to the stimulus of pain or handling, carbon dioxide retention, or pneumothorax (60). Respiratory activity, however, has been described in the absence of such stimuli and in association with improvements in blood gases (2). The duration of the apnea resulting from stimulation of the Hering Breuer inflation reflex varies directly with the inflation volume (40), and, in cats, apnea can be induced by

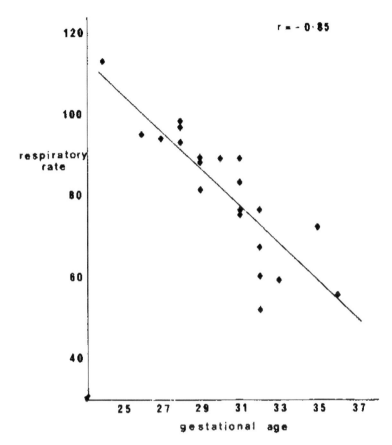

Figure 6 Spontaneous respiratory rate of ventilated infants studied in the first days after birth related to gestational age. The solid line depicts the regression line: Respiratory rate, 223.97–4.71; gestational age, ($P < .01$) $r = -0.85$. (From Ref. 58.)

increasing the delivered volume to at least 5 mL/kg (61). Thus, the difference between the results in infants and those in animal models may be explained by the lower volume, ~2.5 mL/kg, delivered to infants during HFO (62) and the infants' being normocarbic when studied (2).

Patient-Triggered Ventilation

During patient-triggered ventilation (PTV), the infant's respiratory efforts trigger positive pressure inflations. In synchronized intermittent positive pressure venti-lation (SIPPV), otherwise known as assist/control (A/C), any number of inflations can be triggered provided the change in pressure, flow, volume, etc., exceeds the critical trigger level, whereas in synchronized intermittent mandatory ventilation (SIMV), only a preset number of inflations can be triggered regardless of the frequency of the infant's spontaneous respiratory efforts. As, during either SIPPV or SIMV, the infant's respiratory efforts trigger positive pressure inflations it was expected that these ventilatory modes would provoke synchrony with improvements in blood gases. In physiological studies involving infants with acute respiratory distress, PTV compared to conventional ventilation was indeed associated with higher rates of synchrony, better blood gases, and higher tidal volumes; additional advantages were lower rates of work of breathing and fluctuations in blood pressure and cerebral blood flow velocity. Comparison of the different ventilation modes, however, was only made over very short periods, and only relatively mature infants were examined. Subsequent studies have demonstrated that asynchrony does occur during PTV (63). Then PTV is much more likely to fail, that is, the infant develops apnea, irregular triggering, or a metabolic or respiratory acidosis. Asynchrony, inflation extending into expiration, results from a long trigger delay. The trigger delay is the time from the onset of the infant's spontaneous inspiration and the commencement of a positive pressure inflation. The length of the trigger delay is affected by the performance of the ventilator's triggering system (see below) and the nature of the infant's respiratory efforts, which are influenced by the infant's lung function and respiratory drive. For example, a long trigger delay is likely to occur in infants with high airways resistance if a device triggered by a critical change in airflow is employed or in very immature infants with feeble respiratory efforts if an airway pressure trigger is used (64). The use of a ventilator with an airway pressure trigger may explain the lack of superiority of PTV over conventional ventilation in a recently published randomized trial (65). Failure of PTV is also associated with a low triggering rate related to the infant's gestational age, which is more common in immature infants (66). Prolonged inflation times, that is, >0.4 sec, can also reduce the triggering rate by stimulation of the Hering Breuer reflex (67).

In premature infants recovering from RDS, the results of a randomized trial demonstrated that the duration of weaning during conventional ventilation was longer than on SIPPV (68). SIMV compared to SIPPV allows more flexible weaning, as weaning can be by pressure and/or rate reduction. Nevertheless, the results of three randomized trials failed to demonstrate that weaning by SIMV rather than SIPPV was more advantageous (69,70). Indeed, overall there was a tendency for a shorter duration of weaning in infants randomized to SIPPV, particularly if the SIMV rate was reduced below 20 breaths/min (69,70). Oxygen consumption is increased at low levels of ventilator support (71). Thus it seems likely that at least 20 spontaneous breaths/min must be supported by positive pressure inflations to overcome the work of breathing imposed by the endo-tracheal tube.

Pressure Support Ventilation (PSV)

During PSV, the infant triggers a pressure-supported breath at a preset level. The patient determines the duration of the positive pressure inflation, as the triggering device senses not only the beginning but also the end of the infant's inspiratory effort. Inflation is terminated when the inspiratory flow is reduced to a certain level, for example, at 15% of maximum flow when the Draeger Babylog 8000 (Draeger Medical, Luebeck, Germany) is used and at 15–25% of maximum flow when the termination sensitivity of the Bird VIP (Bird Products, Palm Springs, CA) is employed. Employment of PSV thus should eliminate asynchrony. In a group of very immature infants (72), increasing the termination sensitivity to maximum was associated with almost total elimination of asynchrony. The reduction in asynchrony resulted from shortened inflation times as the termination sensitivity was increased but, despite the lower inflation time, volume exchange was maintained. Delivered volume is compromised in certain ventilators when inflation time is reduced (73). The maintenance of delivered volume, as the termination sensitivity was increased, suggests then that this was as a result of an increase in the infant's respiratory efforts. Thus, although PSV may increase the likelihood of synchrony, it is important to determine if preterm infants can compensate for very short inflation times throughout their ventilatory career or whether use of this ventilatory mode should be restricted in infants ready to wean. In addition, whether the lower rate of asynchrony during PSV translates into a reduced rate of airleak needs to be investigated.

Proportional Assist Ventilation (PAV)

Ventilatory support during PTV is synchronized with the beginning and sometimes the end of the infant's inspiration, but during PAV it is synchronized throughout the infant's respiratory cycle. The applied pressure is servocontrolled throughout each spontaneous breath, and increases in proportion to the tidal volume and inspiratory flow generated by the patient. The frequency, timing, and amplitude of lung inflation are controlled by the patient (74). The results of a crossover study (74) indicated that gas exchange might be maintained with smaller transpulmonary pressure swings during PAV than during intermittent mandatory ventilation or PTV. Only 36 infants, however, were studied during three consecutive 45-min periods. Potential problems with PAV could occur if there was a significant leak around the endotracheal tube, inadvertent overcompensation leading to lung overdistension or a lack of responsiveness to apnea or hypoventilation (75).

Volume Guarantee Ventilation (VSV)

During VSV, a preset volume is delivered to the infant, so this mode of ventilation compensates for changes in the mechanical characteristics of the respiratory system. Preliminary studies comparing VSV to conventional ventilation suggest that during conventional ventilation infants be overventilated (76–78). During VSV adequate ventilation was achieved with lower airway pressures than during other ventilatory modes, the likely explanation being that, when VSV is employed, infants contribute more to the volume exchange (76). To date, the physiological studies examining VSV have only been of short term, and it is important to assess whether VSV is a suitable long-term ventilatory mode for preterm infants and, like PSV, it is likely to be most useful in the recovery stage.

V.   Methods of Detecting Respiratory Activity During Mechanical Ventilation

A.   Physiological Recordings

Spontaneous respiratory activity can be recorded using a pressure measuring device in the esophagus, such as a balloon or catheter, to reflect changes in pleural pressure (79), or by monitoring chest wall movements using impedance. Esophageal pressure measurements are inaccurate in infants with chest wall distortion (80). Nevertheless, under such circumstances, the esophageal pressure signal can be used qualitatively to indicate respiratory timing, particularly in relationship to positive pressure inflations. Simultaneous recording of the infant's respiratory activity and changes in airway pressure will reveal if expiration is occurring during positive pressure inflation. An alternative method of detecting active expiration is to record the fluctuations between the maximum and minimum systolic peaks of the arterial blood pressure, active expiration being present when the fluctuations are increased (81).

B.   Clinical Observation

Respiratory patterns may be inaccurately diagnosed if an infant is observed at only one respiratory rate. Selective paralysis, when used with physiological monitoring to detect active expiration, was an effective method of preventing pneumothoraces (46). If, however, clinical observation alone was used, then selective paralysis was no more effective in reducing the incidence of pneumothoraces than paralyzing all infants (82), suggesting that active expiration may have been misdiagnosed. Visually assessing respiratory activity at two different ventilator rates, particularly if changes in transcutaneous oxygen concentrations were also considered, improved diagnostic accuracy (83). Synchrony was diagnosed when the infant's respiratory efforts became less obvious when the ventilator rate was increased, and this was associated with an improvement in oxygenation. Similarly, active expiration was diagnosed when the infant's respiratory efforts became more obvious, or there was poor chest wall expansion or even a downward movement of the chest wall during positive pressure inflation which was associated with impairment of oxygenation when the ventilator rate was reduced. Using such criteria all infants who breathed synchronously were correctly identified by clinical observation and active expiration/asynchrony correctly identified on 88% of occasions (83).

C. Importance of Recording Respiratory Activity During Mechanical Ventilation

During mechanical ventilation, the infant's respiratory efforts may impair gas exchange and/or result in a pneumothorax. It is important, then, to determine whether the infant's inspiratory efforts are in time with each positive pressure inflation. Some infants, however, may expire during each positive pressure inflation. This can be revealed by watching the direction of chest wall movement while timing each positive pressure inflation by listening to the ventilator. A more secure method of detecting active expiration, however, is to simultaneously record airway and esophageal pressure changes (see above). Similarly, successful suppression of respiratory activity by administering sedative/analgesic agents cannot be assumed and will only be accurately assessed if the infant's respiratory efforts are directly monitored.

Recording respiratory activity can identify infants in whom PTV is more likely to fail. PTV is frequently unsuccessful if there is a long trigger delay and in those immature infants who have a weak Hering Breuer reflex (84). The trigger delay can be assessed by simultaneous recording of esophageal and ventilator pressure changes (85). From such recordings, the sensitivity of the triggering system can also be determined, the sensitivity being demonstrated by the proportion of the infant's inspiratory efforts that trigger ventilation inflations. Simultaneous esophageal and airway recordings also highlight when triggering is occurring in expiration, as can occur in very immature infants when an abdominal movement sensor is used as the triggering mechanism (86). There have now been many studies, in both animal models and infants, comparing the performance of different triggering systems. Unfortunately, the majority have concentrated on relatively mature infants with RDS, and it is important to be aware that triggering systems have poorer performance in very immature infants (85). A further limitation of the literature is that different triggering systems with different ventilators have usually been compared and that the ventilators available vary in performance (73). Thus, differences may reflect differences in performance of the triggering system, the ventilator, or both. To correctly identify differences in the performance of triggering systems it is essential to compare them using the same ventilator (64).

VI. Influence of Respiratory Activity on the Outcome of Mechanical Ventilation for Acute Ventilatory Failure

One pattern of respiratory activity, active expiration, has been shown to result in a poor ventilation outcome. Examination of 34 infants on 120 occasions (1) revealed that only one type of respiratory pattern, active expiration, consistently preceded the development of a pneumothorax. The association was confirmed by the results of a trial in which infants demonstrated to be actively expiring were randomly allocated to receive standard therapy and a neuromuscular blocking agent, pancuronium or standard therapy alone (46). Pneumothoraces developed in all of the infants who continued to actively expire, but in only one of those whose active expiratory efforts were inhibited by administration of pancuronium. The likely mechanism of pneumothorax development following active expiration is that the active expiratory efforts opposing positive pressure inflation increase the shearing forces to which the lung is subjected.

It had been postulated (87) that pneumothorax would occur if the infant took a spontaneous breath simultaneously with positive pressure inflation, synchrony, as that combination would generate large transpulmonary pressure swings rupturing the airways or alveoli. Synchrony, however, was shown not to result in air leak but rather had a positive influence on the outcome of ventilation (88). Blood gases improved when synchrony was provoked (88), and this has been an incentive to develop ventilation modes which guaranteed synchrony. Augmented inspirations provoked by positive pressure inflations also do not lead to air leaks (1), but to an improvement in compliance (44).

References

1. Greenough A, Morley CJ, Davis JA. Interaction of spontaneous respiration and artificial ventilation in preterm babies. J Pediatri 1983; 103(5):769–773.
2. Chan V, Greenough A, Dimitriou G. High frequency oscillation, respiratory activity and changes in blood gases. Early Hum Dev 1995; 40:87–94.
3. Hird MF, Greenough A. Spontaneous respiratory effort during mechanical ventilation in infants with and without acute respiratory distress. Early Hum Dev 1991; 25:69–73.
4. Cross KW, Klaus M, Tooley WH, Weiser K. The response of the newborn baby to inflation of the lungs. J Physiol 1960; 151:551–565.
5. Hering E, Breuer J. Die selbsteurung der Amnung durch den nevus vagus sitzber. Sitzungsbericht der kaiserlichen Akademie der Wissenschaften in Wien 1868; 57:672–677.
6. Clark FJ, Von Euler C. On the regulation of depth and rate of breathing. J Physiol 1972; 222:267–295.

7. Bouverot P, Crance JP, Dejours P. Factors influencing the intensity of the Breuer-Hering inspiration-inhibiting reflex. Respir Physiol 1970; 8(3):376–384.

8. Greenough A, Morley CJ, Davis JA. Respiratory reflexes in ventilated premature babies. Early Hum Dev 1983; 8:65–75.

9. Sankaran K, Leahy FN, Cates D, MacCallum M, Rigatto H. Effect of lung inflation on ventilation and various phases of the respiratory cycle in preterm infants. Biol Neonate 1981; 40:160–166.

10. Stark AR, Frantz ID. Prolonged expiratory duration with elevated lung volume in newborn infants. Pediatr Res 1979; 13(4 Part 1):261–264.

11. Guz A, Noble MI, Eisele JH, Trenchard D. The effect of lung deflation on breathing in man. Clin Sci 1971; 40(6):451–461.

12. Hannam S, Ingram DM, Rabe-Hesketh S, Milner AD. Characterisation of the Hering-Breuer deflation reflex in the human neonate. Respir Physiol 2001; 124(1):51–64.

13. Knox CK. Characteristics of inflation and deflation reflexes during expiration in the cat. J Neurophysiol 1973; 36:284–295.

14. Head H. On the regulation of respiration. J Physiol 1889; 10:1–70.

15. Greenough A, Morley CJ, Davis JA. Provoked augmented inspirations in ventilated premature infants. Early Hum Dev 1984; 9(2):111–117.

16. Thach BT, Taeusch HWJ. Sighing in newborn human infants: role of inflation-augmenting reflex. J Appl Physiol 1976; 41(4):502–507.

17. Mead J, Collier C. Relation of volume histories of lungs to respiratory mechanics in anaesthetized dogs. J Appl Physiol 1959; 14:669–678.

18. Glogowska M, Richardson PS, Widdicombe JG, Winning AJ. The role of the vagus nerves, peripheral chemoreceptors and other afferent pathways in the genesis of augmented breaths in cats and rabbits. Respir Physiol 1972; 16(2):179–196.

19. Grunstein MM, Milic-Emili J. Analysis of interactions between central and vagal respiratory control mechanisms in cats. IEEE Trans Biomed Eng 1978; 25(3):225–235.

20. De Winter JP, Merth IT, Berkenbosch A, Brand R, Quanjer PH. Strength of the Hering Breuer inflation reflex in term and preterm infants. J Appl Physiol 1995; 79:1986–1990.

21. Kirkpatrick SML, Olinsky A, Bryan MH, Bryan AC. Effect of premature delivery on the maturation of the Hering-Breuer inspiratory inhibitor reflex in human infants. J Pediatr 1976; 88:1011–1014.

22. Olinsky A, Bryan MH, Bryan AC. Influence of lung inflation on respiratory control in neonates. J Appl Physiol 1974; 36:426–429.

23. Bodegard G, Schwieler GH, Skoglund S, Zetterstrom R. Control of respiration in newborn babies. I. The development of the Hering Bruer inflation reflex. Acta Paediatr Scand 1969; 58:567–571.

24. Fisher JT, Mortola JP, Smith JB, Fox GS, Weeks S. Respiration in newborns. Development of the control of breathing. Am Rev Respir Dis 1982; 125:650–657.

25. Rabbette PS, Costeloe KL, Stocks J. Persistence of the Hering-Breuer reflex beyond the neonatal period. J Appl Physiol 1991; 71:474–480.

26. Greenough A, Pool J. Hering Breuer reflex in young asthmatic children. Pediatr Pulmonol 1991; 11:345–349.

27. Giffin F, Greenough A, Naik S. The Hering-Breuer reflex in ventilated children. Respir Med 1996; 90(8):463–466.
28. Gautier H, Bonora M, Gaudy JH. Breuer-Hering inflation reflex and breathing pattern in anesthetized humans and cats. J Appl Physiol: Respir, Environ Exercise Physiol 1982; 51(5):1162–1168.
29. Polacheck J, Strong R, Arens J, Davies C, Metcalf I, Younes M. Phasic vagal influence on inspiratory motor output in anesthetized human subjects. J Appl Physiol: Respir, Environ Exercise Physiol 1980; 49(4):609–619.
30. Simon PM, Skatrud JB, Badr MS, Griffin DM, Iber C, Dempsey JA. Role of airway mechanoreceptors in the inhibition of inspiration during mechanical ventilation in humans. Am Rev Respir Dis 1991; 144(5):1033–1041.
31. Simon PM, Griffin DM, Landry DM, Skatrud JB. Inhibition of respiratory activity during passive ventilation: a role for intercostal afferents? Respir Physiol 1993; 92:53–64.
32. Widdicombe JG. Respiratory reflexes excited by inflation of the lungs. J Physiol 1953; 123:105–115.
33. Greenough A. The premature infant's respiratory response to mechanical ventilation. Early Hum Dev 1988; 17:1–5.
34. Widdicombe JG. Respiratory reflexes in man and other mammalian species. Clin Sci 1961; 21:163.
35. Chan V, Greenough A. Lung function and the Hering Breuer reflex in the neonatal period. Early Hum Dev 1992; 28:111–118.
36. Simbruner G, Salzer H, Coradello H, Popow C. Respiratory control in premature and mature healthy newborns. Prog Respir Res 1981; 77:35–42.
37. Reynolds LR. Characteristics of an inspiration-augmented reflex in anaesthetized cats. J Appl Physiol 1962; 17:683–688.
38. Taeusch HW, Carson S, Frantz ID, Milic-Emili J. Respiratory regulation after elastic loading and CO_2 rebreathing in normal term infants. J Pediatr 1976; 88(1):102–111.
39. Cherniack NS, Von Euler C, Glogowska M, Homma J. Characteristics and rate of occurrence of spontaneous and provoked augmented breaths. Acta Paediatr Scand 1981; 111:349–360.
40. Younes MP, Vaillancourt P, Milic-Emili J. Interaction between chemical factors and duration of apnoea following lung inflation. J Appl Physiol 1974; 36:190–201.
41. Gerhardt T, McCarthy J, Bancalari E. Effects of aminophylline on respiratory center and reflex activity in premature infants with apnea. Pediatr Res 1983; 7:188–191.
42. Trippenbach T, Zinman R, Milic Emili J. Caffeine effect on breathing pattern and vagal reflexes in newborn rabbits. Respir Physiol 1980; 40:211–215.
43. Laubscher B, Greenough A. Comparative effects of theophylline and caffeine on respiratory function of preterm infants. Early Hum Dev 1998; 50(2):185–192.
44. Greenough A, Morley CJ. Provoked augmented inspirations in preterm ventilated infants. In: Jones CT, Nathanielsz PW, eds. The Physiological Development of the Fetus and Newborn. London: Academic Press, 1985; 263–267.
45. Greenough A, Elias-Jones A, Pool J, Morley CJ. The therapeutic actions of theophylline in preterm ventilated infants. Early Hum Dev 1985; 12:15–22.

46. Greenough A, Wood S, Morley CJ, Davis JA. Pancuronium prevents pneumothoraces in ventilated premature babies who actively expire against positive pressure inflation. Lancet 1984; i:1–3.

47. Rabbette PS, Dezateux CA, Fletcher ME, Costeloe KL, Stocks J. Influence of sedation on the Hering-Breuer inflation reflex in healthy infants. Pediatr Pulmonol 1991; 11(3):217–222.

48. Stark AR. Muscle relaxation in mechanically ventilated infants. J Pediatr 1979; 94(3):439–443.

49. Kelman GR, Kennedy BR. Cardiovascular effects of pancuronium in man. Br J Anaesth 1971; 43(4):335–338.

50. Javorka K, Tomori Z, Zavarska L. Effect of lung inflation on the respiratory frequency and heart rate of premature neonates. Physiol Bohemoslav 1982; 31:129–135.

51. Martin RJ, Nearman HS, Katona PG, Klaus MH. The effect of a low continuous positive airway pressure on the reflex control of respiration in the preterm infant. J Pediatr 1977; 90:976–981.

52. Martin RJ, Okken A, Katona PG, Klaus MH. Effect of lung volume on expiratory time in the newborn infant. J Appl Physiol: Respir, Environ Exercise Physiol 1978; 45(1):18–23.

53. Greenough A, Morley CJ, Pool J. Fighting the ventilator—are fast rates an effective alternative to paralysis? Early Hum Dev 1986; 13:189–194.

54. Hird M, Greenough A. Inflation time in mechanical ventilation of preterm neonates. Eur J Pediatr 1991; 150:440–443.

55. Greenough A, Morley C, Johnson P. An active expiratory reflex in preterm ventilated infants. In: Jones CT, Nathanielsz PW, ed. The Physiological Development of the Foetus and Newborn. London: Academic Press, 1985: 259–263.

56. Greenough A, Greenall F. Performance of respirators at fast rates commonly used in the neonatal intensive care unit. Pediatr Pulmonol 1987; 3(5):357–361.

57. Davies A, Roumy M. The effect of transient stimulation of lung irritant receptors on the pattern of breathing in rabbits. J Physiol 1982; 324:389–401.

58. Greenough A, Greenall F, Gamsu H. Synchronous respiration: which ventilator rate is best? Acta Paediatr Scand 1987; 76:713–718.

59. Thompson WK, Marchak BE, Bryan AC, Froese AB. Vagotomy reverses apnoea induced by high frequency oscillatory ventilation. J Appl Physiol 1981; 51:1484–1487.

60. England SJ, Sullivan C, Bowes G, Onayemi A, Bryan AC. State-related incidence of spontaneous breathing during high frequency ventilation. Respir Physiol 1985; 60(3):357–364.

61. Mautone AJ, Sica AL, Scarpelli EM. Ventilatory control during high frequency oscillation (HFO). Fed Proc 1982; 41:1507.

62. Dimitriou G, Greenough A, Kavvadia V, Laubscher B, Milner AD. Volume delivery during high frequency oscillation. Arch Dis Child Fetal Neonatal Ed 1998; 78:F148–F150.

63. Hird MF, Greenough A. Causes of failure of neonatal patient triggered ventilation. Early Hum Dev 1990; 23:101–108.

64. Dimitriou G, Greenough A, Cherian S. Comparison of airway pressure and airflow triggering systems using a single type of neonatal ventilator. Acta Paediatr 2001; 90:445–447.

65. Baumer JH. International randomized controlled trial of patient triggered ventilation in neonatal respiratory distress syndrome. Arch Dis Child Fetal Neonatal Ed 2000; 82:F5–F10.

66. Mitchell A, Greenough A, Hird M. Limitations of patient triggered ventilation in neonates. Arch Dis Child 1989; 64:924–929.

67. Upton CJ, Milner AD, Stokes GM. The effect of changes in inspiratory time on neonatal triggered ventilation. Eur J Pediatr 1990; 149:648–650.

68. Chan V, Greenough A. Randomised controlled trial of weaning by patient triggered ventilation or conventional ventilation. Eur J Pediatr 1993; 152(1):51–54.

69. Chan V, Greenough A. Comparison of weaning by patient triggered ventilation or synchronous intermittent mandatory ventilation in preterm infants. Acta Paediatr 1994; 83:335–337.

70. Dimitriou G, Greenough A, Giffin F, Chan V. Synchronous intermittent mandatory ventilation modes compared with patient triggered ventilation during weaning. Arch Dis Child 1995; 72(3):F188–F190.

71. Roze JC, Liet JM, Gournay V, Debillon T, Gaultier C. Oxygen cost of breathing and weaning process in newborn infants. Eur Respir J 1997; 10(11):2583–2585.

72. Dimitriou G, Greenough A, Laubscher B, Yamaguchi N. Comparison of airway pressure triggered and airflow triggered ventilation in very immature infants. Acta Paediatr 1998; 87:1256–1260.

73. Dimitriou G, Greenough A. Performance of neonatal ventilators. Br J Intens Care 2000; 10:186–188.

74. Schulze A, Gerhardt T, Musante G, et al. Proportional assist ventilation in low birth weight infants with acute respiratory disease. A comparison to assist/control and conventional mechanical ventilation. J Pediatr 1999; 135:339–344.

75. Schulze A, Schaller P. Proportional assist ventiation: a new strategy for infant ventilation? Neonatal Respir Dis 1996; 6(1):1–10.

76. Herrera CM, Gerhardt T, Everett R, Claure N, Musante G, Bancalari E. Randomized, crossover study of volume guarantee (VG) versus synchronized intermittent mandatory ventilation (SIMV) in very low birth weight (VLBW) infants recovering from respiratory failure. Pediatr Res 1994; 45(4 Part 2):304A.

77. Cheema IU, Ahluwalia JS. Feasibility of tidal volume-guided ventilation in newborn infants: a randomized, crossover trial using the volume guarantee modality. Pediatrics 2001; 107(6):1323–1328.

78. Abubakar KM, Keszler M. Patient-ventilator interactions in new modes of patient-triggered ventilation. Pediatr Pulmonol 2001; 32(1):71–75.

79. Greenough A, Morley CJ. Oesophageal pressure measurements in ventilated preterm babies. Arch Dis Child 1982; 57:851–855.

80. LeSouef PN, Lopes JM, England SJ, Bryan MH, Bryan AC. Influence of chest wall distortion on oesophageal pressure. J Appl Physiol 1983; 55:353–358.

81. Levene MI, Quinn MW. Use of sedatives and muscle relaxants in newborn babies receiving mechanical ventilation. Arch Dis Child 1992; 67:870–873.

82. Shaw NJ, Cooke RWI, Gill AB, Shaw NJ, Saeed M. Randomised trial of routine versus selective paralysis during ventilation for neonatal respiratory distress syndrome. Arch Dis Child 1993; 69:479–482.
83. Greenough A, Greenall F. Observation of spontaneous respiratory interaction with artificial ventilation. Arch Dis Child 1988; 63:168–171.
84. Chan V, Greenough A, Muramatsu K. Influence of lung function and reflex activity on the success of patient triggered ventilation. Early Hum Dev 1994; 37:9–14.
85. Chan V, Greenough A. Neonatal patient triggered ventilators. Performance in acute and chronic lung disease. Br J Intens Care 1993; 3:216–219.
86. Laubscher B, Greenough A, Kavadia V. Comparison of body surface and airway triggered ventilation in extremely premature infants. Acta Paediatr 1997; 86:102–104.
87. Pollitzer MJ, Reynolds EOR, Shaw DG, Thomas RM. Pancuronium during mechanical ventilation speeds recovery of lungs of infants with hyaline membrane disease. Lancet 1981; i:346–348.
88. Greenough A, Pool J, Greenall F, Morley CJ, Gamsu HR. Comparison of different rates of artificial ventilation in preterm neonates with the respiratory distress syndrome. Acta Paediatr Scand 1987; 76:706–712.

20

Respiratory Control in Bronchopulmonary Dysplasia

MIRIAM KATZ-SALAMON

Karolinska Institute and Karolinska Hospital
Stockholm, Sweden

I. Introduction

The markedly improved survival of extremely immature neonates in recent decades has not been without significant costs—~30% of infants with a birth weight <1000 g develop lung injury in form of chronic lung disease (CLD) (1). For the most part, this term is synonymous with bronchopulmonary dysplasia (BPD). The disease has been attributed to respiratory distress that requires therapeutic interventions such as ventilatory support and oxygen therapy. Infants with BPD not only suffer from serious respiratory problems during the neonatal period but are also impaired by prolonged respiratory insufficiency in subsequent years. BPD is a complex disease characterized by stiff lungs, decreased alveolarization, poor lung mechanics, extremely compliant chest wall, and an insufficient muscle mass to sustain adequate ventilation. Together with an inadequate respiratory drive and frequent hypoxemic episodes, these pathological characteristics result in suboptimal growth, poor lung functions, affected cognition, and inferior motor development in the long term. Despite the intensive research in the last decade, the etiology of BPD is still unclear. The pivotal consensus focusing on the key questions regarding BPD has been published recently after a workshop organized by National Institute of Child Health and Human Development (2).

Because of the complexity of the disease this chapter is devoted mainly to respiratory control issues that have bearing on the clinical care of infants with BPD. The short- and long-term outcomes of preterm born infants with BPD are also briefly discussed.

II. Definition and Etiology

The most widely used definitions of BPD have been based predominantly on the duration of oxygen therapy. In the report from the workshop on BPD in 1979, the disease has been defined on the basis of specific radiographic changes in the lungs and the need of oxygen therapy for at least 28 days (3). The results from studies on late pulmonary sequelae of BPD have shown that oxygen therapy at 36 weeks of postmenstrual age has been a significant predictor for long-term respiratory outcome. That led to changes in the definition so the requirement for supplemental oxygen at 36 weeks of postmenstrual age was required for the diagnosis (4). In the report from the recent workshop on BPD (2) a new definition and criteria for grading of the severity of BPD have emerged. The "new" definition uses different criteria for infants born before and after 32 weeks of postmenstrual age, takes into consideration the length and intensity of O_2 supplementation and/or the need for ventilatory support, and disregards radiographic findings (2).

In the 1970s BPD developed in those preterm born infants who were treated with positive pressure ventilation and with high levels of supplemental oxygen for respiratory distress syndrome (RDS). The improvement of ventilatory support in the 1980s increased survival of extremely premature infants and significantly decreased the overall morbidity among those born at later gestation. The introduction of antenatal corticosteroids and surfactant treatment in the late 1980s and early 1990s resulted in the dramatic increase in survival among extremely preterm infants. However, the decline in the mortality among these infants has been paralleled by an increase in the prevalence of BPD (5) (Table 1).

Table 1 Mortality and Incidence of BPD Among VLBW Infants (<1500 g) at Vanderbilt NICU 1976–1990

Time period	Mortality (%)	BPD (%)
1976–1980	26.4	10.6
1981–1985	18.3	21.2
1986–1990	15.9	32.9

Source: Ref. 5.

Furthermore, the improvements in assisted ventilation techniques changed the character of BPD. The "old," classic BPD was characterized by severe alveolar septal and peribronchial fibrosis, squamus metaplasia, and/or hypertensive vascular bed (6–8). These aberrations are not seen in the "new" BPD. However, smooth muscle hypertrophy in the airways and abnormalities in the elastic fibers are seen both in the classic and in the new BPD (9,10). The new BPD is also characterized by alveolar hypoplasia, saccular wall fibrosis, and minimal airway disease (11). Interestingly, the new BPD has been described in newborns with initially no or minimal lung disease who develop increasing need for both ventilatory support and oxygen therapy in the ensuing weeks (12).

The structurally immature and surfactant-deficient lung is extremely susceptible to injury because these alveolar units are prone to collapse. The use of mechanical ventilation to open airways induces lung injury by over-distension of the airways and alveoli. Surfactant treatment prior to initiation of assisted ventilation seems to counteract the atelectasis by promoting more uniform inflation of the lungs (13). The susceptibility to volume trauma due to mechanical ventilation is further potentiated by high chest wall compliance. The following mechanical injury leads to protein and fluid leakage into airways, alveoli, and interstitium; inhibition of surfactant function; and inflammation (14). These processes are reinforced by antenatal exposure to inflammatory mediators and infection (15,11). Since multiple proinflammatory factors are prominent in the airways, the inflammation seems to be a central factor in BPD (16).

Besides the mechanical injury and inflammatory processes, the prolonged oxygen treatment seems to be a significant factor leading to lung damage. Since the antioxidant systems develop as late as during the third trimester, the exposure to hyperoxia leads to an overproduction of superoxide and perhydroxy radicals and results in inflammation and diffuse lung damage (17). Treatment with supplemental oxygen aimed at keeping oxygen saturation between 89% and 94% or between 96% and 99% (18) clearly demonstrated higher prevalence of BPD and retinopathy of prematurity (ROP) in the group of infants with the higher range for saturation.

III. Control of Breathing in BPD

Respiration is regulated by chemical mechanisms, so called chemoreceptors, which monitor PO_2 and PCO_2 and adjust ventilation to maintain blood gases and pH within normal ranges. Rise in PCO_2 and/or decrease in PO_2 augments inspiratory activity and stimulates respiration to facilitate absorption of O_2 and excretion of CO_2 to maintain homeostasis.

A. Peripheral Chemoreceptors

Function and Developmental Aspects

The peripheral chemoreceptors play a crucial role in the defense against hypoxia and in control of breathing (19,20). In healthy infants and in adults a fall in partial pressure of O_2 (PaO_2) elicits a hyperventilatory response, which is mediated predominantly by peripheral chemoreceptors in the carotid bodies and, to a lesser degree, by receptors in the aorta (21). The reactivity to hypoxia is present in the fetus and it responds to an acute O_2 deficiency by cessation of breathing movements (22). At birth, the shift from fetal life to extrauterine air breathing requires resetting of the sensitivity in the peripheral chemoreceptors to higher O_2 levels. During the first few days after birth, the carotid chemoreceptors seem crucial for maintaining adequate respiration but their importance disappears with age; in newborn lambs and piglets the carotid body denervation leads to abnormal breathing pattern, prolonged apneas, and deaths (23,24), while the bilateral denervation of carotid bodies in adult humans (25) does not have any effect on respiratory control.

The study on the maturation of the peripheral chemoreceptors in very prematurely born infants (gestational age 28.8 ± 2.7 weeks) described a marked decrease in the response time to 100% O_2 between 36 and 40 gestational weeks (26).

The function of peripheral chemoreceptors in humans can be examined by measuring changes in ventilation while breathing hypoxic or hyperoxic gas mixtures (see below). Even though the ventilatory response to hyperoxia/hypoxia reflects complex integrated inputs from peripheral chemoreceptors, central nervous system mechanisms, and changes in metabolism, the hypoxic/hyperoxic ventilatory response is predominantly controlled by carotid chemoreceptors. As such, the response mirrors function of these receptors (20).

Methodological Approaches

In clinical tests the hyperoxic exposure to breath-by-breath alternating inhalation of 100% O_2 and air or inhalation of 100% O_2 for at least 30 sec (so-called chemodenervation), is most frequently used. In studies on peripheral chemo-receptor function in infants with RDS or BPD, the exposure to hyperoxia lasting several seconds is preferred owing to maldistribution and reduction in the perfusion area, and the unevenness in the ratio between alveolar ventilation and vascular perfusion (27,28). It seems likely that the structural changes in the dysplastic lung delay the delivery of the hyperoxic stimuli to peripheral chemoreceptors. Infants with BPD need a significantly longer time to reach the peak in oxygenation when breathing 100% O_2 than preterm infants without lung disease (29) (for a short review of the methods, see Ref. 30).

Development of Peripheral Chemoreceptor in BPD

The postnatal adjustment to higher partial pressures of O_2 can be altered when the fetus (31,32) or child is subjected to low PO_2 levels. Infants born at high altitude do not react to hyperoxia by changes in ventilation during the first 5 days of life, but show an adequate response at 2–6 months of age (33). Similarly, the weakest or absent response to oxygen in very preterm infants was found in infants requiring the long-lasting treatment with supplemental O_2 (26), particularly in those suffering from BPD (29,34).

The clinical consequences of defective function of the peripheral chemoreceptors are very serious. In animal models it has been linked with severe disturbances in respiratory control mechanisms (35), an absence of arousal from hypoxia (36), and, in infants, with apparent life-threatening events (37). Furthermore, it has been suggested that absent or attenuated peripheral chemoreceptor function may, at least in part, explain the significantly increased incidence of SIDS in infants with BPD (34,37–39). However, the lack of sensitivity in peripheral chemoreceptors is not permanent. In infants with BPD with absent response to hyperoxia, the response appeared at the mean postnatal age of 14 weeks (range 9–33 weeks) (40). This suggests that infants with BPD are in fact unprotected against hypoxia at the age when they are at highest risk for SIDS (see Fig. 1).

B. Central Chemoreceptors—CO_2 Drive in BPD

Increases in PCO_2 and/or H^+ stimulate central chemoreceptors, located on the ventral surface of the medulla, and give rise to significant cardioventilatory interaction. Even though other areas also react to CO_2, their effect on ventilation is not well established. The action of CO_2 on medullary chemosensitive cells is essential for the maintenance of normal breathing, particularly during deep sleep (41,42). Therefore, the ventilatory response to hypercapnia is often employed in studies of central respiratory control mechanisms (41,43–46). The ventilatory response to CO_2 is the result of an interaction between central and peripheral CO_2 drives, central control mechanisms, CO_2 storage in blood and tissues, and respiratory mechanics.

Methodological Approaches

The ventilatory CO_2 response as a measure of central chemoreceptor activity has been studied either by the *steady-state* or the *rebreathing* method. Both techniques describe the respiratory system controlled predominantly by central chemoreceptors. The ventilatory response to inspired CO_2 is measured when PCO_2 equilibrium at the alveolar, arterial, and central levels is reached, which corresponds to venous CO_2 concentrations. The steady-state procedure is based

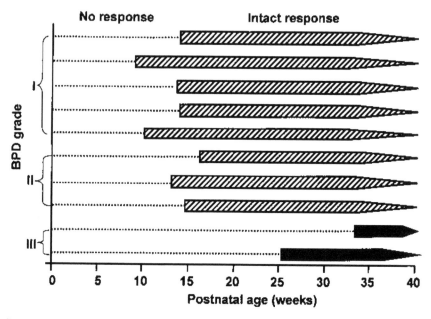

Figure 1 Postnatal age at the appearance of the hyperoxic response in relation to the severity of BPD.

on inhalation of at least three gas mixtures of different CO_2 concentrations (e.g., 2%, 4%, and 6% CO_2 in air). The time necessary to obtain steady state for each mixture varies from 5 to 10 min (47). Thus, the steady-state method is a laborious procedure and therefore seldom used in studies in sleeping infants. In contrast, the rebreathing method, also called the Read method, is much more efficient and therefore preferable (48). The procedure is based on rebreathing from a small bag with a gas mixture initially containing 3–7% CO_2 in oxygen. The procedure lasts only 3–4 min, during which time a marked increase in ventilation occurs. The slope of the regression line describing the relationships between the increase in the end-tidal PCO_2 and the increase in ventilation is used as a measure of the sensitivity of respiratory system to CO_2.

Developmental Aspects

The CO_2 drive has been seen in fetus with significantly increased breathing movements in response to maternal inhalation of 4–6% CO_2. However, the response was only seen during low-voltage electro-oculogram, corresponding to REM sleep (22). After birth the threshold for CO_2 response decreases almost immediately, and the response is seen in all sleep stages (49). The postmenstrual age seems to play a role since preterm infants have lower sensitivity to CO_2 than term infants (46,50–52), but the response increases with advancing postnatal age (50,53). Lower sensitivity to CO_2 in preterm infants has mainly been attributed to low responsiveness of the central chemoreceptors (42,52) and/or to suboptimal respiratory mechanics such as highly compliant chest wall (42,50). This is illustrated in Figure 2 (personal data); the ventilatory response in the same preterm infant at a postconceptional age of 36 and 40 weeks as compared to a full-term infant at 5 days and at 3 months of age. As seen in the figure the preterm infant reacted to CO_2 with an initial increase in ventilation and a subsequent leveling of the ventilatory response. The first part of the response implies well-functioning chemoceptive mechanisms. The second part, the leveling of the response, may be explained by an inability to sustain hyperventilation due to suboptimal respiratory mechanics such as lower lung compliance, fatigue in respiratory muscles, and/or decrease in central drive. Beyond the observations described above, very little can be extrapolated specifically to BPD infants. So far only one study (54) has examined CO_2 response in infants with BPD and compared it with the response in non-BPD preterm infants (with apneas and IVH). A similar ventilatory response to CO_2 was observed in both groups. The serious shortcoming of this study was the use of chloral hydrate that, despite no obvious effect on chemosensitivity (55) might have influenced the infants in different ways and thus secondarily influenced the reported results (56).

IV. Relationships Between Control of Heart Rate and Respiration

Respiration and heart rate (HR) are rhythmic phenomena with distinct intrinsic frequencies that are functionally linked to interactions of oscillating centers in the brainstem. Our knowledge about the control of HR has been based on analysis of HR and HR variability (HRV) in either time or frequency domain. The latter analysis, called spectral analysis, is based on the assumption that control of HR consists of general rhythmic, linear components and nonlinear, spontaneous, and chaotic elements, which give rise to chaotic oscillations and irregularities in HR (57). The periodic components of R-R intervals are defined in terms of low-frequency (LF; 0.02–0.2 Hz), high-frequency (HF; >0.2–1.5 Hz) power spectra and as the ratio between LF and HF (LF/HF). The LF component is influenced by both sympathetic and parasympathetic efferents to the heart, while the HF component is governed predominantly by parasympathetic system. Thus, by investigating HR oscillations in different physiological conditions and sleep states, one may gain a deeper insight into the autonomic control of HR (58). It has been shown that the ratio between LF and HF spectra decreases after 28 postnatal days in healthy newborn infants, suggesting a more pronounced parasympathetic control of HR with postnatal age (59).

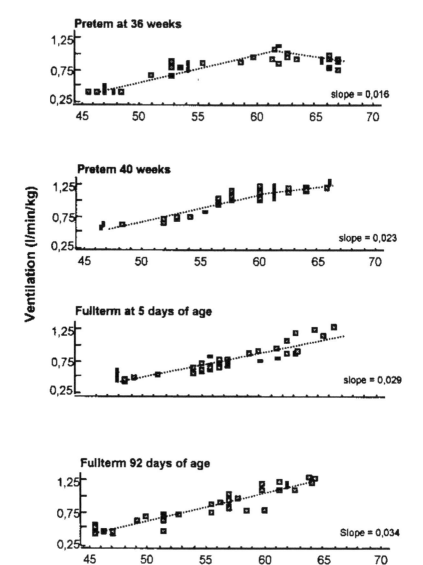

Figure 2 Breath-by-breath changes in ventilation in response to increases in the end-tidal PCO_2 during rebreathing tests in a premature infant (36 and 40 weeks' postconceptional age) and a full-term infant (5 and 92 days).

Spectral analysis of HRV in infants with BPD and infants born at term at the same postnatal age revealed significantly reduced LF spectra in QS and thus lowered LF/HF ratio in BPD infants compared to healthy controls. This suggests a lowered sympaticovagal balance of the autonomic control of HR in infants with BPD. Furthermore, the autonomic control of HR can be modulated by changes in SaO_2; a mild lowering in SaO_2 accelerates HR and changes LF and HF spectra (60). The reduced LF spectra might also imply a reduced baroreceptor activity in these infants (61).

Similarly to HR, the respiratory rhythm consists of basic oscillations in form of inspiratory/expiratory phases. Superimposed on these basic oscillations are frequent ($<0.2\,Hz$) modulations of the amplitude and frequency of the breaths (62,63).

The coupling of breathing and HR rhythms is controlled by a network of interactive processes, is fine-tuned by external stimuli and emotional influences, and changes with age. For example, during first 3 days of life HR oscillations are influenced predominantly by modulations in breath amplitude while in older infants and adults breathing frequency contributes significantly to HR variability (64) at HF spectra, inducing so-called respiratory sinus arrhythmia (RSA).

The coordination between cardiovascular and respiratory systems can be disturbed in different clinical situations. Numerous studies on cardiorespiratory control mechanisms in SIDS suggest some loss of coordination between cardiovascular and respiratory systems and that influences of one system on the other are diminished. Infants who succumb to SIDS show weaker minute-by-minute correlation between cardiac and respiratory measures (65) and reduced respiratory influence on cardiac rate (66,67). Infants with severe or mild recurrent apneas in sleep and infants who have experienced apparent life-threatening events (ALTE) have an adequate ventilatory response but divergent HR response to mild hypercapnia; these infants respond to mild hypercapnia with an adequate increase in ventilation but with a simultaneous decrease in heart rate (68). Since infants with BPD are at significantly higher risk for SIDS (38,69), one can assume similar background mechanisms.

Cardiorespiratory control undergoes maturational changes during first 6 months of life (70). The disturbances in ventilation during sleep, particularly REM sleep, are most frequent during first 6 months of life (71). Furthermore, the observed decrease in the frequency and duration of nighttime desaturations, which is not paralleled by an improvement in respiratory mechanics, might be explained by maturation of the ventilatory control mechanisms (29).

V. Hypoxemia in BPD

Despite long-term oxygen supplementation, infants with BPD usually exhibit varying degrees of hypoxemia and hypercapnia. The rationale for supplemental

O₂ therapy has been to elude the adverse effects of hypoxia while avoiding O_2 toxicity. Until the early 1990s, the clinical recommendation for weaning infants with BPD from supplemental O_2 was set at the average SaO_2 between 88% and 90%. However, the negative effects of suboptimal oxygenation (see below) were described in a number of clinical studies. As a consequence, a baseline oxygenation in air breathing between 93% and 95% is now recommended to justify discontinuation of oxygen treatment.

Nevertheless, future studies are needed to establish the effect of supplemental O_2 therapy on mortality and morbidity in infants with BPD. Studies evaluating oxygen therapy showed that the initiation of O_2 therapy with the prime aim of maintaining optimal oxygenation (saturation >93%) has been associated with a marked decrease of the incidence of sudden unexpected deaths from 11% to 0% among infants with BPD (38,72,73). It is certainly possible that obtaining optimal oxygenation levels in this infant population might favorably improve an overall developmental outcome.

Figure 3 illustrates the etiology and clinical consequences of hypoxia experienced by infants with BPD. Respiration in BPD is characterized by tachypnea and hyperventilation that indicate high respiratory load. As a result of damage in the lung parenchyma, infants with BPD have lower transcutaneous PO_2 and oxygen saturation. That together with blunted chemosensitivity (29)

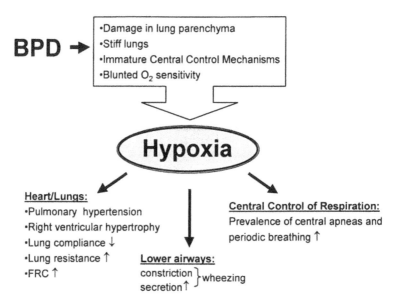

Figure 3 Etiology and clinical consequences of hypoxia in BPD.

makes them susceptible to hypoxia. In fact, infants with BPD, when on ventilatory support, have frequent desaturations that are associated with alveolar hypoxia and an increased pulmonary resistance (74). Also in spontaneously breathing infants with BPD suboptimal oxygenation causes airway constriction and wheezing (75). The latter is the sum result of airway narrowing during hypoxia due to airways hypersensitivity and increased airway secretion. Measurements of lung mechanics during hypoxic episodes demonstrate that lung mechanics in infants with BPD worsened further during hypoxia: lung resistance and FRC increased by $\sim$50% and 26% respectively, and lung compliance decreased by 24% (76). Administration of supplemental oxygen reverses the negative effect of hypoxia and improves the mechanical properties of the lung significantly (75).

Besides its negative effect on lung mechanics, hypoxemia has a marked effect on central control of ventilation as well: it increases both the prevalence of central apneas and the densities of periodic breathing while elevation of saturation above 93% stabilizes the breathing pattern (77). Furthermore, an elevation of mean saturation from 87–91% to 94–96% markedly decreased the incidence of spontaneous desaturations (78).

The positive effect of improved oxygenation in severe BPD with persistent pulmonary hypertension has also been reported. A study on the effect of an increase in inspired oxygen fraction during cardiac catheterization in six infants with BPD showed clearly the therapeutic benefit of supplemental O_2 therapy in the form of a reduction in mean pulmonary artery pressure from 48 by at most 10 mm Hg (79) since the pulmonary vascular bed is highly responsive to supplemental oxygen. Furthermore, right ventricular hypertrophy resolved under treatment with supplemental O_2. More generally, supplemental oxygen therapy facilitates physical growth and development (80).

VI. Respiration During Sleep in BPD

During wakefulness, the respiratory control systems provide an effective control of overall ventilation. Sleep onset and oscillations in sleep states destabilizes breathing by reducing central respiratory drive and responsiveness to changes in the external milieu. The relationships between sleep and respiration are complex: on the one hand, sleep aggravates respiratory symptoms in infants with breathing disorders (for review see 81); on the other hand, respiratory disorders per se change sleep architecture (Fig. 4).

In infants with a variety of respiratory problems, sleep alters mechanical properties of breathing apparatus and chemical drives. That results in an increase of upper-airways resistance and obstruction, and gives rise to apneas and hypoxemic episodes. The system reacts to obstructive apneas and hypoxia with

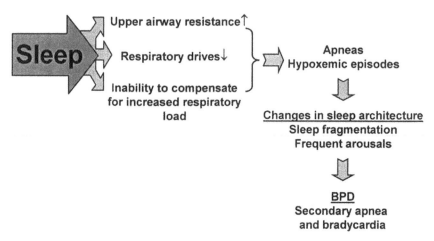

Figure 4   Interactive effects of sleep and respiratory control in lung disease.

arousal, during which saturation is restored to optimal levels. An insufficient propensity to arouse decreases our ability to survive exposures to noxious conditions during sleep.

In infants who suffer from obstructive apneas, sleep is fragmented by frequent arousals. Similarly, in infants with BPD, sleep is characterized by an increased frequency and duration of arousals. These arousals are partly a consequence of obstructive apneas and desaturations that appear predominantly in REM sleep (39). Even though infants with BPD have an intact arousal response to mild hypoxia, the period directly following the arousal is, in as many as one-third of events, characterized by apnea and bradycardia (Fig. 5) that require brief ventilatory assistance to restore normal breathing (39).

Obstructive apneas in BPD infants during sleep increase further work of breathing and aggravate hypoxia. This vicious circle is reinforced by an inability of BPD infants to compensate for respiratory loading.

Greenspan et al. (82) measured respiratory effort in response to applied resistive load in 11 BPD infants and 11 healthy preterm born infants. BPD infants showed no changes in respiratory drive in response to added load-in, whereas healthy preterm infants showed an adequate response in form of increased airway pressure. Besides arousals due to obstructive apneas, sleep fragmentation in BPD patients seems to be directly associated with the levels of oxygenation. Suboptimal oxygenation affects sleep by reducing the number and duration of REM sleep episodes (39,83,84). Interestingly, sleep fragmentation is observed even when mean saturation in sleep is kept above 90% (39). Furthermore, frequent episodes of clinically unexpected arterial oxygen desaturations in sleep are common even when saturation during wakefulness is kept at 90–92% (85). However, when

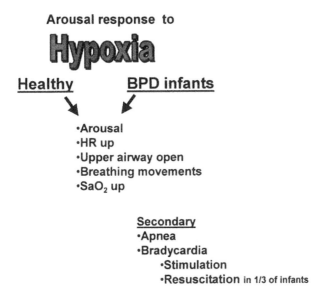

Figure 5 Arousal response to hypoxia in normal and BPD infants. Secondary effects are seen only in BPD infants.

supplemental oxygen levels are further elevated, the frequency of arousals and sleep fragmentation decrease, and the total sleep time and duration of REM sleep periods increase (84).

VII. Respiratory Sequelae in BPD Infants

The neonatal course of very preterm infants is complicated by varying degree of pulmonary problems. Structural and physiological processes alter the elastic and resistive properties of the immature pulmonary system. Restrictive lung (low compliance) is a result of increased interstitial tissue, interstitial fibrosis, or pulmonary edema. Mucosal edema, peribronchial swelling, bronchospasm, and mucous plugging of the airways give rise to an increased resistance in the airways. At 3 months of age minute ventilation is still elevated, indicating abnormal lung function (86). Increased pulmonary resistance and decreased lung compliance contribute to increased work of breathing while low FRC at first 6 months of age mirrors alveolar collapse (86). With age, a parallel lung growth and formation of new alveoli are mirrored by an increase in lung compliance.

Generally, the first 2 years of life are characterized by frequent respiratory illnesses that require hospitalizations (87). Even though symptoms for neonatal injury typical for BPD alleviate with age, in the long term perspective, particularly in infants with severe BPD persisting wheezing, chronic cough and chest congestion restrict physical activities by 7 years of age (88). Incidence of airway hyperactivity in adolescents and young adults with neonatal BPD is high (89). Significantly decreased forced expiratory volumes (90), markedly lower specific airway conductance, and larger residual volume in the presence of normal spirometric measurements (91) have been described as well. The abnormal pulmonary functions, however, are related to severity of BPD since infants with relatively mild BPD had normal respiratory mechanics and diffusing capacity (92).

The long-term studies of respiratory functions in infants with BPD born today are necessary. Despite the pronounced intratest variability in pulmonary mechanics (93), sequential measurements demonstrate age-dependent character-istics of lung mechanics and might provide insight into the postnatal development of respiratory system in BPD.

VIII. Short- and Long-Term Neuromotor and Cognitive Development

Exposure to frequent hypoxic episodes renders infants with BPD to be at high risk for deviations in motor and mental functions (94–96). Long-term sequelae in terms of growth and neurodevelopmental and cognitive outcome have been subject of ongoing concern. The frequency of neurological sequelae among infants with BPD has been reported to be much higher than among very low birth weight (VLBW) infants without chronic lung complications (40% vs. 6%, respectively) (97). In several studies, however, the impaired development of infants with BPD has been linked to intraventricular hemorrhage (IVH) and/or periventricular leukomalacia (PVL) rather than to lung disease per se (96,98–102). Nevertheless, a large cohort study involving 122 infants with BPD, 84 VLBW infants without BPD and 123 full-term infants at 3 years of age revealed that BPD *itself* is a specific high-risk condition affecting predominantly motor performance, while neurological neonatal risk factors (IVH and PVL) and social class have adverse effect on mental development (103). At school age VLBW infants without BPD and infants born at term have significantly better cognitive performance than infants with BPD (104,105).

Whether the severity of BPD affects development is not clear, and opinions are divided. Katz-Salamon et al. (106) described significantly poorer motor performance of volitional movements and lower total sum in the Griffiths test in infants with severe BPD (grade III) at 10 months of age. The deviations in specific skills persisted until school age (107). Severe BPD, as defined by the need for supplemental oxygen therapy after discharge home, was described as a potent risk factor for neurological and motor deficits at school age: 71% of BPD infants as compared to 19% preterm-born infants without BPD had cerebral palsy, subtle neurological signs, and behavioral difficulties. Furthermore, more than half of BPD infants have deviations in gross and fine motor skills (108). On the other hand, Luchi et al. (109) did not find any correlation between the severity of BPD and the neurodevelopmental outcome at 2–4 years of age.

IX. Conclusions

Bronchopulmonary dysplasia, a lung injury in very preterm born infants, is the most common lung disorder in infancy. The complexity of the disease comprises arrest of and/or disturbances in lung development, inadequate oxygenation, suboptimal lung mechanics, and immature respiratory control mechanisms.

The clinical picture is further complicated by the use of a variety of therapeutic strategies that might improve one aspect of the disease but adversely alter another (for example, the use of antenatal or postnatal systemic steroids stimulates lung maturation but affects alveolarization). Despite improvements in the neonatal care of very preterm born infants, BPD, owing to its complexity, may have lifelong consequences. However, one should be aware that the long-term data describing respiratory morbidity pertain to children born before the era of prenatal steroids, surfactant, and high-frequency ventilation. Thus they are not representative of infants with BPD born and cared for today.

Furthermore, studies on neuromotor and cognitive development of infants who suffered from BPD during the neonatal period clearly show that while medical complications are most pronounced in early childhood, the socioeconomic status of the family confounds the outcome at pre- and early school age. More research is needed to improve our knowledge about pathophysiology of BPD. In the final analysis, the therapeutic strategies to promote better long-term health ought to be the primary focus.

References

1. Stevenson DK, Wright LL, Lemons JA, Oh W, Korones SB, Papile LA, Bauer CR, Stoll BJ, Tyson JE, Shankaran S, Fanaroff AA, Donovan EF, Ehrenkrantz RA, Verter J. Very low birth weight outcomes of the National Institute of Child Health and Human Development Neonatal Research Network, January 1993 through December 1994. Am J Obstet Gynecol 1998; 179:1632–1639.
2. Jobe AH, Bancalari E. Bronchopulmonary dysplasia. Am J Respir Crit Care Med 2001; 163:1723–1729.

3. Report of Workshop on Bronchopulmonary Dysplasia, NIH Publication No. 80-1660. Washington; National Institute of Health, 1979.

4. Shennan AT, Dunn MS, Carlisle K, Parker B, Popp R, Pitlick P, Eichler I, Lamm R, Brown B Jr. Abnormal pulmonary outcome in premature infants: prediction from oxygen requirement in the neonatal period. Pediatrics 1988; 82:527–532.

5. Parker RA, Lindstrom DP, Cotton RB. Improved survival accounts for most, but not all, of the increase in bronchopulmonary dysplasia. Pediatrics 1992; 90:663–668.

6. Northway WH, Rosan RC, Porter DY. Pulmonary disease following respirator therapy of hyaline-membrane disease. Bronchopulmonary dysplasia. N Engl J Med 1967; 276:357–363.

7. Becker MJ, Koppe JG. Pulmonary structural changes in neonatal hyaline membrane disease treated with high pressure artificial respiration. Thorax 1969; 24:689–694.

8. Hislop AA, Wigglesworth JS, Desai R, Aber V. The effects of preterm delivery and mechanical ventilation on human lung growth. Early Hum Dev 1987; 15:147–164.

9. Coalson JJ, Winter VT, Siler-Khodr T, Yoder BA. Neonatal chronic lung disease in extremely immature baboons. Am J Respir Crit Care Med 1999; 160:1333–1346.

10. Albertine KH, Jones GP, Starcher BC, Bohnsack JF, Davis PL, Cho SC, Carlton DP, Bland RD. Chronic lung injury in preterm lambs. Disordered respiratory tract development. Am J Respir Crit Care Med 1999; 159:945–958.

11. Clark RH, Gerstman DR, Jobe AH, Moffitt ST, Slutsky AS, Yoder BA. Lung injury in neonates: causes, strategies for prevention, and long-term consequences. J Pediatr 2001; 139:478–486.

12. Charafeddine L, D'Angio CT, Phelps DL. Atypical charonic lung disease patterns in neonates. Pediatrics 1999; 103:759–765.

13. Wada K, Jobe AH, Ikegami M. Tidal volume effects on surfactant treatment responses with the initiation of ventilation in preterm lambs. J Appl Physiol 1997; 83:1054–1061.

14. Dreyfuss D, Saumon G. Ventilator induced lung injury: lessons from experimental studies. Am J Respir Crit Care Med 1998; 157:294–323.

15. Jonsson B, Li Y-H, Noack G, Brauner A, Tullus K. Downregulatory cytokines in tracheobronchial aspirate fluid from infants with chronic lung disease of prematurity. Acta Paediatr 2000; 89:1375–1380.

16. Groneck P, Speer CP. Inflammatory mediators and bronchopulmonary dysplasia. Arch Dis Child 1995; 73:1–3.

17. Frank L. Antioxidants, nutrition, and bronchopulmonary dysplasia. Clin Perinatol 1992; 19:541–562.

18. STOP-ROP Study Group. Supplemental therapeutic oxygen for prethreshold retinopathy of prematurity (STOP-ROP), a randomized, controlled trial. I. Primary outcomes. Pediatrics 2000; 105:295–310.

19. Blanco, CE, Dawes, GS, Hanson, MA and McCooke HB. The response to hypoxia of arterial chemoreceptors in fetal sheep and newborn lambs. J Physiol 1984; 351:25–37.

20. Honda Y. Role of carotid chemoreceptors in control of breathing at rest and in exercise: studies on human subjects with bilateral carotid body resection. Jpn J Physiol 1985; 35:535–544.

21. Marshall JM. Peripheral chemoreceptors and cardiovascular regulation. Physiol Rev 1994; 74: 543–584.
22. Johnston BM, Lagercrantz H. Neural regulation of respiration. In: Gluckman PD, Heyman MA, eds. Perinatal and Pediatric Pathophysiology: A Clinical Perspective. London: E. Arnold, 1993.
23. Bureau MA, Lamarche J, Foulon P, Dalle D. Postnatal maturation of respiration in intact and carotid body–chemodenervated lambs. J Appl Physiol 1985; 59:869–874.
24. Donnelly DF, Haddad GG. Prolonged apnea and impaired survival in piglets after sinus and aortic nerve section. J Appl Physiol 1990; 68:1048–1052.
25. Whipp BJ, Ward SA. Physiologic changes following bilateral carotid-body resection in patients with chronic obstructive pulmonary disease. Chest 1992; 101:656–661.
26. Katz-Salamon M, Lagercrantz H. Hypoxic ventilatory defence in very preterm graduates—attenuation after long oxygen treatment. Arch Dis Child 1994; 70:90–95.
27. Auld PA. Pulmonary physiology of the newborn infants. In: Scarpelli MM, Febiger L, eds. Pulmonary Physiology of the Fetus, Newborn and Child. Philadelphia: W.B. Saunders, 1975.
28. Gorenflo, M, Vogel M, Obalden M. Pulmonary vascular changes in bronchopulmonary dysplasia: a clinicopathologic correlation in short- and long-term survivors. Pediatr Pathol 1991; 11:851–866.
29. Katz-Salamon M, Jonsson B, Lagercrantz H. Blunted peripheral chemoreceptor response to hyperoxia in a group of infants with BPD. Pediatr Pulmonol 1995; 20:101–107.
30. Carrol JL, Donelly DF. Postnatal development of carotic chemoreceptor function. In: Loughlin GM, Carrol JL, Marcus CL, eds. Sleep and breathing in Children. A Developmental Approach. New York: Marcel Dekker, 2000.
31. Hanson MA, Kumar P, Williams BA. The effect of chronic hypoxia upon the development of respiratory chemoreflexes in newborn kitten. J Physiol 1989; 411:563–574.
32. Hertzberg T, Hellström S, Holgert H, Lagercrantz H, Pequignot JM. Ventilatory response to hyperoxia in newborn rats born in hypoxia—possible relationship to carotid body dopamine. J Physiol 1992; 456:645–654.
33. Lahiri S, Brody JS, Motoyama EK, Velasquez TM. Regulation of breathing in newborns at high altitude. J Appl Physiol 1978; 44:673–678.
34. Calder NA, Williams BA, Smyth J, Boon AW, Kumar P, Hanson MA. Absence of ventilatory response to alternating breaths of mild hypoxia and air in infants who have had bronchopulmonary dysplasia: implications for the risk of sudden infant death. Pediatr Res 1994; 35:677–681.
35. Hofer MA. Role of carotid sinus and aortic nerves in respiratory control of infant rats. Am J Physiol 1986; 251:811–817.
36. Fewell JE, Kondo CS, Dascalu V, Filyk SC. Influence of carotic denervation on the arousal and cardiopulmonary response to rapidly developing hypoxemia in lambs. Pediatr Res 1989; 25:473–477.
37. Hunt CE, McCulloch K, Brouillette RT. Diminished hypoxic ventilatory responses in near-miss sudden infant death syndrome. J Appl Physiol 1981; 50:1315–1317.

38. Werthammer J, Brown ER, Neff RK and Taeusch HW. Sudden infant death syndrome in infants with bronchopulmonary dysplasia. Pediatrics 1982; 69:301–304.

39. Garg M, Kurzer S, Bautista D, Keens T. Hypoxic arousal in infants with bronchopulmonary dysplasia. Pediatrics 1988; 82:59–63.

40. Katz-Salamon M, Eriksson M, Jonsson B. Development of peripheral chemoreceptor function in infants with chronic lung disease and initially lacking hyperoxic response. Arch Dis Child 1996; 75:4–9.

41. Sullivan CE. Breathing in sleep. In: Owen J, Barnes CD, eds. Physiology in Sleep. New York: Academic Press, 1980.

42. Moriette G, Van Reempts P, Moore M, Cates D, Rigatto H. The effect of rebreathing CO_2 on ventilation and diaphragmatic electromyography in newborn infants. Respir Physiol 1985; 62:387–397.

43. Cross KW, Hooper JMD, Oppe TE. The effect of inhalation of carbon dioxide in air on the respiration of the full-term and premature infants. J Physiol 1953; 122:264–273.

44. Moriette G, Van Reempts P, Moore M, Yorke K, Rigatto H. Does prematurity or chest distortion imply a mechanic disadvantage to neonates inhaling CO_2? Pediatr Res 1983; 17:28A.

45. Carlo W, Martin RJ, Difiore JM. Differences in CO_2 threshold of respiratory muscles in preterm infants. J Appl Physiol 1988; 65:2434–2439.

46. Cohen G, Henderson-Smart DJ. A modified rebreathing method to study the ventilatory response of the newborn to carbon dioxide. J Dev Physiol 1990; 14:295–301.

47. Kao FF. Regulation of ventilation. In: An Introduction to Respiratory Physiology. Amsterdam: Excerpta Medica, 1974.

48. Read DJC. A clinical method for assessing the ventilatory response to carbon dioxide. Australas Ann Med 1967; 16:20–32.

49. Cohen G, Xu C, Henderson-Smart D. Ventilatory response of the sleeping newborn to CO_2 during normoxic rebreathing. J Appl Physiol 1992; 72:1218–1219.

50. Frantz ID, Adler SM, Thach BT, Taeusch HW Jr. Maturational effects on respiratory responses to carbon dioxide in premature infants. J Appl Physiol 1976; 41:41–45.

51. Krauss AN, Waldman S, Auld PAM. Diminished response to carbon dioxide in premature infants. Biol Neonate 1976; 30:216–223.

52. Rigatto H, Brady JP, De la Torre R. Chemoreceptor reflexes in preterm infants. II. The effect of gestational and postnatal age on the ventilatory response to inhaled carbon dioxide. Pediatrics 1975; 55:614–620.

53. Guthrie RD, Standaert TA, Hodson WA, Woodrum DA. Sleep and maturation of eucapnic ventilation and CO_2 sensitivity in the premature primate. J Appl Physiol 1980; 48:347–354.

54. Anwar M, Marotta F, Fort MD, Mondestin H, Mojica C, Walsh S, Hiatt M, Hegyi T. The ventilatory response to carbon dioxide in high risk infants. Early Hum Dev 1993; 35:183–192.

55. Lee MH, Olsen GD, McGilliard KL, Newcomb JD, Sunderland CO. Chloral hydrate and the carbon dioxide chemoreceptor response: a study of puppies and infants. Pediatrics 1982; 70:447–450.

56. American Thoracic Society, European Respiratory Society. Respiratory function measurement in infants: symbols, abbreviations, and units. Am J Respir Crit Care Med 1995; 151:2041–2057.
57. Patzak A, Schluter B, Orlow W, Mrowka R, Gerhardt D, Schubert E, Persson PB, Barschdorff D, Trowitzsch E. Linear and nonlinear properties of heart rate control in infants at risk. Am J Physiol 1997; 273:540–547.
58. Montano N, Ruscone TG, Porta A, Lombardi F, Pagani M, Malliani A. Power spectrum analysis of heart rate variability to assess the changes in sympathovagal balance during graded orthostatic tilt. Circulation 1994; 90:1826–1831.
59. Mrowka R, Patzak A, Schubert E, Persson P. Linear and non-linear properties of heart rate in postnatal maturation. Cardiovasc Res 1996; 31:447–454.
60. Filtchev SI, Curzi-Descalova L, Spassov L, Kauffmann F, Trang HTT, Gaultier C. Heart rate variability during sleep in infants with bronchopulmonary dysplasia. Chest 1994; 106:1711–1716.
61. Pagani M, Lombardi S, Guzzetti S, Rimoldi O, Furlan R, Pizzinelli P, Sandrone G, Malfatto G, Dell'Orto S, Piccaluga E. Power spectral analysis of heart rate and arterial pressure variabilities as a marker of sympatho-vagal interaction in man and conscious dog. Circ Res 1986; 59:178–193.
62. Hathorn MK. Analysis of periodic changes in ventilation in new-born infants. J Physiol 1978; 285:85–99.
63. Aarimaa T, Valimaki IA. Spectral analysis of impedance respirogram in newborn infants. Biol Neonate 1988; 54:188–194.
64. Dykes FD, Ahmann PA, Baldzer K, Carrigan TA, Kitney R, Giddens DP. Breath amplitude modulations of heart rate variability in normal full term neonates. Pediatr Res 1986; 20:301–308.
65. Schechtman VL, Harper RM, Kluge KA, Wilson AJ, Southall DP. Correlations between cardiorespiratory measures in normal infants and victims of sudden infant death syndrome. Sleep 1990; 13:304–317.
66. Kluge KA, Harper RM, Schechtman VL, Wilson AJ, Hoffman HJ, Southall DP. Spectral analysis assessment of respiratory sinus arrhythmia in normal infants and infants who subsequently died of sudden infant death syndrome. Pediatr Res 1988; 24:677–682.
67. Schechtman VL, Harper RM, Kluge KA, Wilson AJ, Hoffman HJ, Southall DP. Heart rate variation in normal infants and victims of the sudden infant death syndrome. Early Hum Dev 1989; 19:167–181.
68. Katz-Salamon M, Milerad J. The divergent ventilatory and heart rate cardiac responses to moderate hypercapnia in infants with apparent life threatening events (ALTE) and recurrent apnoeas of other causes. Arch Dis Child 1998; 79:231–236.
69. Wierenga H, Brand R, Geudeke T, Van Geijn HP, Van der Harten H, Verloove-Vanhorick P. Prenaral risk factors for cot death in very preterm and small for postconceptual age infants. Early Hum Dev 1990; 23:15–26.
70. Patzak A, Lipke K, Orlow W, Mrowka R, Stauss H, Windt E, Persson PB, Schubert E. Development of heart rate power spectra reveals neonatal peculiarities of cardiorespiratory control. Am J Physiol 1996; 271:1025–1032.

71. Gaultier C. Respiratory adaptation during sleep in infants. Lung 1990; (suppl):905–911.

72. Gray PH, Rogers Y. Are infants with bronchopulmonary dysplasia at risk for sudden infant death syndrome? Pediatrics 1994; 93:774–777.

73. Poets CF. When do infants need additional inspired oxygen—a review of current litterature. Pediatr Pulmonol 1998; 26:424–428.

74. Durand M, McEvoy C, MacDonald K. Spontaneous desaturations in intubated very low birth weight infants with acute and chronic lung disease. Pediatr Pulmonol 1992; 13:136–142.

75. Tay-Uyboco JS, Kwiatkowska K, Cates DB, Kavanagh L, Rigatto H. Hypoxic airway constriction in infants of very low birth weight recovering from moderate to severe bronchopulmonary dysplasia. J Pediatr 1989; 115:456–459.

76. Teague WG, Pian MS, Heldt GP, Tooley WH. An acute reduction in the fraction of inspired oxygen increases airway constriction in infants with chronic lung disease. Am Rev Respir Dis 1988; 137:861–865.

77. Sekar KC, Duke J. Sleep apnea and hypoxemia in recently weaned premature infants with and without bronchopulmonary dysplasia. Pediatr Pulmonol 1991; 10:112–116.

78. McEvoy C, Durand M, Hewlett V. Episodes of spontaneous desaturations in infants with chronic lung disease at two different levels of oxygenation. Pediatr Pulmonol 1993; 15:140–144.

79. Abman SH, Wolfe RR, Accurso FJ, Koops BL, Bowman MC, Wiggins JW. Pulmonary vascular response to oxygen in infants with severe bronchopulmonary dysplasia. Pediatrics 1985; 85:80–84.

80. Moyer-Mileur LJ, Nielson DW, Pfeefer KD, Witte MK, Chapman DL. Eliminating sleep-associated hypoxemia improves growth in infants with bronchopulmonary dysplasia. Pediatrics 1996; 98:779–783.

81. Gaultier C. Effects of breathing during sleep in children with chronic lung disease In: Loughlin GM, Carroll JL, Marcus CL, eds. Sleep and Breathing in Children. New York: Marcel Dekker, 2001.

82. Greenspan JS, Wolfson MR, Locke RG, Allen JL, Shaffer TH. Increased respiratory drive and limited adaptation to loaded breathing in bronchopulmonary dysplasia. Pediatr Res 1992; 32:356–359.

83. Sher MS, Richardson GA, Salerno DG, Day NL, Guthrie RD. Sleep architecture and continuity measures of neonates with chronic lung disease. Sleep 1992; 15:195–201.

84. Harris MA, Sullivan CE. Sleep pattern and supplementary oxygen requirements in infants with neonatal chronic lung disease. Lancet 1995; 345:831–832.

85. Zinman R, Blanchard PW, Vachon F. Oxygen saturation during sleep in patients with bronchopulmonary dysplasia. Biol Neonate 1992; 61:69–75.

86. Gerhardt T, Hehre D, Feller R, Reifenberg L, Bancalari E. Serial determination of pulmonary function in infants with chronic lung disease. J Pediat 1987; 110:448–455.

87. Kitchen WH, Ford GW, Doyle LW, Rickards AL, Kelly EA. Health and hospital readmission of very-low-birth-weight children. Am J Dis Child 1990; 144:213–218.

88. Gross SJ, Iannuzzi DM, Kveselis DA, Anbar RD. Effect of preterm birth on pulmonary function at school age: a prospective controlled study. J Pediatr 1998; 133:188–192.

89. Smyth JA, Tabachnik E, Duncan WJ, Reilly BJ, Levison H. Pulmonary function and bronchial hyperreactivity in long-term survivors of bronchopulmonary dysplasia. Pediatrics 1981; 68:336–340.

90. Northway WH, Moss RB, Carlisle KB, Parker BR, Popp RL, Pitlick PT, Eichler I, Lamm RL, Brown BW. Late pulmonary sequelae of bronchopulmonary dysplasia. N Engl J Med 1990; 323:1793–1799.

91. Hakulinen AL, Heinonen K, Lansimies E, Kiekara O. Pulmonary function and respiratory morbidity in school-age children born prematurely and ventilated for neonatal respiratory insufficiency. Pediatr Pulmonol 1990; 8:226–232.

92. Hakulinen AL, Jarvenpaa AL. Turpeinen M. Sovijarvi A. Diffusing capacity of the lung in school-aged children born very preterm, with and without bronchopulmonary dysplasia. Pediatr Pulmonol 1996; 21:353–360.

93. Nickerson BG, Durand DJ, Kao LC. Short-term variability of pulmonary function tests in infants with bronchopulmonary dysplasia. Pediatr Pulmonol 1989; 6:36–41.

94. Aylward GP, Pfeiffer SI. Perinatal complications and cognitive/neuropsychological outcome. In: Gray JW, Dean RS, eds. Neuropsychology of Perinatal Complications. New York: Springer-Verlag, 1991.

95. Goldstein RF, Thompson RJ Jr, Oehler JM, Brazy JE. Influence of acidosis, hypoxemia and hypotension on neurodevelopmental outcome in very low birth weight infants. Pediatrics 1995; 95:238–243.

96. Gray PH, Burns YR, Mohay HA, O'Callahan MJ, Tudehope D. Neurodevelopmental outcome of preterm infants with bronchopulmonary dysplasia. Arch Dis Child 1995; 73:128–134.

97. Skidmore MD, Rivers A, Hack M. Increased risk of cerebral palsy among very low-birthweight infants with chronic lung disease. Dev Med Child Neurol 1990; 32:325–332.

98. Lifschitz MH, Seilheimer DK, Wilson GS, Williamson WD, Thurber SA, Desmond MM. Neurodevelopmental status of low birth weight infants with bronchopulmonary dysplasia requiring prolonged oxygen supplementation. J Perinatol 1987; 7:127–132.

99. Leonard CH, Clyman RI, Piecuch RE, Juster RP, Ballard RA, Behle MB. Effect of medical and social risk factors on outcome of prematurity and very low birth weight. J Pediatr 1990; 116:620–626.

100. Teberg AJ, Pena I, Finello K, Aguilar T, Hodgman JE. Prediction of neurodevelopmental outcome in infants with and without bronchopulmonary dysplasia. Am J Med Sci 1991; 301:369–374.

101. Landry SH, Fletcher JM, Denson SE, Chapieski ML. Longitudinal outcome for low birth weight infants: effects of intraventricular hemorrhage and bronchopulmonary dysplasia. J Clin Exp Neuropsychol 1993; 15:205–218.

102. Gerner EM, Katz-Salamon M, Hesser U, Soderman E, Forssberg H. Psychomotor development at 10 months as related to neonatal health status: the Stockholm Neonatal Project. Acta Paediatr 1997; 419(suppl):37–43.

103. Singer L, Yamashita T, Lilien L, Collin M, Baley J. A longitudinal study of developmental outcome of infants with bronchopulmonary dysplasia and very low births weight. Pediatrics 1997; 100:987–993.

104. Hughes CA, O'Gorman LA, Shyr Y, Schork MA, Bozynska MEA, McCormick MC. Cognitive performance at school age of very low birth weight infants with bronchopulmonary dysplasia. J Dev Behav Pediatr 1999; 20:1–8.

105. Robertson CMT, Etches PC, Goldson E, Kyle JM. Eight-year school performance, neurodevelopmental, and growth outcome of neonates with bronchopulmonary dysplasia: a comparative study. Pediatrics 1992; 89:365–372.

106. Katz-Salamon M, Gerner EM, Jonsson B, Lagercrantz H. Early motor and mental development in very preterm infants with chronic lung disease. Arch Dis Child 2000; 83:1–6.

107. Böhm B, Katz-Salamon M. Cognitive development of preterm children with chronic lung disease at $5\frac{1}{2}$ years of age. (Submitted.)

108. Majnemer AR, Riley P, Shevell M, Birnbaum R, Greenstone H, Coates AL. Severe bronchopulmonary dysplasia increases risk for later neurological and motor sequelae in preterm survivors. Dev Med Child Neurol 2000; 42:53–60.

109. Luchi JM, Bennet FC, Jackson JC. Predictors of neurodevelopmental outcome following bronchopulmonary dysplasia. Am J. Dis Child 1991; 45:813–817.

21

Gastroesophageal Reflux and Related Diseases

TAHER OMARI

University of Adelaide and Women's and Children's Hospital
Adelaide, South Australia, Australia

I. Introduction

Physiological gastroesophageal reflux (GER), or benign feed-related regurgitation, is common in infants and usually resolves spontaneously by 6 months of age. Gastroesophageal reflux disease (GERD), however, affects <10% of infants and can cause varying degrees of morbidity from irritability, feeding problems, and intolerance to failure to thrive and respiratory complications, including exacerbation of chronic lung diseases and initiation of apnea episodes. In this way, infant GERD is considered to be clinically different from GERD in older children and adults in whom chest pain or frequent "heartburn" is a more common symptom. In the adult and older child, long-term exposure of the esophagus to acid and pepsin results in esophagitis, dysmotility (altered peristalsis and reduced lower esophageal sphincter pressure), and anatomical changes (strictures, hiatus hernia, Barrett's esophagus).

The occurrence, frequency, and extent of GER are above all else influenced by the motor mechanisms responsible for gastroesophageal competence, esophageal volume clearance, and gastric emptying. Factors that influence physiological GER in the infant do so by altering these basic mechanisms. In GER disease, these mechanisms are altered sufficiently to cause a pathological increase in the occurrence of GER and greater esophageal exposure to acid and pepsin. In infants, compared to adults, GER is more frequently low acid (pH >4) owing to regular milk feeding. The occurrence of supraesophageal GER is also more likely due to a proportionately shorter esophagus and lower ratio of esophageal to gastric volume; hence, the likelihood of an interaction of low-acid refluxate with pharyngeal and laryngeal structures is increased. Such interactions will initiate neural reflexes that are protective against aspiration, and these protective mechanisms are also, paradoxically, a potential cause of apnea triggering.

II. Gastrointestinal Motility

The term *gastrointestinal motility* refers to the integration of neural control mechanisms and gastrointestinal smooth muscle contraction to enable the purposeful movement of foodstuffs through the gastrointestinal lumen. This process begins with swallowing, which is initiated in response to posterior propulsion of mouth contents toward the pharynx by the lingual musculature. Pharyngeal swallowing enables food to be propelled through the upper esophageal sphincter (UES) and into the esophageal body, and esophageal contraction further propels the food bolus through the lower esophageal sphincter (LES) into the stomach. In the stomach food is mixed with gastric secretions and emptied in a regulated fashion into the duodenum, where the bulk of chemical digestion and nutrient absorption occur.

With respect to mechanisms of gastroesophageal reflux and clearance of the refluxate, the regions of most interest include the pharynx, UES, esophageal body, LES, and the stomach. Motility of the upper GI tract has now been well characterized in infants owing to the development of micromanometric techniques, for direct measurement of peristaltic and sphincter pressures, and noninvasive tests such as breath tests for measurement of gastric emptying and electrogastrography (EGG) for measurement of gastric pacemaker activity.

A. Esophageal Peristalsis

Swallowing initiates primary persitaltic esophageal contractions, which can be measured as pressure wave sequences propagated in an aboral direction along the length of the esophageal body (Fig. 1). Normal primary esophageal peristalsis has been recorded in the human premature infant from 26 weeks' gestation and older (1–3). The human premature infant also exhibits frequent esophageal body contractions that are not triggered by swallowing and are propagated in a retrograde, synchronous, or incomplete fashion (Fig. 1) (1–3). Similar, "swallow-unrelated" esophageal motor activity has been observed in adults, but these events are less common and are usually associated with occurrence of the migrating motor complex of the small intestine (4). Swallow-unrelated pressure wave sequences appear to be a characteristic feature of the motility of the

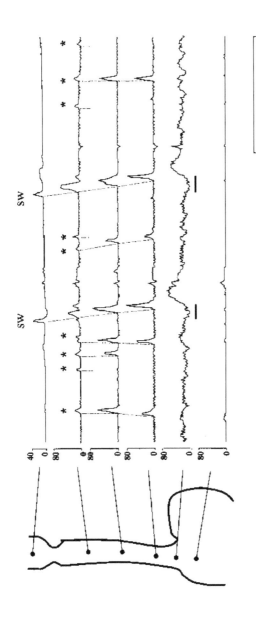

Figure 1 An example tracing of "typical" esophageal motility in the premature infant. Two pharyngeal swallows (sw) initiate primary peristalsis and LES relaxation (bars). Nine swallow-unrelated pressure waves can also been seen (asterisks); these are usually nonperistaltic (synchronous, incomplete, and retrograde) in sequence.

immature esophagus, and occur as a background to what appears to be normal, mature, "swallow-induced" peristalsis. Hence, although a feature of prematurity, they do not appear to impair esophageal function.

B. Sphincter Competence

Upper esophageal sphincter pressure is generated predominantly by tonic contraction of the cricopharyngeus muscle. With swallowing, the cricopharyngeus muscle is inhibited, producing relaxation, and the UES is then opened by the pressure of the food bolus and the superior excursion of the hyoid and larynx (5,6). Premature infants exhibit UES resting tone and UES relaxation in response to dry swallow (7). The magnitude of UES resting pressure is dependent on behavioral state with periods of apparent "comfort" associated with significantly lower UES pressures than periods of activity and apparent "discomfort," or abdominal straining (7). These findings are consistent with the effect of behavior and arousal reported in older children and adults (5,6,8). Measurements of UES relaxation interval, which corresponds closely to the physiological opening and closing of the UES (6), also appear similar to those recorded in healthy adult subjects [7].

The LES functions as a physical esophagogastric antireflux barrier and comprises two sphincter mechanisms—the intrinsic smooth muscle sphincter, and the crural diaphragm, which provides extrinsic support and squeeze. The two sphincter components work together and contribute to LES pressure. Early reports concluded that premature infants have poor LES tone owing to immaturity of sphincter control mechanisms (9–12). However, more recently it has been shown that premature infants have a LES that generates tonic pressures that are sufficiently higher than intragastric pressure to maintain effective esophagogastric competence (5–10 mm Hg) (1–3,13,14).

The LES relaxes with swallow to allow passage of a food bolus. This "swallow-related" relaxation lasts for 3–6 sec during which the LES pressure drops to within 2–4 mmHg of intragastric pressure. Swallow-related relaxation (Fig. 1) is well developed in the premature infant (3). In addition to swallow related relaxation, the LES exhibits transient LES relaxation (TLESR). TLESR is part of the normal belch mechanism required for venting gas from the stomach to prevent gastrointestinal bloating (15). TLESR is also the major mechanism of reflux triggering (15) (refer to Sec. III. B).

C. Gastric Emptying

Gastric emptying in neonates is generally considered a function of fluid (milk) flow across the pylorus; however, upon acidification, milk does separate into semisolid curd and liquid whey fractions. The presence of milk in the fundus stimulates gastric contraction that empties the milk into the duodenum. In premature infants as young as 30 weeks' gestation, gastric half-emptying times have been shown to vary from 17 to 72 min dependent on the feed volume, type, and caloric content where emptying is slowed by higher volumes and greater coloric content and is slower for formula-fed infants than breast milk (16,17). One recent EGG study reported a significantly higher proportion of abnormal gastric pacemaker activity in infants <29 weeks' gestation, but older infants were essentially normal (18).

Studies in adults have shown that gastric motility is highly complex and that in the fed state the spatial and temporal coordination of fundic tone, antral contraction, and pyloric contraction changes substantially over time. During the early phase of gastric emptying, proximal gastric tone provides the driving force for gastric emptying and phasic contractions of the pylorus, known as isolated pyloric pressure waves (IPPWs), serve to regulate flow of gastric contents through the gastric outlet. In addition, coordinated patterns of propagated antral pressure wave sequences facilitate mixing and pumping gastric contents into the duodenum (19). Evaluations of antral motility in premature infants have also shown that patterns of antral and pyloric motility are well developed by 30 weeks (20).

III. Gastroesophageal Reflux

Gastroesophageal reflux is the retrograde flow of gastric contents (gas or acidic/nonacidic liquid) into the esophagus. GER can manifest as gas, liquid, or a combination of liquid and gas, the liquid being either acidic (pH <4), low-acidic (pH 4–7), or nonacidic (pH ≥7) depending on the timing relative to feeding. Immediately after feeding GER is nonacidic and then becomes gradually more acidic during the postprandial period (Fig. 2). Gastric secretory capacity in premature infants appears to be well developed, as they have the ability to acidify gastric contents to pH <4 by 25 weeks' gestation (21). However, infants feed more frequently than adults, buffering intragastric pH such that infants fed at shorter intervals have higher intragastric pH and less acid reflux (22).

Figure 2 indicates that very few acid GER episodes (pH <4) and mostly low-acid GER episodes (pH 4–7) are recorded by pH probe in the first 2 h after feeding. The relatively recent development of combined multichannel intraluminal impedance catheters has allowed all forms of reflux (gas, liquid, acid, nonacid) to be precisely measured in infants. Impedance studies have shown that >70% of GER episodes occur during the first 2 h after feeding and are nonacidic (23). Nonacid GER can also be measured by intraluminal manometry where GER episodes produce a characteristic "common-cavity episode," which is an abrupt sustained equalization of intragastric, LES, and esophageal pressures. This equalization occurs subsequent to flow of liquid and/or gas from the stomach into the esophagus. Like the impedance studies, manometry in prema-

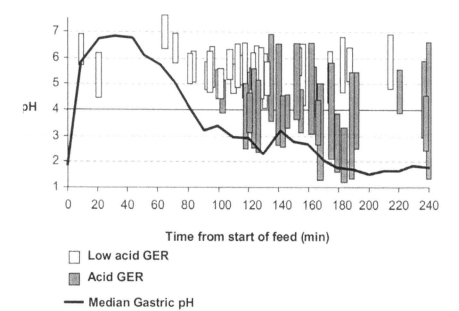

Time from start of feed (min)

☐ Low acid GER

▨ Acid GER

━━ Median Gastric pH

Figure 2 Correlation of acid GER and intragastric pH. Bars show the extent of esophageal pH change (from basal pH to nadir) during 57 acid GER episodes, recorded in 14 breast-fed premature infants at 35–37 weeks' gestation. Acid GER was defined as an esophageal pH drop of >1 pH unit with a nadir pH >4 (low acid GER) or a nadir pH <4 (acid GER). Median gastric pH determined by three pH sensors located in the stomach.

ture infants has shown that ~70% of common cavities recorded in the first 2 h after feeding are not associated with an esophageal pH drop (2). These observations clearly highlight the limitation of pH probes alone for measurement of GER where almost all GER episodes occurring in the early postprandial period are not identified.

A. Mechanisms of GER Triggering

The likelihood of reflux occurring is dictated by both the pressure gradient between the stomach and the esophagus (positive in the stomach with respect to the esophagus), and the pressure at the esophagogastric junction, which forms the antireflux barrier. The gastroesophageal pressure gradient is changing constantly, usually increasing with each inspiration and/or abdominal straining event. The basal pressure at the gastroesophageal junction is generated by both tonic contraction of the LES and the extrinsic "squeeze" of the crural diaphragm;

this physical pressure barrier protects against reflux and is maintained as long as LES pressure exceeds intragastric pressure. GER will occur if either LES pressure is low (<5 mm Hg) or absent (e.g., during LES relaxation) or if gastric pressure rises sufficiently to surpass LES pressure (eg during abdominal straining events).

As previously mentioned, healthy infants, including premature infants, have a competent LES. Therefore most GER events are associated with relaxation of the LES. A number of motor mechanisms of GER triggering have been identified, including predominantly failed peristalsis, multiple swallowing, and TLESR (2) (Fig. 3). Common to all of these reflux-related motor events is the temporary absence or inhibition of LES pressure coupled with the absence or inhibition of esophageal peristalsis.

B. Transient LES Relaxation

TLESR is by far the most common mechanism of GER triggering in normal subjects and has been described in all age groups from 26-week-old premature infants through to adults. Compared to normal swallow-related LES relaxations, TLESRs occur independently of pharyngeal swallowing, are prolonged in duration (>10 sec), relax more completely (lower nadir), and are associated with inhibition of the esophageal body and crural diaphragm. The inhibition of the crural diaphragm is critically important for reflux to occur, as crural squeeze pressures alone are often sufficient to prevent reflux during prolonged periods of absent LES pressure (24).

Physiologically, TLESRs serve to vent gases from the stomach during belching to prevent gastrointestinal bloating (15,24). TLESRs are also stimulated in response to a meal, being most common in the early postprandial period and reducing in frequency over time (Fig. 4). Although fewer in number, TLESRs occurring later postprandially trigger proportionately more acid GER (Fig. 4). The meal-induced stimulation of TLESRs is primarily due to gastric distension (25). Distension of the proximal stomach with nonmeal stimuli such as air insufflation or balloon inflation will similarly induce TLESRs (26–28). By this we can infer that the occurrence of TLESRs is dependent upon the size of the meal and (probably) the rate of gastric emptying which serves to regulate the degree and duration of gastric distension.

Neurophysiologically, TLESRs occur via a vagovagal reflex initiated by stretch-sensitive receptors located in the smooth muscle of the stomach wall; the greatest concentration of these receptors is likely to be in the cardia of the stomach, which is the region most sensitive to TLESR triggering (28). The stretch-sensitive sensory nerve fibers of the afferent arm of the reflex pathway terminate in the brainstem (nucleus tractus solitarius) and ultimately synapse with vagal motor neurones (dorsal motor nucleus of the vagus nerve and nucleus ambiguous) projecting to the LES, esophagus, pharynx, and crural diaphragm.

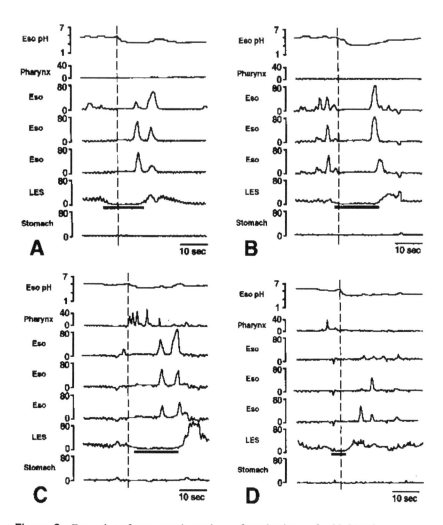

Figure 3 Examples of manometric tracings of mechanisms of acid GER in premature infants: spontaneous TLESR (A), TLESR occurring after esophageal body contraction (B), multiple swallows (C), and peristaltic failure (D). Dotted lines indicate the onset of GER episodes. Black bars indicate duration of LESR. (From Ref. 2.)

The brainstem structures implicated in the reflex collectively form the neural pattern generator, which exquisitely choreographs the complex series of events that manifest as a TLESR (24) (Fig. 5).

A range of neurotransmitters, including acetylcholine (ACh), cholecystokinin (CCK), gamma-amino-butyric acid (GABA), glutamate, nitric oxide (NO),

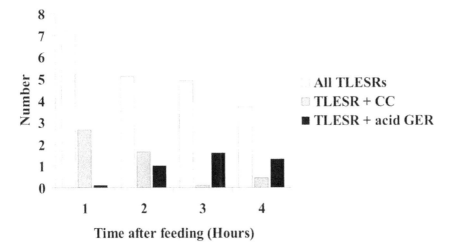

Figure 4 Postprandial occurrence of TLESRs, TLESRs with common cavities (nonacid GER), and TLESRs with acid GER. Data from 10 premature infants at 37–39 weeks' gestation.

and opioids, have been immunohistochemically and pharmacologically implicated in the TLESR reflex pathway. These are believed to act either peripherally, regulating excitability of the stretch receptor, or centrally, regulating signal transduction and/or activation of vagal motor neurones (24).

That premature infants have TLESRS with the same characteristics (duration, nadir pressure) as those described in adults (3) indicates that the basic neurological mechanisms underlying TLESRs are well developed in these infants.

C. Mechanisms of GER clearance

Peristalsis serves to clear the esophagus of its contents (collectively known as esophageal volume clearance) and therefore is important in both feeding and in the clearing of gastroesophageal refluxate. Normal primary (swallow-related) peristalsis has been recorded in the human premature infant, and, when recorded in conjunction with esophageal pH, primary peristalsis effectively facilitates rapid esophageal volume clearance of acid gastroesophageal refluxate as indicated by the resolution of esophageal pH from <4 to >4 (2). Secondary peristalsis is usually initiated in response to the abrupt sustained increase in intraesophageal pressure (common cavity), which accompanies all reflux episodes. The secondary peristaltic pressure wave is usually synchronous and leads to termination of the common cavity episode (2). Any refluxate remaining in the esophageal lumen is

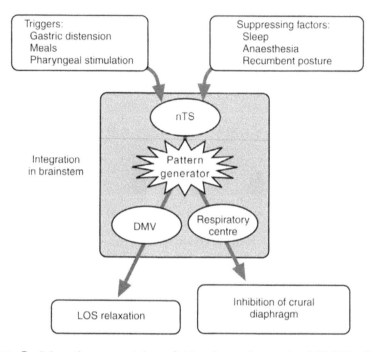

Figure 5 Schematic representation of triggering and control of TLESR. Gastric distension activates mechanoreceptors in the proximal stomach and send signals to the brainstem centers (DMV, dorsal motor nucleus of the vagus; nTS, nucleus of the tractus solitarius) via vagal afferent pathways. The structured sequence of resultant motor events and consistent and complex pattern of activation suggest that it occurs in a programmed manner, thought to be controlled by a pattern generator within the region of the vagal nuclei. (From Ref. 24.)

then cleared by primary peristalsis, whereby swallows trigger pressure wave sequences propagated down the body of the esophagus at a velocity of ~3 cm/sec (2).

Impedance studies have shown that the bulk of refluxate is rapidly cleared from the oesophageal lumen. In the case of acid reflux however, it usually takes longer to remove all acid residues and return esophageal pH to prereflux values. Swallowed saliva plays an important role in buffering postreflux acid residues. The frequency of swallowing and type of pressure wave sequence propagated are important in determining the effectiveness of peristalsis for esophageal volume clearance and acid residue clearance. In infants, increased swallowing and peristalsis are the normal responses to GER; studies that have directly compared preterm infants with newborn full-term infants suggest that, in the newly born,

GER stimulates swallowing, but only 40% of these swallows trigger esophageal peristalsis, leading to slower clearance. In the preterm infant at term age, a higher proportion of swallows trigger peristalsis, leading to more effective esophageal clearance (29). This suggests that a degree of maturation of clearance mechanisms occurs in the early postnatal period.

IV. Pathophysiology of GER Disease

A. Normal Values for GER: Physiological vs. Pathological

Reflux disease is typically characterized by a greater-than-normal exposure of the esophageal lumen to acid and pepsin and/or an association of reflux episodes with symptoms. In older infants and children, extended distal esophageal pH monitoring has proven to be an effective clinical tool for the recognition of pathological degrees of esophageal acid exposure, establishment of associations between symptoms and the occurrence of GER and to evaluate the effectiveness of antireflux therapy. In the preterm and term infant, however, there are no consistent and uniformly accepted "gold standard" pH monitoring criteria for GERD. Some studies have applied adult pH monitoring reflux index (% time pH <4) criteria (i.e., >5%) to confirm the clinical diagnosis of GERD in premature infants (30,31), one of these (31) indicating that infants selected in this way have increased acid oropharyngeal aspirates, which may in itself be useful diagnostically.

Normative data in term infants asymptomatic of GER suggest that 95th percentile of reflux index scores decreases from 13% in the first month of life to 8% at 1 year of age (32). Twenty-four-hour esophageal pH monitoring studies in asymptomatic premature infants have reported mean reflux indices in this group with a high degree of variability, ranging from 0.7% to 11.9% (33–37). The applicability of extended pH monitoring to term and preterm infants remains controversial, but given the difficulties in performing endoscopic evaluations in such small infants, is the only diagnostic test available. In different centers, the reflux index cutoff considered to be indicative of pathological GER has ranged from 5% to 12%.

B. Role of TLESRs in GERD

The evidence for the role of TLESRs in the pathophysiology of pediatric GER disease is now unequivocal. TLESRs were originally described in children with GERD by Werlin et al. (38), and a number of studies have now reported that 34–100% of acid GER episodes recorded in infants and children with GERD are triggered by this mechanism (39–42). This is also the case in preterm infants where TLESRs trigger 50–100% of acid GER episodes (43). It is now well established that TLESR is the single most common mechanism underlying GER in GERD at all ages.

In the absence of normal data from healthy children, it is unclear whether GERD in children is characterized by either a higher rate of TLESR or a greater incidence of GER episodes during TLESR. Studies in adults have been inconclusive on this issue, as studies have recorded both a higher rate of TLESRs (25) and a greater incidence of GER episodes during TLESRs (44,45). Studies in infants agree with the latter observation that there is a greater incidence of GER during TLESR (43) (Fig. 6). This suggests that infants with reflux disease may

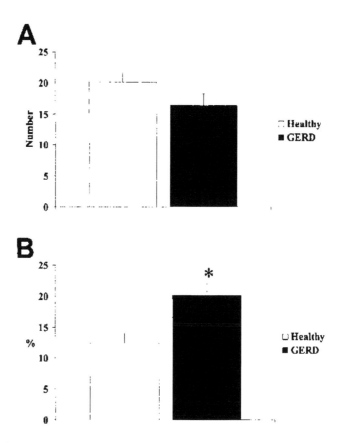

Figure 6 Number of TLESRs (A) and proportion of TLESRs (B) associated with acid GER during the period from 0 to 4 h after feeding in preterm and term infants with GER disease. GERD is characterized by a higher proportion of acid GER in association with TLESR. Data from 36 infants at 33–40 weeks' gestation comprising 22 health controls and 14 infants with GERD.

have anatomical or functional differences that increase the likelihood of liquid (rather than gas) reflux during TLESR.

To date, only pH criteria have been used to detect (acid) GER in infants with GER disease; however, as previously discussed, these criteria cannot accurately detect nonacid GER during the early postprandial period. Nonacidic liquid GER is likely to be of great importance in neonatal reflux disease as it occurs during the period of time that is usually associated with most putative "reflux-related" events, especially apnea and regurgitation. The precise role of nonacidic liquid reflux in the pathophysiology of infant GERD still requires further evaluation, particularly the role of nonacidic supraesophageal reflux, occurring in the early postprandial period, which may be responsible for initiating reflex apnea.

C. Role of Esophageal Dysmotility in GERD

Esophageal dysmotility leading to delayed esophageal clearance appears to be less important in the pathophysiology of infant GERD than it is in older children and adults. Infants do not exhibit esophageal dysmotility in relation to GERD (40). Sondheimer et al. (46) reported few motility defects in infants with GERD, but found that these infants swallowed less frequently, particularly during sleep. Studies in older children with GERD do indicate delayed clearance of acid reflux due to higher incidence of "nonspecific esophageal motility defects," which become more prevalent with increasing severity of disease. Severe pediatric GERD with reflux esophagitis is also associated with a 30–50% decrease in pressure wave amplitude (41), indicating that the contractile strength of the esophagus is also impaired.

D. Delayed Gastric Emptying

Hillemeier and colleagues (47) first reported delayed gastric emptying in pediatric GERD, and since then a number of studies have reported both normal (48–52) and delayed (39,53–57) gastric emptying in infants and children with GERD. EGG studies indicate that there is a higher proportion of abnormal EGG patterns in children with GERD (51,58). The precise role of delayed GE in the pathophysiology of GERD is still unclear. Delayed GE may exacerbate GER by prolonging gastric distension and increasing the frequency of transient LES relaxation; however attempts to correlate gastric emptying with acid GER have been unsuccessful (37,48). Despite these conflicting observations, impaired gastric motor function leading to delayed gastric emptying is apparent in a few well-defined subgroups of patients at the severe end of the reflux spectrum— particularly those with failure to thrive and/or vomiting when associated with neurological or respiratory disease (47,53,57,59).

E. Straining

Previous studies in children with GERD indicate that abdominal straining and GER are often associated (38). Several different straining patterns can be identified, including sustained strains (associated with defecation or movement), and transient strains (associated with inspiration/expiration or cough). Straining results in a simultaneous, sometimes rapid increase/decrease in gastric, LES, and esophageal pressures. During straining the extrinsic LES support rendered by the crural diaphragm and the fact LES pressure changes to a similar extent as intragastric pressure help maintain the antireflux barrier (24). Hence, GER episodes that occur during straining usually occur when LES pressure is low or absent either as the result of sphincter incompetence or even during LES relaxation. In infants and children, TLESRs occurring during straining are more likely to trigger acid GER than TLESRs that are not associated with straining (43). It is likely that straining exacerbates GER during TLESR because both LES tone and crural diaphragm tone are inhibited by the TLESR reflex.

A further straining pattern that has been described is transient abdominal pressure increases caused by sudden contraction of the diaphragm and abdominal respiratory muscles. This event causes a sudden elevation (or spike) of gastric pressure, which provides a driving force for active expulsion of gastric contents. This appears to be the major mechanism of common postprandial regurgitation or "spitting up" (61). As shown in Figure 7, esophageal manometric studies in infants suggest that during these events the LES relaxes completely several seconds prior to straining and regurgitation. Strain-related regurgitation episodes such as these are responsible for 5% of acid GER episodes in infants (2).

V. Respiratory Disease and GER

A. Methylxanthine Therapy

Methylxanthines (aminophylline, theophylline, and caffeine) are potent bronchodilators and CNS respiratory stimulants, and are commonly used in the treatment of chronic obstructive pulmonary diseases, asthma, and apnea. Methylxanthines also appear to exacerbate GER. Studies in premature and term infants with apnea or at risk of sudden infant death syndrome (35,62–63) have shown that methylxanthine therapy augments esophageal acid exposure recorded by esophageal pH probe. These findings have largely been attributed to the fact that methylxanthines are known to stimulate gastric acid secretion and to inhibit LES tone (64–66). Other specific effects of methylxanthines on esophageal function per se have not been investigated. One study has indicated that theophylline therapy may also augment the frequency of transient LES relaxations in healthy premature infants (3), but this observation was not supported by a similar study of infants with chronic lung disease (67).

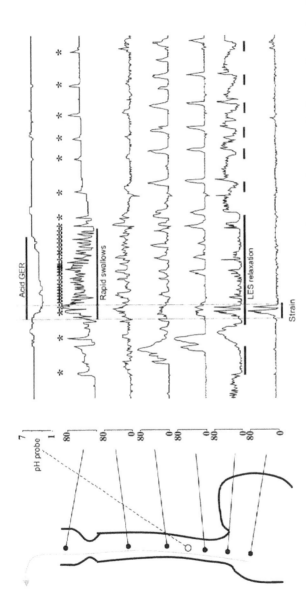

Figure 7 An example tracing of esophageal motility during a regurgitation event. The LES relaxes completely several seconds prior to straining, which forces gastric content out of the esophagus. Acid exposure to the esophagus is indicated by a drop in esophageal pH; supraesophageal exposure is indicated by very rapid swallowing, which initiates frequent peristalsis and clearance of esophageal refluxate. Frequent swallowing persists after esophageal clearance is complete, indicating the persistent pharyngeal exposure to refluxate. An identical motor pattern is seen irrespective of the acidity of refluxate.

B. Respiratory Effort

As previously mentioned, the abdominothoracic pressure gradient provides the driving pressure for GER to occur, but intragastric pressure must exceed the pressure at the LES for GER triggering. Two dominant factors influence the abdomino-thoracic pressure gradient, respiratory effort and abdominal straining (see Sec. IV.E above).

With increased respiratory effort, such as is the case in chronic lung disease, the abdominothoracic pressure gradient is increased (i.e., intrathoracic pressures become more negative and intragastric pressures become more positive). It is important to recognize that this increase in pressure gradient alone is insufficient to overcome LES pressure and trigger GER, and TLESR is still the predominant mechanism of GER in these infants (67). However, the association of GER with TLESR is much more likely because, owing to higher intragastric pressures, the LES does not need to relax as completely to trigger a GER episode.

C. Reflux and Apnea

Apnea is a major problem in infants with the incidence being inversely proportional to gestational age (68). Frequent apnea and bradycardia, particularly with feeding, is a common clinical correlate of GERD which may (69–71) or may not (72) improve with antireflux therapy. However, the precise role of GER in the pathophysiology of apnea is still unclear. Apnea with feeding and/or due to GER may result through one of three predominate mechanisms: poor coordination of suck and swallow with breathing; neural reflex mechanisms initiated by chemical stimulation of the larynx and pharynx; or neural reflex mechanisms initiated by esophageal distension.

Anatomically, the laryngeal inlet is located higher in the pharynx in the infant than in the adult, and the epiglottis extends into the nasopharynx, separating the respiratory passages and digestive conduit (73). This anatomical arrangement reduces the risk of aspiration and limits laryngeal stimulation during feeding and after reflux. Swallowing also plays an important protective role in clearing the pharynx of residues and in turn limiting or preventing aspiration and/or stimulation of laryngeal chemoreflexes (see below). Swallowing is commonly observed during regurgitation and GER episodes where swallowing and primary peristalsis serve to clear the pharynx and esophagus of gastric refluxate (see Fig. 7). Neonates possess a normal airway protective mechanism which is triggered prior to pharyngeal swallowing (74). Although protective against aspiration, this respiratory inhibition can itself lead to apnea episodes if suck, swallow, and breathing are not adequately coordinated, as is the case in the newborn or preterm infant [75].

The laryngeal chemoreflex is a protective mechanism preventive against aspiration. Sensory nerve endings at the laryngeal opening, located in the narrow interarytenoid space, are stimulated by contact with fluid; this triggers a series of centrally mediated responses including swallowing, cessation of breathing, bronchoconstriction, and coughing. The sensory endings that initiate the reflex are thought to be chemoreceptors rather than mechanoreceptors because the receptors are more sensitive to water than to an equal volume of saline. The laryngeal chemoreflex is more readily initiated in preterm infants than in term infants, which may explain why apnea is a greater problem in premature infants (76).

The esophagoglottal closure reflex is one of a number of reflex responses that can be initiated by esophageal distension, including secondary esophageal peristalsis, UES closure, and UES relaxation. The esophagoglottal closure reflex results in adduction of the vocal cords and narrowing the interarytenoid space and therefore is thought to provide airways protection. The sensory endings that initiate the reflex are mechanoreceptors located in the body of the esophagus. The threshold for initiation of the reflex is high (requiring balloon distension), and the reflex is therefore unlikely to be initiated during most GER episodes but is more likely to occur during episodes of abrupt esophageal distension, such as that which occurs during vomiting (77).

GER may be a direct or indirect trigger for apneic episodes via the mechanisms described above, or, alternatively, the likelihood of GER occurring may be exacerbated by a transient increase in the gastroesophageal pressure gradient resulting from airways obstruction. Studies that have evaluated the temporal association between reflux and apnea have required prolonged simultaneous monitoring of both reflux and respiratory events. Such studies have produced conflicting findings of either little or no association (78–85) or an association (86–91) between apnea and GER. Two studies have evaluated these associations using impedance methods. Wenzl et al. (91) reported that 29.7% of apnea episodes were temporally associated (within ±30 sec) with GER of which 77.6% were nonacidic (64). In contrast, Peter et al. (85) found that the frequency of apnea during GER was no different from the frequency of apnea occurring independently of GER, suggesting that the majority of temporal associations were random associations rather than cause and effect. A small minority of apnea episodes were, however, associated with supraesophageal GER, and in these circumstances apnea usually occurred after GER, suggesting a potential link between the two.

It is clear from these recent investigations that a high proportion of GER episodes are missed using standard pH monitoring and that supraesophageal reflux, which may be an important precursor to the initiation of apnea reflexes, may not be adequately measured using standard methodologies. In light of these new observations, the diagnosis of GERD in the neonate and our assumptions regarding the relationship of GER and apnea may need reexamination.

References

1. Omari T, Benninga M, Barnett C, Haslam R, Davidson G, Dent J. Characterisation of esophageal body and lower esophageal sphincter motor function in the very premature neonate. J Pediatr 1999; 135(4):517–521.
2. Omari TI, Barnett C, Snel A, Goldsworthy W, Haslam R, Davidson G, Kirubakaran C, Bakewell M, Fraser R, Dent J. Mechanisms of gastroesophageal reflux in healthy premature infants. J Pediatr 1998; 133:650–654.
3. Omari TI, Miki K, Davidson G, Fraser R, Haslam R, Goldsworthy W, Bakewell M, Dent J. Characterisation of relaxation of the lower oesophageal sphincter in healthy premature infants. Gut 1997; 40:370–375.
4. Janssens J, Annese V, Vantrappen G. Bursts of non-deglutative simultaneous contractions may be a normal oesophageal motility pattern. Gut 1993; 34:1021–1024.
5. Cook I, Dent J, Shannon S, Collins S. Measurement of upper esopageal sphincter pressure: effect of acute emotional stress. Gastroenterology 1987; 93:526–532.
6. Kahrilas P, Dodds W, Dent J, Haeberle B, Hogan W, Arndorfer R. Effect of sleep, spontaneous gastroesophageal reflux and a meal on upper esophageal sphincter pressure in normal human volunteers. Gastroenterology 1987; 92:466–471.
7. Omari T, Snel A, Barnett C, Davidson G, Haslam R, Dent J. Measurement of upper esophageal sphincter tone and relaxation during swallowing in premature infants. Am J Physiol 1999; 277(4):G862–G866.
8. Willing J, Furukawa Y, Davidson GP, Dent J. Stain induced augmentation of upper esophageal sphincter pressure in children. Gut 1994; 35:159–164.
9. Boix-Ochoa J, Canals J. Maturation of the lower oesophagus. J Pediatr Surg 1976; 11:749–756.
10. Gryboski J. Suck and swallow in the premature infant. Pediatrics 1969; 43:96–102.
11. Gryboski J, Thayer W, Spiro H. Esophageal motility in infants and children. Pediatrics 1963; 31:382–395.
12. Gryboski J, Thayler W, Spiro H. Esophageal motility in infants and children. Pediatrics 1983; 31:382–395.
13. Newell S, Sarkar P, Durbin G, Booth I, McNeish A. Maturation of the lower oesophageal sphincter in the preterm baby. Gut 1988; 29:167–172.
14. Omari TI, Miki K, Fraser R, Davidson G, Haslam R, Goldsworthy W, Bakewell M, Kawahara H, Dent J. Esophageal body and lower esophageal sphincter function in healthy premature infants. Gastroenterology 1995; 109:1757–1764.
15. Mittal R, Holloway R, Penagini R, Blackshaw L, Dent J. Transient lower esophageal relaxation. Gastroenterology 1995; 109:601–610.
16. Cavill B. Gastric emptying in preterm infants. Acta Paediatr Scand 1979; 68:725–730.
17. Newell SJ, Chapman S, Booth IW. Ultrasonic assessment of gastric emptying in the preterm infant. Arch Dis Child 1993; 69:32–36.
18. Cucchiara S, Salvia G, Scarcella A, Rapagiolo S, Borrelli O, Boccia G, Riezzo G, Ciccimarra F. Gestational maturation of electrical activity of the stomach. Dig Dis Sci 1999; 44:2008–2013.

19. Sun WM, Hebbard GS, Malbert CH, Jones KL, Doran S, Horowitz M, Dent J. Spatial patterns of fasting and fed antro-pyloric pressure waves in humans. J Physiol 1997; 503:455–462.

20. Hassan B, Butler R, Davidson G, Benninga M, Haslam R, Barnett C, Dent J, Omari T. Patterns of antropyloric motility in fed healthy preterm infants. Arch Dis Child 2002; 87(2):F95–99.

21. Hyman PE, Clarke DD, Everett SL, Sonne B, Stewart D, Harada T, Walsh JH, Taylor IL. Gastric acid secretory function in preterm infants. J Pediatr 1985; 106(3):467–471.

22. Mitchell DJ, McLure BG, Tubman TRJ. Simultaneous monitoring of gastric and oesophageal pH reveals limitations of conventional oesophageal pH monitoring in milk fed infants. Arch Dis Child 2001; 84:273–276.

23. Skopnik H, Silny J, Heiber O, Schulz J, Rau G, Heimann G. Gastroesophageal reflux in infants: evaluation of a new intraluminal impedance technique. J Pediatr Gastroenterol Nutr 1996; 23(5):591–598.

24. Holloway RH. The anti-reflux barrier and mechanisms of gastro-oesophageal reflux. Baillieres Clin Gastroenterol 2000; 14(5):681–699.

25. Holloway RH, Kocyan P, Dent J. Provocation of transient lower esophageal sphincter relaxations by meals in patients with symptomatic gastroesophageal reflux. Dig Dis Sci 1991; 36:1034–1039.

26. Holloway RH, Hongo M, Berger K, McCallum RW. Gastric distension: a mechanism for post-prandial gastroesophageal reflux. Gastroenterology 1985; 89:779–784.

27. Boeckxstaens GE, Hirsch DP, Fakhry N, Holloway RH, D'Amato M, Tytgat GNJ. Involvement of cholecystokinin-A receptors in transient lower esophageal sphincter relaxations triggered by gastric distension. Am J Gastroenterol 1998; 93:1823–1828.

28. Franzi SJ, Martin CJ, Cox MR, Dent J. Response of canine lower esophageal sphincter to gastric distension. Am J Physiol 1990; 259:G380–G385.

29. Jeffery HE, Ius D, Page M. The role of swallowing during active sleep in the clearance of reflux in term and preterm infants. J Pediatr 2000; 137:545–548.

30. Ewer A, James M, Tobin J. Prone and left lateral positioning reduce gastro-oesophageal reflux in preterm infants. Arch Dis Child Fetal Neonatal Ed 1999; 81:F201–F205.

31. James M, Ewer A. Acid oro-pharyngeal secretions can predict gastro-oesophageal reflux in preterm infants. Eur J Pediatr 1999; 80:F174–F177.

32. Vandenplas Y, Sacre-Smits L. Continuous 24-hour esophageal pH monitoring in 285 asymptomatic infants 0–15 months old. J Pediatr Gastroenterol Nutr 1987; 6:220–224.

33. Sutphen J, Dillard V. Effects of maturation and gastric acidity on gastroesophageal reflux in infants. Am J Dis Child 1986; 140:1062–1064.

34. Ng S-Y, Quak S-H. Gastroesophageal reflux in preterm infants: norms for extended distal esophageal pH monitoring. J Pediatr Gastroenterol Nutr 1998; 27:411–414.

35. Newell S, Booth I, Morgan M, Durbin G, McNeish A. Gastro-oesophageal reflux in preterm infants. Arch Dis Child 1989; 64:780–786.

36. Jeffery H, Page M. Developmental maturation of gastro-oesophageal reflux in preterm infants. Acta Paediatr. 1995; 84:245–250.
37. Ewer A, Durbin G, Morgan M, Booth I. Gastric emptying and gastro-oesphageal reflux in preterm infants. Arch Dis Child 1996; 75:F117–F121.
38. Werlin S, Dodds W, Hogan W, Arndorfer R. Mechanisms of gastroesophageal reflux in children. J Pediatr 1980; 97:244–249.
39. Mahony MJ, Migliavacca M, Spitz L, Milla PJ. Motor disorders of the oesophagus in gastro-oesophageal reflux. Arch Dis Child 1988; 63:1333–1338.
40. Cucchiara S, Bortolotti M, Minella R, Auricchio S. Fasting and postprandial mechanisms of gastroesophageal reflux in children with gastroesophageal reflux. Dig Dis Sci 1993; 38:86–92.
41. Cucchiara S, Staiano A, Di Lorenzo C, De Luca G, della Rocca A, Auricchio S. Pathophysiology of gastroesophageal reflux and distal esophageal motility in children with gastroesophageal reflux disease. J Pediatr Gastroenterol Nutr 1988; 7:830–836.
42. Kawahara H, Dent J, Davidson G. Mechanisms responsible for gastroesophageal reflux in children. Gastroenterology 1997; 113:399–408.
43. Omari TI, Barnett CP, Benninga MA, Lontis R, Goodchild L, Haslam RR, Dent J, Davidson GP. Mechanisms of gastro-oesophageal reflux in preterm and term infants with reflux disease. Gut 2002; 51(4):475–479.
44. Mittal R, McCallum R. Characteristics and frequency of transient relaxations of the lower esophageal sphincter on patients with reflux esophagitis. Gastroenterology 1988; 95:593–599.
45. Sifrim D, Holloway J, Silney J, Tack J, Lerut A, Janssens J. Composition of the post prandial refluxate in patients with gastroesophageal reflux disease. Am J Gastro-enterol 2001; 96(3):647–655.
46. Sondheimer JM. Clearance of spontaneous gastroesophageal reflux in awake and sleeping infants. Gastroenterology 1989; 97:821–826.
47. Hillemeier AC, Lange R, McCallum R, Seashore J, Gryboski J. Delayed gastric emptying in infants with gastroesophageal reflux. J Pediatr 1981; 98:190–193.
48. Jolley SG, Leonard JC, Tunell WP. Gastric emptying in children with gastro-esophageal reflux. J Pediatr Surg 1987; 22:923–926.
49. Euler AR, Byrne WJ. Gastric emptying times of water in infants and children: comparison of those with and without reflux. J Pediatr Gastroenterol Nutr 1983; 2:595–598.
50. Jackson PT, Glasgow JFT, Thomas PS, Carre IJ. Children with gastroesophageal reflux with or without partial thoracic stomach (hiatal hernia) have normal gastric emptying. J Pediatr Gastroenterol Nutr 1989; 8:37–40.
51. Seigl A, Mayr J, Huber A Uray E. Postprandial tachygastria in frequent in infants with gastroesophageal reflux. Pediatr Surg Int 1998; 13:569–571.
52. Billeaud C, Guillet J, Sandler B. Gastric emptying in infants with and without gastro-oesophageal reflux according to the type of milk. Eur J Clin Nutr 1990; 44:577–583.
53. Hillemeier AC, Grill B, McCallum R, Gryboski J. Esophageal and gastric motor abnormalities in gastroesophageal reflux during infancy. Gastroenterology 1983; 84:741:746.

54. Guillet J, Wynchank S, Christophe E, Basse-Cathalinat B, Ducassou D, Blanquet P. Gastro-oesophageal reflux and gastric emptying of liquids in paediatric patients. Int J Nucl Med Biol 1984; 11:254–258.

55. Di Lorenzo C, Piepsz A, Ham H, Cadranel S. Gastric emptying with gastro-oesophageal reflux. Arch Dis Child 1987; 62:449–453.

56. Papaila JG, Wilmont D, Grosfeld JL, Rescorla FJ, West KW, Vane DW. Increased incidence of delayed gastric emptying in children with gastroesophageal reflux. Arch Surg 1989; 124:933–936.

57. LiVoti G, Tulone V, Bruno R, Cataliotti F, Iacono G, Cavataio F, Balsamo V. Ultrasonography and gastric emptying: evaluation in infants with gastroesophageal reflux. J Pediar Gastroenterol Nutr 1992; 14:397–399.

58. Cucchiara S, Salvia G, Borrelli O, Ciccimarra E, Az-Zeqeh N, Rapagiolo S, Minella R, Campanozzi A, Riezzo G. Gastric electrical dysrythmias and gastric emptying in gastroesophageal reflux disease. Am J Gastroenterol 1997; 92:1103–1107.

59. Andres JM, Mathias JR, Clench MH, Davis RH. Gastric emptying in infants with gastroesophageal reflux. Dig Dis Sci 1988; 33:393–399.

60. Kawahara H, Dent J, Davidson G, Okada A. Relationship between straining, transient lower esophageal sphincter relaxation, and gastroesophageal reflux in children. Am J Gastroenterol 2001; 96(7):2019–2025.

61. Orenstein S, Dent J, Deneault L. Regurgitant reflux vs non regurgitant reflux is preceded by rectus abdominis contraction in infants. Neurogastroenterol Motil 1994; 6:271–277.

62. Vandenplas Y, De Wolf D, Sacre L. Influence of xanthines on gastroesophageal reflux in infants at risk for sudden infant death syndrome. Pediatrics 1986; 77:807–810.

63. Sacre L, Vandenplas Y. Xanthines in apnea of premature infants. Influence on gastroesophageal reflux. Arch Fr Pediatr 1987; 44:383–385.

64. Forster L, Trudeau W, Goldman A. Bronchodilator effects on gastric acid secretion. JAMA 1979; 241:2613–2615.

65. Stein M, Towner T, Weber R. The effect of theophylline on the lower esophageal sphincter pressure. Ann Allergy 1980; 45:238–241.

66. Berquist W, Rachelefsky G, Kadden M, Seigel S, Katz R, Mickey M. Effect of theophylline on gastroesophageal reflux in normal adults. J Allergy Clin Immunol 1981; 67:407–411.

67. Omari T, Barnett C, Snel A, Davidson G, Haslam R, Bakewell M, Dent J. Mechanisms of gastro-oesophageal reflux in premature infants with chronic lung disease. J Pediatr Surg 1999; 34(12):1–5.

68. Bontarline-Young H, Smith C. Respiration of full-term and of premature infants. Am J Dis Child 1953; 80:753.

69. Bauman NM, Sandler AD, Smith RJ. Respiratory manifestations of gastroesophageal reflux disease in pediatric patients. Ann Otol Rhinol Laryngol 1996; 105(1):23–32.

70. Burton DM, Pransky SM, Katz RM, Kearns DB, Seid AB. Pediatric airway manifestations of gastroesophageal reflux. Ann Otol Rhinol Laryngol 1992; 101(9):742–749.

71. Sindel BD. Neonatal apnea casebook. Gastroesophageal reflux (GER)-associated apnea. J Perinatol 1999; 19(1):77–79.
72. Kimball AL, Carlton DP. Gastroesophageal reflux medications in the treatment of apnea in premature infants. J Pediatr 2001; 138:355–360.
73. Laitman J, Reidenberg J. Specialization of the human upper respiratory and upper digestive systems as seen through comparative and developmental anatomy. Dysphagia 1993; 8:318–325.
74. Koenig JS, Davies AM, Thach BT. Coordination of breathing, sucking, and swallowing during bottle feedings in human infants. J Appl Physiol 1990; 69:1623–1629.
75. Mathew OP. Respiratory control during nipple feeding in preterm infants. Pediatr Pulmonol 1988; 5:220–224.
76. Thach BT. Reflex associated apnea in infants: evidence for a laryngeal chemoreflex. Am J Med 1997; 103(5A):120S–124S.
77. Lang IM, Medda BK, Shaker R. Mechanisms of reflexes induced by esophageal distension. Am J Physiol Gastrointest Liver Physiol 2001; 281(5):G1246–G1263.
78. De Ajuriaguerra M, Radvanyi-Bouvet MF, Huon C, Moriette G. Gastroesophageal reflux and apnea in prematurely born infants during wakefulness and sleep. Am J Dis Child 1991; 145(10):1132–1136.
79. Tirosh E, Jaffe M. Apnea of infancy, seizures, and gastroesophageal reflux: an important but infrequent association. J Child Neurol 1996; 11(2):98–100.
80. Arad-Cohen N, Cohen A, Tirosh, E. The relationship between gastroesophageal reflux and apnea in infants. J Pediatr 2000; 137(3):321–326.
81. Paton JY, MacFadyen U, Williams A, Simpson H. GOR and apnoeic pauses during sleep in infancy—no direct relation. Eur J Pediatr 1990; 149:680–686.
82. Sacre L, Vandenplas Y. Gastroesophagea reflux associated with respiratory abnormalities during sleep. J Pediatr Gastroenterol Nutr 1989; 9:28–33.
83. Walsh JK, Farrell MK, Keenan WJ, Lucas M, Kramer M. Gastroesophageal reflux in infants: relation to apnea. J Pediatr 1981; 99:197–201.
84. Kahn A, Rebuffat E, Sottiaux M, Dufour D, Cadranel S, Reiterer K. Lack of temporal relation between acid reflux in the proximal oesophagus and cardiorespiratory events in sleeping infants. Eur J Pediatr 1992; 151:208–212.
85. Peter CS, Sprodowski N, Bohnhorst B. Gastroesophageal reflux and apnea of prematurity: no temporal relationship. Pediatrics 2002 (in press).
86. Herbst JJ, Book LS. Gastroesophageal reflux causing respiratory distress and apnea in newborn infants. J Pediatr 1979; 95(5):763–768.
87. Spitzer AP, Boyle JT, Tuchman DN, Fox WW. Awake apnea associated with gastroesophageal reflux: a specific clinical syndrome. J Pediatr 1984; 104:200–205.
88. Leape L, Holder TM, Franklin JD, Amoury RA, Ashcroft KW. Respiratory arrest in infants secondary to gastroesophageal reflux. Pedatrics 1977; 60(6):924–928.
89. Gomes H, Lallemand P. Infant apnea and gastroesophageal reflux. Pediatr Radiol 1992; 22:8–11.
90. Menon AP, Schefft GL, Thach BT. Apnea associated with regurgitation in infants. J Pediatr 1985; 106:625–629.
91. Wenzel TG, Schenke S, Peschgens T, Silny J, Heimann G, Skopnik H. Association of apnea and nonacid gastroesophageal reflux in infants: investigations with the intraluminal impedance technique. Pediatr Pulmonol 2001; 31:144–149.

22

Airway Disorders in the Newborn

OOMMEN P. MATHEW

Brody School of Medicine at East Carolina University
Greenville, North Carolina, U.S.A.

I. Introduction

The respiratory tract is a complex structure and is generally divided into the upper and lower airways. From the physiologic standpoint, the intrathoracic portion of the airways is defined as the lower airways, and the extrathoracic portion as the upper airways. Besides serving as an air conduit during breathing, the respiratory tract participates in several important physiologic functions, such as deglutition, olfaction, humidification, vocalization, and airway protection. Our understanding of upper-airway physiology and pathophysiology has increased substantially over the past two decades. Obstructive sleep apnea and sudden infant death syndrome (SIDS) have served as the impetus for this increased interest. The focus of this chapter is on disorders of airway patency in the neonate. Several unique problems in airway maintenance faced by the neonates are discussed in detail in subsequent sections.

II. Maintenance of Airway Patency

Activity of the muscles of the upper airway plays an important role in the maintenance of upper airway patency. For a detailed discussion of control of upper airway muscle activity during development, the reader is referred to

Chapter 5, by Dr. Gauda. A thorough knowledge of normal airway anatomy is a prerequisite for understanding the pathophysiology of airway disorders. The upper airway, which extends from the nose or mouth to the extrathoracic portion of the trachea, is a complex structure with some areas being fairly rigid, other areas being very soft and collapsible. It also contains several valvelike structures that add to the complexity in function. For example, some segments of the nose have rigid bony or cartilaginous support, whereas others depend primarily on the action of dilator muscle activity. The pharynx, on the other hand, is the most collapsible portion of the upper airway (Fig. 1). It can be divided into three regions: velopharynx, oropharynx, and hypopharynx. The pharynx has little bony or cartilaginous support and is primarily surrounded by muscles. The hyoid bone, which is located anterior to the epiglottis, is literally suspended by several groups of muscles (1,2). The anterior, posterior, and lateral walls of the oropharynx are formed by a number of structures. The soft palate, tongue, and lingual tonsils form the anterior wall of the oropharynx. The superior, middle, and inferior constrictor muscles form the posterior wall of the oropharynx and hypopharynx. Several muscles form the lateral walls, including the hyoglossus, styloglossus, stylohyoid, stylopharyngeus, palatoglossus, palatopharyngeus, and the pharyngeal constrictors (superior, middle, and inferior). The styloglossus, stylohyoid, and stylopharyngeus muscles arise from the styloid process, and the hypoglossus, middle constrictor, and stylohyoid muscles insert on the hyoid bone. The lateral pharyngeal walls are complex structures made up of a number of muscles with varying functions. The activity of these muscles plays an important role in maintaining pharyngeal airway patency as well. The larynx has multiple bony, cartilaginous, and muscular components. Thyroid, cricoid and arytenoid cartilages form the skeleton of the larynx connecting the pharynx to the trachea (Fig. 2). The activity of intrinsic muscles such as the cricoarytenoid and thyroarytenoid determine the size of the laryngeal lumen; the extrinsic laryngeal muscles control the location of the larynx.

Patency of the airway depends on several factors, and the relative significance of these factors varies from one segment to the next. These dependent variables include cross-sectional area, compliance, and pressure-flow dynamics. Cross-sectional area is an important determinant of airflow resistance. Nasal resistance in infants, for example, accounts for nearly one-half of the total airway resistance (3). Deviated nasal septum, mucosal edema, or nasal congestion can alter the nasal resistance markedly. Compliance characteristics of the airway walls are another important determinant of airway patency. A highly compliant pharyngeal airway decreases in size when subjected to subatmospheric pressure. Upper-airway dilator muscle activity increases the rigidity of these walls and the cross-sectional area of the lumen. Vascularity of the tissue and mucosal factors also contributes to airway wall rigidity. Micrognathia can influence pharyngeal airway patency adversely by decreasing cross-sectional area. Although several

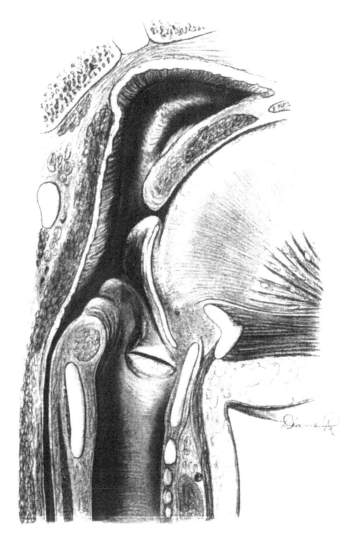

Figure 1   Drawing of paramedian section of the pharynx, larynx and posterior portion of the mouth in an infant. (Bosma, 1986.)

models have been proposed to describe the pressure-flow relationship in the upper airway, none are very satisfactory. Changes in airflow characteristics, changes in cross-sectional area during breathing, and the series of valves each having its own pressure-flow characteristics may explain this. Craniofacial abnormalities or increases in the size of upper-airway soft-tissue structures may narrow the

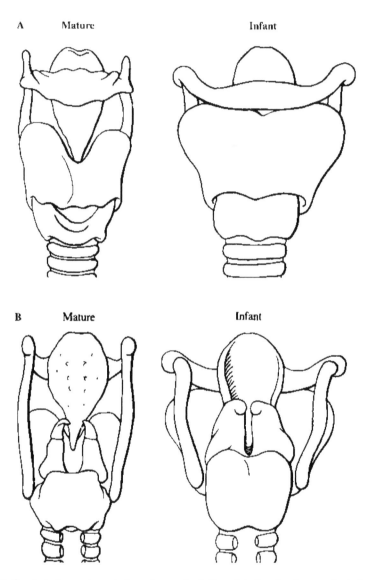

Figure 2 Anterior and posterior views of adult and infant hyolaryngeal skeletons. (Bosma, 1986.)

upper-airway lumen, predisposing the airway to collapse. In the majority of sleep apnea patients, airway closure during sleep occurs in the retropalatal and retroglossal regions (4,5).

III. Airway Imaging Studies

Endoscopy has been the most valuable diagnostic procedure in the evaluation of pediatric airway disorders (6). Radiologic evaluation of the airway has been used as a screening tool and as an adjunct to endoscopy. In recent years noninvasive airway imaging has fast become the procedure of choice. Airway imaging modalities in the adult include acoustic reflection, fluoroscopy, nasopharyngoscopy, cephalometry, computerized tomography (CT), and magnetic resonance imaging (MRI). Some of these techniques have limited usefulness in the neonate. The ideal imaging study should be not only highly accurate but also noninvasive and inexpensive. Radiation should be avoided or limited whenever possible.

A. Acoustic Reflection

Acoustic reflection is a noninvasive technique and has been used primarily as a research tool. It is based on the analysis of sound waves reflected from the respiratory system (7–9). It has no role in the evaluation of airway in the newborn.

B. Cephalometry

Cephalometry is a standardized lateral radiograph of the head and neck. It is widely available, easily performed, and relatively inexpensive. It is useful in quantifying skeletal and soft-tissue structures in patients (10,11). It has limited clinical utility in the neonate; it may be useful in neonates with craniofacial abnormalities such as micrognathia.

C. Airway Fluoroscopy

Airway fluoroscopy provides a quick, safe, and noninvasive way of evaluating the entire airway (12–16). Compared to the newer technologies, fluoroscopy is widely available and relatively inexpensive. It is a useful adjunct to flexible fiberoptic nasolaryngoscopy, particularly in the workup of neonatal stridor. A fixed lesion can be seen throughout the respiratory cycle, whereas a functional lesion changes during breathing. Airway fluoroscopy is useful not only in demonstrating dynamic lesions such as tracheobronchomalacia but also in correlating its severity, extent, and location when compared to other simple radiographic modalities. The sensitivity of airway fluoroscopy is reported to be 100% for oropharyngeal collapse, 80% for subglottic lesions, 73% for tracheal lesions, and

75% for bronchial causes of airway obstruction (17). It is less sensitive for supraglottic and glottic lesions.

D. Functional Swallowing Studies

Dysphagia often complicates the clinical course of infants with congenital structural abnormalities of the upper airway as well as neuromuscular disorders. Evaluation of the swallowing mechanism may yield important diagnostic information about upper-airway dysfunction. Modified barium swallow or video-fluoroscopy of swallowing, largely developed at the Johns Hopkins University Swallowing Center, is especially suited for this purpose (1,18). Preterm neonates with apnea and bradycardia constituted a large portion of the patients evaluated at this center. Immature feeding skills and respiratory functions predispose the preterm neonates to aspiration (19). Since feeding-related apnea and bradycardia are primarily maturational disorders, videofluoroscopy is not widely used for this purpose in other centers unless these symptoms persist. One of the most important aspects of this examination is that the effect of proposed feeding intervention, such as thickening feeds, could be documented during the procedure.

E. Computed Tomography

CT accurately determines airway cross-sectional area in the supine position. It is widely available and relatively expensive, and exposes the infant to radiation. Images are obtained in the axial plane only. CT is superior to MRI for evaluating craniofacial structures. Three-dimensional image reconstructions of the airway and bony skeleton by CT may also be helpful in planning the surgical approach (20,21). However, soft-tissue contrast resolution of MRI is superior to CT (21).

F. Magnetic Resonance Imaging

MRI is the ideal modality for imaging the airway because it provides excellent upper-airway and soft-tissue resolution, accurately determines cross-sectional area and volume, and allows imaging in the axial, sagittal, and coronal planes. It can be performed during wakefulness and sleep without radiation (21–23). MRI is available in most hospitals; however, it remains expensive.

G. Dynamic Imaging During Respiration

Dynamic upper-airway imaging has been performed during respiration with CT, MRI, and nasopharyngoscopy (24–27). The respiratory changes in the upper-airway geometry have been documented with excellent temporal and spatial resolution using electron beam CT (26). Four distinct phases of breathing have been recognized during wakefulness. At the onset of inspiration, there is an increase in upper-airway lumen, presumably reflecting the action of upper airway dilator muscles. The size of the lumen is maintained relatively constant during the remainder of inspiration, suggesting a balance between upper-airway collapsing and dilating forces. At the beginning of expiration, the airway enlarges again, reflecting the effects of positive intraluminal pressure. The largest airway caliber is seen at the beginning of expiration. There is a rapid reduction in upper-airway size toward the end of expiration. The airway may be particularly vulnerable to collapse at the end of expiration because it is no longer kept open by upper-airway dilating muscle activity or positive intraluminal pressure. The respiratory-related changes in the upper airway lumen demonstrated in CT studies (26) were noted predominantly in the lateral dimension, indicating that the lateral walls play an important role in modulating airway caliber. However, no such data are available in the neonates.

A significant increase in the size of the upper-airway lumen is seen with the application of nasal continuous positive airway pressure (CPAP) in normal subjects and patients with obstructive sleep apnea (28–30). With the aid of CT, Kuna and colleagues demonstrated that upper airway dilatation was greatest in the lateral dimension with the application of CPAP (29). Others have recently confirmed this finding (22). Although similar data are lacking in the newborn, it is likely that the reduction in mixed and obstructive apnea observed with nasal CPAP application has a similar basis (31).

IV. Disorders of Airway Patency

Airway disorders can be classified as those causing complete obstruction and those causing incomplete or partial obstruction. In some cases, the cause of airway obstruction is anatomical. Choanal atresia is an excellent example of complete anatomic obstruction, whereas obstructive sleep apnea is an example of intermittent complete functional obstruction. Stridor, on the other hand, is typical of an incomplete airway obstruction. These episodes often occur intermittently in infants with an underlying anatomic abnormality. Although both congenital and acquired lesions can cause airway disorders in the neonate, the focus of this chapter is on congenital abnormalities. Some of these disorders may manifest soon after birth, whereas others may become symptomatic after many months or even years.

The respiratory tract continues to undergo growth and development following birth. Irregular breathing patterns are common in neonates. This is a reflection of immaturity of the nervous system at birth. Usually these irregular breathing patterns are benign and improve over time. However, these abnormalities are more pronounced in premature infants and are the focus of several chapters. The majority of the episodes of apnea in premature infants are associated with upper-airway obstruction. Airway closure is seen not only in mixed and obstructive apnea but also in some central apneas (32). There are several significant differences in respiratory control between infants and adults; these issues have been addressed in the preceding chapters, especially in those chapters on chemical and neural control of breathing. In addition to control abnormalities, there are anatomic differences between the airways of the neonate and those of the older child or adult. The laryngeal lumen, for example, is much smaller in the neonate (Fig. 3). Furthermore, although neonates are capable of oral breathing (as in crying), they are preferential nose breathers at rest. Ability for sustained oral breathing is not established for several weeks in these infants.

A detailed discussion of all airway disorders is beyond the scope of this chapter. Therefore, I have decided to focus on three congenital disorders: choanal atresia, Pierre Robin sequence, and laryngotracheomalacia. These conditions represent common airway disorders among neonates; they involve abnormalities of different segments of the airways and represent different degrees of severity. Among acquired airway disorders in the neonate, subglottic stenosis is the most common lesion. Numerous conditions associated with airway disorders in the newborn are listed below; others are given in Table 1. Airway management in the delivery room is addressed separately, because it presents some unique challenges of its own.

A. Airway Management in the Delivery Room

Management of the airway is an important part of resuscitation in the delivery room. In most nondepressed infants, it consists of suctioning the oropharynx and the nose and positioning of the infant to avoid flexion of the head and neck. On the other hand, management of the airway in the delivery room is more critical in the depressed infant. Following oropharyngeal suction, if cutaneous stimulation of the infant is unsuccessful in initiating or sustaining breathing, positive pressure ventilation with bag and mask must be initiated. Since the tone of upper-airway muscles is diminished or absent, the position of the head and neck is particularly important (Fig. 4). In the absence of muscle tone, the upper-airway remains occluded in the human infant when the head is flexed, and remains open when slightly extended (34). Positioning of the infant and obtaining a good seal are the two key factors in determining a successful outcome of positive pressure ventilation. Good chest movement ensures that these two factors are adequately addressed. Endotracheal intubation may be attempted in the unresponsive infant if skilled personnel are available.

Airway management in the delivery room can be particularly difficult in a small subset of infants. In these cases, the difficulty is often due to obstruction at the level of the pharynx or larynx, either from extrinsic causes, as in space-occupying lesions, or from intrinsic causes as in laryngeal atresia. Although rare,

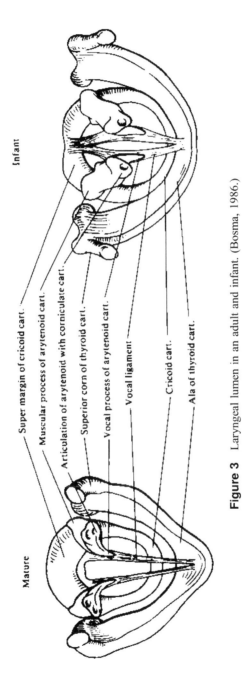

Figure 3 Laryngeal lumen in an adult and infant. (Bosma, 1986.)

Table 1 Laryngeal and Tracheal Causes of Neonatal Stridor

Location	Specific Diagnosis
Laryngeal	
supraglottic	bifid epiglottis, floppy epiglottis, laryngeal saccular cysts, supraglottic web, anomalous cuneiform cartilage
glottic	laryngomalacia, laryngeal paralysis, laryngeal web, posterior laryngeal cleft
subglottic	Stenosis (congenital or acquired), hemangioma
Tracheal	
tracheal stenosis	generalized tracheal hypoplasia, funnellike stenosis, short segmental stenosis
complete tracheal rings	stovepipe trachea
tracheal compression	complete vascular rings, anomalous innominate artery, pulmonary artery sling, intrathoracic tumors
tracheomalacia	congenital or acquired

infants with potential airway obstruction are being recognized antenatally with increasing frequency because of widespread use of prenatal ultrasound. The space-occupying lesions, which can occlude the upper airway at birth, are often diagnosed prenatally because they interfere with in utero swallowing and result in polyhydraminos. These include epignathus, teratoma, dermoid, epulis, macroglossus, and encephalocele (35–39). Epignathus is a teratomalike tumor arising from the palate or pharynx, and is the most commonly reported oropharyngeal lesion. A higher incidence has been seen among female infants.

Extrinsic compression from cervical masses may also result in airway obstruction. Cervical teratoma, cystic hygroma, and goiter comprise the vast majority of these lesions (40). When these conditions are diagnosed in utero, a prenatal MRI may be helpful in delineating the mass.

In some of these cases, difficulty in airway management can be expected at birth. These infants should be delivered in an institution where physicians experienced in difficult airway management are available (41). The team should consist of perinatologist, neonatologist, anesthesiologist, and pediatric or ENT surgeon. Because of expected airway management problems, a cesarean section under general anesthesia should be considered to optimize survival and, whenever possible, delivery should wait until a mature lung profile can be assured. Generally infants are delivered before anesthesia depresses the newborn infant. In these infants with compromised airway, however, respiratory depression from general anesthesia may be an advantage. It prevents the fetus from attempting to breathe at birth when a tracheotomy might be required. Placental circulation can be maintained while the airway is being secured either by

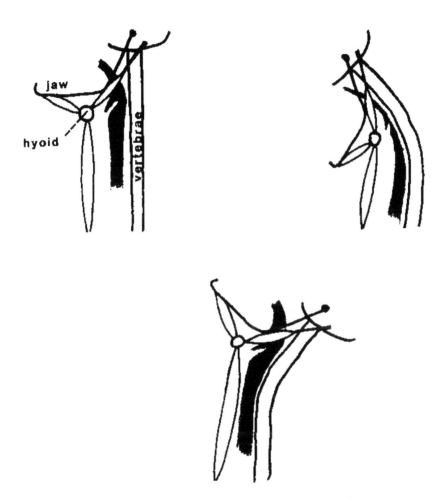

Figure 4 Effect of head position on pharyngeal airway lumen. Neutral, flexed, and extended head positions are shown. Airway narrows during head flexion. (Olson et al., 1988.)

intubation or by tracheotomy. Use of this ex utero intrapartum treatment (EXIT) procedure (42–44) can be potentially life saving.

On rare occasions, difficulty in airway management arises unexpectedly. When there are no personnel in the delivery suite skilled in emergency airway management, physicians skilled in tracheotomy and/or fiberoptic tracheal intubation should be contacted immediately, while attempting to secure an airway. When the difficulty in airway management is due to space-occupying lesions, and intubation is not possible, a small endotracheal tube inserted nasally and placed in the posterior pharynx may improve oxygenation (41). When this method is used as the mode of ventilation, inserting a nasogastric tube through the other nostril into the stomach can prevent abdominal distension. For intrinsic lesions such as laryngeal atresia, percutaneous transtracheal ventilation may be attempted as a temporizing measure, while preparing for tracheotomy. Percutaneous transtracheal ventilation involves the insertion of a large (10- or 12-gauge) catheter through the cricothyroid membrane to permit oxygenation. There are several important considerations regarding the oxygen source for percutaneous transtracheal ventilation and variations in the technique for patients of various ages. The reader is referred elsewhere to review these important principles (45). Once the airway is secured, ventilation and oxygenation should be evaluated using pulse oximetry and arterial blood gases. Other associated defects, including congenital heart disease, may be seen in a small percentage of infants. Further diagnostic studies can be performed once the infant is stabilized. Because of unexpected presentation, these lesions tend to be fatal. However, with increasing number of lesions being diagnosed prenatally, the number of survivors of these rare disorders is increasing.

B. Disorders of the Nose and Nasopharynx

Nasal obstruction at birth can cause central cyanosis and represents a potentially life-threatening condition. Causes of neonatal nasal obstruction include choanal atresia, encephalocele, hemangioma, dermoid cyst, dacryocystocele, nasal septum deviation, hematoma, and nasal glioma. Choanal patency is routinely checked in the delivery room by introducing a catheter through each nostril. However, the catheter may cause trauma to the nasal mucosa.

Choanal Atresia

Choanal atresia occurs in approximately 1 in 8000 births. The atresia is unilateral in the majority of cases and is seen more often in female infants (46–48). In nearly half the cases other congenital anomalies are present, and these anomalies occur more frequently in bilateral choanal atresias. Other anomalies observed include craniofacial anomalies, polydactylism, congenital heart diseases, coloboma of the iris, external ear malformation, esophageal atresia, TE fistula, craniosynostosis, meningocele, and mental retardation. These anomalies may be part of a syndrome such as Treacher Collins syndrome or CHARGE association (49–51).

Nasal placodes develop on the inferior part of frontonasal prominence as bilateral oval thickenings of the surface ectoderm during the fourth week. As the face develops, nasal placodes become depressed forming nasal pits, which subsequently deepen forming the primitive nasal sacs. The nasal sacs are initially separated from the oral cavity by oronasal membrane. This membrane ruptures during the sixth week. There are several theories about the embryogenesis of choanal atresia (48,52). These include the failure of rupture of the bucconasal membrane, and misdirection of mesodermal flow by local factors leading to malrotation of the burrowing nasal pits. The anatomic deformities observed include a narrow nasal cavity, lateral bony obstruction by the lateral pterygoid plate, medial obstruction by a thickened vomer, and a membranous obstruction. Choanal atresia was believed to be bony in 90% and membranous in 10%. Unlike earlier reports, more recent studies using CT classify the anatomy as bony, mixed bony-membranous, or pure membranous (53). These studies show that the incidence of pure bony lesion is <30%. The vast majority of atresias are mixed bony-membranous; pure membranous atresia is very rare (53).

Neonates with bilateral choanal atresia have a characteristic presentation. They are symptomatic at rest and exhibit marked retractions without any air movement. Their symptoms improve with crying. However, marked variability in symptoms has been noted among these infants. Although once considered obligatory nose breathers, neonates are now recognized as preferential nose breathers. Intermittent oronasal breathing has been well documented even in preterm infants (54). Intermittent oral breathing may explain, at least in part, the variability in observed symptoms. Unilateral atresia may go undetected in the neonatal period but become symptomatic later during upper respiratory infection.

Functional patency of the nose can be tested in a number of ways. These include holding a thin wisp of cotton fibers, listening to breath sounds, looking for frosting on a mirror, installing a colored solution into the nose and gently blowing air into each nasal cavity with Politzer bag. Nasal obstruction can be confirmed clinically when a feeding tube cannot be passed through the nose into the pharynx. However, one should be cautious in making a diagnosis of choanal atresia, if the infant did not exhibit any signs of distress around the time of birth but develops these symptoms later, especially if they have been suctioned vigorously in the delivery room. Mucosal edema of the nose can present with similar signs and symptoms. A simple clinical maneuver to check choanal patency has been suggested as an alternative to passing the nasogastric tube (55). With the left little finger, the examiner gently keeps the newborn's mouth closed while the thumb obstructs the left nostril. The stethoscope's membrane is held by the right hand just under the right nostril detecting the gentle sound of airflow. This maneuver is then repeated on the opposite side. These authors claim that the "nasal airflow test" has never failed to demonstrate choanal patency (55).

Oropharyngeal airway or orotracheal intubation is a must in suspected cases of bilateral choanal atresia. Once a stable airway is established and the site of obstruction bypassed, further investigations can be undertaken to establish the diagnosis. If mucosal edema is suspected, no attempt should be made to pass a nasopharyngeal tube for 48–72 h. Although choanogram can be helpful in establishing the diagnosis, the imaging of choice is computerized tomography (47,48,56). Images in the orbitotragal plane often yield the best results. Secretions in the nose may give a falsely thickened appearance of the atretic segment. The application of a decongestant or suctioning before the CT reduces secretions. Thickness of the bone and the degree of stenosis are important for surgical planning. Other related diagnoses that should be entertained include posterior choanal stenosis and anterior nasal stenosis or stenosis of the pyriform aperture (41,57).

For patients with bilateral atresia, definitive surgery should be performed before discharge from the hospital (41,48,58). Transnasal and transpalatal approaches have been utilized. Transantral or transseptal approaches are not suitable for the neonate. A period of stenting with silastic tubing is routinely used, most surgeons recommending postoperative stenting for 4–6 weeks, followed by serial endoscopy with dilatation and removal of granulation tissue. Major reported disadvantages of transpalatal repair are the potential effect on palatal growth and subsequent cross bite deformity. The incidence of cross bite has been reported as high as 50% in the operated group, compared to 4% in the control group (59). In recent years lasers have been used to repair choanal atresia (48). No case-controlled data are available comparing different types of laser or comparing the laser with conventional surgery in the management of choanal atresia. Restenosis is a well-recognized but uncommon complication.

C. Disorders of the Oropharynx

Compromise of the oropharyngeal airway can occur in the neonate for a variety of reasons, some of which have been discussed already. Since neonates cannot adequately control their head and neck position, even neck flexion can result in airway obstruction (60). This problem is exacerbated in infants with hypotonia. From a clinical standpoint, one should be vigilant about airway obstruction while caring for infants with hypotonia. These include premature infants, infants with hypoxic ischemic encephalopathy, infants with neuromuscular diseases, and infants with trisomy 21 and other syndromes. Oropharyngeal and cervical masses causing airway obstruction are discussed under delivery room management. Narrowing of the oropharyngeal airway can occur with macroglossia. It presents as tongue protrusion from muscular hypertrophy (Beckwith-Wiedemann syndrome), vascular malformations (hemangiomas or lymphangiomas), systemic disorders (hypothyroidism and the mucopolysaccharidoses), or tumors (61). Pharyngeal airway obstruction also occurs in infants with micrognathia. Pierre Robin sequence is an excellent example of such a condition and is discussed below.

Pierre Robin Sequence (PRS)

Although the triad of cleft palate, micrognathia, and airway obstruction was described earlier, Robin was the first to report the association of micrognathia with glossoptosis. Cleft palate was subsequently added to his original description (62). This triad was known as *Pierre Robin syndrome* until the term *Pierre Robin anomalad* was introduced in mid-1970s (63,64). The currently accepted term, *Pierre Robin sequence*, was proposed by an international working group (65). The widely accepted incidence is 1 : 8500 varying from 1 : 2000 to 1 : 30,000 (66,67).

Infants with PRS are classified into two major categories: nonsyndromic and syndromic. The majority of infants is nonsyndromic (68) and has the potential for normal growth and development. The facial features are often typical with a flattened base of the nose and micrognathia. A U-shaped palatal cleft is characteristic of PRS. Syndromic patients have poorer prognosis for normal growth and development even with early intervention.

Life-threatening respiratory distress and severe feeding difficulties are seen among newborns with glossoptosis. Marked anteroposterior mandibular deficiency is invariably present at birth. An objective definition of micrognathia can be helpful in the diagnosis of glossoptosis and possible airway obstruction. The Jaw Index was developed for this purpose (69). The Jaw Index quantifies maxillomandibular discrepancy in the newborn. A linear relationship between mandibular growth and gestational age or biparietal diameter is normally seen. The jaw index is three to four times greater in infants with PRS. Recently, a jaw index for the fetus, validated by postnatal measurements, has also been reported (70). However, one should be aware that the jaw index is calculated differently in the fetus. The fetal jaw index had 100% sensitivity and 98% specificity in diagnosing micrognathia and is superior to subjective estimate from the fetal profile (70).

Mandibular catchup growth occurs during infancy and early childhood in patients with PRS (71,72). Mandibular growth potential is better if intrauterine positioning is the cause of the mandibular deficiency. If there is an intrinsic growth disturbance, as in many syndromic PRS, self-correction may not occur (73,74). In others, "partial mandibular catchup growth" may be seen (73). Because of limited data, it is difficult to predict the outcome with certainty in any given infant.

Airway obstruction has been recognized as an important part of the clinical symptomatology. Posterior displacement of the floor of the mouth and tongue by retrognathia was believed to be the cause of airway obstruction. Other symptoms such as failure to thrive and cor pulmonale resulting from airway obstruction were soon recognized. Large negative pressure swings during the inspiratory efforts were subsequently confirmed (75,76).

It is now generally accepted that airway obstruction is multifactorial in nature. Both anatomic and neuromuscular components such as retroposition of the mandible and diminished effectiveness of the genioglossus muscle have been implicated (77). Varying degrees of neuromuscular impairment have been reported in the genioglossus and other pharyngeal muscles. Delorme and coworkers emphasized the inadequacy of muscular insertions of the tongue on the anterior mandible (78). They proposed the controversial view that the retruded mandible is the result, not the cause, of the tongue position. Evaluation of the activity of genioglossus, the main tongue muscle, by intramuscular electromyograms revealed respiratory activity that was modulated by airway mechanoreceptors and chemoreceptors (79). This respiratory modulation in micrognathic infants was qualitatively similar to that observed in normal neonates and children (79). When pharyngeal airway stability was tested by nasal mask occlusions (to increase negative pharyngeal airway pressures during inspiration), midinspiratory pharyngeal obstructions developed in both normal and micrognathic infants (80). However, airway obstructions were more frequent in micrognathic infants (80). The mechanism of airway obstruction was studied using flexible fiberoptic nasopharyngoscopy (77). On the basis of endoscopic findings, four types of obstructions were identified. The posterior movement of the tongue contacting the posterior pharyngeal wall constituted type 1; posterior movement of the tongue compressing the soft palate against the posterior pharyngeal wall constituted type 2. The lateral pharyngeal walls moved medially in type 3, and the pharynx constricted in a sphincteric manner in type 4. The mechanism of obstruction was either type 1 or 2 in 80% of cases studied (77). Taken together, these findings suggest that the genioglossus muscle is less effective in micrognathic infants in counteracting the effects of negative pressure generated during inspiration either because of its intrinsic properties or because of its mechanical disadvantage.

Medical Management

Clinical symptoms are less severe in the prone position. Prone placement of the infant relies on gravity to displace the tongue anteriorly. It may be useful for infants with mild symptoms. However, it does not allow observation of retractions, the major symptom of upper-airway obstruction. A nasopharyngeal airway placed transnasally into the pharynx may be used either as a temporizing measure (7–10 days) or as a form of chronic treatment (several weeks). A single nasopharyngeal tube with an internal diameter of 3.0 mm is advanced until good air movement is observed. The positioning of this tube above the larynx but below the base of the tongue is not easy. In addition to air flowing through its lumen, air movement can occur at the side as well. Nasopharyngeal airway is often appropriate in the early management of airway problems until clinical issues are sorted out. Gavage feeding through a nasogastric tube is recommended during this period (81). Controlled endotracheal intubation is appropriate when positioning and nasopharyngeal tubes have not been successful. Although it provides adequate temporary relief, it has significant disadvantages as well. Intubation using standard laryngoscopes is difficult at best and occasionally impossible. In emergency situations, pulling the tongue forward with toothed forceps or suture may improve airway patency.

Surgical Management

A variety of surgical interventions to relieve airway obstruction have been described over the years (81–83). However, the vast majority of these procedures are seldom used nowadays, with the exception of tracheotomy. If positioning and nasopharyngeal tube fail, prolonged endotracheal intubation or tracheotomy are the two viable options. Other, rarely used surgical procedures include glossopexy, mandibular distraction osteogenesis, and subperiosteal release of the floor of the mouth.

Tracheotomy. Tracheotomy bypasses the pharyngeal obstruction and is usually reserved for patients who have failed other forms of airway management. Frequency and severity of the clinical symptoms are important determinants. Most infants can be successfully decannulated between 3 and 18 months.

Tongue-Lip Adhesion and Other Glossopexy Procedures. The lip-to-tongue adhesion procedure was designed to alleviate upper airway obstruction by correcting abnormal tongue positioning. In this procedure the mucosal surface under the tongue over the alveolus and onto the lower lip is denuded, and the tongue is then sutured in place in a more anterior position. It has significant failure rate. A modified glossopexy procedure is most commonly used today (84). A nasogastric tube, left in place for 2–3 days, is used for feeding while the tissues are healing. Development of speech is of concern in patients undergoing glossopexy. Speech development at age 18 months in these patients is equivalent to that of patients with cleft palate and their syndrome-matched counterparts (85).

Mandibular Distraction Osteogenesis. A definitive structural resolution of micrognathia is provided by mandibular distraction osteogenesis with correction of both hard and soft tissue deformities (86). Internal or external devices can be used for mandibular distraction osteogenesis. Initially, an osteotomy is performed and the segments are fixed with a distraction device. Postoperatively, a fibrovascular bridge is allowed to form at the osteotomy site. The appliance is then activated. Once the desired lengthening is obtained, 4–6 weeks is allowed for consolidation. The distraction device is then removed. This procedure is technically more difficult than other alternatives and requires good compliance from the parents.

Subperiosteal Release of the Floor of the Mouth. Through a submental incision, the periosteum of the inferior border of the mandible is incised up to the mandibular angle. This procedure releases the geniohyoid, genioglossus, and mylohyoid muscles from their attachment to the mandible, allowing the development of a new and more favorable equilibrium (78). Endotracheal intubation is maintained for 1–2 weeks. Limited experience with this procedure suggests that it may have a role in selected patients (87).

Syndromes with PRS

Syndromes associated with PRS include Stickler syndrome, velocardiofacial syndrome, and Treacher Collins syndrome. All three syndromes have auto-somal-dominant inheritance with variable expression. Stickler syndrome is a connective tissue dysplasia (71). The craniofacial spectrum ranges from normal facial appearance to midfacial flattening, prominent eyes, epicanthal folds, depressed nasal bridge, long philtrum, and small chin (67). The mandibular morphology is characterized by a short ramus and notching of the body. Velocardiofacial syndrome includes typical facies, prominent nose, retrognathic mandible, cardiovascular anomalies, palatal cleft, velopharyngeal insufficiency, and learning disability. Patients with Treacher Collins syndrome have a convex facial profile with prominent nasal dorsum and a retrusive mandible. Malar hypoplasia, antimongoloid slanting of the palpebral fissure, and cleft palate with or without cleft lip are also seen (82). Its prevalence is equal in males and females.

D. Larynx/Trachea

Complete obstruction of the larynx or trachea such as laryngeal atresia and tracheal agenesis manifests itself in the delivery room. Therefore, the airway disorders originating from this segment of the airway and becoming symptomatic subsequently tend to be either partial or intermittent complete obstruction. Stridor is a common symptom of partial airway obstruction and can be defined as a variably pitched respiratory sound caused by tissue vibration due to turbulent airflow through a narrow tube (88,89). Stridor is not normal in neonates; therefore, whenever stridor is noted in neonates, it should be watched closely. In some cases, stridor may require immediate airway intervention. The most common laryngeal and tracheal lesions causing stridor in infants are listed in the Table 1.

The clinical presentation of stridor varies considerably in neonates. In most cases, these infants are mildly tachypneic (90). Small caliber of the airway and the less rigid supporting cartilage make the airway in the newborn inherently more vulnerable to the effects of partial narrowing (91). Changes in the laryngeal lumen during development are substantial (Fig. 5). Distinctive vibratory patterns produced in this narrowed segment are transmitted to the surrounding soft tissues (92). Volume, pitch, and phase are three important characteristics. Loud stridor generally indicates a significant narrowing of the airway. However, a sudden decrease in volume in cases of progressively worsening stridor can signify impending airway collapse (91). In general, high-pitched stridor is caused by obstruction at the level of the glottis (93), low-pitched stridor by supralaryngeal lesions; intermediate pitch usually signifies obstruction below the glottis (94).

On the basis of its timing within the respiratory cycle, stridor can be classified as inspiratory, expiratory, or biphasic. Stridor produced by the collapse of nonrigid soft tissues is usually inspiratory, with laryngomalacia being the most common cause (95). Obstructive lesions of the nasopharynx and oropharynx typically produce a low-pitched stridor similar to snoring. Biphasic stridor results from fixed obstruction at the level of the glottis or below (93,95,96). Vocal cord paralysis and subglottic stenosis account for the majority of biphasic stridor in neonates (91,93). Tracheomalacia and bronchomalacia often produce an expiratory stridor (94,97).

History is an important part of the evaluation of stridor in the neonatal period, including birth history, reason for and duration of intubation, and any suspected intubation trauma (94,98). Additionally, the age at the onset of stridor, its duration, association with precipitating events (crying or feeding) or position (prone, or supine), quality and nature of crying, and presence of other symptoms (cough, aspiration, or drooling) should be sought and documented. Stridor present since birth is most commonly caused by laryngomalacia, congenital subglottic stenosis, vocal fold paralysis, or vascular compression of the trachea (95,97,99). Stridor present only during agitation and crying is likely to be due to unilateral vocal fold paralysis (99).

Severity of the stridor can be assessed rapidly during the physical examination by observing the heart rate, respiratory rate, oxygen saturation, and skin color. Use of accessory muscles, nasal flaring, and chest wall retractions are useful in assessing the severity as well. When the stridor is severe enough to warrant transfer, experienced personnel, utilizing pulse oximetry and cardiorespiratory monitoring, should transport the infant. Consultation with/or referral

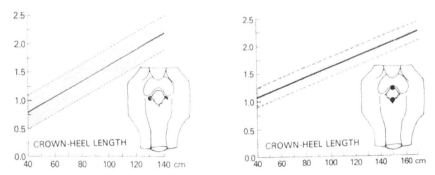

Figure 5   Changes in laryngeal lumen with body growth. Mean and standard deviation of maximal transverse (left) and vertical (right) dimensions are shown. (Bosma, 1986.)

to an otolaryngologist experienced in the evaluation of stridor in infants is indicated in most cases.

Laryngomalacia

As mentioned earlier, laryngomalacia is the most frequent cause of stridor in infants (102). Stridor often begins in the neonatal period, is inspiratory in nature, and progresses in severity over a period of several months. It is usually benign and typically resolves within 12–18 months. Retractions, tachypnea, and feeding difficulties are seen in severe cases. Agitation or supine positioning may exacerbate the symptoms, whereas positioning the infant in the prone position or on the side may relieve the stridor. Although the exact cause(s) of laryngomalacia is not clear, an altered embryologic development of the larynx is the most likely etiology (102). No inherent cartilaginous abnormality has been demonstrated in histological studies.

History and physical examination are sufficient in making a tentative diagnosis. Flexible laryngoscopy, however, is the gold standard, and the typical findings are an omega-shaped epiglottis, redundant aryepiglottic folds, and excessive tissue in the supra-arytenoid area that may prolapse into the laryngeal inlet during inspiration. In some cases laryngomalacia may be site specific, primarily posterior laryngomalacia with prolapse of the supra-arytenoid tissue, or anterior laryngomalacia with prolapse of the anterior aspect of the aryepiglottic folds and epiglottis into the airway.

In general, the treatment of laryngomalacia is supportive. In the majority of patients, laryngomalacia resolves spontaneously over time and no surgical intervention is required. Parental counseling, reassurance, and prone or side positioning of the infant are often enough. Acute upper-respiratory infection may precipitate admission to the hospital. In some infants symptoms may be severe enough to cause feeding difficulties, apnea, cyanosis, and failure to thrive, symptoms warranting surgical intervention. In the past, tracheotomy was the procedure of choice. Epiglottoplasty represents an alternative to tracheotomy. In fact, epiglottoplasty or supraglottoplasty is now considered the surgical procedure of choice. Epiglottoplasty is performed endoscopically and involves the excision of redundant mucosa over the lateral edges of the epiglottis, aryepiglottic folds, arytenoids, and corniculate cartilages. Results of this procedure are very encouraging (102). Conservative resection minimizes the likelihood of complications, such as supraglottic stenosis or aspiration. A secondary procedure may be performed if symptoms are not adequately relieved.

Tracheomalacia

Tracheomalacia may occur with laryngomalacia or bronchomalacia. Two types of tracheomalacia are recognized: primary and secondary. Inherent structural weakness causes primary tracheomalacia. In secondary tracheomalacia, the collapse may be due to extrinsic compression by a mass or vascular structure. Secondary tracheomalacia occurs in conditions such as tracheoesophageal fistula, laryngotracheoesophageal cleft, vascular compression, or compression by mediastinal masses. Patients with tracheomalacia may present with minimal symptoms or severe life-threatening airway obstruction. The classic symptom of tracheomalacia is expiratory stridor, which may be present at birth. Primary tracheomalacia has a good prognosis. The expiratory stridor is usually of mild or moderate severity, and demonstrates gradual improvement over time. In contrast, secondary tracheomalacia may cause persistent symptoms even after the external compressive factor is corrected. Sometimes the stridor may not be apparent until the infant develops respiratory tract infections.

Endoscopy confirms the diagnosis of tracheomalacia. The tracheobronchial tree is more collapsible in a newborn than in an adult. Tracheomalacia is defined as collapse of the trachea on expiration, which results in >10–20% obstruction of the airway (103,104). The abnormal shape of the tracheal lumen is diagnostic of fixed tracheomalacia. Findings in dynamic tracheomalacia are subtle. When examined endoscopically, the normally round airway lumen appears flattened with reduction in the anteroposterior dimension. During expiration, this weak area collapses further. Plain static radiographs may reveal areas of collapse, but airway fluoroscopy invariably provides better functional detail. Evidence of vascular compression may be seen on barium swallow. MRI and echocardiography may be warranted in cases of suspected vascular compression. Acquired tracheomalacia is often seen in infants with severe bronchopulmonary dysplasia. The treatment of tracheomalacia depends on the severity of symptomatology. No intervention is necessary in mild cases. It often resolves within the first 2 years of life. Surgical decompression of the trachea may improve symptoms significantly when the underlying problem is related to airway compression. Surgical procedures that have been attempted include placement of internal and external tracheal stents, segmental resection, and cartilage grafting (105).

Subglottic stenosis

Subglottic stenosis in the neonate can be either congenital or acquired. Acquired stenosis is primarily a complication of prolonged intubation. Other well-recognized risk factors include traumatic intubation, multiple intubations, and bacterial colonization of the endotracheal tube. Extubation failure and postextubation stridor are often the first clinical signs. At present subglottic stenosis is an infrequent complication of endotracheal intubation in very low birth weight infants. The estimated incidence of subglottic stenosis in the 1980s varied from 1% to 8% among intubated infants. The reported incidence decreased to 0– 2% in the 1990s (105,106). Improvement in the management of ventilated infants is primarily responsible for this reduced incidence. Less severe complications are still common. Endoscopic evaluation is still the cornerstone in the diagnosis of subglottic stenosis. It can be classified into four grades (107): grade I, up to 50% obstruction; grade II, from 51% to 70%; grade III, >70% with any detectable lumen; and grade IV, with no lumen.

Detailed examination of the subglottis is often better performed with a rigid endoscope under general anesthesia. Airway imaging may be helpful in selected cases. Infants with occasional symptoms of stridor without retractions or feeding difficulties can be managed conservatively. Infants with stage I and some stage II stenosis fall in this category. Surgical treatment options include anterior cricoid split, tracheotomy, endoscopic resection, and laryngotracheal reconstruction.

Anterior Cricoid Split

The underlying premise is to avoid tracheotomy in these low birth weight infants with subglottic stenosis. However, it should be limited to acquired subglottic stenosis in the absence of significant glottic, supraglottic, or tracheal obstructions. Therefore, patient selection is extremely important. Infants with severe chronic lung disease, especially those requiring high peak pressures, are not good candidates for this procedure. Criteria for patient selection have been established (108). These include extubation failure on at least two occasions secondary to subglottic laryngeal pathology and weight >1500 g. To avoid serious complications, anterior cricoid split must only be performed in a setting with a high level of medical and nursing skills (109).

Endoscopic Management

Surgical intervention with an endoscope is often performed with a CO_2 laser. This is generally reserved for mild cases of isolated subglottic stenosis (108). The CO_2 laser is a useful adjunct during laryngotracheal reconstruction as well.

Tracheotomy

This is often the initial step in caring for a neonate with severe subglottic stenosis. It allows the infant time to recover from chronic lung disease and gain weight while awaiting laryngotracheal reconstruction. However, one must be aware of the fact that tracheotomy has some morbidity and mortality risk for these infants. They may develop delays in language skills as well. Early airway reconstruction is therefore attractive.

Laryngotracheal Reconstruction

Laryngotracheal reconstruction has become the standard of care for symptomatic subglottic stenosis in the pediatric age group. A variety of techniques of laryngotracheal reconstruction have been described (108). Anterior cartilage grafts with a tracheotomy is generally indicated for isolated anterior subglottic stenosis. The concept of single-stage procedure is appealing because of the advantages of immediate tracheotomy decannulation or even the avoidance of a tracheotomy. These advantages must be weighed against the potential for airway complications. There is no uniform agreement concerning the management of these patients in the immediate postoperative period (108). The options include heavy sedation, pharmacologic paralysis, and management while awake.

V. Summary

The airway is a vital part of the respiratory system. Besides serving as a conduit for gas exchange, it participates in several important functions. Patency of the airway is actively maintained in certain segments of the airway such as the oropharynx. It is easily compromised in the neonate with positional changes as well as with physiological changes such as sleep. Congenital and acquired lesions may further compromise the narrow airway of the newborn infant. These lesions may result in partial or total obstruction of the airway. Airway disorders involving different segments of the airways are discussed in greater detail to illustrate the differences with particular attention being paid on airway imaging studies. Clinical management of these infants is also discussed.

Acknowledgments

I want to thank Drs. Marcus Albernaz, Alex Robertson, and Art Kopelman for their suggestions.

References

1. Donner MW, Bosma JF, Robertson DL. Anatomy and physiology of the pharynx. Gastrointest Radiol 1985; 10:196–212.
2. Bosma JF. Anatomy of the Infant Head. Baltimore: Johns Hopkins, 1986.
3. Lacourt G, Polgar G. Interaction between nasal and pulmonary resistance in newborn infants. J Appl Physiol 1971; 30:870–873.
4. Hudgel DW. Variable site of airway narrowing among obstructive sleep apnea patients. J Appl Physiol 1986; 61:1403–1409.
5. Suto Y, Matsuo T, Kato T, Hori I, Inoue Y, Ogawa S, Suzuki T, Yamada M, Ohta Y. Evaluation of the pharyngeal airway in patients with sleep apnea: value of ultrafast MR imaging. AJR 1993; 160:311–314.
6. Berkowitz RG. Neonatal upper airway assessment by awake flexible laryngoscopy. Ann Otol Rhinol Laryngol 1998; 107:75–80.
7. Fredberg JJ, Wohl ME, Glass, GM, Dorkin HL. Airway area by acoustic reflections measured at the mouth. J Appl Physiol 1980; 48:749–758.

8. Hoffstein V, Zamel N, Phillipson, EA. Lung volume dependence of pharyngeal cross-sectional area in patients with obstructive sleep apnea. Am Rev Respir Dis 1984; 130:175–178.

9. Rivlin J, Hoffstein V, Kalbfleisch J, McNicholas W, Zamel N, Bryan AC. Upper airway morphology in patients with idiopathic obstructive sleep apnea. Am Rev Respir Dis 1984; 129:355–360.

10. Guilleminault C, Riley R, Powell N. Obstructive sleep apnea and abnormal cephalometric measurements. Implications for treatment. Chest 1984; 86:793–794.

11. Lowe AA, Fleetham JA, Adachi S, Ryan CF. Cephalometric and computed tomographic predictors of obstructive sleep apnea severity. Am J Orthod Dentofacial Orthop 1995; 107:589–595.

12. Katsantonis GP, Walsh JK. Somnofluoroscopy: its role in the selection of candidates for uvulopalatopharyngoplasty. Otolaryngol Head Neck Surg 1986; 94:56–60.

13. Suratt PM, Dee P, Atkinson RL, Armstrong P, Wilhoit SC. Fluoroscopic and computed tomographic features of the pharyngeal airway in obstructive sleep apnea. Am Rev Respir Dis 1983; 127:487–492.

14. Fernbach SK, Brouillette RT, Riggs TW, Hunt CE. Radiologic evaluation of adenoids and tonsils in children with obstructive sleep apnea: plain films and fluoroscopy. Pediatr Radiol 1983; 13:258–265.

15. Gibson SE, Myer CM 3rd, Strife JL, O'Connor DM. Sleep fluoroscopy for localization of upper airway obstruction in children. Ann Otol Rhinol Laryngol 1996; 105:678–683.

16. Schlesinger AE, Hernandez RJ. Radiographic imaging of airway obstruction in pediatrics. Otolaryngol Clin North Am 1990; 23:609–637.

17. Wiet GJ, Long FR, Shiels WE II, Rudman DT. Advances in pediatric airway radiology. Otolaryngol Clin North Am 2000; 33:15–28.

18. Kramer SS. Radiologic examination of the swallowing impaired child. Dysphagia 1989; 3:117–125.

19. Stevenson RD, Allaire JH. The development of normal feeding and swallowing. Pediatr Clin North Am 1991; 38:1439–1453.

20. Kauczor HU, Wolcke B, Fischer B, Mildenberger P, Lorenz J, Thelen M. Three-dimensional helical CT of the tracheobronchial tree: evaluation of imaging protocols and assessment of suspected stenoses with bronchoscopic correlation. AJR 1996; 167:419–424.

21. Hoffman EA, Gefter WB. Multimodality imaging of the upper airway: MRI, MR spectroscopy, and ultrafast x-ray CT. Prog Clin Biol Res 1990; 345:291–301.

22. Abbey NC, Block AJ, Green D, Mancuso A, Hellard DW. Measurement of pharyngeal volume by digitized magnetic resonance imaging. Effect of nasal continuous positive airway pressure. Am Rev Respir Dis 1989; 140:717–723.

23. Rodenstein DO, Dooms G, Thomas Y, Liistro G, Stanescu DC, Culee C Aubert-Tulkens G. Pharyngeal shape and dimensions in healthy subjects, snorers, and patients with obstructive sleep apnoea. Thorax 1990; 45:722–727.

24. Badr MS, Toiber F, Skatrud JB, Dempsey J. Pharyngeal narrowing/occlusion during central sleep apnea. J Appl Physiol 1995; 78:1806–1815.

25. Launois SH, Feroah TR, Campbell WN, Issa FG, Morrison D, Whitelaw WA, Isono S, Remmers JE. Site of pharyngeal narrowing predicts outcome of surgery for obstructive sleep apnea. Am Rev Respir Dis 1993; 147:182–189.

26. Schwab RJ, Gefter WB, Pack AI, Hoffman EA. Dynamic imaging of the upper airway during respiration in normal subjects. J Appl Physiol 1993; 74:1504–1514.

27. Brasch RC, Gould RG, Gooding CA, Ringertz HG, Lipton MJ. Upper airway obstruction in infants and children: evaluation with ultrafast CT. Radiology 1987; 165:459–466.

28. Brown IB, McClean PA, Boucher R, Zamel N, Hoffstein V. Changes in pharyngeal cross-sectional area with posture and application of continuous positive airway pressure in patients with obstructive sleep apnea. Am Rev Respir Dis 1987; 136:628–632.

29. Kuna ST, Bedi DG, Ryckman C. Effect of nasal airway positive pressure on upper airway size and configuration. Am Rev Respir Dis 1988; 138:969–975.

30. Ryan CF, Lowe AA, Li D, Fleetham JA. Magnetic resonance imaging of the upper airway in obstructive sleep apnea before and after chronic nasal continuous positive airway pressure therapy. Am Rev Respir Dis 1991; 144:939–944.

31. Miller MJ, Carlo WA, Martin RJ. Continuous positive airway pressure selectively reduces obstructive apnea in preterm infants. J Pediatr 1985; 106:91–94.

32. Milner AD, Boon AW, Saunders RA, Hopkin IE. Upper airways obstruction and apnoea in preterm babies. Arch Dis Child 1980; 55:22–25.

33. Olson LG, Fouke JM, Hoekje PL, Strohl KP. A biomechanical view of upper airway function In: Mathew OP, Sant'Ambrogio G, eds. Respiratory Function of the Upper Airway. New York: Marcel Dekker, 1988: 359–389.

34. Wilson SL, Thach BT, Brouillette RT, Abu-Osba YK. Upper airway patency in the human infant: influence of airway pressure and posture. J Appl Physiol 1980; 48:500–504.

35. Krespi YP, Husain S, Levine TM, Reede DL. Sublabial transseptal repair of choanal atresia or stenosis. Laryngoscope 1987; 97:1402–1406.

36. Lodeiro JG, Feinstein SJ, McLaren RA, Shapiro SL. Antenatal diagnosis of epignathus with neonatal survival. A case report. J Reprod Med 1989; 34:997–999.

37. Maeda K, Yamamoto T, Yoshimura H, Itoh H. Epignathus: a report of two neonatal cases. J Pediatr Surg 1989; 24:395–397.

38. Senyuz OF, Rizalar R, Celayir S, Oz F. Fetus in fetu or giant epignathus protruding from the mouth. J Pediatr Surg 1992; 27:1493–1495.

39. Todd DW, Votava HJ, Telander RL, Shoemaker CT. Giant epignathus. A case report. Minn Med 1991; 74:27–28.

40. Liechty KW, Crombleholme TM. Management of fetal airway obstruction. Semin Perinatol 1999; 23:496–506.

41. Weintraub AS, Holzman IR. Neonatal care of infants with head and neck anomalies. Otolaryngol Clin North Am 2000; 33:1171–1189.

42. Levine AB, Alvarez M, Wedgwood J, Berkowitz RL, Holzman I. Contemporary management of a potentially lethal fetal anomaly: a successful perinatal approach to epignathus. Obstet Gynecol 1990; 76:962–966.

43. Mychaliska GB, Bealer JF, Graf JL, Rosen MA, Adzick NS, Harrison MR. Operating on placental support: the ex utero intrapartum treatment procedure. J Pediatr Surg 1997; 32:227–230.

44. Liechty KW, Crombleholme TM, Weiner S, Bernick B, Flake AW, Adzick NS. The ex utero intrapartum treatment procedure for a large fetal neck mass in a twin gestation. Obstet Gynecol 1999; 93:824–825.

45. Eckmann DM. Transtracheal oxygen delivery. Crit Care Clin 2000; 16:463–472.

46. Guzzetta PC, Anderson KD, Eichelberger MR. General surgery. In: Avery GB, Fletcher MA, MacDonald MD, eds. Neonatology: Pathophysiology and Management of the Newborn. Philadelphia: Lippincott: 1994:918–919.

47. Benjamin B. Evaluation of choanal atresia. Ann Otol Rhinol Laryngol. 1985; 94:429–432.

48. Keller JL, Kacker A. Choanal atresia, CHARGE association, and congenital nasal stenosis. Otolaryngol Clin North Am 2000; 33:1343–1351.

49. Amir R, Dunham ME. Bilateral choanal atresia associated with nasal dermoid cyst and sinus: a case report and review of the literature. Int J Pediatr Otorhinolaryngol 2001; 58:81–85.

50. Duncan NO 3rd, Miller RH, Catlin FI. Choanal atresia and associated anomalies: the CHARGE association. Int J Pediatr Otorhinolaryngol 1988; 15:129–135.

51. Harris J, Robert E, Kallen B. Epidemiology of choanal atresia with special reference to the CHARGE association. Pediatrics 1997; 99:363–367.

52. Hengerer AS, Strome M. Choanal atresia: a new embryologic theory and its influence on surgical management. Laryngoscope 1982; 92:913–921.

53. Brown OE, Pownell P, Manning SC. Choanal atresia: a new anatomic classification and clinical management applications. Laryngoscope 1996; 106:97–101.

54. Miller MJ, Carlo WA, Strohl Kp, Fanaroff AA, Martin RJ. Effect of maturation on oral breathing in sleeping premature infants. J Pediatr. 1986; 109:515–519

55. Capasso A, Capasso L, Raimondi F, Perri D, Paludetto R. A nontraumatic and inexpensive clinical maneuver to check nasal patency at birth. Pediatrics. 2001; 107:214.

56. Crockett DM, Healy GB, McGill TJ, Friedman EM. Computed tomography in the evaluation of choanal atresia in infants and children. Laryngoscope 1987; 97:174–183.

57. Brown OE, Myer CM 3rd, Manning SC. Congenital nasal pyriform aperture stenosis. Laryngoscope 1989; 99:86–91.

58. Josephson GD, Vickery CL, Giles WC, Gross CW. Transnasal endoscopic repair of congenital choanal atresia: long-term results. Arch Otolaryngol Head Neck Surg 1998; 124:537–540.

59. Freng A. Subperiosteal early resection of the mid-palatal suture. A morphological study in twelve patients operated for choanal atresia. Scand J Plast Reconstr Surg 1979; 13:289–293.

60. Stark AR, Thach BT. Mechanisms of airway obstruction leading to apnea in newborn infants. J Pediatr 1976; 89:982–985.

61. Vogel JE, Mulliken JB, Kaban LB. Macroglossia: a review of the condition and a new classification. Plast Reconstr Surg 1986; 78:715–723.

62. Robin P. Glossoptosis due to atresia and hypotrophy of the mandible. Am J Dis Child 1934; 48:541.
63. Hanson JW, Smith DW. U-shaped palatal defect in the Robin anomalad: developmental and clinical relevance. J Pediatr 1975; 87:30–33.
64. Cohen MM. The Robin anomalad—its specificity and associated syndromes. J Oral Surg 1976; 34:587–593.
65. Sadewitz VL. Robin sequence: changes in thinking leading to changes in patient care. Cleft Palate Craniofac J 1992; 29:246–253.
66. Bush PG, Williams AJ. Incidence of Robin anomalad (Pierre Robin syndrome). Br J Plast Surg 1983; 36:434–437.
67. Gorlin RJ, Cohen MM, Levin LS. Syndromes of the Head and Neck. New York: Oxford University Press, 1990.
68. Shprintzen RJ. Pierre Robin, micrognathia, and airway obstruction: the dependency of treatment on accurate diagnosis. Int Anesthesiol Clin 1988; 26:64–71.
69. Van der Haven I, Mulder JW, Van der Wal KG, Hage JJ, De Lange–De Klerk ES, Haumann TJ. The jaw index: new guide defining micrognathia in newborns. Cleft Palate Craniofac J 1997; 34:240–241.
70. Paladini D, Morra T, Teodoro A, Lamberti A, Tremolaterra F, Martinelli P. Objective diagnosis of micrognathia in the fetus: the jaw index. Obstet and Gynecol 1999; 93:382–386.
71. Glander K, Cisneros GJ. Comparison of the craniofacial characteristics of two syndromes associated with the Pierre Robin sequence. Cleft Palate Craniofac J 1992; 29:210–219.
72. Vegter F, Hage JJ Mulder JW. Pierre Robin syndrome: mandibular growth during the first year of life. Ann Plast Surg 1999; 42:154–157.
73. Figueroa AA, Glupker TJ, Fitz MG, BeGole EA. Mandible, tongue and airway in Pierre Robin sequence: a longitudinal cephalometric study. Cleft Palate Craniofac J 1991; 28:425–434.
74. Amaratunga NA. A comparative clinical study of Pierre Robin syndrome and isolated cleft palate. Br J Oral Maxillofac Surg 1989; 27:451–458.
75. Fletcher MM, Blum SL, Blanchard CL. Pierre Robin syndrome pathophysiology of obstructive episodes. Laryngoscope 1969; 79:547–560.
76. Cozzi F. Glossoptosis as cause of apnoeic spells in infants with choanal atresia. Lancet 1977; 2(8042):830–831.
77. Sher A. Mechanisms of airway obstruction in Robin sequence: implication for treatment. Cleft Palate Craniofac J 1992; 29:224–231.
78. Delorme RP, Larocque Y, Caouette-Laberge L. Innovative surgical approach for the Pierre Robin anomalad: subperiosteal release of the floor of the mouth musculature. Plast Reconstr Surg 1989; 83:960–964.
79. Roberts JL, Reed WR, Mathew OP, Thach BT. Control of respiratory activity of the genioglossus muscle in micrognathic infants. J Appl Physiol 1986; 61:1523–1533.
80. Reed WR, Roberts JL, Thach BT. Factors influencing regional patency and configuration of the human infant upper airway. J Appl Physiol 1985; 58:635–644.
81. Singer L, Sidoti EJ. Pediatric management of Robin sequence. Cleft Palate Craniofac J 1992; 29:220–223.

82. Posnick JC. Treacher Collins syndrome: perspectives in evaluation and treatment. J Oral Maxillofac Surg 1997; 55:1120–1133.

83. St.-Hilaire H, Buchbinder D. Maxillofacial pathology and management of Pierre Robin sequence. Otolaryngol Clin North Am 2000; 33:1241–1256.

84. Argamaso RV. Glossopexy for upper airway obstruction in Robin sequence. 1992; 29:232–238.

85. LeBlanc SM, Golding-Kushner KJ. Effect of glossopexy on speech sound production in Robin sequence. Cleft Palate Craniofac J 1992; 29:239–245.

86. McCarthy JG, Schreiber J, Karp N, Thorne CH, Grayson BH. Lengthening of the human mandible by gradual distraction. Plast Reconstr Surg 1992; 89:1–8.

87. Caouette-Laberge L, Plamondon C, Larocque Y. Subperiosteal release of the floor of the mouth in Pierre Robin sequence: experience with 12 cases. Cleft Palate Craniofac J 1996; 33:468–472.

88. Nowlin JH, Zalzal GH. The stridorous infant. Ear Nose Throat J 1991; 70:84–88.

89. Mancuso RF. Stridor in neonates. Pediatr Clin North Am 1996; 43:1339–1356.

90. Perkins JA, Sie KC, Milczuk H, Richardson MA. Airway management in children with craniofacial anomalies. Cleft Palate Craniofac J 1997; 34:135–140.

91. Holinger LD. Etiology of stridor in the neonate, infant and child. Ann Otol Rhinol Laryngol 1980; 89:397–400.

92. Ferguson JL, Neel HB 3rd. Choanal atresia: treatment trends in 47 patients over 33 years. Ann Otol Rhinol Laryngol 1989; 98:110–112.

93. Grundfast KM, Harley E. Vocal cord paralysis. Otolaryngol Clin North Am 1989; 22:569–597.

94. Richardson MA, Cotton RT. Anatomic abnormalities of the pediatric airway. Pediatr Clin North Am 1984; 31:821–834.

95. Belmont JR, Grundfast K. Congenital laryngeal stridor (laryngomalacia):etiologic factors and associated disorders. Ann Otol Rhinol Laryngol 1984; 93:430–437.

96. Ferguson CF. Congenital abnormalities of the infant larynx. Otolaryngol Clin North Am 1970; 3:185–200.

97. Backer CL, Ilbawi MN, Idriss FS, DeLeon SY. Vascular anomalies causing tracheoesophageal compression. Review of experience in children. J Thorac Cardiovasc Surg 1989; 97:725–731.

98. Pransky SM, Grundfast KM. Differentiating upper from lower airway compromise in neonates. Ann Otol Rhinol Laryngol 1985; 94:509–515.

99. Parnell FW, Brandenburg JH. Vocal cord paralysis. A review of 100 cases. Laryngoscope 1970; 80:1036–1045.

100. Rimell FL, Shapiro AM, Meza MP, Goldman S, Hite S, Newman B. Magnetic resonance imaging of the pediatric airway. Arch Otolaryngol Head Neck Surg 1997; 123:999–1003.

101. Wiatrak BJ. Congenital anomalies of the larynx and trachea. Otolaryngol Clin North Am 2000; 33:91–110.

102. Zalzal GH, Anon JB, Cotton RT. Epiglottoplasty for the treatment of laryngomalacia. Ann Otol Rhinol Laryngol 1987; 96:72–76.

103. Benjamin B. Tracheomalacia in infants and children. Ann Otol Rhinol Laryngol 1984; 93:438–442.

104. Walner DL, Loewen MS, Kimura RE. Neonatal subglottic stenosis—incidence and trends. Laryngoscope 2001; 111:48–51.
105. Mair EA, Parsons DS, Lally KP, Van Dellen AF. Comparison of expandable endotracheal stents in the treatment of surgically induced piglet tracheomalacia. Laryngoscope 1991; 101:1002–1008.
106. Choi SS, Zalzal GH. Changing trends in neonatal subglottic stenosis. Otolaryngol Head Neck Surg 2000; 122:61–63.
107. Myer CM, O'Connor DM, Cotton RT. Proposed grading system for subglottic stenosis based on endotracheal tube sizes. Ann Otol Rhinol Laryngol 1994; 103:319–323.
108. Cotton RT. Management of subglottic stenosis. Otolaryngol Clin North Am 2000; 33:111–130.
109. Zeitouni AG, Manoukian J. Severe complications of the anterior cricoid split operation and single-stage laryngotracheoplasty. Ann Otol Rhinol Laryngol 1994; 103:723–725.

23

SIDS and the Newborn Infant

JEAN M. SILVESTRI and DEBRA E. WEESE-MAYER

Rush Children's Hospital
Chicago, Illinois, U.S.A.

I. Introduction

The incidence of sudden infant death syndrome (SIDS) has continued to decrease into the 21st century. However, sudden infant death syndrome remains a leading cause of infant mortality. In 1992 the American Academy of Pediatrics (AAP) recommended that infants sleep nonprone to reduce the risk of SIDS (1). After examining further epidemiological evidence, the recommendation was revised in 1996 to "Back to Sleep" as the preferred sleep position to reduce the risk of SIDS (2). These landmark public health interventions divide studies into the pre– and post–Back to Sleep eras. Identification of sleep position has become critical in understanding any epi-demiological or physiologic studies. Infant position has also been critical in newborn respiratory physiology especially in the preterm infant. The epidemiology of SIDS, with emphasis on the modifiable risk factors of prone sleep position and cigarette smoking, contrasting the pre– and post–Back to Sleep eras, as well as understanding mechanisms that may explain these risk factors as they relate to the infant in the newborn and special care nurseries will be the focus of this review.

II. Definition and Risk Factors

Sudden infant death syndrome is defined as the "sudden death of an infant under one year of age, which remains unexplained after a thorough case investigation, including performance of a complete autopsy, examination of the death scene, and review of the clinical history" (3). Risk factors that have been identified in both the pre– and post–Back to Sleep eras include prone sleep position, soft sleeping surface, maternal smoking during pregnancy, overheating, poor prenatal care, young maternal age, male gender, prematurity, and low birth weight (4–6). Other characteristics regarding SIDS include observations that the majority of deaths occur unobserved during nighttime sleep and to mothers with higher parity. Also breastfeeding, which has many other benefits and thus is promoted in our newborn and special care nurseries, does not have an independent protective effect on reducing the risk of SIDS (7). The lack of a dose-response effect suggests that the earlier observations of a protective effect may be a marker of the lifestyle of mothers who chose to breastfeed (6). In the United States, African-Americans and American Indians have consistently higher rates of SIDS. In England, the Confidential Enquiry for Stillbirths and Deaths in Infancy (CESDI) study identified a strong association of SIDS and other sudden unexpected infant deaths with extreme poverty, socioeconomic deprivation, unemployment, and a high degree of "social chaos" (7).

III. Age at Presentation

SIDS is rare in the newborn nursery and the first month of life. From the CESDI study (which did not include deaths under 7 days), 5% of SIDS deaths were of infants aged 1–4 weeks. From the Avon study ~2–3% of sudden deaths under 1 year of age occurred at <7 days of life (P.J. Fleming, personal communication, 2001). SIDS has been reported in the literature in full-term infants in newborn nurseries as a rare event in the pre–Back to Sleep era (8,9). The peak incidence of SIDS is between 2 and 4 months of age and then declines with >95% of deaths occurring in the first 6 months of life.

IV. Gestational Age

A. SIDS and the Preterm Infant

Prematurity and low birth weight are also risk factors for SIDS, with increasing risk for greater immaturity and lower birth weight. However, the age at death may differ by 4–6 weeks between preterm and term infants. In a restricted analysis of a large cohort of infants with appropriately classified gestational ages, preterm infants died at a later postnatal age but at a younger postconceptional age than term infants, which implies an altered peak of vulnerability for the preterm infant (10). In evaluating two large cohorts of infants in the pre– and post–Back to Sleep eras in the United States, African-American infants and infants born at <1000 g had an increased relative risk compared to non-Hispanic white infants weighing

>2500 g (11). A comparison of SIDS deaths in the pre– and post–Back to Sleep era demonstrates that there has been a decline in SIDS rates across all gestational and birth weight categories (12). This implies that the reduction of prone sleep has been effective in reducing SIDS in preterm and low birth weight infants as well as term infants. However, prematurity and low birth weight still remain risk factors for SIDS, and ethnic/racial differences are even more apparent.

B. SIDS and the Term Infant

Other aspects of the newborn period are associated with an increased risk of SIDS. In the CESDI study, SIDS infants had a higher chance of needing resuscitation at birth as well as being admitted to a special care baby unit (7). This factor remained significant after preterm infants were excluded from the analysis.

V. Modifiable Risk Factors for SIDS

A. Prone Sleep Position

In terms of modifiable risk factors, prone sleeping has been consistently implicated as a risk factor for SIDS. Although less of a risk than prone sleeping, side sleeping also has an increased risk for SIDS. It is in part related to the inherent instability with the infant likely to roll into the prone position, but there may be other mechanisms related intrinsically to the side position (7,13). Even in countries where there is a low incidence of SIDS and a low incidence of prone positioning in the Back to Sleep era, prone sleeping continues to be a major risk factor, with a large number of deaths associated with the prone position (14,15). In the United States as the rate of SIDS has decreased, so has the rate of prone sleeping; however, there is a marked racial and ethnic disparity in sleep position. In the most recent publication of the National Sleep Position Study, prone sleep decreased to 17% among white infants as compared to 32% among black infants (16). Further, studies have demonstrated that the incidence of prone sleep increased from 1 to 3 months of age just at the time of the peak incidence of SIDS (17), suggesting that parents are not understanding the importance of avoiding prone sleeping as it relates to SIDS.

Although SIDS is rare in the newborn period and first month of life, the birth hospitalization is the ideal time for critical education and preparation of the family to understand the risk reduction process. Despite evidence that prone positioning is one of the major risk factors for SIDS, hospitals have not consistently placed newborns on their backs to sleep in the newborn nursery (18). Nurses cited that side positioning was an acceptable alternative (18). Also, mothers who saw their infants placed prone in the hospital intended to place their infants prone at home. Thus, it is imperative for physicians and neonatal nurses not only to know the potential SIDS risk factors, but also to educate parents and infant caretakers since physician and neonatal nurse recommendations significantly increase the probability of supine placement of infants (16).

Why Is Prone Sleep a Risk Factor for SIDS Among Term Infants?

Diaphragm thickness

An ultrasound study in 16 healthy term infants demonstrated that the diaphragm is thicker (and thus shorter) at both end expiratory and inspiratory volumes when in the prone position (19). Thus the diaphragm is placed at a mechanical disadvantage with regard to a potential environmental stressor when an infant is in the prone position.

Sleep Characteristics by Position

Khan et al. (20) examined the differences in sleep characteristics between prone and supine positioning among 34 term infants who routinely slept prone and 34 infants who routinely slept supine. Prone-positioned infants demonstrated a significant increase in sleep duration and non REM sleep and a significant decrease in the number and duration of arousals, regardless of their routine sleep position (20). Galland et al. (21) reported full awakenings in response to the tilt test to be common in active sleep, but significantly less in the prone position (15% of prone as compared to 54% supine) among 37 healthy term infants at 2–4 months of age.

Physiologic Measures of Heart Rate and Temperature by Position

Skadberg and Markestad (22) reported higher heart rates and peripheral skin temperature in REM and NREM sleep in the prone as compared to supine position among 32 term infants studied at 2.5 and 5 months of age. Galland et al. reported reduced heart rate variability in REM and NREM sleep among 37 healthy infants at 2–4 months of age in the prone position as compared to supine (21).

Ventilatory and Arousal Responses by Position

Galland et al. reported that prone positioning altered the ventilatory sensitivity to mild asphyxia (5% carbon dioxide, 13.5% oxygen) only during active sleep among 53 infants studied at 3 months of age as compared to supine (23). Ventilatory responses were unaffected by sleep position in the newborn period. In contrast to their prior studies, older infants were twice as likely to arouse as newborns, and prone positioning increased the chances of arousal.

Physiologic and Arousal Responses to Auditory and Nasal Air Jet Stimulus by Sleep Position

Among 20 term healthy infants (age 8–15 weeks) presented with an auditory challenge during REM sleep, there were significantly fewer changes in heart rate, heart rate drops, less heart rate variability, and fewer and shorter central apneas in the prone as compared to the supine position (24). Auditory arousal thresholds during REM sleep were higher in prone as compared to supine among 22 healthy term infants age 4–12 weeks (25). Arousal to air jet stimulation was reduced in the prone position among 24 healthy term infants studies at 2–3 weeks and 2–3 months, but unchanged when studied at 5–6 months (26).

Arousal Responses to Obstructive Apnea by Position

Reduced behavioral arousals after an obstructive apnea have been seen in 20 preterm and term infants aged 3–13 weeks sleeping prone (31.3%) as compared to supine (57.5%) as well as a significantly delayed time to arousal after an obstructive apnea in the prone position (10.5 sec) as compared to supine (8 sec) (27).

In summary, there are several studies that aid in our understanding why prone sleep may be associated with a higher risk of SIDS. The prone position in healthy term infants affects anatomy, sleep architecture, cardiorespiratory parameters, and autonomic function as reflected in heart rate variability and ventilatory and arousal responses.

Why Is Prone Sleep a Risk Factor for SIDS Among Preterm Infants?

Although preterm infants are at higher risk of SIDS, it has been controversial in the NICU as to when to recommend the supine position as the preferred sleep position for the convalescing preterm infant. In 1996 the AAP included asymptomatic preterm infants in the recommendation of nonprone sleep.

Advantages of Prone Sleep

There are several publications that address the advantages of the prone position in the ill preterm infant (28–30). In the convalescing preterm infant, the prone position improves oxygenation, reduces chest wall asynchrony (31), reduces the incidence of apnea and periodic breathing (32), and reduces energy expenditure (33).

Apnea, Bradycardia, and Desaturation by Position

In a study of 22 preterm infants studied at 31.9 ± 3 weeks PCA, no significant difference was found in the incidence of apnea ≥ 15 sec, heart rate <90 bpm, and hemoglobin saturation $>90\%$ between the prone and supine positions (34). In a study of 16 older preterm infants with a PCA of 36.5 ± 0.6 weeks, there was no apnea <15 sec, apnea with bradycardia and/or desaturation, or difference in the amount of periodic breathing in either prone or supine position (35).

Sleep Characteristics by Position

Among 23 preterm infants at 31–36 weeks PCA, prone sleep was associated with a 79% increase in quiet sleep and a 71% decrease in awake time, with increases in quiet sleep in the prone position found in the first hour postfeeding and near the end of the interfeed interval (36). Thus, sleep position can alter sleep state organization in the preterm infant, and the effect of feeding may play a role.

Physiologic, Ventilatory, and Arousal Responses by Position

Increased arousals were found in the supine position (36). Among 19 healthy convalescing preterm infants (postconceptional age $\sim 35 \pm 1$ weeks), the supine position was associated with a significantly higher respiratory rate and lower hemoglobin saturation than prone (37). An attenuated response to hypercapnia was seen in the supine position as compared to prone; however, significance depended on the methodology of measurement. Among 16 convalescing preterm infants (postconceptional age 36.5 ± 0.6 weeks), more awakenings were seen in all sleep states in the supine than in the prone position (35). However, sleep duration, percent sleep state, and arousal as defined as body movement ≥ 10 sec, cry, or eye opening ≥ 5 sec, were unaffected by position. In quiet sleep maximal heart rate and heart rate variability were higher in the supine than the prone position. Older premature infants (n = 9) of 31–35 weeks gestation studied at 36 weeks, 2–3 weeks and 2–3 months postterm demonstrated no state-related difference in arousal threshold to nasal air jet stimulation at 36 weeks or 2–3 weeks; however, at 2–3 months arousal was higher in quiet sleep than in active sleep (38). This study did not provide detail of sleep position.

As in the term infant, the prone position in preterm infants affects sleep architecture, cardiorespiratory parameters, and ventilatory and arousal responses.

How Does Prone Positioning Interact with Other Factors in the Sleep Environment?

Term Infants

Prone positioning may interact with other factors in the sleep environment such as soft bedding and temperature, resulting in physiologic compromise. Among 11 term infants studied prone in the laboratory, all infants slept face down for variable periods of time but more often after a cold stimulus than after a warm stimulus (39). When in the face-down position, all had impaired ventilation; in addition, rebreathing was increased on soft bedding. Observations in the home environment of 10 healthy prone sleeping infants confirm that infants often sleep in the face-straight-down or in the face-near-straight-down position (40). However, only a small subset of these (3% of face-near-straight-down and 14% face-straight-down) positions are associated with airway obstruction. Thus prone positioning in concert with environmental stressors and potentially defective arousal responses in the prone position could lead to SIDS in vulnerable infants.

Preterm Infants

Among 15 prone sleeping preterm infants (PCA 40 ± 1 weeks) nearing hospital discharge, it was observed that they seldom turned their heads during sleep and rarely demonstrated the face-near-straight-down or face-straight-down position (41). This is in contrast to the term infant and may provide insight into the age of risk of death in SIDS.

The dilemma still exists owing to a lack of substantial acute and longitudinal studies to identify the effect of sleep position on sleep and cardiorespiratory physiology as infants are discharged from the NICU. Many of the studies are flawed by small numbers of infants at different gestational ages and other known and unknown variables that may interact in the experimental design, such as clothing, feeding, intrauterine cigarette smoke exposure, time of study (day vs. night), variations in neonatal intensive care, and caretaker interface. The impact of factors that the preterm infant experiences such as chronic prone sleeping, prior apnea and bradycardia, IVH of any degree, and intrauterine smoke exposure is also unclear. All of these factors may place stress on key physiological systems as they are developing, and may ultimately lead to alterations in the development of these same systems that can result in maladaptation to an environmental stress.

Possible Complications of Prone Sleeping

Concern for Aspiration

A primary concern among medical and nursing personnel has been the risk of aspiration with supine positioning. Nurses cited risk of aspiration as the largest barrier in placing infants supine in the newborn nursery (18). There has been no increase in infant deaths attributable to aspiration in the United Kingdom with the change from prone to supine sleeping (42). There is evidence that infants who are prone are at greater risk of choking if they are sleeping face down.

Swallow Mechanics

When term (n = 14) and preterm (n = 9 with apnea) infants are presented with small boluses of normal saline delivered to the oropharynx, swallows and obstructed breaths occurred frequently, and cough and prolonged apnea infrequently (43). Prolonged apnea was more common in preterm infants. In addition, postmortem data demonstrate that when supine, pooling of fluid occurs in the piriform fossae when fluid is introduced in the pharynx, and the path of flow was dependent on head position—face up or face to side. When term (n = 5) and preterm (n = 7) infants studied at term are presented with pharyngeal fluid infusions (n = 229) in the supine position, swallowing rather than apnea was the primary defense mechanism (44). Swallowing was related to the volume infused. Spontaneous swallows were influenced by sleep state, being more frequent in active sleep. Sleep state did not effect swallowing (occurrence or frequency) after fluid infusion. Without an increase in significant apnea, there is protection from laryngeal chemoreflex stimulation, and the response is dependent on intact swallowing. In contrast to the prior study, where apnea was common in preterm infants, this may reflect a maturational response of the preterm infant. Multiple infusions (n = 164) of small amounts of water (0.4 mL) in 10 term infants studied at 3–5 days of age evoked swallowing (95%) and arousal (54%). In active sleep, there was a significant decrease in swallowing and breathing, but not arousal in prone as compared to supine (45). These studies indicate that airway protective mechanisms are reduced in prone sleep and may suggest that different receptors are activated at the pharyngeal or laryngeal level depending on sleep position (prone vs. supine).

There may be interaction with an inhibitory effect of other factors such as smoking and the influence of nicotine. Term (n = 12) and preterm (n = 11) infants studied at term did not differ in spontaneous swallowing rates when supine in active sleep, and had little swallowing in quiet sleep (46). In active sleep term infants increased swallows/min as a result of GER and preterm infants did not, but they had a larger proportion of pharyngeal propagated swallows. In summary, position and sleep state influence pharyngeal and laryngeal airway defenses that are all influenced by maturation with younger infants being more vulnerable.

B. Cigarette Smoke

Exposure to cigarette smoke is a modifiable risk factor in SIDS. Smoking was identified as a major risk factor for SIDS in studies in the pre–Back to Sleep era (4), and it remains a strong independent risk factor in the post–Back to Sleep era with a dose-response effect (7,13,47). In addition, passive exposure has been identified as a risk factor with a dose-response relationship between number of hours of exposure and increased risk (7,47). In a large population-based study among different ethnic groups in the United States, after controlling for other risk factors, smoking remained a strong risk factor for SIDS even in the low-risk groups of Hispanics and Asian and Pacific Islanders, with the risk increasing with the number of cigarettes smoked (48).

Why is Cigarette Smoking a Risk Factor for SIDS?

Animal Models

Animal models of nicotine infusions in the developing lamb have demonstrated an attenuated response to hypoxia, an increased response to hyperoxia (49), delayed arousal to hypoxia in quiet sleep, and a lower level of hypoxemia to initiate arousal as well as an attenuated ventilatory response to hypoxemia (50). Nicotine may alter responses with a direct effect on carotid body chemoreceptors and central processing of carotid body chemoreceptor discharge in addition to cortical activation mechanisms.

Human Infant: Pathology, Respiratory Physiology, and Arousal

Poor fetal growth and altered nervous system development (51,52) are well-known sequelae of smoking during pregnancy. In the human infant a correlation between smoke exposure during pregnancy and brainstem gliosis associated with hypoxic-ischemic events has been observed in SIDS infants (53). Prenatal smoke exposure has correlated with an increase in frequency and length of obstructive apneas in newborns and infants (54). Infants of smoking mothers had less auditory habituation and orientation to noise while awake than controls (55). Physiologic studies have demonstrated in some cases altered ventilatory and arousal responses in infants of smoking mothers. Deficient hypoxia awakening responses were found in 13 term infants of smoking mothers studied at 8–12 weeks of age as compared to 34 control infants (56). However, ventilatory responses to hypoxia and hypercapnia were similar whether mothers smoked or not.

On the other hand, another study demonstrated attenuated responses to hypoxia in six term infants of smoking mothers as compared to nine control infants who were studied between 2 and 12 months of age (57). Among newborns and infants 4–21 weeks of age whose mothers smoked during pregnancy, a decreased arousal to an auditory stimulus was observed (58). In addition, behavioral awakenings occurred less frequently in infants of smokers, emphasizing the impact of exposure before birth.

In a study that controlled and matched for confounding factors such as social class, maternal age, parity, feeding, birth weight, gestational age, and gender, no significant differences were found in respiratory timing or control during nighttime sleep among 17 term infants of smoking mothers and 23 controls studied at 8–12 weeks of age (59). One presumes these infants were supine, but this is not explicitly stated in the study. In addition, the change in end-tidal oxygen level when 40% oxygen was used was higher in the smoking group as compared to controls. This information may provide further understanding regarding mechanisms and warrants further study.

Human Infant: Heart Rate Response

Spectral analyses of heart rate evaluated by sleep state revealed that infants of smoking mothers (n = 18) had significantly lower high-frequency (HF) and normalized HF powers and higher LF/HF ratios than nonsmokers (n = 18) in REM sleep. Values did not reach significance in non REM sleep. Infants were studied supine at 6–16 weeks. No differences were found in sleep characteristics (60). Heart rate responses were altered in apparently healthy-appearing term newborn infants (23 smoking mothers and 23 controls) exposed to hypoxia and hypercarbia (61). Overall, heart rate decreased in response to hyperoxia and increased in response to hypoxia and hypercarbia, and the change was correlated to the change in ventilation. The number of cigarettes smoked by the mother was associated with sharper heart rate declines and smaller heart rate rises. For all infants, the heart rate response lagged behind the ventilatory response, and the lag was significantly longer among the smoke-exposed infants.

Although nicotine appears to have a consistent effect on arousal, there is not a consistent effect on respiratory responses to oxygen in the developing human. Limitations of these studies are related to the small sample size, variable amount of smoke exposure in both the infants of smoking mothers and controls, as well as quantification of passive smoke exposure, day vs. night studies, and other epidemiologic factors.

VI. Summary

Although modifiable risk factors may act independently, they can interact with each other and other risk factors. The preterm infant discharged from the special care nursery is particularly vulnerable, both epidemiologically and physiologically. It is the combination of an acute stressor with the individual vulnerability and a developmental immaturity of the infant that may result in death. In understanding future directions in SIDS research, there is a need to further understand the biologic mechanisms underpinning the risk factors—which in some cases such as prone position and smoking are strong enough to imply causality. However, how does one explain the infant who dies of SIDS and does not have risk factors?

After 15 years of investigation of brainstems of 52 infants who died of SIDS compared to acute and chronic controls, a map has emerged of the neuropathology and neurotransmitters of the ventral medulla (62). Decreased muscarinic, kainite, and serotonergic receptor binding have been identified in the arcuate nucleus as well as decreased serotonergic receptor binding in nucleus raphe obscurus. It is postulated that SIDS or a subset of SIDS is a result of this abnormality in the medulla and related sertonergic neurons including the caudal raphe and the arcuate nucleus. This can cause a failure in homeostatic mechanisms in that a vulnerable infant may be unable to respond to a potentially life-threatening environmental stressor and result in a SIDS death. This medullary serotonergic defect hypothesis requires further verification and validation, in addition to identification of underlying cellular and molecular mechanisms. These need to be translated to implement pathophysiologic studies of cardiorespiratory control in the human infant. Because the serotonergic system does not play a key role in the autonomic nervous system (ANS), a system considered to be dysfunctional among infants who have succumbed to SIDS, the role of the serotonergic system relative to the ANS will need to be further delineated. Other insights may be uncovered as other investigators explore the underlying genetic basis of SIDS such as defects in polymorphisms in the serotonin transporter gene (63).

Until a better understanding of the mechanisms of SIDS is elucidated, it is the responsibility of all health care professionals to educate infant caretakers about modifiable SIDS risk factors that can reduce the risk of SIDS. An opportunity for this educational process exists at the birth of the infant, either in the newborn nursery or in the epidemiologically high-risk special care nursery. If health care providers can model sleep position and a safe sleep environment, there is great potential to further reduce the incidence of prone sleeping and SIDS risk. In addition, efforts to reduce smoke exposure to fetuses and infants may be one of the most important interventions to substantially lower the incidence of SIDS.

References

1. American Academy of Pediatrics Task Force on Infant Positioning and SIDS. Positioning and SIDS. Pediatrics 1992; 89:1120–1126.
2. Task Force on Infant Positioning and SIDS. Positioning and sudden infant death syndrome (SIDS): update. Pediatrics 1996; 98:1216–1218.
3. Willinger M, James LS, Catz C. Defining the sudden infant death syndrome (SIDS): deliberations of an expert panel convened by the National Institutes of Child Health and Human Development. Pediatr Pathol 1991; 11:677–684.
4. Hoffman HJ, Hillman LS. Epidemiology of the sudden infant death syndrome: maternal, neonatal, and postneonatal risk factors. In: Hunt CE, ed. Apnea and SIDS: Clinics in Perinatology. Philadelphia: W.B. Saunders, 1992: 717–737.
5. Ponsonby AL, Dwyer T, Gibbons LE, Cochrane JA, Wang YG. Factors potentiating the risk of sudden infant death syndrome associated with the prone position. N Engl J Med 1993; 329:377–382.
6. Fleming PJ, Blair PS, Bacon C, Bensley D, Smith I, Taylor E, Berry J, Golding J, Tripp J. Confidential Enquiry into Stillbirths and Deaths Regional Coordinators and Researchers. Environments of infants during sleep and risk of the sudden infant death syndrome: results of 1993–5 case-control study for confidential enquiry into stillbirths and deaths in infancy. BMJ 1996; 313:191–195.
7. Fleming P, Blair P, Platt MW, Smith I, Chantler S. The case-control study: results and discussion. In: Fleming P, Blair P, Bacon C, Berry J, eds. Sudden Unexpected Deaths in Infancy. London: Her Majesty's Stationery Office, 2000; 13–96.
8. Polberger S, Svenningsen NW. Early neonatal sudden infant death and near death of fullterm infants in maternity wards. Acta Pædiatr Scand 1985; 74:861–866.
9. Burchfield DJ, Rawlings DJ. Sudden deaths and apparent life-threatening events in hospitalized neonates presumed to be healthy. Am J Dis Child 1991; 154:1319–1322.

10. Malloy MH, Hoffman HJ. Prematurity, sudden infant death syndrome, and age of death. Pediatrics 1995; 96:464–471.

11. Pollack HA, Frohna JG. A competing risk model of sudden infant death syndrome incidence in two US birth cohorts. J Pediatr 2001; 138:661–667.

12. Malloy M, Freeman DH. Birth weight– and gestational age–specific sudden infant death syndrome mortality: United States, 1991 versus 1995. Pediatrics 2000; 105:1227–1231.

13. Oyen N, Markestad T, Skaerven R, Irgens LM, Helwig-Larsen K, Alm B, Norvenius G, Wennergen G. Combined effects of sleeping position and prenatal risk factors in sudden infant death syndrome: the Nordic epidemiological SIDS study. Pediatrics 1997; 100:613–621.

14. Skadberg BT, Morild I, Markestad T. Abandoning prone sleeping: effect on the risk of sudden infant death syndrome. J Pediatr 1998; 132:340–342.

15. L'Hoir MP, Engelberts AC, Van Well GT, McClelland S, Westers P, Dandachli T, Mellenbergh GJ, Wolters WH, Huber J. Risk and preventive factors for cot death in the Netherlands, a low incidence country. Eur J Pediatr 1998; 157:681–688.

16. Willinger M, Ko CW, Hoffman HJ, Kessler RC, Corwin MJ. Factors associated with caregivers' choice of infant sleep position, 1994–1998: the National Infant Sleep Position Study. JAMA 2000; 283:2135–2142.

17. Lesko SM, Corwin MJ, Vezina RM, Hunt CE, Mandell F, McClain M, Heeren T, Mitchell AA. Changes in sleep position during infancy: a prospective longitudinal assessment. JAMA 1998; 280:336–340.

18. Hein HA, Pettit SF. Back to Sleep: good advice for parents but not for hospitals? Pediatrics 2001; 107:537–539.

19. Rehan VK, Nakashima JM, Gutman A, Rubin LP, McCool FD. Effects of the supine and prone position on diaphragm thickness in healthy term infants. Arch Dis Child 2000; 83:234–238.

20. Kahn A, Groswasser J, Sottiaux M, Rebuffat E, Franco P, Dramaix M. Prone or supine body position and sleep characteristics in infants. Pediatrics 1993; 91:1112–1115.

21. Galland BC, Reeves G, Taylor BJ, Bolton DPG. Sleep position, autonomic function, and arousal. Arch Dis Child Fetal Neonatal Ed 1998; 78:F189–F194.

22. Skadberg BT, Markestad T. Behaviour and physiologic responses during prone and supine sleep in early infancy. Arch Dis Child 1997; 76:320–324.

23. Galland BC, Bolton DPG, Taylor BJ, Sayers RM, Williams SM. Ventilatory sensitivity to mild asphyxia: prone versus supine sleep position. Arch Dis Child 2000; 83:12–128.

24. Franco P, Groswasser J, Sottiaux M, Broadfield E, Kahn A. Decreased cardiac responses to auditory stimulation during prone sleep. Pediatrics 1996; 97:174–178.

25. Franco P, Pardou A, Hassis S, Lurquin P, Groswasser J, Kahn A. Auditory arousal thresholds are higher when infants sleep in the prone position. J Pediatr 1998; 132:240–243.

26. Horne RSC, Ferens D, Watts AM, Vitkovic J, Lacey B, Andrew S, Cranage SM, Chau B, Adamson T. The prone sleeping position impairs arousability in term infants. J Pediatr 2001; 138:811–816.

27. Groswasser J, Simon T, Scaillet S, Franco P, Kahn A. Reduced arousals following obstructive apneas in infants sleeping prone. Pediatr Res 2001; 49:402–406.
28. Kurlak LO, Ruggins NR, Stephenson TJ. Effect of nursing position on incidence, type, and duration of clinically significant apnoea in preterm infants. Arch Dis Child 1994; 71:F16-F19.
29. McEvoy C, Mendoza ME, Bowling S, Hewlett V, Sardesai S, Durand M. Prone positioning decreases episodes of hypoxemia in extremely low birth weight infants (1000 grams or less) with chronic lung disease. J Pediatr 1997; 130:305–309.
30. Wolfson MR, Greenspan JS, Deoras KS, Allen JL, Shaffer TH. Effect of position on the mechanical interaction between the rib cage and abdomen in preterm infants. J Appl Physiol 1992; 72:1032–1038.
31. Martin RJ, Herrell N, Rubin D, Fanaroff A. Effect of supine and prone positions on arterial oxygen tension in the preterm infant. Pediatrics 1979; 63:528–531.
32. Heimler R, Langlois J, Hodel DJ, Nelin LD, Sasidharan P. Effect of positioning on the breathing pattern of preterm infants. Arch Dis Child 1992; 67:312–314.
33. Masterson J, Zucker C, Schulze K. Prone and supine positioning effects on energy expenditure and behavior of low birth weight neonates. Pediatrics 1987; 80:689–692.
34. Keene DJ, Wimmer JE, Mathew OP. Does supine positioning increase apnea, bradycardia, and desaturation in preterm infants? J Perinatol 2000; 1:17–20.
35. Goto K, Mirmiran M, Adams M, Longford R, Baldwin R, Boeddiker MA, Ariagno R. More awakening and heart rate variability during supine sleep in preterm infants. Pediatrics 1999; 103:603–609.
36. Myers M, Fifer WP, Schaeffer L, Sahni R, Ohira-Kist K, Stark RI, Schulze KF. Effects of sleeping position and time after feeding on the organization of sleep/wake states in prematurely born infants. Sleep 1998; 21:343–349.
37. Martin RJ, DiFiore JM, Korenke CB, Randal H, Miller MJ, Brooks LJ. Vulnerability of respiratory control in healthy preterm infants placed supine. J Pediatr 1995; 127:609–614.
38. Horne RSC, Sly DJ, Cranage SM, Chau B, Adamson TM. Effects of prematurity on arousal from sleep in the newborn infant. Pediatr Res 2000; 47:468–474.
39. Chiodini BA, Thach BT. Impaired ventilation in infants sleeping facedown: potential significance for sudden infant death syndrome. J Pediatr 1993; 123:686–692.
40. Waters KA, Gonzalez A, Jean C, Morielli A, Brouillette RT. Face-straight-down and face-near-straight-down positions in healthy term infants. J Pediatr 1996; 128:616–625.
41. Constantin E, Waters KA, Morielli A, Brouillette RT. Head turning and face-down positioning in prone-sleeping premature infants. J Pediatr 1999; 134:558–562.
42. Fleming PJ. Understanding and preventing sudden infant death syndrome. Curr Opin Pediatr 1994; 6:158–162.
43. Pickens DL, Schefft GL, Thach BT. Pharyngeal fluid clearance and aspiration preventive mechanisms in sleeping infants. J Appl Physiol 1989; 66:1164–1171.
44. Page M, Jeffrey HE. Airway protection in sleeping infants in response to pharyngeal fluid stimulation in the supine position. Pediatr Res 1998; 44:691–698.

45. Jeffrey HE, Megevand A, Page M. Why the prone position is a risk for sudden infant death syndrome. Pediatrics 1999: 104:263–269.
46. Jeffrey HE, Ius D, Page M. The role swallowing during active sleep in the clearance of reflux in term and preterm infants. J Pediatr 2000; 137:545–548.
47. Blair PS, Fleming PJ, Bensley D, Smith I, Bacon C, Taylor E, Berry J, Golding J, Tripp J. Smoking and the sudden infant death syndrome: results from 1993–5 case-control study for confidential inquiry into stillbirths and deaths in infancy. BMJ 1996; 313:195–198.
48. MacDorman MF, Cnattingius S, Hoffman HJ, Kramer MS, Haglund B. Sudden infant death syndrome in the United States and Sweden. Am J Epidemiol 1997; 146:249–257.
49. Milerad J, Larsson H, Lin J, Sundell HW. Nicotine attenuates the ventilatory response to hypoxia in the developing lamb. Pediatr Res 1995; 37:652–660.
50. Hafström O, Milerad J, Asokan N, Poole SD, Sundell HW. Nicotine delays arousal during hypoxemia in lambs. Pediatr Res 2000; 47:646–652.
51. Slotkin TA, Lappi SE, McCook EC, Lorber BA, Seidler FJ. Loss of neonatal hypoxia tolerance after prenatal exposure: implications for sudden infant death syndrome. Brain Res Bull 1995; 38:69–75.
52. Kinney HC, O'Donnell TJ, Kriger P, White FW. Early developmental changes in [^{3}H]nicotine binding in the human brainstem. Neuroscience 1993; 55:1127–1138.
53. Storm H, Nylander G, Saugstad OD. The amount of brainstem gliosis in sudden infant death syndrome (SIDS) victims correlates with maternal cigarette smoking during pregnancy. Acta Pædiatr 1999; 88:13–18.
54. Kahn A, Groswasser J, Sottiaux M, Kelmanson I, Rebuffat E, Franco P, Dramaix M, Wayenberg JL. Prenatal exposure to cigarettes in infants with obstructive sleep apneas. Pediatrics 1994; 93:778–783.
55. Saxton DW. The behavior of infants whose mothers smoke during pregnancy. Early Hum Dev 1978; 2:363–369.
56. Lewis KW, Bosque M. Deficient hypoxia awakening response in infants of smoking mothers: possible relationship to sudden infant death syndrome. J Pediatr 1995; 127:691–699.
57. Ueda Y, Stick SM, Hall G, Sly PD. Control of breathing in infants born to smoking mothers. J Pediatr 1999; 135:226–232.
58. Franco P, Groswasser J, Hassid S, Lanquart JP, Scaillet S, Kahn A. Prenatal exposure to cigarette smoking is associated with a decrease in arousal in infants. J Pediatr 1999; 135:34–38.
59. Poole KA, Hallinan H, Beardsmore CS, Thompson JR. Effect of maternal smoking on ventilatory responses to changes in inspired oxygen levels in infants. Am J Respir Crit Care Med 2000; 162:801–807.
60. Franco P, Chabanski S, Szliwowski H, Dramaix M, Kahn A. Influence of maternal smoking on autonomic nervous system in healthy infants. Pediatr Res 2000; 47:215.
61. Søvik S, Lossius K, Walløe L. Heart rate response to transient chemoreceptor stimulation in term infants is modified by exposure to maternal smoking. Pediatr Res 2001; 49:558–565.

62. Kinney HC, Filiano JJ, White WF. Medullary serotonergic network deficiency in the sudden infant death syndrome: review of a 15-year study of a single dataset. J Neuropathol Exp Neurol 2001; 60:228–247.
63. Narita N, Narita M, Takashima S, Nakayama M, Nagai T, Okado N. Serotonin transporter gene variation is a risk factor for sudden infant death syndrome in the Japanese population. Pediatr 2001; 107:690–692.

AUTHOR INDEX

Italic numbers give the page on which the complete reference is listed.

A

Aarimaa T, 459, *469*
Abbassi S, 282, *291*, 300, *313*, 384, 385, *391*
Abbey NC, 500, 501, *518*
Abboud EL, 93, *108*
Abdiche M, 162, *177*
Abend M, 192, *205*, 281, *290*, 343, *352*
Aber V, 453, *466*
Abman SH, 461, *470*
Abrams RM, 130, *144*
Abroms IF, 358, *369*
Absood A, 59, *77*
Abu-Osba YK, 62, *78*, 126, *141*, 211, 215, 305, 309, *314*, *316*, 379, *390*, 502, *519*
Abu-Shaweesh J, 86, 88, *105*
Abu-Shaweesh JM, 86, 92, *105*, *107*
Abubakar KM, 442, *448*
Abuektteish F, 212, *215*
Accurso FJ, 461, *470*
Adachi S, 499, *518*
Adam E, 397, *405*
Adams JA, 218, 219, *231*, 298, *311*
Adams L, 280, 283, *289*
Adams M, 529, 530, *537*

Adams MA, 416, *422*
Adams MM, 162, *178*
Adamson JS, 323, *331*
Adamson T, 529, *536*
Adamson TM, 344, *352*, 530, *537*
Adcock JJ, 71, *80*
Adderley R, 412, 413, *421*
Adkins JC, 396, 397, *405*
Adler SM, 85, 86, *104*, 344, *352*, 457, *468*
Adolph EF, 19, 24, *33*
Adriaensen D, 59, 60, *76*, *77*
Adrian S, 308, *316*
Adrien J, 152, *174*
Adzick NS, 505, *520*
Affonso DD, 162, *178*
Agani FH, 89, *106*
Agostoni E, 61, *77*, 246, *268*, 298, *311*, 360, *370*
Aguilar T, 464, *471*
Ahlborn V, 229, *235*
Ahlstrom H, 306, *314*
Ahluwalia JS, 442, *448*
Ahmann PA, 459, *469*
Aina A, 117, 125, *138*, 365, 366, 367, *371*
Ainsworth DM, 184, *203*

541

SUBJECT INDEX

A

Adenosine receptor, 135
Airway fluoroscopy, 499–500
Airway imaging, 499–501
Airway innervation, 39–81
  density of, 56, 59
  neural crest–derived cells, 40–43, 45
  vagus nerve, 44, 57
Airway management, 502–506
Airway occlusion pressure, 213
Airway patency, 495–499
Airway protective reflex, 214
Airway smooth muscle, 39, 41, 46, 54
ALTE, 237, 260
Alveolar ventilation, 183
Anterior horn cell disease, 413–415
Aortic chemoreceptors, 99
Apnea, 11, 92–94, 116–118, 125,
    134–136, 295–316
  central, 93, 116, 274–276, 305
  definition, 273–274
  differential diagnosis, 277–281
  immunization, 181
  mixed, 93, 116–118, 274–276
  obstructive, 93, 116–118, 274–276

  outcome, 286–287
  periodic breathing, 259–261
  pulmonary edema, 280
  types, 117, 274–275
Apnea of prematurity, 254, 295–316,
    355
  anemia, 308, 345
  arousal, 309
  caffeine, 320–323
  CPAP, 347–348
  diaphragm fatigue, 302–304
  doxapram, 323–325
  GE reflux, 299–302, 325–326, 338,
    488–490
  and lung volume, 298–299
  methylxanthines, 317–325
  pharmacotherapy, 317–333
  resolution of, 365–368
  temporal relationship, 282–284,
    295–298
  termination of, 309
  theophylline, 317–320, 323
  upper airway obstruction, 304–306
Arnold–Chiari malformation, 411–413
Arousal, 90–91, 129–130, 250, 309, 396,
    413

Milton Keynes UK
Ingram Content Group UK Ltd.
UKHW020004071024
449327UK00031B/2646